ANNALS OF THE NEW YORK ACADEMY OF SCIENCES

VOLUME 155, ART. 3 PAGES 657–1031

December 30, 1968

LEUKOCYTE CHEMISTRY AND MORPHOLOGY CORRELATED WITH CHROMOSOME ANOMALIES*

Consulting Editors and Conference Cochairmen

ARNOLD R. KAPLAN AND MARGARET A. KELSALL

CONTENTS

Introduction. *By* ARNOLD R. KAPLAN

Part I. Chromosome Studies

Relevance of Meiotic Studies in Human Chromosome Identification. *By* M. FRACCARO, MAJ HULTÉN, AND J. LINDSTEN 664

Chromosome Studies in Normal Human Subjects. *By* SAJIRO MAKINO, AKIO A. AWA, AND MOTOMICHI SASAKI 679

The Interrelationship of Sex Chromosome Constitution and Phenotype in the Syndrome of Gonadal Dysgenesis and Its Variants. *By* AKIRA MORISHIMA AND MELVIN M. GRUMBACH 695

Biochemical Changes in Chromosomal Abnormalities. *By* DAVID YI-YUNG HSIA, HENRY L. NADLER, AND LING-YU SHIH 716

Virus-Induced Chromosome Changes. *By* PERTTI AULA, WARREN W. NICHOLS, AND ALBERT LEVAN 737

Chromosome Polyploidization in Human Leukocytes Induced by Radiation. *By* CARLOS E. NASJLETI AND HERBERT H. SPENCER 748

Autoantibodies in Down's Syndrome and Gonadal Dysgenesis. *By* PHILIP J. FIALKOW AND IRENE A. UCHIDA 759

Chromosome Abnormalities in Anemias. *By* GERALD E. BLOOM AND LOUIS K. DIAMOND 770

Genetics in Acute Lymphatic Leukemia in Childhood. *By* J. JEFFREY MCCULLOUGH, MELVYN T. KOROBKIN, AND WILLIAM KRIVIT 777

Familial Aggregates of the 21-Trisomy Syndrome. *By* HANS ZELLWEGER 784

Heredity and Carcinoma. *By* H. T. LYNCH, D. E. ANDERSON, A. J. KRUSH, AND A. L. LARSEN 793

Genetic Studies of Diseases Associated with Chromosomal Aberrations. *By* RICHARD H. OSBORNE 801

* This series of papers is the result of a conference entitled Leukocyte Chemistry and Morphology Correlated with Chromosome Anomalies, held by The New York Academy of Sciences on November 3, 4, and 5, 1966.

Part II. Leukocytes in Genetic Anomalies

Neutrophil Nuclei and the Sex-Chromosome Complement. *By* Ursula Mittwoch ... 804

Neutrophils in the 13(D_1)-Trisomy Syndrome. *By* E. R. Huehns, M. Lutzner, and F. Hecht ... 811

The Chediak-Higashi Anomaly and the Aleutian Trait in Mink: Homologous Defects of Lysosomal Structure. *By* D. B. Windhorst, J. G. White, A. S. Zelickson, C. C. Clawson, P. B. Dent, B. Pollara, and R. A. Good ... 818

Morphology of Leukocytic Hypergranulation in Batten's Disease. *By* Sheila Donahue, Itaru Watanabe, and Wolfgang Zeman ... 847

Detection of Heterozygotes in Batten's Disease. *By* A. D. Merritt, S. A. Smith, J. C. Strouth, and W. Zeman ... 860

Biochemical Genetics of Glucose-6-Phosphate Dehydrogenase Variation. *By* Akira Yoshida, George Stamatoyannopoulos, and Arno G. Motulsky ... 868

Chromosomal Aberrations and Suppression of Leukocyte Mitosis Induced *In Vitro* by a Circulating Factor Associated with Acute Infectious Hepatitis. *By* Barbara Mella and David J. Lang ... 880

The Metabolic Pattern and Phagocytic Function of Leukocytes from Children with Chronic Granulomatous Disease. *By* Beulah Holmes, Arthur R. Page, Dorothy B. Windhorst, Paul G. Quie, James G. White, and Robert A. Good ... 888

Part III. Leukocyte Alkaline Phosphatase

The Regulation of Leukocyte Alkaline Phosphatase. *By* F. Rosner, S. L. Lee, F. S. Schultz, and P. C. Gorfien ... 902

Leukocyte Alkaline Phosphatase Cytochemistry: Applications and Methods. *By* Leonard S. Kaplow ... 911

Isozymes of Human Leukocyte Alkaline Phosphatase. *By* Richard B. Lyons, David D. Weaver, and James H. Beck ... 948

Leukocyte Alkaline Phosphatase Activity Test for Pregnancy. *By* Charles T. Stubblefield ... 972

Leukocytic Alkaline Phosphatase in Myeloproliferative Syndrome. *By* W. J. Mitus and K. A. Kiossoglou ... 976

Leukocyte Alkaline Phosphatase in the Infant. *By* Richard T. O'Kell ... 980

Part IV. Neutrophils in 21 Trisomy and the Leukemias

The Philadelphia Chromosome and Leukocyte Alkaline Phosphatase in Chronic Myelocytic Leukemia and Related Disorders. *By* Stephen Krauss ... 983

Leukocyte Alkaline Phosphatase in Chronic Granulocytic Leukemia of Childhood. *By* Robert B. Rosen and Hiroshi Nishiyama ... 992

Karyotypes of Human Cultured Cell Clones and Their Alkaline Phosphatase Activity. *By* L. De Carli, Fiorella Nuzzo, A. Silvana Santachiara-Benerecetti, and J. Morrow ... 1003

Abnormal Leukokinetics in 21 Trisomy. *By* W. J. Mellman, S. O. Raab, F. A. Oski, and T. A. Tedesco ... 1020

Leukocyte Alkaline Phosphatase in the 21-Trisomy (Down's) Syndrome. *By* Aaron A. Alter and Stanley L. Lee ... 1023

Concluding Remarks. *By* Margaret A. Kelsall ... 1028

INTRODUCTION

Arnold R. Kaplan

Laboratory of Medical Genetics, Cleveland Psychiatric Institute
Cleveland, Ohio

This meeting could not have occurred without much work, cooperation, and kind consideration by many individuals. We also want to acknowledge our personal appreciation to all the conference participants: to Admiral Schanze, Mrs. Eunice T. Miner, and their staff at The New York Academy of Sciences; to Doctor Edward N. Hinko, Director of Research at the Cleveland Psychiatric Institute; to Miss Wilma Powell of the Laboratory of Medical Genetics, and Mrs. Lois Soucie of the Laboratory of Cytology, at the Cleveland Psychiatric Institute.

The common interests of the participants in this conference are the etiology of chromosome anomalies and the pathologies associated with them.

Inductions of chromosome anomalies have been associated with various factors: genetically-transmitted pathological conditions; infectious agents; radiation; and numerous chemical agents. Vast amounts of available data have led to a variety of different concepts and different investigative approaches.

There have been reports of family clusters and of community clusters with leukemia, with other malignancies, and with malformations associated with cytogenetic abnormalities.

The high correlation between increasing maternal age and increasing incidence of the autosomal aneuploidy involved in Down's syndrome has been well established.[1–7] The association between increasing maternal age and increasing incidence of an anomaly is not confined to Down's syndrome, but has also been observed for pregnancies terminating in miscarriage;[8] for stillbirths, placenta praevia, anencephaly, hydrocephaly, spina bifida,[9] and for pregnancies producing normal infants who develop leukemia later in childhood.[10] Epidemiological studies of Down's syndrome, which have shown annual fluctuations in incidence, multiannual periodicity, and regional clustering, may be interpreted as indicating the possible relevance of a virus or other infectious agent.[11,12] Periodic fluctuations in incidence, which are characteristic of recurrent epidemics,[13] have also been reported for other congenital anomalies, such as anecephaly, spina bifida, and hydrocephaly.[12–16]

There have been numerous well-documented reports of familial clusterings of leukemia[17–21] and of other malignancies.[22–24] There have also been reports of seasonal variation in leukemia incidence.[25–27]

The observations of associations between Down's syndrome and leukemia incidence[20–32] suggest an etiological relationship between the two conditions. Similarly, associations have been observed between the congenital aneuploidies involved in Klinefelter's syndrome and leukemia and other malignancies.[33,34] Increased incidence of cancer in general has been observed in families in which chronic lymphocytic leukemia and lymphosarcoma had occurred.[35]

Observations on patients with Bloom's syndrome[36,37] and on patients with Fanconi's syndrome[38–40] have indicated abnormally high frequencies of chromosomal abnormalities in their somatic cells. There were also strikingly increased incidences of malignancies in the same patients. These reports suggest that the two diseases, each of which may involve simple Mendelian genetic transmission, induce abnormal frequencies of chromosomal rearrangements in the somatic cells of affected individuals.[41]

Abnormally high frequencies of chromosome breaks have been observed in patients with serum hepatitis[42] and in patients with aseptic meningitis.[43,44]

The induction of chromosome breaks by viruses has been well documented.[45–47] Recently, it has been shown that a specific virus, adenovirus 12, may be incorporated into the genetic material of a specific host cell and transform the normal cell into a malignant-type cell.[48]

Chromosome anomalies in circulating leukocytes have been found in patients following their subjection to x-irradiation,[49–51] to gamma ray and proton exposure,[52] and to therapeutic doses of radioactive iodine.[53,54]

Chromosome breakages have been induced by numerous chemical compounds, and these effects have been extensively documented.[55–60] Homologous lymphocyte extracts have been shown to induce hyperploidy in tissue culture fibroblasts.[61] The latter observation may be related to the increased frequency of thyroid autoantibodies observed in mothers who bore children affected with Down's syndrome.[62]

The discovery of the Philadelphia chromosome in patients with chronic myelogenous leukemia[63,64] has been extensively corroborated.[65–75] In addition, a significant minority of the patients with chronic myelogenous leukemia have been found to manifest various aneuploid abnormalities,[76] with some cells showing chromosome numbers ranging from 47 to 55.

Differences have been observed in alkaline phosphatase activity[77] and in the distribution patterns of lysosomes[78] in different strains of cultured cells. There have been numerous investigations of possible associations between alkaline phosphatase activity and the G(21/22)-trisomy genotype and between alkaline phosphatase activity and the occurrence of the Philadelphia chromosome. Other associations have been reported among morphological and biochemical variables of the leukocytes, other traits, certain congenital anomalies, certain malignancies, and epidemiological variables.

Improved insights regarding etiology may be derived through studying relationships involved in the various concurrences: in cells; in individuals; in families; and in communities. We will, in this conference, discuss chromosomal characteristics, and we will explore associations between clinico-pathological, genetical, cytological, biochemical, and other variables.

References

1. Carter, C. D. & K. A. Evans. 1961. Risk of parents who have had one child with Down's syndrome (mongolism) having another child similarly affected. Lancet **ii:** 785–788.
2. Oster, J. 1956. The causes of mongolism. Danish Med. Bull. **3:** 158–164.
3. Penrose, L. S. 1954. Observations on the aetiology of mongolism. Lancet **ii:** 267, 505–509.
4. Penrose, L. S. 1954. Mongolian idiocy (mongolism) and maternal age. Ann. N. Y. Acad. Sci. **57:** 494–502.
5. Penrose, L. S. 1955. Parental age and mutation. Lancet **ii:** 269, 312–313.
6. Penrose, L. S. 1961. Mongolism. Brit. Med. Bull. **17:** 184–189.
7. Penrose, L. S. 1961. Mongolism. *In* Clinical Aspects of Genetics. F. A. Jones, Ed. Pitman Publishing Co., Ltd. London, England.
8. Shapiro, S. 1962. A life table of pregnancy terminations and correlates of fetal loss. Milbank Mem. Fund Quart. **40:** 7–45.
9. Parson, P. A. 1962. Maternal age and development variability. J. Exp. Biol. **39:** 251–260.

10. STEWARD, A., J. WEBB & D. HEWITT. 1958. Survey of childhood malignancies. Brit. Med. J. **i:** 1495–1508.
11. COLLMANN, R. D. & A. STOLLER. 1962. A survey of mongoloid births in Victoria, Australia, 1942–1957. Amer. J. Pub. Health **52:** 813–829.
12. COLLMANN, R. D. & A. STOLLER. 1962. A survey of mongolian and congenital anomalies of the central nervous system in Australia. New Zealand Med. J. **61:** 24–32.
13. GORDON, J. E. 1962. Chickenpox: an epidemiological review. Amer. J. Med. Sci. **244:** 362–389.
14 ALTER, M. 1962. Anencephalus, hydrocephalus, and spina bifida epidemiology, with special reference to a survey in Charleston, S. C. Arch. Neurol. **7:** 411–422.
15. GUTHKELCH, A. N. 1962. Studies in spina bifida cystica. III. Seasonal variations in the frequency of spina bifida births. Brit. J. Prevent. Soc. Med. **16:** 159–162.
16. SLATER, B. C. S., G. I. WATSON & J. C. MCDONALD. 1964. Seasonal variation in congenital abnormalities. Brit. J. Prevent. Soc. Med. **18:** 1–7.
17. ANDERSON, R. C. 1951. Familial leukemia: a report of leukemia in five siblings, with a brief review of the genetic aspects of this disease. Amer. J. Dis. Child. **81:** 313–322.
18. KOLMEIER, K. H. & E. D. BAYRD. 1963. Familial leukemia: report of instance and review of the literature. Proc. Mayo Clinic **38:** 523–531.
19. STEINBERG, A. G. 1957. A genetic and statistical study of acute leukemia in children. *In* Proceedings of The Third National Cancer Conference, 1956. : 353–356. J. B. Lippincott Co., Ltd., Philadelphia.
20. VIDABAEK, A. 1947. Heredity in Human Leukemia and Its Relation to Cancer. H. K. Lewis & Co., Ltd., London.
21. VIDABAEK, A. 1958. Familial leukemia. Acta Path. Microbiol. Scand. **44:** 372–376.
22. OLIVER, C. P. 1958. Studies on human cancer families. Ann. N. Y. Acad. Sci. **71:** 1198–1212.
23. LYNCH, H. T., M. W. SHAW, C. W. MAGNUSON, A. L. LARSEN & A. J. KRUSH. 1966. Hereditary factors in cancer. Arch. Intern. Med. **117:** 206–212.
24. TOKUHATA, G. K. & A. M. LILIENFELD. 1963. Familial aggregation of lung cancer in humans. J. Nat. Cancer Inst. **30:** 289–312.
25. FRAUMENI, J. F., JR. 1963. Seasonal variation in leukemia incidence. Brit. Med. J. **ii:** 5369.
26. LEE, J. A. H. 1963. Seasonal variation in leukemia incidence. Brit. Med. J. **ii:** 623.
27 SWAN, A. 1963. Seasonal variation in leukemia incidence. Brit. Med. J. **ii:** 1063–1064.
28. KRIVIT, W. & R. A. GOOD. 1956. Simultaneous occurrence of leukemia and mongolism. Amer. J. Dis. Child. **91:** 218–222.
29. KRIVIT, W. & R. A. GOOD. 1957. Simultaneous occurrence of mongolism and leukemia: report of a nationwide survey. Amer. J. Dis. Child. **94:** 289–293.
30. MERRITT, D. H. & S. J. HARRIS. 1956. Mongolism and acute leukemia. Amer. J. Dis. Child. **92:** 41–44.
31. STEWART, A. M. & D. HEWITT. 1959. The epidemiology of human leukemia. Brit. Med. Bull. **15:** 73–77.
32. WALD, N., W. H. BORGES, C. C. LI, J. H. TURNER & M. C. HARNOIS. 1961. Leukemia associated with mongolism. Lancet **i:** 1228.
33. ROBINSON, L. R. 1966. Neoplastic liability in Klinefelter's syndrome. Brit. J. Psychiat. **112:** 713–715.
34. MILLER, R. W. 1966. Relation between cancer and congenital defects in man. New Engl. J. Med. **275:** 87–93.
35. MORGANTI, C. & A. CRESSERI. 1954. Nouvelles recherches génétiques sur les leucémies. Sang **25:** 421–453.
36. GERMAN, J. 1964. Cytological evidence for crossing-over *in vitro* in human lymphoid cells. Science **144:** 298–301.
37. GERMAN, J., R. ARCHIBALD & D. BLOOM. 1965. Chromosomal breakage in a rare and probably genetically determined syndrome of man. Science **148:** 506.
38. SCHROEDER, T. M., F. ANSCHÜTZ & A. KNOPP. 1964. Spontane Chromosomenaberrationen bei familiärer Panmyelopathie. Humangenetik **1:** 194–196.
39. BLOOM, G. E., S. WARNER, P. S. GERALD & K. DIAMOND. 1966. Chromosome abnormalities in constitutional aplastic anemia. New Engl. J. Med. **274:** 8–14.
40. SCHMID, W., K. SCHÄRER, T. BAUMANN & G. FANCONI. 1965. Chromosomenbrüchigkeit bei der familiären Panmyelopathie (Typus Fanconi). Schweiz. Med. Wschr. **95:** 1461–1464.
41. DE GROUCHY, J. 1966. Genetic diseases, chromosome rearrangements, and malignancy. Ann. Intern. Med. **65:** 603–607.

42. AYA, T. & S. MAKINO. 1966. Notes on chromosome abnormalities in cultured leucocytes from serum hepatitis patients. Proc. Japan Acad. **42:** 648–653.
43. MAKINO, S., K. YAMADA & T. KAJII. 1965. Chromosome aberrations in leukocytes of patients with aseptic meningitis. Chromosoma **16:** 372–380.
44. MAKINO, S., T. AYA, T. IKEUCHI & S. KASAHARA. 1966. A further study of chromosomes in cultured leukocytes from aseptic meningitis patients. Proc. Japan Acad. **42:** 270–274.
45. AULA, P. 1965. Virus-associated chromosome breakage. *In* Ann. Acad. Scient, Series A. IV, Biologica. Suomalainen Tiedeakatemia, Helsinki.
46. NICHOLS, W. W. & A. LEVAN. 1965. Measles associated with chromosomes breakage. Arch. Ges. Virus-forsch. **16:** 168–174.
47. NICHOLS, W. W., A. LEVAN, P. AULA & E. NORBY. 1964. Extreme chromosome breakage induced by measles virus in different *in vitro* systems. Preliminary communications. Hereditas **51:** 380–382.
48. FUJINAGA, K. & M. GREEN. 1966. The mechanism of viral carcinogenesis by DNA mammallian viruses: viral-specific RNA in polyribosomes of adenovirus tumor and transformed cells. Proc. Nat. Acad. Sci. **55:** 1567–1574.
49. TOUGH, I. M., K. E. BUCKTON, A. G. BAIKIE & W. M. COURT-BROWN. 1960. X-ray-induced chromosome damage in man. Lancet **ii:** 849–851.
50. STEWARD, J. S. S. & A. R. SANDERSON. 1961. Chromosomal aberration after diagnostic X-irradiation. Lancet **i:** 978–979.
51. NASJLETI, C. E., J. M. WALDEN & H. H. SPENCER. 1966. Polyploidization and aberration of human chromosomes induced *in vitro* and *in vivo* with ionizing radiations. J. Nuclear Med. **7:** 159–176.
52. BENDER, M. A. & P. C. GOOCH. 1962. Persistent chromosome aberrations in irradiated human subjects. Radiat. Res. **16:** 44–53.
53. BOYD, E., W. W. BUCHANAN & B. LENNOX. 1961. Damage to chromosomes by therapeutic doses of radioiodine. Lancet **i:** 977–978.
54. MACINTYRE, M. N. & B. M. DOBYNS. 1962. Anomalies in chromosomes of the circulating leukocytes in man following large doses of radioactive iodine. J. Clin. Endocrin. & Metab. **22:** 1171–1181.
55. KIHLMAN, B. A. 1962. The production of chromatid aberrations with 5-fluorodeoxyuridine alone and in combination with X-rays and 8-ethoxycaffeine. Caryologia **15:** 261–277.
56. KIHLMAN, B. A., W. W. NICHOLS & A. LEVAN. 1963. The effects of deoxyadenosine and cytosine arabinoside on the chromosomes of human leukocytes *in vitro*. Hereditas **50:** 139–143.
57. HSU, T. C., R. M. HUMPHREY & C. E. SOMERS. 1964. Response of Chinese hamster and L cells to 2-deoxy-5-fluoro uridine and thymidine. J. Nat. Cancer Inst. **32:** 839–855.
58. COHEN, M. & M. W. SHAW. 1964. Effects of mitomycin C on human chromosomes. J. Cell. Biol. **23:** 386–395.
59. BELL, S. & S. WOLFF. 1964. Studies on the mechanism of the effect of fluorodeoxyuridine on chromosomes. Proc. Nat. Acad. Sci. **51:** 195–202.
60. AHNSTRÖM, G. & A. T. Natarajan. 1965. Mechanism of chromosome breakage–a new theory. Hereditas **54:** 379–388.
61. FIALKOW, P. J. & S. M. GARTLER. 1965. Effect of human leukocyte extracts on mitosis of human fibroblasts *in vitro*. J. Clin. Invest. **44:** 1046.
62. FIALKOW, P. J., I. A. UCHIDA, F. HECHT & A. G. MOTULSKY. 1965. Increased frequency of thyroid autoantibodies in mothers of patients with Down's syndrome. *Lancet* **ii:** 868–870.
63. NOWELL, P. C. & D. A. HUNGERFORD. 1960. Chromosome studies on normal and leukemic human leukocytes. J. Nat. Cancer Inst. **25:** 85–109.
64. BAIKIE, A. G., W. M. COURT-BROWN, K. E. BUCKTON, D. G. HARNDEN, P. A. JACOBS & I. M. TOUGH. 1960. A possible specific chromosome abnormality in human chronic myeloid leukemia. Nature **188:** 1165–1166.
65. NOWELL, P. C. & D. A. HUNGERFORD. 1961. Chromosome studies in human leukemia. II. Chronic granulocytic leukemia. J. Nat. Cancer Inst. **27:** 1013–1035.
66. NOWELL, P. C. & D. A. HUNGERFORD. 1964. Chromosome changes in human leukemia and a tentative assessment of their significance. Ann. N. Y. Acad. Sci. **113:** 654–662.
67. SANDBERG, A. A., T. ISHIHARA, L. H. CROSSWHITE & T. S. HAUSCHKA. 1962. Comparison of chromosome constitution in chronic myelocytic leukemia and other myeloproliferative disorders. Blood **20:** 393–423.

68. SANDBERG, A. A., T. ISHIHARA, T. MIWA & T. S. HAUSCHKA. 1961. The *in vivo* chromosome constitution of marrow from 34 human leukemias and 60 nonleukemic controls. Cancer Res. **21**: 678–689.
69. TOUGH, I. M., W. M. COURT-BROWN, A. G. BAIKIE, K. E. BUCKTON, D. G. HARNDEN, P. A. JACOBS & J. A. WILLIAMS. 1962. Chronic myeloid leukaemia: cytogenetic studies before and after splenic irradiation. Lancet **ii**: 115–120.
70. TOUGH, I. M., P. A. JACOBS, W. M. COURT-BROWN, A. G. BAIKIE & E. R. D. WILLIAMSON. 1963. Cytogenetic studies on bone marrow in chronic myeloid leukemia. Lancet **i**: 844–846.
71. LEVAN, A., W. W. NICHOLS & A. NORDÉN. 1963. A case of chronic myeloid leukemia with two stemlines in the blood. Hereditas **49**: 433–441.
72. TRUJILLO, J. M. & S. OHNO. 1963. Chromosomal alteration of erythropoietic cells in chronic myeloid leukemia. Acta Haemat. **29**: 311–316.
73. FREI, E., J. H. TJIO, J. WHANG & P. P. CARBONE. 1964. Studies of the Philadelphia chromosome in patients with chronic myelogenous leukemia. Ann. N. Y. Acad. Sci. **113**: 1073–1080.
74. HAMMOUDA, F., D. QUAGLINO & F. G. J. HAYHOE. 1964. Blastic crisis in chronic granulocytic leukemia. Cytochemical, cytogenetic, and autoradiographic studies in four cases. Brit. Med. J. **i**: 1275–1281.
75. MAKINO, S. & A. A. AWA. 1964. Chromosome breakages in four chronic myeloid leukemia patients. Hereditas **52**: 253–264.
76. TJIO, J. H., P. P. CARBONE, J. WHANG & E. FREI. 1966. The Philadelphia chromosome and chronic myelogenous leukemia. J. Nat. Cancer Inst. **36**: 567–584.
77. DE CARLI, L., J. J. MAIO & F. NUZZO. 1963. Approach to the cytogenetics of mammammalian cells *in vitro*. *In* Genetics Today, Vol. 1, S. J. Geerts, Ed. : 311–312. Pergamon Press, Ltd., London.
78. YAMAMOTO, K. 1965. Distribution of lysosomes in cultured cells and ascites tumor cells. J. Faculty Science, Hokkaido University, Series VI, Zoology **15**: 693–698.

PART I. CHROMOSOME STUDIES

RELEVANCE OF MEIOTIC STUDIES IN HUMAN CHROMOSOME IDENTIFICATION

M. Fraccaro

Euratom Unit for Human Radiation and Cytogenetics
University of Pavia, Pavia, Italy

and

Maj Hultén and J. Lindsten

Department of Endocrinology and Metabolism
Karolinska Hospital, Stockholm, Sweden

INTRODUCTION

Identification of normal mitotic chromosomes is an important and interesting cytological exercise although at present void of genetic interest, because no autosomal linkage group has been established in man. Analysis of mitotic karyotypes can be performed with different techniques that have varying degrees of resolution. None of these techniques is final per se and optimal results should be obtained only by their combined use. Analytical methods at our disposal are essentially:

1) Visual morphological analysis aided by use of estimates of metrical characters such as absolute and relative total length of chromosome arms, arm ratios, centromeric indexes, and similar characters. The possibility of automating all or part of this type of analysis is being actively considered by several groups. Combined use of automated scanning procedures and computers (Ruddle, 1964) should help to eliminate a major part of the human effort in this field.

2) Analysis of differentials in the chronology and patterns of DNA replication at the level of whole chromosomes and/or parts of chromosomes. Asynchrony of DNA replication is usually extreme in the case of the sex chromosomes in most species (FIGURE 1). In addition, critical use of replication patterns is undoubtedly a major aid in identification of autosomal pairs (Schmid, 1963; German, 1964).

3) Analysis of the ultrastructure of whole chromosomes or of sections of them by the use of electron microscopy. The results obtained by this method up to now have been rather disappointing when used for the identification of single chromosomes (Barnicot & Huxley, 1961). However it should be more useful in its application to problems of chromosome topology within the cell. Electron microscope autoradiography should result in greatly improved resolution in the type of analysis mentioned in (2).

4) Various types of analyses that we could call generically "biophysical." Among these, quoting at random: differential sensitivity of chromosome structures to physical or chemical agents which modify and/or interfere with their components; chemical composition and other characteristics of isolated chromosomes; and immunological properties of chromosomes. There is ample scope for the ingenuity of the experimental cell biologist in devising a wide range of similar approaches. Identification of abnormal chromosomes requires the same battery of technical procedures as used in the identification of normal chromosomes, but with the additional difficulties posed by the problems of phenotype-

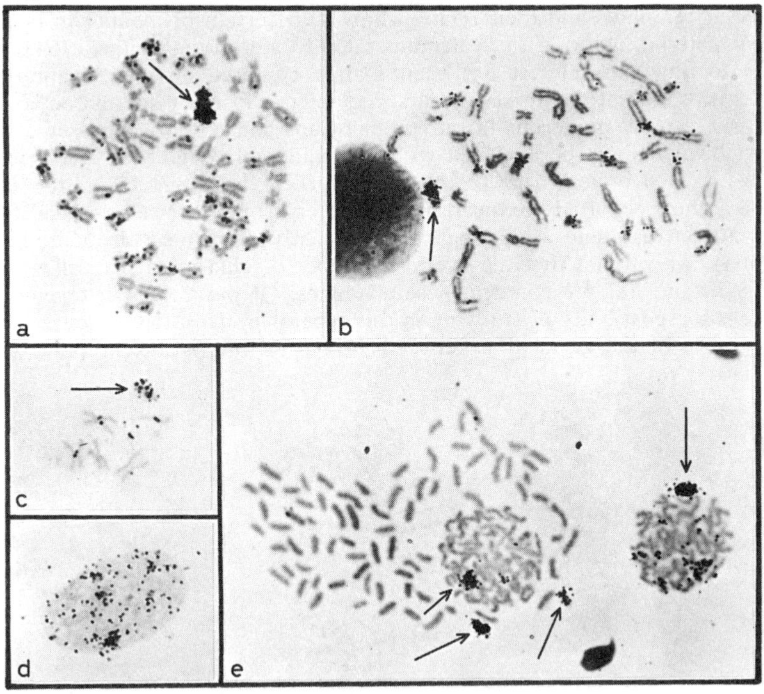

FIGURE 1. Examples of asynchrony in the replication of chromosomal DNA. Autoradiographs after labeling with tritiated thymidine. a) Human female mitotic blood cell labeled *in vitro.* Arrow indicates a late replicating X chromosome. b) Heteroploid metaphase of an ovarian cancer cell labeled *in vitro.* Blocks of late replication and an entire late replicating chromosome (arrow). c) Metaphase of a male embryonic cell of *Drosophila melanogaster* cultured *in vitro.* Late replicating Y chromosome (arrow). From Barigozzi *et al.,* 1966. d) Labeled nucleus from a culture of male mouse kidney cells. Multiple heteropycnotic masses are labeled. e) Squash preparation from a mouse testis. Spermatogonial cells labeled *in vivo.* Late-replicating Y chromosomes (arrows).

karyotype relationships. The nature and origin of abnormal chromosomes usually remain unknown or at best presumptive on the basis of mitotic studies alone. Meiotic studies are a powerful and often decisive diagnostic tool for identification of abnormal chromosomes and for interpretation of pathological situations. In this paper we present some of our experience in this field.

Normal Meiotic Chromosomes

The meiotic chromosomes of the human male are technically easy to study, the only limitation being that of access to suitable material, namely, tiny biopsy fragments from testicles. We routinely obtain successful preparations by a modification (Hultén *et al.,* 1966a) of the air-drying method of Evans *et al.* (1964), in which all stages of the two meiotic divisions are usually seen (FIGURE 2), although in varying proportions. It should be noted that the old squash technique is still useful if one is interested in obtaining a large number of spermatogonial mitoses. Cells in pachytene are generally numerous, though not usually spread out enough to permit an analysis of all individual bivalents. The behavior of nucleolar remnants and their relationships with certain bivalents can be studied in this material, (FIGURE 3) as demonstrated by Ferguson-Smith (1964).

Up to now our interest has been mainly centered on identification of the bivalents as seen at diakinesis and first metaphase. Primary spermatocytes in this stage are usually numerous in our preparations and the size and shape of individual bivalents can be analyzed with a considerable degree of precision, (FIGURE 4) as first indicated by the classical work of Ford and Hamerton (1956). These authors reported the mean number of chiasmata per cell as usually higher than 50, an estimate which has been recently confirmed by McIlree *et al.* (1966a), who found that the average number of chiasmata per cell varied between 50 and 58. We confirm these estimates. Of paramount cytogenetic relevance is the possibility of studying in this type of preparation the morphological appearance of the association between the X and the Y chromosomes (Hultén

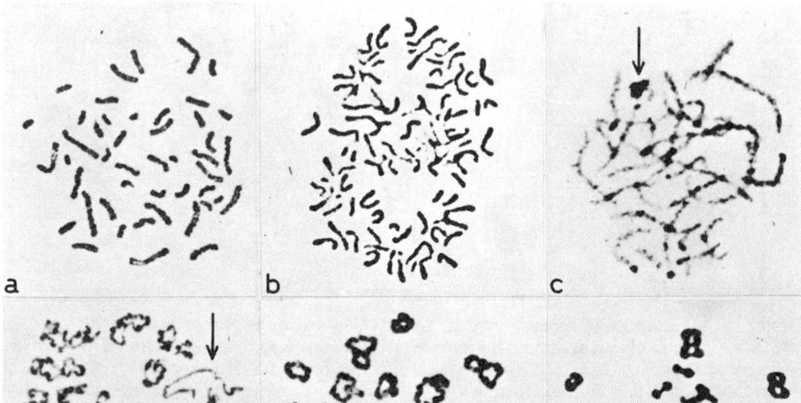

FIGURE 2. Different types of cell divisions from air-dry preparations of a human testis. Spermatogonial metaphase (a) and anaphase (b). Pachytene (c). Diakinesis–first metaphase (d to g). Second metaphase (h) and anaphase (i). Arrows point to sex chromosomes. (Rearranged from Lindsten & Hultén, 1966).

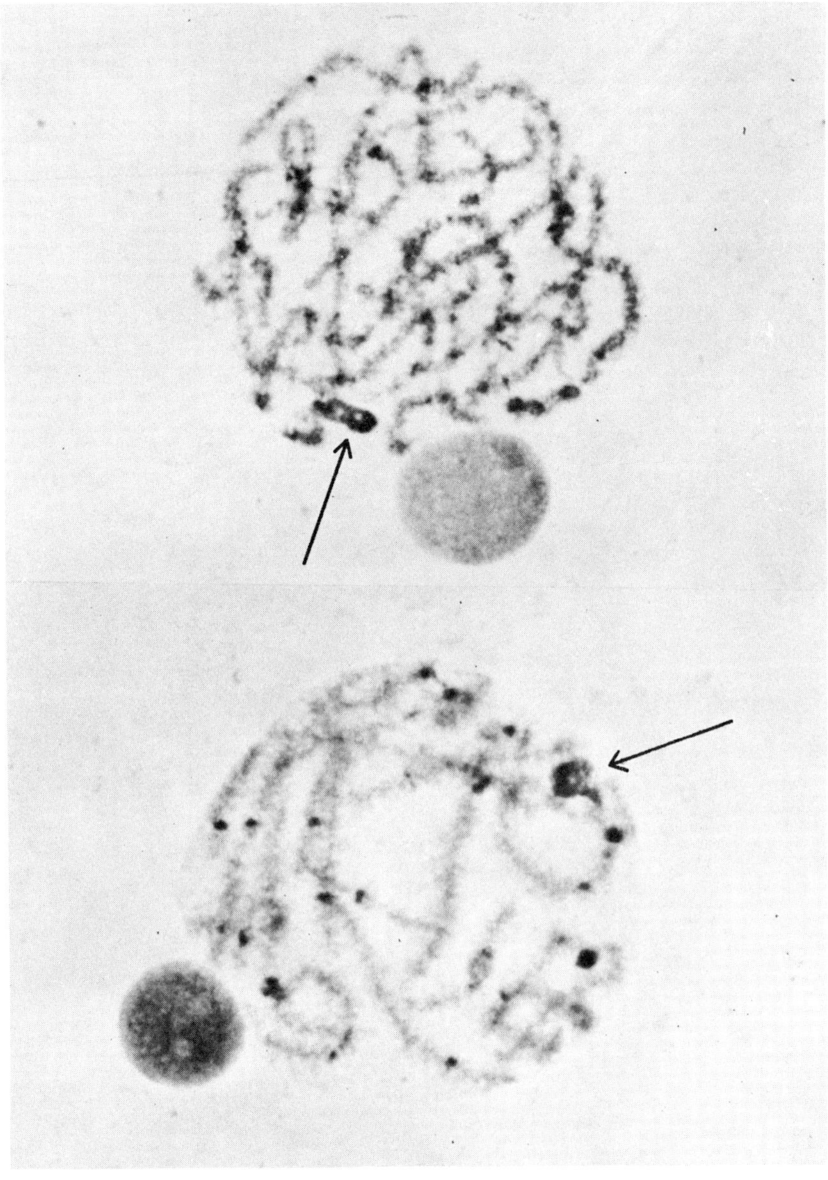

FIGURE 3. Cells in pachytene (arrows point to sex bivalent).

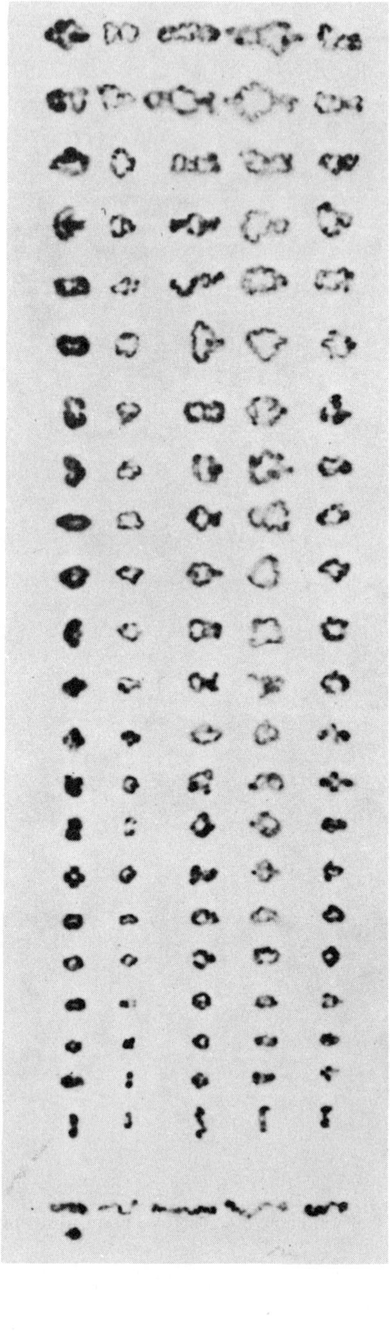

FIGURE 4. Meiotic karyotypes from five cells in diakinesis and first metaphase. The 22 autosomal bivalents are arranged in decreasing order of size. The sex bivalents are at the extreme right.

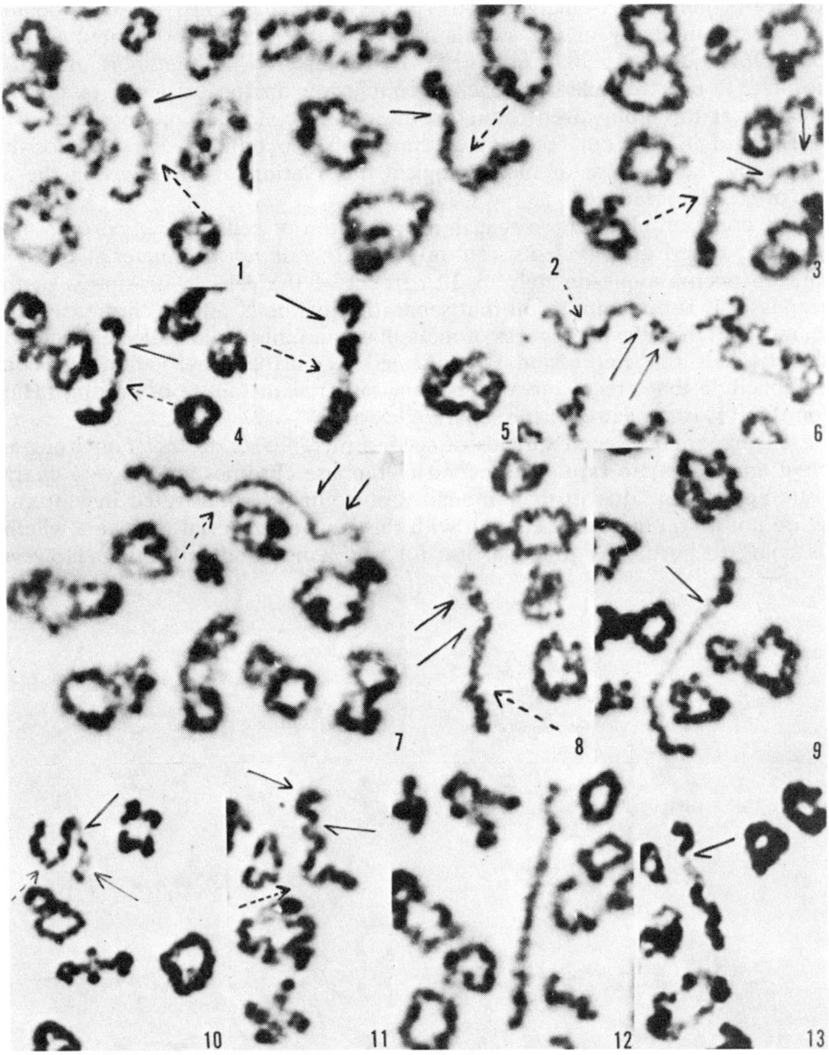

FIGURE 5. Details from 13 cells in diakinesis showing the terminal association between X and Y. Solid arrows point to the presumptive location of the centromere of the Y, incomplete arrows to the point of association, and broken arrows to the presumptive location of the centromere of the X. (From Hultén, 1966a).

et al., 1966a). The terminal type of association of the XY bivalent has, since its first identification, posed the problem of the eventual existence of a short pairing segment between the two homologous sections, and therefore that of the existence of partial sex-linkage in our species (Haldane, 1936). After a detailed study of the modality of the association, we have recently postulated (Hultén *et al.* 1966a) that the long arm of Y is associated with the short arm of X (FIGURE 5), but we failed to reach a conclusion on the existence of chiasma formation at this point even though some of the configurations observed were suggestive of it. It is our feeling that the problem is difficult, if not impossible, to solve by the exercise of morphological observation of this type, in the absence of genetic evidence.

It is a common observation that in a proportion of cells the sex chromosomes appear separated as univalents (FIGURE 2g). In our *normal* material this phenomenon occurs approximately in 20 percent of the cells in diakinesis or first metaphase. It is our impression that separation of the X and Y chromosomes is seen more often at the later stages of metaphase and this could indicate precocious disjunction. If this impression is confirmed by further observation, we could then conclude that precocious disjunction, rather than failure of pairing (Hamerton, 1961), is the cause of the separated X and Y.

In our experience, good spreads of second metaphases are not numerous and second anaphases are rare. The second metaphase chromosomes have a characteristic appearance due to their modality of coiling, as illustrated in FIGURE 6. We are not as yet confident enough with this type of material to decide whether it is going to be of any practical use for problems of identification. However,

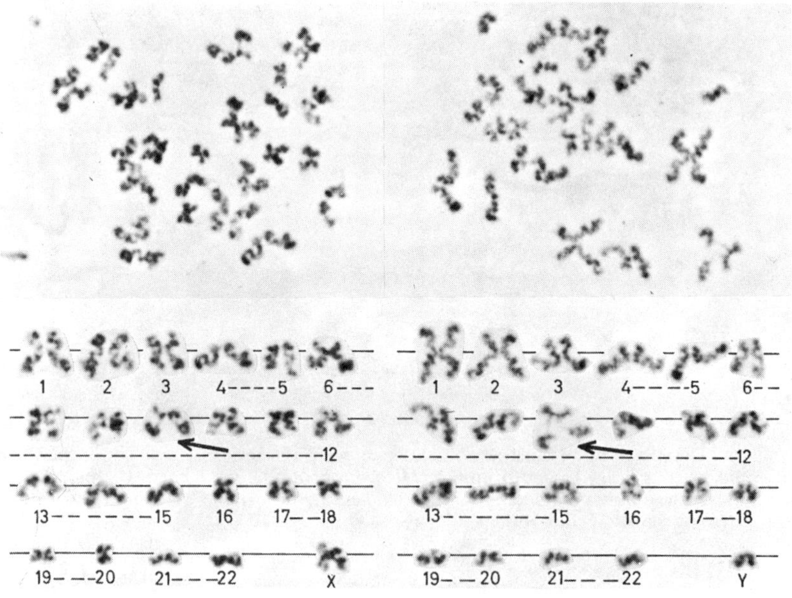

FIGURE 6. X chromosome bearing (left) and Y chromosome bearing (right) secondary spermatocytes in metaphase and their haploid karyotypes. Arrows point to a characteristic elongated secondary constriction.

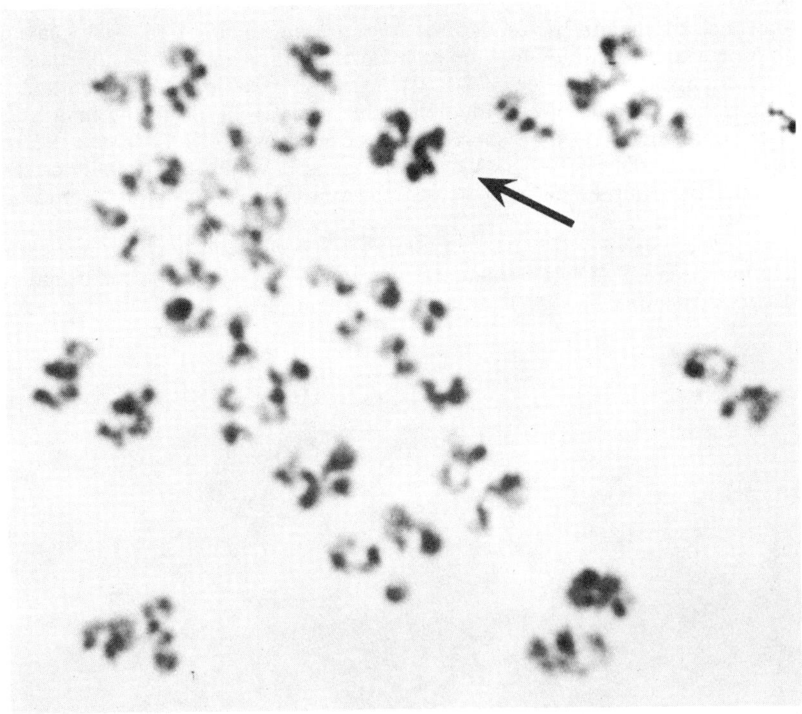

FIGURE 7. Metaphase of a secondary spermatocyte. Arrow points to the single heteropycnotic X chromosome.

we should point out that in second metaphase karyotypes, we do not usually see clear satellites on the acrocentric chrosomes, but an extremely obvious and very extended "secondary constriction" on the long arm of a C-group chromosome, probably No. 9. The presence of a single intensely heteropycnotic chromosome in both X bearing and Y bearing secondary spermatocytes (FIGURE 7) is characteristic, but not constant. Thus, we confirm the observation made by Ohno (1962) in a single subject. Numerical analysis of a large number of metaphases and anaphases of the second meiotic division should permit an estimate of the relative frequency of spermatids which are aneuploid as a consequence of nondisjunction. Such an analysis is in progress on our accumulating material.

Examination of the meiotic chromosomes of any given human female is at present practically impossible. However, when access to the ovary is practical, it is relatively easy to isolate single eggs and, as shown by Edwards (1965), to manipulate them *in vitro* (FIGURE 8). This new method should reveal in the near future the morphological appearance of the chromosomes in several stages of human female meiosis.

In conclusion, we think that detailed study of normal meiotic chromosomes is still required for a better definition of their appearance and behavior. This is an essential preliminary to the use of meiotic configurations as a diagnostic tool for the identification of chromosome abnormalities.

Meiotic Chromosomes in the Diagnosis of Chromosome Abnormalities

Relevance of meiotic investigations for an assessment of the role played by chromosome abnormalities in human male infertility and subfertility has been recently discussed by McIlree *et al.,* (1966b). These authors concluded that such studies are bound to be of considerable value both as an aid in the management of male subfertility and as a source of basic information on meiosis. We have found meiotic studies of diagnostic and prognostic value in any individual who is a carrier of a numerical or structural chromosome abnormality. Some examples follow:

Case 1 (See also Hultén *et al.,* 1966b): A 19-year-old male referred for investigation because of slight mental retardation and various defects including left-sided gynecomastia, renal aplasia, persistent deciduous teeth, and an ab-

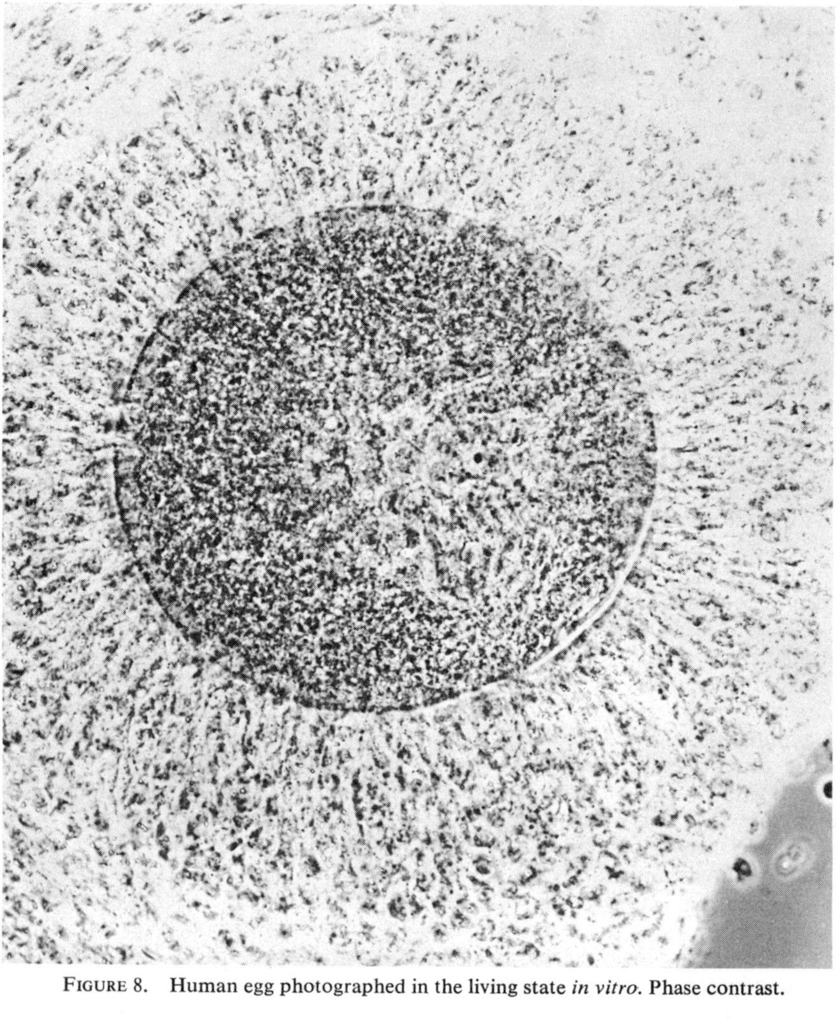

FIGURE 8. Human egg photographed in the living state *in vitro*. Phase contrast.

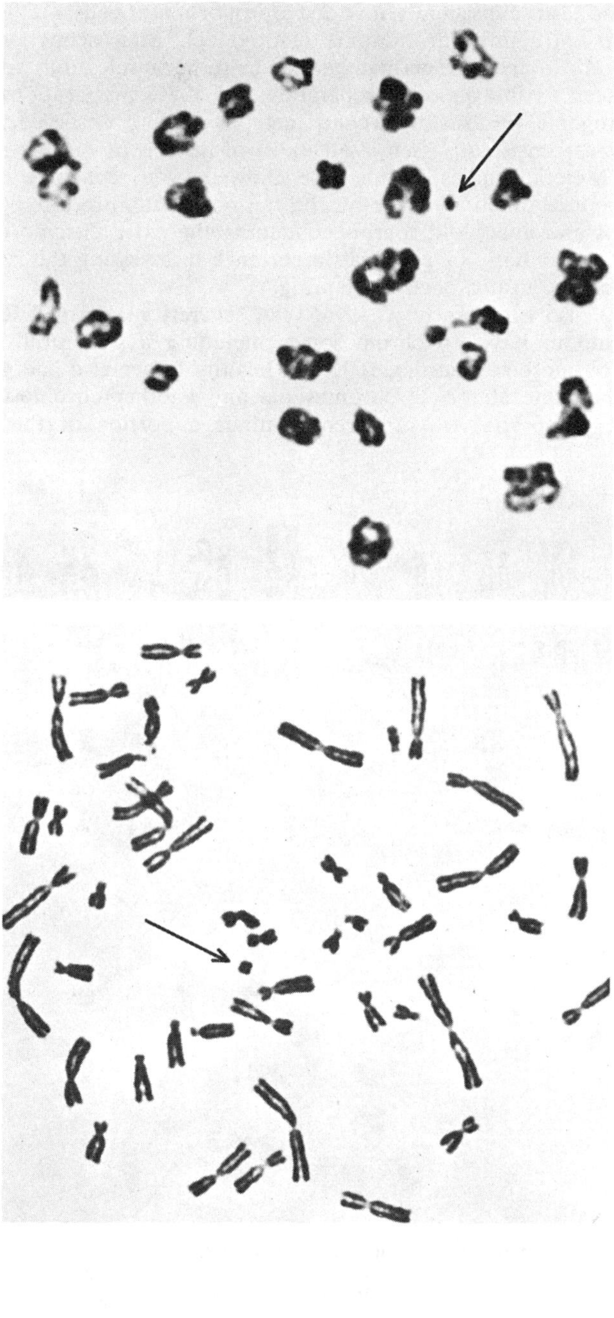

FIGURE 9. Mitotic blood cell (left) and metaphase of the first meiotic divition (right) from *Case 1*. Arrow indicate the tiny extra chromosome.

normal electroencephalogram. Somatic sexual development was normal. On examination, the patient displayed a lack of interest in sexual activity and it was impossible to obtain seminal fluid. Analysis of mitotic cells from cultures of blood, skin, and testis consistently revealed a proportion of cells with 47 chromosomes plus an extra tiny chromosome (FIGURE 9). Microscopy of the testis showed scant and defective spermatogenesis in some tubules, but sperms were occasionally seen in the meiotic preparations. In these preparations all stages from spermatogonial mitosis to second metaphase were observed. The extra chromosome was consistently seen in all stages of meiosis in varying proportions (FIGURE 9). Meiotic studies in this case allowed us to conclude that, if the patient can produce functioning sperms, he can potentially produce both euploid normal sperms and aneuploid sperms containing the extra chromosome. Thus, the studies are potentially of practical importance in assessing the risk of chromosomal imbalance in prospective offspring.

Case 2 (See also Lindsten *et al.*, 1965): A severely malformed female newborn was found to have 46 chromosomes including a structurally abnormal metacentric chromosome (FIGURE 10). Her healthy father also had 46 chromosomes with the same abnormal chromosome and another chromosome in the medium-sized group that was apparently minus a portion of the long arm.

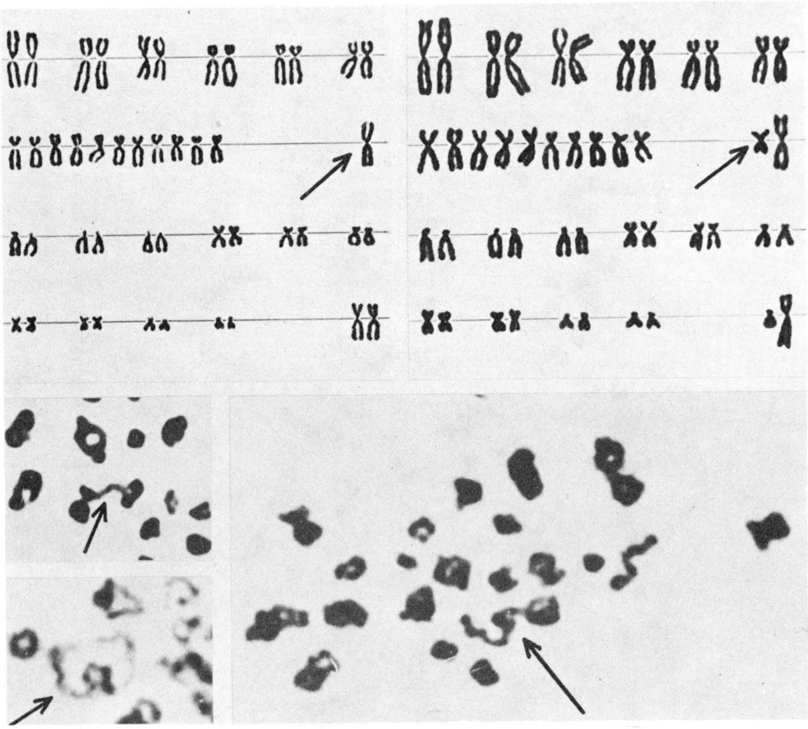

FIGURE 10. *Case 2*. Mitotic unbalanced karyotype of the malformed girl (top left) and balanced karyotype of her healthy father (top right). Quadrivalent configurations (arrows) in her father's primary spermatocytes. (Rearranged from Lindsten *et al.*, 1965).

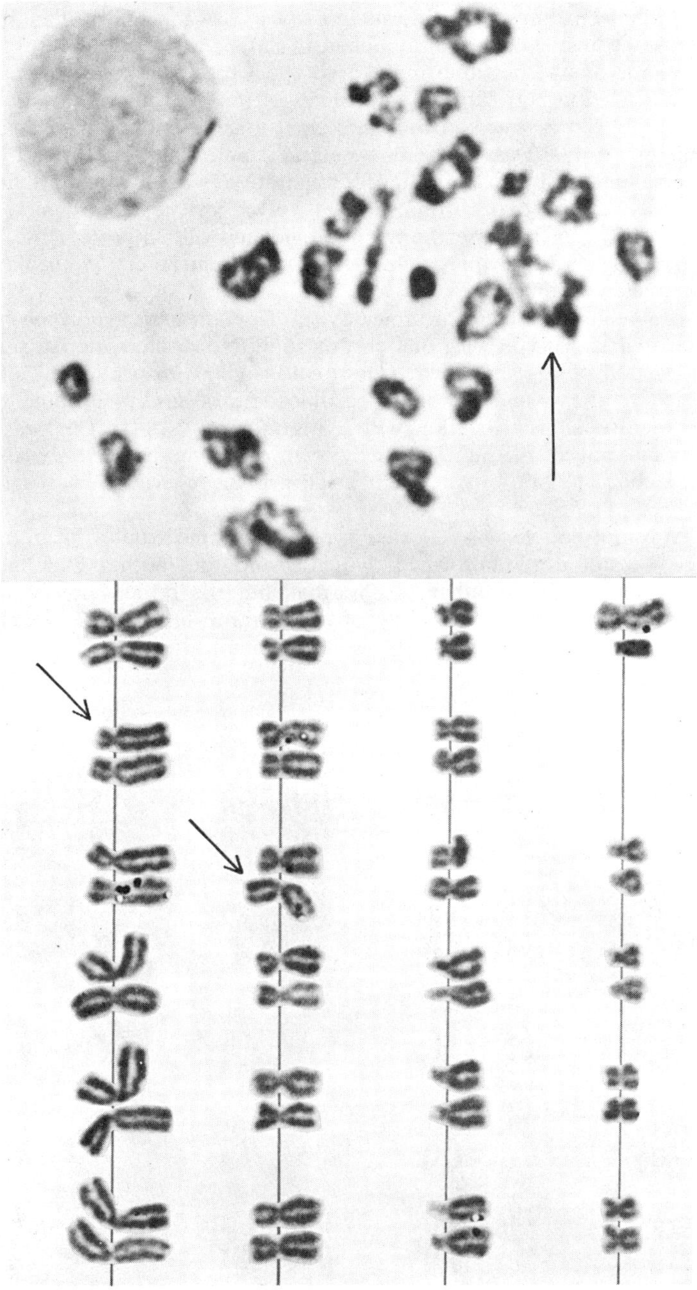

FIGURE 11. *Case 3*. Mitotic karyotype (left) and diakinesis in a primary spermatocyte of the healthy father of a case with the *cri du chat* syndrome. Arrows point to the translocated mitotic chromosomes and to the quadrivalent configuration.

(FIGURE 10). The infant's brother, grandmother, and half-aunt had the same abnormal karyotype as found in her father. The most plausible interpretation of this set of familial chromosome abnormalities was that the malformed subject was a carrier of a translocation in an unbalanced state, whereas the healthy members of the family with the abnormal karyotype were carriers of a balanced reciprocal translocation between two autosomes of the C group. Analysis of the father's meiotic chromosomes showed that this interpretation was the correct one. At diakinesis only 22 associations were consistently counted instead of the normal 23 bivalents and one abnormal configuration was obviously a quadrivalent, composed of the two chromosomes involved in the reciprocal translocation (FIGURE 10). In this case the meiotic evidence was important mainly to reach a firm diagnosis of reciprocal translocation, already very plausible from study of the somatic chromosomes.

Case 3: The healthy father of a typical case of *cri du chat* syndrome had in turn an abnormal karyotype with one chromosome No. 5 characteristically deficient of a portion of the short arm (FIGURE 11). Close inspection of a set of karyotypes led to the suspicion that a chromosome of group C could be involved in a reciprocal translocation with the abnormal No. 5. This was fully confirmed by an analysis of the man's meiotic chromosomes, which revealed the presence of a characteristic quadrivalent in all primary spermatocytes analyzed (FIGURE 11).

Case 4: A young couple was selected for chromosome studies because they had produced a stillborn, malformed daughter and the mother had had one spontaneous abortion. The mother was normal, but the father showed a very slight abnormality in that the short arm of one chromosome No. 2 was shorter

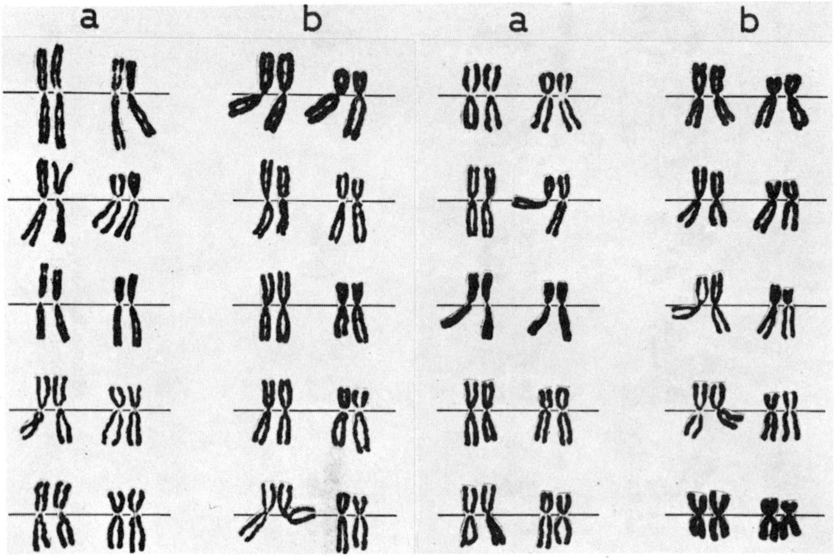

FIGURE 12. Chromosomes No. 1 and No. 2 from ten cells of normal controls (a) and from *Case 4* (b).

than usual. This was rather evident in some cells but in others it was very slight and in some hardly detectable, as seen from the array of normal controls and abnormal cells shown in FIGURE 12. A similar abnormality was detected in three other members of the family. It would have required an ingenuity we do not possess to interpret correctly this abnormality of the somatic chromosomes. However, a testicular biopsy from the father yielded 50 analyzable cells in diakinesis or first metaphase, all of them demonstrating a normal XY bivalent and one characteristic quadrivalent (FIGURE 13). Judging from the shape and size of the quadrivalent, chromosome No. 2 and one chromsome in the group 6–12 seemed to be involved in a reciprocal translocation. All individuals with the abnormal mitotic karyotype could thus be considered as translocation carriers. Therefore, in this instance analysis of the meiotic chromosomes had an absolute diagnostic value. Furthermore, this family provided some evidence for a possible localization of the genes for the Kidd blood group on one of the autosomes involved in the translocation (Hultén *et al.*, 1966c).

Concluding Remarks

In conclusion, our experience indicates that meiotic studies in the human male are relevant to several problems of chromosome identification both in normal and abnormal conditions. We hope to have demonstrated that, beside their scientific relevance, they are of practical importance not only in connection with

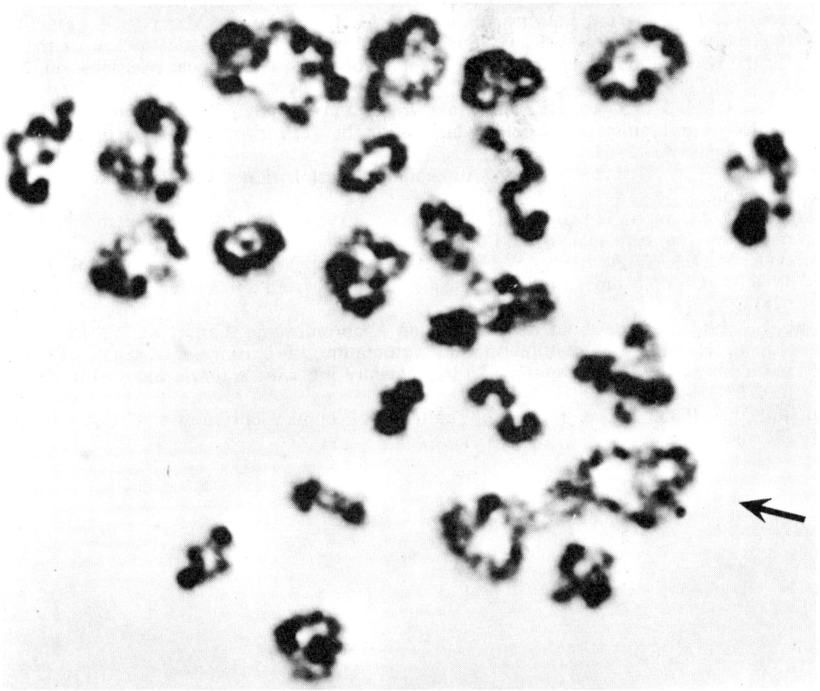

FIGURE 13. Diakinesis of a primary spermatocyte from *Case 4*. Note 22 associations instead of the normal 23 bivalents and the obvious quadrivalent configuration (arrow).

management of male infertility but also during investigation of any carrier of a numerical or structural chromosomal abnormality which can be transmitted to prospective offspring. However, such studies cannot become a routine procedure, at least not before it is demonstrated that a testis biopsy is absolutely harmless in its immediate and long-term consequences.

References

Barigozzi, C., S. Dolfini, M. Fraccaro, G. R. Raimondi & L. Tiepolo. 1966. In vitro study of the DNA replication patterns of somatic chromosomes of *Drosophila melanogaster*. Expt. Cell Res. **43:** 232–234.

Barnicot, N. A. & H. E. Huxley. 1961. The electron microscopy of unsectioned human chromosomes. Ann. Hum. Genet. **25:** 253–258.

Edwards, R. G. 1965. Maturation in vitro of human ovarian oöcytes. Lancet **ii:** 926–929.

Evans, E. P., G. Breckon & C. E. Ford. 1964. An air-drying method for meiotic preparations from mammalian testes. Cytogenetics **3:** 289–294.

Ferguson-Smith, M. A. 1964. The sites of nucleolus formation in human pachytene chromosomes. Cytogenetics **3:** 124–134.

Ford, C. E. & J. L. Hamerton. 1956. The chromosomes of man. Nature **178:** 1020–1023.

German, J. 1964. Identification and characterization of human chromosomes by DNA replication sequence. Symp. Int. Soc. Cell. Biol. **3:** 191–207.

Haldane, J. S. B. 1936. A search for incomplete sex-linkage in man. Ann. Eugen. **7:** 28–57.

Hamerton, J. L. 1961. Sex chromatin and human chromosomes. Int. Rev. Cytol. **12:** 1–68.

Hultén, M., J. Lindsten, L. Ming Pen-Ming & M. Fraccaro. 1966 a. The XY bivalent in human male meiosis. Ann. Hum. Genet. **30:** 119–123.

Hultén, M., J. Lindsten, M. Fraccaro, A. Mannini & L. Tiepolo. 1966 b. Extra minute chromosome in somatic and germ-line cells of the same person. Lancet **ii:** 22–24.

Hultén, M., J. Lindsten, L. Ming Pen-Ming, M. Fraccaro, A. Mannini, L. Tiepolo, E. B. Robson, A. Heiken & K. G. Tillinger. 1966 c. Possible localization of the genes for the Kidd blood group on an autosome involved in a reciprocal translocation. Nature **211:** 1067–1068.

Lindsten, J., M. Fraccaro, H. P. Klinger & P. Zetterqvist. 1965. Meiotic and mitotic studies of a familial reciprocal translocation between two autosomes of group 6–12. Cytogenetics **4:** 45–64.

Lindsten, J. & M. Hultén. 1966. Autosomala translokationer hos människa. Obstetrik & Gynekologi, Stockholm **3:** 1–29.

McIlree, M. E., W. S. Tulloch & J. E. Newsam. 1966 a. Studies on human meiotic chromosomes from testicular tissue. Lancet **i:** 679–682.

McIlree, M. E., W. H. Price, W. M. Court Brown, W. S. Tulloch & J. E. Newsam. 1966 b. Chromosome studies on testicular cells from 50 subfertile men. Lancet **ii:** 69–71.

Ohno, S. 1962. More about the mammalian X chromosome. Lancet **ii:** 152–153.

Ruddle, F. H. 1964. Quantitation and automation of chromosomal data with special reference to the chromosomes of the Hamshire pig (*Sus scrofa*). Symp. Int. Soc. Cell. Biol. **3:** 273–305.

Schmid, W. 1963. DNA replication patterns of human chromosomes. Cytogenetics **2:** 175–193.

CHROMOSOME STUDIES IN NORMAL HUMAN SUBJECTS

Sajiro Makino, Akio A. Awa, and Motomichi Sasaki
Zoological Institute, Hokkaido University
Sapporo, Japan

Introduction

Chromosome studies of normal human subjects have been carried out in conjunction with those of congenital malformations and developmental defects of various types including sex anomalies. It has been generally emphasized that more information on the so-called normal condition of human chromosomes is indispensable for better understanding and establishment of criteria in determining the normal pattern. Efforts hitherto have been devoted to the characterization of individual chromosomes at metaphase by many investigators,[10,12,16,26,28,33,39] particularly with autoradiographic techniques.[2,7,8,14,15,23,24] In this monograph identification and characterization of individual chromosomes in man are presented in detail by other cytogeneticists from various vantage points. Their data and results of our project, hopefully, will contribute greatly to the growth of knowledge in human cytogenetics and will form an important and fundamental foundation.

First, it is desirable to survey the natural occurrence of chromosomally anomalous individuals in a given population following the current standard nomenclature of human chromosomes.[11,38] Current literature indicates that the aim of a survey of this nature is focused upon (1) the postnatal or adult population and (2) the prenatal population. Most subjects used for the former investigations are derived from cultured leukocytes, and those for the latter from spontaneous and induced abortions. The cytogenetic study group in Edinburgh has been undertaking an exhaustive survey of chromosomes in adults, providing valuable information on the types and frequency of karyotypically abnormal individuals in adult populations.[5,6] A similar scheme of chromosome survey in randomly collected induced abortuses has been carried out extensively in our laboratory for the past several years.[16–18,20,32] However, a question arises whether the study group in a given area is really representative of the general population. In addition, differences in techniques, tissues or organs for study, and evaluation of data by investigators are factors in forming intricate conclusions which sometimes offer obstacles for any generalization in studies of this nature.

It is worth mentioning that, in general, chromosome anomalies in subjects from spontaneous abortions and stillbirths occur more frequently than those from induced abortions or adults. However, there has been a lack of criteria for the standardization of definition, classification, and terminology for aborted subjects. The "Standardization of Procedures for Chromosome Studies in Abortion" recommended by the scientific group of the World Health Organization is particularly useful in this field of investigation.[35]

In addition, it also seems feasible to study the behavior of chromosomes in the course of gametogenesis in both normal and abnormal individuals in relation to the etiology of chromosome abnormalities in man. Gametes with certain abnormal chromosome constitutions may have little or no fertilizability, eventually leading to miscarriages or malformations. However, there are certain cases with abnormal chromosome constitutions transmitted intact from parent to offspring. It is necessary to investigate the meiotic behavior in cells from carriers with such abnormal chromosomes.

Taking the above views into consideration, this report presents the chromosome conditions in (1) induced abortuses, (2) male germ cells in phenotypically normal and abnormal subjects, and (3) individuals of different ethnic groups in Japan. Variation in size of the Y chromosome is given as supplementary information in normal human subjects.

Chromosomes in 358 Cases of Induced Abortuses

Since 1958, we have been engaged in a chromosome survey of induced abortuses collected randomly from several public and private hospitals distributed in the city of Sapporo. The chromosomal data so far obtained from a total of 358 cases have been previously published: 41 cases by Makino and Sasaki,[18] 135 cases by Makino *et al.*,[17] 42 cases by Makino *et al.*[20] and 140 cases by Sasaki *et al.*[32] We will present some generalized aspects of the chromosome conditions in the above 358 induced abortuses.

Aborted specimens used for this study were mostly prepared for tissue culture according to current routine methods. For embryos in early gestational stages, the whole body was used for culturing. For specimens in late developmental stages, cultures were set up from portions of the body as well as organs including lung, liver, kidney, and skin. Chromosome slides were made mainly from cells in the primary culture and occasionally from those of the second to the 44th subculture by water pretreatment, squash, or air-drying methods. Some of the fresh samples were prepared immediately for chromosome observations (for details, see references 17, 18, 20 and 23).

Chromosomally Normal Abortuses

As given in TABLE 1, 351 of 358 abortuses showed a normal human complement of 46 chromosomes (XX in females and XY in males) in nearly 95 percent of observed cells. Losses or gains of chromosomes from the diploid number of 46 were noted with a frequency of 5.25 percent or 543 out of a total of 10,148 cells. Such numerical variations of chromosomes, particularly as seen in the hypodiploid range, were ascribed in part to artifacts caused by technical procedures. Hypodiploid cells were most frequent, tetraploid cells next, and triploid cells had the lowest incidence.

It should be noted here that three out of 351 chromosomally normal abortuses showed an unusually high incidence of chromosome breakage of 21, 36, and 30 percent frequency, respectively (FIGURE 1). Environmental factors altering embryonic development such as ionizing radiation, viral infection, and drug admin-

TABLE 1

CHROMOSOME NUMBER DISTRIBUTION IN CHROMOSOMALLY NORMAL FETUSES

	Chromosome Count							Total
351 cases	<45	45	46	47	>47	≅69	≅92	
Number of cells counted	111	164	9,605	64	14	7	183	10,148
Percent of total cells	(1.09)	(1.52)	(94.65)	(0.63)	(0.14)	(0.07)	(1.80)	

istration may be accepted as possible causes for the observed chromosome breakage. Alternatively, certain intrinsic or genetically determined factors in the embryo may also increase chromosome breakage. In this connection, the chromosome abnormality was studied in cultured leukocytes from the mother of one of the above three cases. Her cultures provided no genetic evidence for a high incidence of chromosome breakage.

Chromosomally Abnormal Abortuses

Chromosome abnormalities were found in seven specimens among the 358 abortuses. Of them, one case was characterized by a structural anomaly of the autosomes, and the remaining six cases showed sex-chromosome abnormalities (TABLE 2). Gestational age of those abortuses ranged from 6–12 weeks. They showed no gross anatomical or developmental anomalies with one exception showing autosomal abnormalities whose external characters remained obscure. Most of the seven mothers from whom the above specimens were taken had neither a history of exposure to ionizing radiation, drugs, nor any recognizable viral disease since the preceding menstrual period. However, one of the mothers

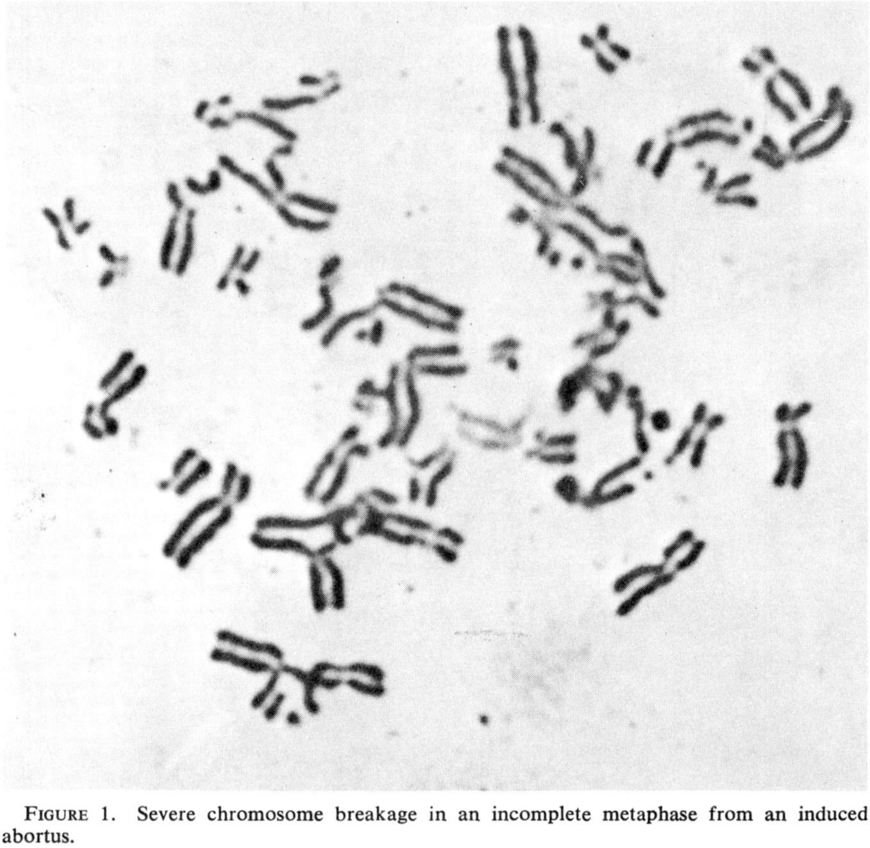

FIGURE 1. Severe chromosome breakage in an incomplete metaphase from an induced abortus.

TABLE 2

CHROMOSOME COUNTS IN SEVEN CHROMOSOMALLY ABNORMAL FETUSES

Gestation (Weeks)	Tissue	Chromosome Count					Total Cells	Sex Chromatin	Chromosome Constitution
		<45	45	46	47	90			
9–12	Whole Embryo	0	49	0	0	1	50	?	45, XY (D-D translocation)
8	Whole Embryo	0	0	0	14	0	14	++	47, XXX
9	Whole Embryo	0	6	28	0	0	34	–	{46, XY {45, XO
8	Whole Embryo	1	0	7	7	0	15	+	{47, XXY {46, XY
8	Whole Embryo	0	1	12	0	0	13	?	46, X+long Y
10	Whole Embryo	2	29	50	1	0	82	+	{46, XX {45, XO
6	Head	0	21	0	0	0	21	–	45, XO

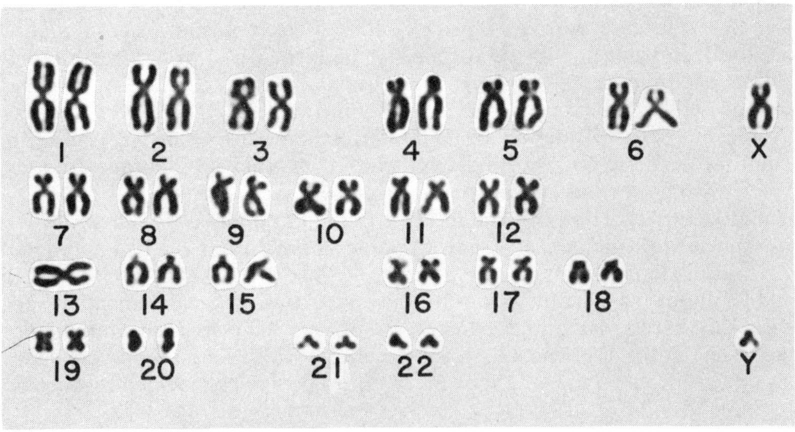

FIGURE 2. Karyotype of a cell with 45 chromosomes showing a D-D translocation in an induced abortus.

had received Salvarsan® therapy for syphilis. At present, a direct relationship between therapy and manifestation of an abnormal chromosome condition in the abortuses has remained undetermined. Four of the above seven mothers had had two or more induced abortions in the past and one had had 12 such occasions. In the remaining three, one had had no previous induced abortion and no obstetric record was available for the other two mothers. The results of chromosome counts and analysis are presented in TABLE 2.

In the first case, all of the cells in the diploid range possessed 45 chromosomes, and one cell had a duplicated chromosome number, 90. Sex chromosome constitution was of XY type, indicating male chromosomal sex. An unusually large metacentric chromosome was present and two chromosomes were missing from the D group (FIGURE 2). The first interpretation of this chromosome aberration was that a reciprocal triple translocation occurred among three of the chromosomes in the D group, leading to the subsequent formation of one large metacentric and one acrocentric with a large satellite. A second possibility was that the translocation took place between two of the chromosomes in the D group.

In the second case, 47 chromosomes with XXX sex chromosome constitution were scored in all of the observed cells (FIGURE 3a). The presence of three X chromosomes was confirmed by the finding that a certain number of cells showed two sex-chromatin bodies.

Sex chromosome mosaicism was observed in three of the seven chromosomally abnormal cases: 46, XY/45, XO in the third, 47, XXY/46, XY in the fourth, (FIGURE 3b, c), and 46, XX/45, XO in the sixth cases, respectively. No autosomal aberrations were detected in these cases.

The fifth case had an unusually long Y chromosome in every metaphase plate examined. The Y corresponded in length approximately to chromosome No. 17. The autosomes and the X chromosome appeared normal.

The seventh case showed 45 chromosomes with an XO sex chromosome constitution and was identical to typical Turner's syndrome cases. The sex-chromosome pattern of this case was in agreement with the results of the sex-chromatin test which was negative in both the cultured and noncultured embryonic cells.

In the present data, a 1.7 percent incidence of chromosome abnormalities is obtained if the case with an unusually long Y chromosome is excluded. However, the frequency in the occurrence of abnormalities would be raised by the addition of three cases showing an unusually high incidence of chromosome breakage and by the case with the long Y, approximating 2.8 percent.

A recent recommendation by WHO[35] for standardization of procedures for chromosome studies in abortion has pointed out that the average frequency of subjects with abnormal karyotypes is 19 percent with a range from 2–65 percent in spontaneous abortions on the basis of the data obtained by different investigators. The overall incidence of chromosome anomalies at birth is estimated as 1 in 240 individuals or about 0.4 percent.[3] Court-Brown *et al.*[5,6] have suggested that (1) about 0.5 percent of adults show structural rearrangements of chromosomes, (2) between 2 and 3 percent of subjects have structural anomalies confined to one autosome, and (3) among males between 2 and 3 percent show well-marked variations in the length of the Y chromosome as revealed by chromosome

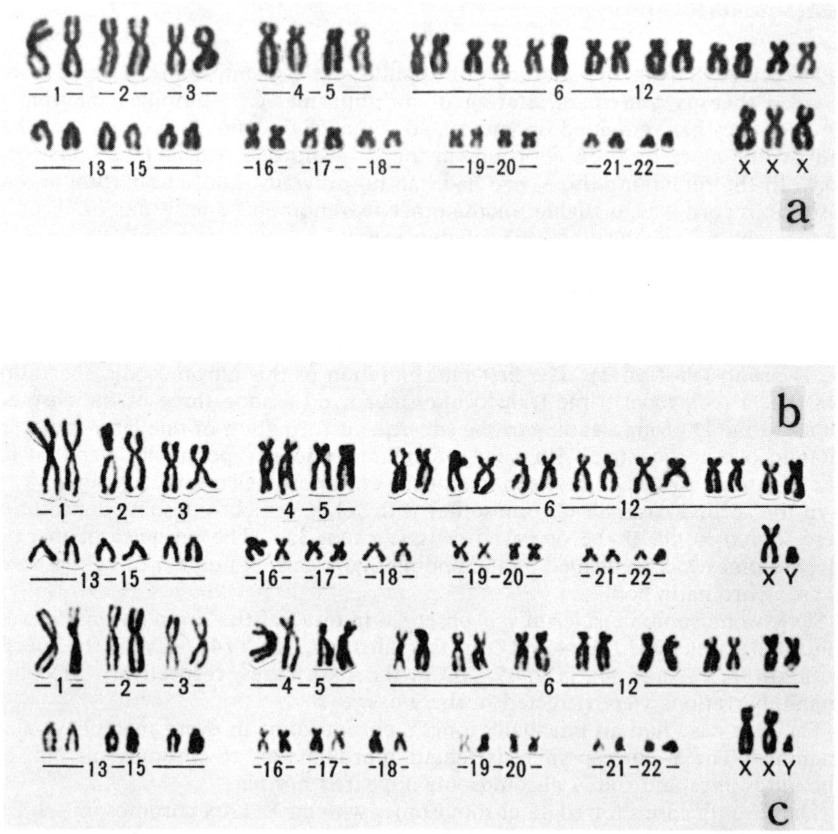

FIGURE 3. (a) Karyotype from an induced abortus with XXX chromsomes (47 chromosomes). (b) and (c) Karyotypes from an induced abortus showing 46,XY and 47,XXY mosaicism.

studies in leukocyte cultures from approximately 1,000 cases, including 438 cases of randomly chosen adults.

Upon comparing the present data with those reported by the above investigators, it is evident that the incidence of chromosomally abnormal specimens from induced abortion is far less frequent than that from spontaneous abortion. However, a decisive conclusion for similarity and/or dissimilarity between prenatal and postnatal populations should be delayed until basic criteria by chromosomal assessment common to both populations are established. In order to study the chromosome conditions in prenatal subjects, attention should be directed primarily to the hygienic and maternal environments. Medical treatments such as contraceptives, induced abortions, and ionizing radiation given to the mothers or women before conception may influence gametogenesis or embryo development with consequent formation of genotypically as well as phenotypically abnormal individuals. Epidemics of various diseases, of viral origin in particular, also may constitute a cause of chromosomal anomalies in embryos.

Among 358 cases so far studied, the chromosomal sex was determined in a total of 322 induced abortuses. The sex ratio was 77.9, with a significant excess of females over male (181 ♀ : 141 ♂ ; TABLE 3). As seen in TABLE 3, lower sex ratios were observed in abortuses obtained between the 5th to 16th weeks: 58.2, 66.4, and 77.3 for 5 to 8, 9 to 12, and 13 to 16 weeks of gestation, respectively; the remaining cases were too few to assess for statistical analysis.

A general tendency similar to our results has been found by Carr[3] in his chromosome study on 200 successfully cultured cases of spontaneous abortions, and by Moore and Hyrniuk[22] in a nuclear-sexing study on abortuses in early stages of gestation. The vast majority of results, however, has offered contradictory evidence to our results, showing a male preponderance, revealed mainly by sex-chromatin tests on subjects obtained from ectopic gestations, therapeutic abortions, and spontaneous abortions.[36] The reason for these discrepancies is obscure at present. It seems too difficult to draw any decisive conclusion from the present status of knowledge, since many factors and variables affect the prenatal sex ratio. However, it should be mentioned that one of the most convincing ways to determine sex is by chromosome analysis if care is taken to obtain chromosome preparations devoid of bacterial contamination, poor growth of cultures, etc.

TABLE 3

SEX RATIO OF INDUCED ABORTUSES BY KARYOTYPE ANALYSIS

Gestation (Weeks)	Chromosomal Sex		Total Cases	Sex Ratio
	Female	Male		
4	6	4	10	
5–8	55	32	87	58.2
9–12	72	48	120	66.4
13–16	22	17	39	77.3
17–20	2	9	11	
21–24	2	1	3	
25–28	2	1	3	
Unspecified	20	29	49	
Total Cases	181	141	322	77.9

Meiotic Chromosomes in Human Males

Increased knowledge of human somatic chromsomes in association with structural as well as numerical aberrations of chromosomes as possible causes of phenotypic anomalies in man demand an investigation of chromosome conditions in germ cells of both sexes to see if any possible chromosome aberrations are correlated with abnormalities in postzygotic subjects.

Out of 25 testicular biopsies from patients with epididymitis, prostate cancer, undescended testes, and infertility, 19 specimens were used for chromosome observations. The patients ranged in age from 4 to 79 years. In addition, meiotic behavior of chromosomes was studied in testicular biopsies from two subjects with Down's syndrome. Results of these studies have been given elsewhere by Sasaki[20,30] and by Sasaki and Makino.[31] Findings from the above investigations are summarized as follows:

(1) Polyploid cells were found in a considerable number in every stage (FIGURE 4). Occurrence of these cells was fairly consistent irrespective of age differences. Giant spermatozoa were not infrequent. It is possible that a triploid zygote with either XXY or XXX sex chromosome constitution would be produced if a diploid spermatozoon fertilized a normal haploid ovum. It is interesting that the frequency of polyploidy in primary spermatocytes was considerably lower than those in spermatogonia or secondary spermatocytes. The reason for such a low incidence of polyploidy in primary spermatocytes is unknown.

(2) Presence of a supernumerary chromosome (or chromosomes) was not demonstrated in 16 cases in which detailed analysis was available. However, it was postulated that the smallest autosomal bivalents tended to segregate precociously in the course of the first meiotic division.

(3) Testicular biopsies from a patient, aged 45, with Down's syndrome showed

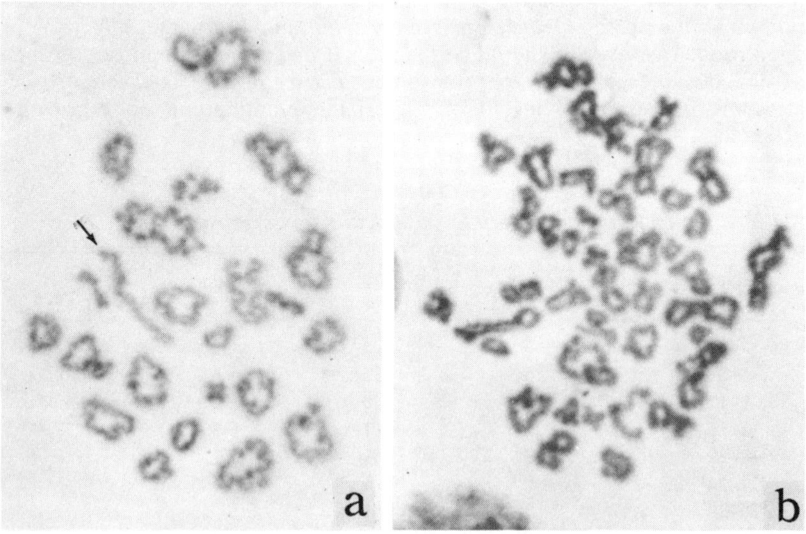

FIGURE 4. (a) A primary spermatocyte with haploid number of bivalents. An arrow indicates an XY-bivalent. (b) A primary spermatocyte with diploid number of bivalents. × 1,400; orig. mag. × 2,000.

that there were 47 chromosomes in spermatogonia as well as in cultured leukocytes, whereas primary spermatocytes showed an XY bivalent and 22 autosomal elements consisting of 21 bivalents and a trivalent. This evidence seems to favor the view by Miller *et al.*,[21] who observed 23 chromosomal elements suggestive of the existence of a trivalent in the first spermatocytes from four patients with typical 21-trisomy (Down's) syndrome. It is a matter of special attention that the seminiferous tubules of our 45-year-old patient contained no mature spermatozoa. However, a recent study on another male with Down's syndrome, aged 17, revealed the existence of mature spermatozoa indistinguishable from those of normal individuals, although detailed studies of meiotic chromosomes were unfortunately unavailable because of unfavorable material. Spermatogenesis may possibly proceed in an ordinary manner in relatively young individuals with Down's syndrome. It may be that cessation of spermatozoa formation is associated with earlier senescence in Down's syndrome patients.

Ultimate knowledge of the chromosome conditions in human meiotic cells will be achieved by the accumulation of sufficient data from female germ cells in addition to those from males.

Chromosomes in Ainu, Oroke, and Gilyak

Chromosome conditions of relatively cosmopolitan populations have been a matter of special attention among cytogeneticists. Because of the isolated environments of certain groups of people with different anthropological or ethnic features, it is dubious if generalized findings of human cytogenetics are applicable to these people. Some of these ethnic groups may disappear in the future. In this view, a chromosome study on such isolated groups as Ainu, Oroke and Gilyak, who are different ethnically but live among the Japanese, was undertaken by the authors in collaboration with Dr. D.A. Hungerford. Detailed accounts of this project will be given elsewhere by Hungerford *et al.* (in preparation).

Table 4 represents the chromosome constitutions of 29 individuals from the above three different ethnic groups. It is apparent from the Table that the chromosomes of these people were principally the same both numerically and morphologically as those of cosmopolitan populations. A relatively high incidence of aneuploid cells was found in older women. A similar tendency has been described by Court-Brown *et al.*[5]

Aberrations in Length of the Y Chromosome

Since the first report by Bender and Gooch,[1] cytogenetic investigations have provided some evidence of abnormality of the Y chromosome in man.[9,19] The human Y chromosome can be identified fairly easily in spreadout metaphase plates without karyotype analysis on the basis of the following criteria: (1) acrocentric configuration with a size slightly longer than G group chromosomes, (2) sister chromatids lying parallel, (3) positive heteropycnosis, (4) presence of a secondary constriction, (5) absence of satellites, (6) late DNA-replicating pattern revealed by autoradiography, and (7) peripheral location in the metaphase plate.

Some instances of structural abnormalities of the Y chromosome have been reported. There are cases with a metacentric Y chromosome interpreted as the isochromosome for the long arm of the Y, or as a pericentric inversion of the

TABLE 4

CHROMOSOME COUNTS IN AINU, OROKE, AND GILYAK

Ethnic Group	Case Number	Purity	Age (Sex)
Ainu	25	Pure(?)	12 (M)
	29	Pure	21 (M)
	28	Pure	26 (M)
	12	F_1	28 (M)
	2	Pure	44 (M)
	6	Pure(?)	51 (M)
	7	Pure(?)	56 (M)
	14	Pure	58 (M)
	26	Pure	62 (M)
	1	Pure	64 (M)
	10	Pure	64 (M)
	11	Pure	68 (M)
	12 cases		46.2*
	24	Pure(?)	11 (F)
	3	Pure(?)	16 (F)
	9	Pure(?)	37 (F)
	31	S × A†	48 (F)
	4	Pure	57 (F)
	27	Pure	58 (F)
	32	Pure§	61 (F)
	16	Pure	64 (F)
	19	Pure	64 (F)
	8	Unknown	64 (F)
	30	Pure§	65 (F)
	15	Pure	66 (F)
	5	Pure(?)	72 (F)
	13 cases		52.5*
	25 cases		49.5*
Oroke	35	?	39 (M)
	34	?	41 (M)
	33	?	29 (F)
	3 cases		36.3*
Gilyak	36	?	59 (F)

M=male, F=female.

* Average age.

† F_1 between Saghalien Ainu and Ainu.

‡ Two of these cells had 47 chromosomes that were not identical in karyotype.

§ Saghalien Ainu.

TABLE 4 (continued)

Chromosome Count						Total	Number of Cells Karyo-typed
<44	45	46	47	48	49		
–	2	28	–	–	–	30	7
–	1	29	–	–	–	30	8
–	1	29	–	–	–	30	6
–	–	2	–	–	–	2	–
–	1	37	1	–	–	39	3
1	1	37	1	–	–	40	6
1	1	20	–	–	–	22	1
–	–	19	–	1	–	20	2
–	2	28	–	–	–	30	5
–	2	28	–	–	–	30	4
1	1	14	–	–	–	16	2
–	–	19	1	–	–	20	1
3	12	290 (93.9%)	3	1	0	309	
–	1	32	–	–	–	33	4
–	1	54	–	–	–	55	7
–	–	14	–	–	–	14	1
–	1	34	–	–	–	35	3
–	1	23	–	–	–	24	5
–	–	29	–	–	1	30	8
–	1	27	2	–	–	30	6‡
–	–	5	–	–	–	5	–
1	3	25	2	1	–	32	4
1	1	20	–	–	–	22	2
–	2	12	–	–	–	14	3
–	2	9	–	–	–	11	–
–	4	34	2	–	–	40	3
2	17	318 (92.2%)	6	1	1	345	
5	29	608 (93.0%)	9	2	1	654	
–	1	29	–	–	–	30	3
1	–	29	–	–	–	30	5
–	2	28	–	–	–	30	3
1	3	86 (95.6%)	0	0	0	90	
–	2	27 (90.0%)	1	–	–	30	4

Y, as assumed from the size of the altered Y chromosome.[13] Deletion of the long arm is also an aberration found in the Y chromosome. Some characteristics of the Y chromosome from recent studies are that the male-determining genes may be situated on the short arm,[13,25] or, otherwise, close to the centromere,[19,24] and that the variability in size and shape of the Y chromosome suggests its relative genetic inertness.

While studying human subjects in the normal and abnormal categories, we obtained 24 individuals with the abnormal Y chromosome.[19,25] Most subjects considered here showed the unusually long Y chromosome (FIGURE 5a) but two subjects showed an extremely short (FIGURE 5b) or comparatively short Y chromosome. Familial investigations on subjects with the long Y chromosome suggested that the unusual length of the Y was an inherited character, transmitted from father to son, and usually had nothing to do with the altered phenotype. In contrast, neither the minute nor the short Y chromosome was detected in any of fathers of the present subjects, though there is evidence of a familial transmission of the deleted Y.[24]

The variation in the length of the Y chromosome was quantitated by the estimation of the Y/F value, i.e., the ratio of the length of the Y to the average length of chromosomes in the F group. According to the above estimation, the typical Y lay in the Y/F value of 0.87, whereas the value exceeded 1.00 in the abnormally long Y chromosome.

Although the abnormality of the Y chromosome may not always be associated with specific phenotypic anomalies, there is evidence that the abnormal Y appears to be rather frequently in association with neuropsychiatric diseases.[37] Such a tendency could be merely coincidental. Price *et al.*[27] have reported nine males, who have criminal records and are considered to be mentally retarded, with an XYY sex chromosome complement, though the Y abnormality is a numerical rather than a structural change.

Recently Cohen *et al.*[4] have compared the variation in the length of the Y in 100 males derived from five different racial and ethnic subgroups. One of the interesting findings is that the mean length of the Japanese Y chromosome is significantly greater than that of other groups such as Asiatic Indians, American Negroes, Jews of Eastern European extraction, and non-Jews of Anglo-Saxon origin.[4] It should be noted however that, as suggested by Cohen *et al.*[4] and by many others, differences in mean length of the Y can be seen among groups, as well as among the individuals within each group, and occasionally the cells within each individual.[19] Court-Brown *et al.*[5] have recently described well-marked variations in the length of the Y with a frequency of between two and three percent in adult males.

General Remarks

With the data presently available, we can draw the general conclusion that there are always present, in a certain percentage, individuals having abnormal chromosome constitutions in the general population. Recent information has shown a high incidence of chromosome abnormalities in specimens from spontaneous abortions. This fact strongly suggests that a certain proportion of individuals with abnormal chromosome constitutions may be lost in certain developmental stages due to genetic imbalance. The rest of the individuals may, however, develop in a more or less ordinary manner with subsequent livebirth, since many adults have been found with various autosomal and sex-chromosomal anomalies.

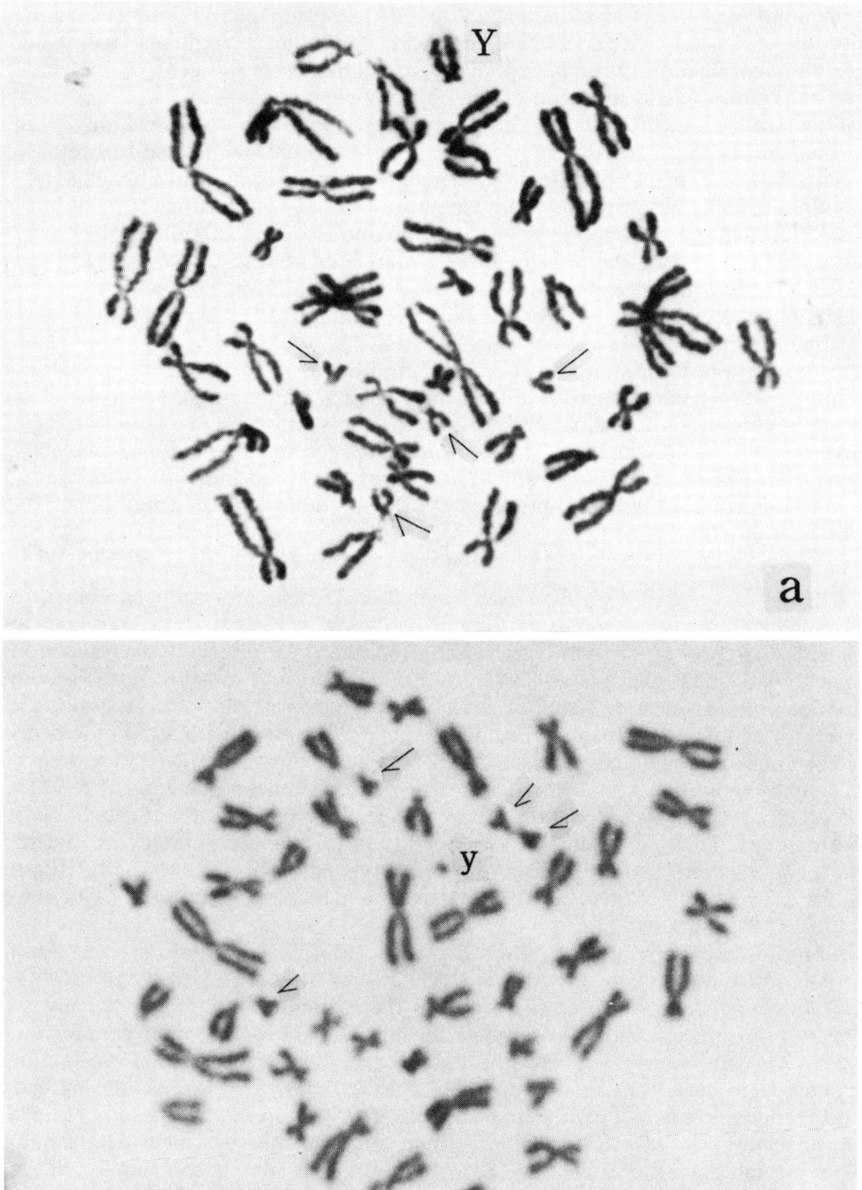

FIGURE 5. (a) Metaphase showing the unusually long Y chromosome. (b) Metaphase with the extremely minute Y. Arrows in both (a) and (b) indicate chromosomes 21–22.

Many cases of phenotypic anomalies have been reported that are not associated with any detectable chromosome abnormality; these are probably caused by technical handicaps or by poor handling of material. Accumulation of knowledge by improved cytogenetic, biochemical, and other techniques, will facilitate the identification of various phenotypic anomalies at the gene or molecular level in relation to the structure of the chromosomes.

Furthermore, identifiable chromosome alterations do not always imply abnormal phenotypes or malformations if the chromosome abnormality occurs in a genetically balanced condition, i.e., a balanced translocation of chromosomes. Examples of this nature have been presented in recent literature.

By contrast, it seems apparent that identifiable chromosomal changes or aberrations alone are not the sole etiological cause of congenital and clinical disorders. There are cases diagnosed as congenital syndromes, in which the disorders may be caused by environmental or physiological factors other than chromosomal changes.

Although there are many obstacles and limitations in the available techniques in human cytogenetics, there is a need for a large scale investigation of the chromosome conditions in induced abortuses to assess the general cytogenetic features in fetal life. Apparently, it is still premature to make any conclusive statement from the present data on the incidence of abnormal individuals in relation to developmental stages of abortuses. Further studies are in progress on this project.

Summary

Chromosome conditions were investigated in 358 cases of induced abortuses. Overall incidence of chromosome abnormalities was 1.7 percent. Among cases studied, chromosome abnormalities were found in six subjects: one case confined to autosomal changes and five cases with abnormal sex-chromosome combinations involving three cases of sex-chromosome mosaicism. In addition, one case with an unusually long Y chromosome and three cases with a high incidence of chromosome breakage were observed. The sex ratio so far determined chromosomally in 322 abortuses is 181 ♀ : 141 ♂, or 77.9, with an excess of females.

Polyploid cells occurred consistently in male meiotic cells through every spermatogenetic stage, though less frequently in primary spermatocytes. Formation of a trivalent, usually not seen in phenotypically normal males, was found in the primary spermatocytes derived from a patient with typical 21-trisomy (Down's) syndrome.

Chromosomes in subjects of three isolated and different ethnic groups, Ainu, Oroke, and Gilyak, were investigated. There was no evidence for chromosome alteration, specific to each ethnic group in these populations: their chromosome constitutions are basically the same as those of Japanese and other people.

Subjects with unusual Y chromosomes were described. Most of the abnormalities were variations in the length of the Y, the Y/F value usually exceeds 1.00 for long Y cases. There were two cases with a short Y chromosome, one of extremely minute size. Evidence presented suggests that the male determining genes or factors are situated on a region proximal to the centromere of the shorm arm of the Y chromosome. The unusual length of the Y chromosome is inherited from the father.

Acknowledgments

Cytogenetic studies on Ainu, Oroke, and Gilyak in a Japanese population were carried out with the cooperation of Dr. David A. Hungerford and his colleagues at the Institute for Cancer Research, Philadelphia, Pa., U.S.A. We wish to express our sincere thanks to Dr. Hungerford for his permission to cite unpublished chromosomal data on these subjects in this report. We acknowledge with cordial thanks Drs. T. Ikeuchi, Y. Kikuchi, J. Muramoto, Y. Nakagome, M. S. Sasaki, H. Shimba, T. Sofuni, N. Takagi, K. Yamada, and M. C. Yoshida for their collaboration and for offering their chromosome data for use in the present paper.

References

1. Bender, M. A. & P. C. Gooch. 1961. An unusually long Y Chromosome. Lancet **ii:** 463–464.
2. Bender, M. A. & D. M. Prescott. 1962. DNA synthesis and mitosis in cultures of human peripheral leukocytes. Exp. Cell Res. **27:** 221–229.
3. Carr, D. H. 1965. Chromosome studies in spontaneous abortions. Obst. Gynec. **26:** 308–326.
4. Cohen, M. M., M. W. Shaw & J. W. MacCluer. 1966. Racial differences in the length of the human Y chromosome. Cytogenetics **5:** 34–52.
5. Court-Brown, W. M., K. E. Buckton, P. A. Jacobs, I. M. Touch, E. V. Kuenssberg & J. D. E. Knox. 1966. Chromosome studies on adults. Eugenics Lab. Mem., Galton Lab., Univ. London **42:** 1–91.
6. Court-Brown, W. M., P. A. Jacobs & M. Brunton. 1965. Chromosome studies on randomly chosen men and women. Lancet **ii:** 561–562.
7. German, J. L. 1962. DNA synthesis in human chromosomes. Trans. N. Y. Acad. Sci. **24:** 395–407.
8. German, J. L. 1962. The pattern of DNA synthesis in the chromosomes of human blood cells. J. Cell Biol. **20:** 37–56.
9. Gripenberg, U. 1964. Size variation and orientation of the human Y chromosome. Chromosoma (Berlin) **15:** 618–629.
10. Hamerton, J. L. 1961. Sex chromatin and human chromosomes. Int. Rev. Cytol. **12:** 1–61.
11. Human Chromosome Study Group. 1960. A proposed standard system of human mitotic chromosomes. Lancet **i:** 1063–1065.
12. Hungerford, D. A. 1964. Observations on the morphology and behavior of normal chromosomes. *In* Mammalian Cytogenetics and Related Problems in Radiology. : 133–155. Pergamon Press, Inc., New York.
13. Jacobs, P. A. & A. Ross. 1966. Structural abnormalities of the Y chromosome in man. Nature **210:** 352–354.
14. Kikuchi, Y. & A. A. Sandberg. 1964. Chronology and pattern of human chromosome replication. I. Blood leukocytes of normal subjects. J. Nat. Cancer Inst. **32:** 1109–1143.
15. Kikuchi, Y. & A. A. Sandberg. 1965. Chronology and pattern of human chromosome replication. II. Autoradiographic behavior of various Y and X chromosomes. J. Nat. Cancer Inst. **34:** 795–813.
16. Makino, S. 1964. Chromosomal studies in normal human subjects and in 300 cases of congenital disorders. Parts I–III. Cytologia **29:** 13–31; 125–150; 233–262.
17. Makino, S., Y. Kikuchi, M. S. Sasaki, M. Sasaki & M. Yoshida. 1962. A further survey of the chromosomes in the Japanese. Chromosoma (Berlin) **13:** 148–162.
18. Makino, S. & M. Sasaki. 1961. A study of somatic chromosomes in a Japanese population. Am. J. Hum. Genet. **13:** 47–63.
19. Makino, S. & N. Takagi. 1965. Some morphological aspects of the abnormal human Y chromosome. Cytologia **30:** 274–292.
20. Makino, S., K. Yamada & T. Sofuni. 1963. A supplementary note on the somatic chromosomes in Japanese. Proc. Japan Acad. **39:** 131–135.
21. Miller, O. J., U. Mittwoch & L. S. Penrose. 1960. Spermatogenesis in man with special reference to aneuploidy. Heredity **14:** 456.
22. Moore, K. L. & W. Hyrniuk. 1960. Sex diagnosis of early human abortions by the chromatin method. Anat. Rec. **136:** 247 (Abstr.).
23. Morishima, A., M. M. Grumbach & J. H. Taylor. 1962. Asynchronous duplication of human chromosomes and the origin of sex chromatin. Proc. Nat. Acad. Sci. U.S.A. **48:** 756–763.

24. MULDAL, S. & C. H. OCKEY. 1961. Muscular dystrophy and deletion of Y chromosome. Lancet **ii**: 601.
25. NAKAGOME, Y., M. SASAKI, I. MATSUI, M. KAWAZURA & Y. FUKUYAMA. 1965. A mentally retarded boy with a minute Y chromosome. J. Pediat. **67**: 1163–1167.
26. PATAU, K. 1960. The identification of individual chromosomes, especially in man. Amer. J. Hum. Genet. **12**: 250–276.
27. PRICE, W. H., J. A. STRONG, P. B. WHATMORE & W. F. MCCLEMONT. 1966. Criminal patients with XYY sex-chromosome complement. Lancet **i**: 565–566.
28. SAKSELA, E. & P. C. MOORHEAD. 1962. Enhancement of secondary constrictions and the heterochromatic X in human cells. Cytogenetics **1**: 225–244.
29. SASAKI, M. 1964. Notes on polyploidy in human male germ cells. Proc. Japan Acad. **40**: 553–557.
30. SASAKI, M. 1965. Meiosis in a male with Down's syndrome. Chromosoma (Berlin) **16**: 652–657.
31. SASAKI, M. & S. MAKINO. 1965. The meiotic chromosomes of man. Chromosoma (Berlin) **16**: 637–651.
32. SASAKI, M., S. MAKINO, J. MURAMOTO, T. IKEUCHI & H. SHIMBA. 1967. A chromososome survey of induced abortuses in a Japanese population. Chromosoma (Berlin) **20**: 267–283.
33. SASAKI, M. S. & S. MAKINO. 1963. The demonstration of secondary constrictions in human chromosomes by means of new techniques. Amer. J. Hum. Genet. **15**: 23–33.
34. SCHMID, W. 1963. DNA replication patterns of human chromosomes. Cytogenetics **2**: 175–193.
35. STANDARDIZATION OF PROCEDURES FOR CHROMOSOME STUDIES IN ABORTION. 1966. Bull. WHO **34**: 765–782.
36. STEVENSON, A. C. 1966. Sex chromatin and the sex ratio in man. *In* The Sex Chromatin. : 263–276. W. B. Saunders Co. Philadelphia, Pa.
37. TAKAGI, N., T. KATO & S. MORITA. 1964. Chromosome studies in 10 congenital neuropsychiatric patients. Proc. Japan Acad. **40**: 674–678.
38. THE LONDON CONFERENCE ON THE NORMAL HUMAN KARYOTYPE. 1963. Cytogenetics **2**: 264–268.
39. YUNIS, J. J. 1965. Human Chromosome Methodology. Academic Press, Inc. New York, N. Y.

THE INTERRELATIONSHIP OF SEX CHROMOSOME CONSTITUTION AND PHENOTYPE IN THE SYNDROME OF GONADAL DYSGENESIS AND ITS VARIANTS*

Akira Morishima and Melvin M. Grumbach
Department of Pediatrics, University of California San Francisco Medical Center, San Francisco, Calif.

Recent work in a number of laboratories has considerably advanced our understanding of the vagaries of the syndrome of gonadal dysgenesis or Turner's syndrome. The syndrome of gonadal dysgenesis may be used as a model to illustrate the effects of variants of a sex chromosome abnormality on the clinical expression of a disorder, in this case the typical Turner's phenotype. In examining the interrelationship of sex chromosomes and phenotype, it is of value first to consider briefly some unique properties of human sex chromosomes recently discovered.

Evidence adduced from detection of abnormal sex chromosome constitution in man indicates that the Y chromosome has potent testis-determining genes, a property similar to that demonstrated in the mouse by Welshons and Russell.[1] Presence of a Y chromosome leads to differentiation of the primordial gonad as a testis, even in individuals with an XXXXY sex chromosome constitution[2–4] and its lack in the XO individual precludes testicular differentiation. On the other hand, survival of oogonia and oocytes and hence development of a normal ovary, unlike the mouse, appear to require two normal X chromosomes in man. True hermaphrodism and a few patients with an apparent XO sex chromosome constitution who experienced spontaneous menstruation,[6] including one who gave birth to a normal child,[6,7] are exceptions to this generalization. Here the situation is complex and other explanations may be advanced (see later discussion).

Fixed Differentiation Hypothesis of X Chromosome Behavior; Lyon Hypothesis

The possibility that homologous alleles on a pair of chromosomes might behave in an ambivalent manner has only recently received consideration. However, it is now recognized that in the human there is a striking differential behavior of the two X chromosomes in female somatic cells, which has led to the concept of the "fixed differentiation" hypothesis of X chromosome behavior,[8–10,17,42] and the "inactive-X" theory of Lyon.[11–13] This discordant behavior has been attributed to heterochromatinization of all X chromosomes but one in diploid somatic nuclei. We suggested that the heterochromatinized X chromosome in man has the following characteristics:[8–10,17] (1) precocious condensation in prophase and interphase nuclei, giving rise to the sex chromatin body of Barr; (2) late completion of DNA replication during the synthetic period of interphase, as assessed by the pattern of incorporation of tritiated thymidine; and (3) suppression of the activity of genes located on the heterochromatinized portions of the X chromosome. Evidence obtained in the mouse[11–13] on the mode of expression of X-lined genes controlling coat color led Lyon to advance the "inactive-X" theory of dosage compensation in female mice with its genetic implications.[11] To explain the mosaic patterns observed in the expression of these loci, Lyon assumed random inactivation of either the maternally or the paternally derived X choromosome in an early stage of embryological development; once the change is induced, the descendants of each cell maintain that state. That one of the two X chromosomes in human females is genetically in-

* This study was supported by grants from the National Foundation and the National Institute of Child Health and Human Development, NIH, USPHS.

activated is strongly supported by the demonstration of two populations of cells in the female heterozygous for the X-linked gene controlling the enzyme glucose-6-phosphate dehydrogenase.[14–16]

Based on the evidence in man, we proposed that a large portion of one of the two X chromosomes in normal females (and any X chromosomes in excess of one when multiple X chromosomes are present in the complement) becomes heterochromatinized during the late blastocyst stage; once this differentiation takes place, the characteristic properties of each X chromosome are fixed and transmitted to the cell progeny. Either the maternally or paternally derived X chromosome may become heterochromatinized in individual cells.[8–10,17,42] When a structurally abnormal X chromosome is present in the complement, however, preferential heterochromatinization of the heteromorphic X chromosome occurs.[17]

Evidence presented in support of the "fixed differentiation" hypothesis of human X chromosome behavior includes: (1) observation of sex chromatin-positive nuclei in XO cell lines isolated in tissue culture from a patient with XO/XX/XXX sex chromosome mocaisism;[8] (2) finding that one of the two X chromosomes in normal females continues DNA replication after all other chromosomes in the complement have completed DNA synthesis;[9] (3) lack of a late replicating X chromosome in cells with XY and XO sex chromosome constitution;[9] (4) the observation that the maximum number of sex chromatin bodies per diploid nucleus is the same as the number of late-replicating X chromosomes in patients with XXX, XXY, XXXXX, and XX^I sex chromosome constitution (X^I denotes presumptive isochromosome for the long arm of the X chromosome) and in XO/XX/XXX mosaicism;[8,9,17] (5) the observation that the late-replicating X chromosome frequently lies at the periphery of the metaphase figures, in a position consistent with the characteristic peripheral location of sex chromatin;[9,17] (6) preferential late replication of the heteromorphic X chromosome when present in the complement, as was observed in cells with XX^I sex chromosome constitution;[17] (7) detection of heavy labeling of sex chromatin in interphase nuclei when pulse-labeled with tritiated thymidine in vitro and then fixed immediately,[17,18] which suggested that DNA replication may proceed in the heterochromatic segments of the X chromosome without requiring prior uncoiling; and (8) the observation that in females, erythrocyte glucose-6-phosphate dehydrogenase activity is not raised over normal males, XO individuals, or patients with X chromosome polysomy.[10,17].

Heterochromatinization of major portions of all X chromosomes in excess of one in any given cell provides an explanation for the relatively minor phenotypic changes produced by extra X chromosomes, in contrast to the strikingly severe changes usually associated with trisomy for an autosome as small as chromosome No. 21. It should be emphasized, however, that inactivation does not involve the entire X chromosome. There are compelling reasons to believe that the heterochromatinized X chromosome in human beings is not completely inactive genetically and that in the female two X chromosomes are necessary for normal development. Two populations of erythrocytes have not been found in females, heterozygous for the X-linked blood group Xg, suggesting that this locus which seems to be on the short arm of the X chromosome is not inactivated.[19–21] (This finding, however, has been questioned in a recent report).[22] Further, individuals with XO or XXY constitutions, for example, are not normal, indicating that there are gene loci on the heterochromatic X chromosome expressing a gene dosage effect. Observation of incorporation of tritium-labeled thymidine in scattered areas of the heterochromatinized X chromosome of human females during the early synthetic period of interphase may also be a reflection of genic activity in these areas.[9,23–25]

Prevalence of Sex Chromosome Abnormalities

The incidence of sex chromosome abnormality among live-born infants is remarkably high, accounting for approximately one-half of all chromosomal aberrations. Based on surveys of sex chromatin, the incidence of seminiferous tubule dysgenesis (Klinefelter's syndrome) is approximately 2.1 per 1,000 live-born males, whereas the incidence of the syndrome of gonadal dysgenesis is 0.4 per 1,000 and that of XXX females is 1.2 per 1,000 live-born females.[26] Furthermore, prevalence of XO gonadal dysgenesis among spontaneously aborted fetuses appears to be over five percent.[27] Explanation for the frequency of sex chromosome aberrations may be attributable in part to the heterochromatinization of the X chromosome (and possibly of the Y chromosome). In the salivary gland chromosomes of *Drosophila melanogaster,* heterochromatin has the tendency to exhibit indiscriminate pairing with other heterochromatic regions and the heteropycnotic segment may break easily.[28–29] Thus, chromosomes comprised largely of heterochromatin may more frequently stick together and lead to nondisjunction or heterochromatic recombination subsequent to chromosomal breakage. On the other hand, genetic inactivation associated with heterochromatinization may render the X chromosome abnormality less deleterious to the embryo than those involving autosomes. Thus, they allow the fetus to survive and result in more frequent detection. Most autosomes or autosomal segments involved in human chromosomal aberrations complete DNA synthesis relatively late in the synthetic period of the cell cycle, although not as late as the heterochromatic X. The short arm of No. 5, a major portion of Y, No. 13, No. 18, and No. 21 chromosomes are some examples.[9,23,24]

Sex chromosomes, especially the X chromosome, are involved in a variety of chromosome aberrations, including structural alterations and mosaicism. A wide spectrum of sex chromosome abnormalities has been described in patients with the syndrome of gonadal dysgenesis, a syndrome in which phenotypic expression is also highly variable.[21,30,35] Thus, these patients provide a model for studying the role of sex chromosomes on gonadogenesis and stature, and on the manifestations of extragenital somatic anomalies. In this report we correlate the karyotype and the phenotype observed in over 80 patients with the syndrome of gonadal dysgenesis and its variants studied in our laboratory, and consider the modifying effects of sex chromosomes on the phenotype in light of our observations and other relavant studies.

Syndrome of Gonadal Dysgenesis with XO Sex Chromosome Constitution

Approximately 80 percent of patients with the gonadal dyngenesis syndrome have sex chromatin-negative interphase nuclei.[36] Most of them have an XO sex chromosome constitution in their diploid cells, as originally reported by Ford *et al.*[37] The typical form of this syndrome was first defined clinically by Turner.[38] Cardinal features are a female phenotype, short stature, rudimentary streak gonads, sexual infantilism, and a variety of associated somatic anomalies.[35,39] The most common associated defects include a typical facies; a shield-like chest; low hair line over the back of the neck; webbed neck in about one-half; coarctation of the aorta in about one-fifth; cubitus valgus; congenital lymphedema or its residual, such as puffiness of the dorsum of the fingers, short fourth metacarpal; high arched palate; various skeletal abnormalities; microthelia; hypoplastic nails;

and cutaneous (including an excessive number of pigmented nevi and a tendency to keloid formation), ocular, otic, and renal abnormalities. The incidence of mental retardation is increased, but the deficiency is generally mild. Although all of these associated somatic anomalies rarely occur in one individual, combination of these defects is sufficiently characteristic to produce the Turner's phenotype.

Of 62 patients with an XO sex chromosome constitution studied in our laboratory, all had normal female external genitalia. None had achieved stature greater than −2½ standard deviations (SD) from the mean height for normal females by the time they reached school age. In those who had reached pubertal age, sexual infantilism, except for sparse pubic hair, was invariably present. Three features, namely phenotype, short stature, and sexual infantilism, were the most consistent characteristics associated with an XO sex chromosome constitution.

An exception to this generalization is one report of an XO individual who produced a normal child.[6,7] Ferguson-Smith[34] recently reviewed the available reports on 117 patients with XO sex chromosome constitution and found seven patients who had experienced at least one eposide of spontaneous menstruation. However, whether these episodes represented ovulatory or anovulatory uterine bleeding was not known, and, furthermore, in most cases the possibility of undetected sex chromosome mosaicism was not convincingly excluded. Alternatively, selective nondisjunction in XO germ cells,[35,40] giving rise to XX cells, could explain the spontaneous menstruation seen in XO individuals.

Syndrome of Gonadal Dysgenesis with X Chromosome Mosaicism

In contrast to the typical form of gonadal dysgenesis in which an XO sex chromosome constitution is present, approximately 20 percent of patients with this syndrome have sex chromatin-positive interphase nuclei.[36,39] This group of patients usually has either a structurally abnormal X chromosome or, more commonly, sex chromosome mosaicism involving an XO cell line.[4]

Among the latter group, six patients with XO/XX and three patients with XO/XX/XXX mosaicism were found in our survey. It is noteworthy that the presence of an XX cell population was demonstrated in the skin biopsy specimens but not in the cultured peripheral leukocytes of one patient with an XO/XX mosaicism. Similarly, in one patient with an XO/XX/XXX mosaicism, the presence of an XX and XXX cell populations was not detected in the first two skin culture specimens and was only found in the third skin biopsy specimen and in the peripheral leukocytes.[8,42] In another individual with an XO/XX/XXX mosaicism, repeated blood cultures failed to reveal presence of the XX cell line.[43] The percentage of interphase cells with a sex chromatin body in these nine patients, as well as the frequency of duplicate sex chromatin masses in cases with XO/XX/XXX mosaicism, varied greatly from one individual to another and in different tissues (buccal mucosa, vaginal mucosa, skin epithelium, and monolayer cells of cultured skin samples) from the same individual. For example, in one patient with an XO/XX/XXX mosaicism, no double sex chromatin masses were found in over 700 nuclei in buccal smears, while duplicate Barr bodies were present in 15 percent of the nuclei of cultured monolayer cells derived from a skin biopsy. These findings demonstrate that chromosome constitution may vary in different tissues and even in different regions of the same tissue when mosaicism is present, emphasizing the difficulties in detecting and, especially, excluding mosaicism.

Clinical features in these nine patients were more variable than the group with XO sex chromosome constitution. Only one of the cardinal signs of the syndrome of gonadal dysgenesis, normal female external genitalia, occurred in all patients. Two individuals, ten years and 13 years of age, were of normal height for their age. Of seven patients who had reached pubertal age, four had developed varying degrees of spontaneous feminization and regular menstrual periods had ensued in two. Associated somatic defects in these patients were generally milder and more variable than in chromatin-negative XO individuals. For example, in one patient with an XO/XX/XXX sex chromosome mosaicism, short stature, multiple pigmented nevi, mild deformity of the helix, slightly high-arched palate, and broad chest and hands were the only somatic abnormalities. On the other hand, a large number of somatic defects including coarctation of the aorta was present in one individual with an XO/XX mosaicism who was of normal height and in whom regular menstrual periods occurred at puberty. Obvious lymphedema was not present in any of the nine patients, although it has been recorded in 39 percent of reported XO individuals.[34] Webbed neck, which occurs in about one-half of the XO patients, was found only in two out of the nine patients with XO/XX or XO/XX/XXX sex chromosome mosaicism. Of interest is the finding of a goiter and hypothyroidism in one patient with an XO/XX/XXX mosaicism in which a high titer of circulating thyroid antibodies was present.

There was no clinical feature which distinguished between the patients with XO/XX and XO/XX/XXX mosaicism; both exhibited modifying effects on the typical Turner's phenotype from that of patients with XO sex chromosome constitution. However, the phenotype of some patients with such mosaicism was indistinguishable from typical Turner's phenotype. It has been pointed out that the clinical expressions in three reported cases of XO/XXX sex chromosome mosaicism were similar to those of XO/XX and XO/XX/XXX mosaics;[34] the XXX cell line would be expected to exert a normalizing influence, since nonmosaic XXX individuals usually do not appear to be distinguishable clinically from normal females except for mental retardation.

Syndrome of Gonodal Dysgenesis with a Structurally Abnormal X Chromosome

Three types of structural alterations of the X chromosome have been reported in association with the syndrome of gonadal dysgenesis. These are isochromosomes, partial deletion of either the long arm or the short arm, or both, and a ring chromosome. In our series, seven of the 16 sex chromatin-positive patients with gonadal dysgenesis syndrome were found to have a structurally abnormal X chromosome.

Two patients had one normal X chromosome and one abnormally large metacentric chromosome. The heteromorphic chromosome was interpreted as an isochromosome for the long arm of an X chromosome (X^I) from its morphology and late completion of DNA replication, as assessed by the autoradiographic pattern of incorporation of tritiated thymidine. An isochromosome for the long arm of an X chromosome is presumed to arise by a transverse division of an X chromosome at or near the centromere resulting in duplication of the long arm and deletion of the short arm.[44] Study of interphase cells of the two patients with an XX^I sex chromosome constitution revealed a sex chromosome body which was larger than that seen in normal females in about 40 percent of the nuclei.

Both of these individuals showed normal female external genitalia and short stature, but the associated somatic anomalies were few and not striking. At puberty, minimum but definite feminization occurred in both, although no uterine bleeding ensued, and the urinary excretion of gonadotropins eventually became elevated. One patient developed an euthyroid goiter, which proved to be Hashimoto's thyroiditis on biopsy. Circulating thyroid antibodies were detected in the patient and her mother.

All reported cases of gonadal dysgenesis with an XX^{I} sex chromosome constitution had short stature.[5,21,32,45–47] Feminization has been rarely observed.[5,34] Although most of the somatic defects, except for lymphedema of Bonnevie-Ullrich type[48] and coarctation of the aorta, have been described in these patients, occurrence of each anomaly appears to be less frequent than in XO individuals.

Evidence presented suggests that shortness of stature, impaired ovarian function, and most somatic defects of Turner's syndrome are associated with an XX^{I} sex chromosome constitution, but the isochromosome X has some modifying effect both on the ontogeny of the rudimentary streak gonads and on the clinical manifestation of the typical Turner's phenotype.

In addition to the XX^{I} sex chromosome constitution, an isochromosome for the long arm of an X chromosome has been reported in association with X chromosome mosaicism, which includes XO/XX^{I} [5,21,30,32,49] and $XO/XX^{I}/XX^{I}X^{I}$ [5,50] mosaicisms. That structurally abnormal X chromosomes are predisposed to mitotic errors is exemplified by detection of highly complex mosaicism in two of our patients. In one patient, the mosaicism consisted of six different cell populations, $XO/X^{I}O/XX/XX^{I}/XXX/XXX^{I}$, and in the other, five different cell lines, $XO/X^{I}O/XX/XX^{I}/XXX^{I}$, were found. Clinical manifestations in these two patients were similar to those seen in patients with XX^{1} sex chromosome constitution.

The second type of structural alteration, a deletion of an X chromosome, was found in an 18-year-old girl. Her sex chromosomes consisted of a normal X chromosome and an acrocentric chromosome of a length similar to that of the long arm of a normal X chromosome. This acrocentric chromosome lay frequently at the periphery of metaphase figures, a characteristic location for a heterochromatinized X chromosome, and completed its DNA replication late in the synthetic period of interphase. Thus, the sex chromosome constitution of this patient was interpreted to be XX^{SD} (XX^{SD} denotes deletion of the short arm of an X chromosome) with a deletion of a major portion of the short arm of one X chromosome. In interphase cells, a few percent of the nuclei had a sex chromatin body which was distinctly smaller than that in normal females. The patient was very short in addition to having a number of characteristic somatic anomalies of the syndrome of gonadal dysgenesis, but she did not have webbed neck, lymphedema, or coarctation of the aorta. Spontaneous feminization occurred at puberty and she had experienced repeated episodes of uterine bleeding. Evidence of ovulation was obtained on several occasions. Breasts and uterus were of adult size and the vaginal mucosa showed a good estrogenic effect.

Reported cases with a deletion of the short arm of an X chromosome include a few patients with an XO/XX^{SD} mosaicism,[5,34] two with an XX^{SD} constitution,[51,52] and another with an $XO/XX^{SD}/XM$ mosaicism (M denotes a minute chromosome).[53] Clinical finding in these individuals may be indistinguishable from those of XO individuals.

Probable deletion of the long arm of an X chromosome has been reported in a few patients with either XX^{LD} constitution (X^{LD} denotes deletion of the long arm of an X chromosome),[32,54,55] XO/XX^{LD} [21,30,32] or XX/XX^{LD} [54] mosaicism, or XX^{SI} constitution (X^{SI} denotes presumptive isochromosome for the short arm of an X chromosome).[34] These individuals are commonly of normal height with a few somatic anomalies, but they usually have rudimentary streak gonads.

A minute sex chromosome, with or without mosaicism, has been described in patients with some features of the gonadal dygenesis syndrome .Whether these fragment chromosomes are derivatives of an X or a Y chromosome cannot be established with certainty at present.[21,30,32,56–58] However, in some patients there was ambiguous differentiation of the external genitalia or hypertrophy of the clitoris, suggesting that in these individuals the minute choromosome quite likely arose from a Y chromosome.[21,56–58]

Another type of structural abnormality of an X chromosome was found in two of our patients who had an XO/XX^{R} mosaicism (X^{R} denotes a ring chromosome derived from an X chromosome). The abnormal chromosome was a ring-shaped monocentric chromosome of variable size which had the characteristic DNA replication pattern of a heterochromatinized X chromosome. In a small portion of interphase, a small sex chromatin body was observed. Both patients were short in stature and had phenotypic features of the gonadal dysgenesis syndrome. However, in one patient the associated somatic anomalies were few and mild. She became well feminized at puberty and experienced repeated episodes of anovulatory uterine bleeding. The second patient was too young to permit an assessment of gonadal function. This patient had both thyrotoxicosis and Hashimoto's thydoiritis. Circulating thyroid antibodies were detected in the patient, her normal maternal grandmother, mother, and sister.

An X ring chromosome has been reported in three females with mosaicism of XO/XX^{R},[59] $XO/XX/XX^{R}$,[60] and $XO/XX^{R}/XX^{R}X^{R}$[61] types. In addition to shortness of stature, some of the somatic features of the syndrome of gonadal dysgenesis were present in all. The two adult patients with XO/XX^{R} and $XO/XX^{R}/XX^{R}X^{R}$ mosaicism were well-feminized and had regular menstrual periods. An XO/XS^{R} mosaicism (S^{R} denotes a small ring-shaped sex chromosome derived from either an X or a Y chromosome) has been found in a sex chromatin-negative phenotypic female with short stature and bilateral streak gonads but with few other somatic anomalies.[21]

A ring chromosome is presumed to arise by breakage of a chromosome at both sides of the centromere with subsequent reunion of the two proximal broken ends. The chromosomal material of the two terminal ends of the breakage is lost from the nucleus, so that inevitably a ring chromosome is deleted of varying portions of the ends of both arms of the original chromosome. The size of such deletions is difficult, if not impossible, to estimate because of the known instability of ring chromosomes, which tend to give rise to larger and smaller ring-shaped chromosomes[62] and to undergo mitotic errors resulting in mosaicism. These characteristics of a ring chromosome complicate the task of assessing the modifying effect of an X ring chromosome on the XO phenotype. However, it is significant that three out of four postadolescent patients, in whom no XX cell population was detected, had well-developed female secondary sexual characteristics and had either repeated anovulatory uterine bleedings or regular menstrual periods. This observation suggests that a minor deletion of the terminal ends of an X chromosome does not lead to the development of streak gonads. The patient with an $XO/XX^{R}/XX^{R}X^{R}$ mosaicism, for example, was found to have primordial and graafian follicles, although few in number.

Variants of Sex Chromatin-Negative Gonadal Dysgenesis: XO/XY Mosaicism

Highly variable phenotypic expression is encountered in patients with XO/XY sex chromosome mosaicism,[33–35,63] who illustrate well the modifying influence of a Y chromosome on the XO phenotype; many individuals with an XO/XY mosaicism do not have the classical features of the syndrome of gonadal dysgenesis.

In our series, nine patients were found to have XO/XY mosaicism. Sex chromatin-negative interphase nuclei were present in all.

One patient, a 16-year-old girl, exhibited clinical features of the syndrome of gonadal dysgenesis, including shortness of stature (3.1 standard deviations below the mean height for females), multiple pigmented nevi over the trunk, broad hands, puffiness of the dorsum of the fingers, and sexual infantilism except for sparse pubic hair. External genitalia were entirely feminine but immature. No signs of virilization or the presence of a urogenital sinus were detected. Although her gonads were not explored, detection of elevated levels of urinary gonadotropins and failure to find signs of feminization of masculinization strongly suggested the absence of functional gonads. Presence of a uterus was documented by rectal examination and by induction of withdrawal bleeding after estrogen administration (TABLE 1).

Three similar cases of XO/XY mosaicism have been described in patients with or without shortness of stature.[51,64] Thus, individuals with XO/XY mosaicism may exhibit bilateral streak gonads, sexual infantilism, female external genitalia, and varying numbers of somatic anomalies of Turner's phenotype. These individuals represent a variant of the sex chromatin-negative form of the syndrome of gonadal dysgenesis.

Seven of our nine patients with XO/XY mosaicism exhibited ambisexual development of the external genitalia, including phallic enlargement, presence of a urogenital sinus, and varying degrees of labio-scrotal fusion. Excretion of urinary gonadotropins was elevated and signs of virilization were present in one patient who had reached puberty. Shortness of stature was noted in five patients who were younger than five years of age; the height of the two older individuals was approximately two standard deviations below the mean value for height of normal females of the same age. Associated somatic defects were generally fewer and milder than in patients with XO sex chromosome constitution, but again, wide individual variation was noted. For example, the associated anomalies were limited to slight epicanthal folds and a high-arched palate in one patient, while in another epicanthal folds, low-set and malformed ears, "fish" mouth, high-arched palate, short neck, low hair line, loose skin folds in the back of the neck, and widely spaced nipples were present. Lymphedema of the extremities and coarctation of the aorta were not present in any of the nine patients. The gonads of the seven patients who had varying degrees of ambiguous differentiation of the external genitalia were found in the mesosalpinx in the position of the ovary. These gonads showed a spectrum of histological findings, ranging from testes with numerous well-formed seminiferous tubules containing a normal complement of germinal cells through dysgenetic testes to vestigial streak gonads. It is noteworthy that in one of the seven patients in this group with ambiguous external genitalia, both gonads were represented by small testes which lacked a well-developed tunica albuginea but which had the normal structure of an immature testis with a normal complement of spermatogonia. In three other individuals, both gonads were also represented by testicular tissues. This ob-

TABLE 1

GENITAL STRUCTURES IN NINE PATIENTS WITH XO/XY SEX CHROMOSOME MOSAICISM

Patient	External Genitalia	Urogenital Sinus	Phallic Enlargement	Gonads	Genital Ducts: Female	Genital Ducts: Female (uterus)	Genital Ducts: Male
S.McL.	Female	–	–	Rt. streaks?	Rt. fallopian tube?	uterus	Rt. –
				Lt. streak?	Lt. fallopian tube?		Lt. –
I.S.	Ambiguous	+	+	Rt. testis	Rt. fallopian tube	uterus	Rt. vas deferens
				Lt. streak	Lt. fallopian tube		Lt. –
R.I.	Ambiguous	+	+	Rt. not found	Rt. fallopian tube	uterus	Rt. –
				Lt. streak	Lt. fallopian tube		Lt. –
R.S.	Ambiguous	+	+	Rt. dysgenetic testis	Rt. fallopian tube	vestigial uterus	Rt. vas deferens
				Lt. dysgenetic testis	Lt. fallopian tube		Lt. –
K.H.	Ambiguous	+	+	Rt. dysgenetic testis	Rt. fallopian tube	uterus	Rt. vas deferens
				Lt. dysgenetic testis	Lt. fallopian tube		Lt. vas deferens
A.A.	Ambiguous	+	+	Rt. dysgenetic testis	Rt. fallopian tube	uterus	Rt. –
				Lt. dysgenetic testis	Lt. fallopian tube		Lt. –
J.S.	Ambiguous	+	+	Rt. dysgenetic testis	Rt. –		Rt. vas deferens
				Lt. dysgenetic testis	Lt. –		Lt. vas deferens
B.A.	Ambiguous	+	+	Rt. dysgenetic testis	Rt. fallopian tube	uterus	Rt. vas deferens
				Lt. streak	Lt. fallopian tube		Lt. –
M.L.	Male	–	Normal penis	Rt. streak	Rt. fallopian tube	vestigial uterus	Rt. –
				Lt. testis	Lt. –		Lt. vas deferens

servation points out that a vestigial streak gonad on one side and a testis on the contralateral side as suggested by others,[65,66] is not an invariable feature of the XO/XY sex chromosome mosaicism. Genital ducts of these seven patients were represented by a Fallopian tube and/or a vas deferens with or without a normal or a vestigial uterus (TABLE 1).

The ninth patient with an XO/XY mosaicism was an eight-year-old boy who was seen because of an unilateral cryptorchidism. External genitalia were entirely masculine in appearance. Penis size was normal and the urethral meatus opened at its tip. The left testis was normal in size and was located in a well-formed scrotum. Biopsy of this testis revealed normal testicular tissue with a normal complement of germinal cells. On the right side, a vestigial streak gonad was found in an inguinal hernial sac together with a rudimentary Fallopian tube and uterus (TABLE 1). By 13 years of age, the left scrotal testis had enlarged and the patient showed a normal male pubertal development. Although not short in stature, he exhibited a few minor associated somatic defects of the syndrome of gonadal dysgenesis.

To examine the effect of a Y chromosome on the XO phenotype, several other reports are of interest. XO/XY mosaicism has been reported in a patient with extragenital features of Turner's syndrome who had bilateral testes and hypospadias.[67] XO/XYY sex chromosome mosaicism has been found in a patient with the typical features of the syndrome of gonadal dysgenesis[51] and in a patient with normal stature who had bilateral dysgenetic gonads.[60] Two cases of suspected XY^I constitution (Y^I denote a presumptive isochromosome for the long arm of a Y chromosome) have been reported.[32,68a] No obvious features of Turner's syndrome were present in these patients except for sexual infantilism. In one patient, both gonads were represented by rudimentary streaks.[32] An abnormal metacentric Y chromosome, similar to that of Y^I in morphology, has been described in two male patients without Turner's features and was interpreted by the authors to have arisen as a consequence of pericentric inversion.[68a] Other complex karyotypes include: (1) $XO/XY^I/XY^IY^D$ (Y^D denotes deletion of part of a Y chromosome) found in a male pseudohermaphrodite;[69] (2) XX^I/XX^Iy (y denotes a morphologically abnormal Y chromosome) seen in a patient with Turner's phenotype and undescended testes;[70] and (3) $XO/XY^D/XXXY^D$ mosaicism detected in an individual with an enlarged clitoris and the typical signs of the syndrome of gonadal dysgenesis.[71]

Origin of XO Sex Chromosome Constitution

A commonly held concept of the origin of an XO sex chromosome constitution involves nondisjunction or anaphase lagging of an X chromosome during gametogenesis, giving rise to a gamete nullisomic for a sex chromosome.[33] Such a gamete is postulated to be involved in fertilization with a normal X chromosome-bearing gamete of the opposite sex, thus leading to a zygote with an XO sex chromosome constitution. By contrast, we have suggested previously that XO individuals may arise more frequently than is generally supposed from a mitotic error of a sex chromosome during the first cleavage division in a fertilized ovum.[72] If an X chromosome from a normal female zygote or a Y chromosome from a normal male zygote is lost during the first cleavage division by anaphase lagging, an individual with an XO sex chromosome constitution will result. Evidence for this contention is as follows: (1) The high incidence of sex chromosome mosaicism in patients with sex chromatin-positive gonadal dysgenesis suggests that errors in segregation of the sex chromosomes during early embryonic development occur rather frequently. (2) XO/XY mosaicism has been found in over 20 reported patients[33,34] and in the nine individuals in the present study, suggesting a rather frequent loss of a Y chromosome during an early cleavage division. (3) No association with advanced parental age at conception has been observed in the syndrome of gonadal dysgenesis,[73] in sharp contrast to other common chromosomal disorders of man including XXY seminiferous tubule dysgenesis and autosomal trisomy syndromes, of which increased frequency has been associated with advanced maternal age. (4) The increased incidence of twin births among sibships of XO individuals suggests a relative prevalence of abnormal cleavage divisions in these families.[74] (5) Russell's extensive studies[75] in both spontaneously occurring and irradiation-induced XO mice indicate that irradiation shortly after fertilization is most effective in the induction of XO mice, and that the XO constitution is a consequence mainly of loss of the paternally derived sex chromosome in a zygote between fertilization and completion of the first cleavage division. (6) The finding of a monozygotic twin of an XO patient who was a normal XY male.[76] The evidence suggests that sex-chromatin-negative XO gonadal dysgenesis may arise not only from an error in segregation of a sex chromosome during meiosis in a germ cell of a parent, but frequently as a consequence of a sex chromosome loss between the time of fertilization and the completion of the first cleavage division.[35]

In considering the origin of sex chromosome abnormalities in man, the relationship between the syndrome of gonadal dysgenesis and autoimmune thyroid disease is of interest. Demonstration of Hashimoto's thyroiditis in three of our juvenile patients who had XX^{I} constitution, XO/XX/XXX and XO/RR^{R} mosaicism, respectively, suggests an increased incidence of autoimmune thyroiditis in the syndrome of gonadal dysgenesis.[77] A similar association in adult patients with XX^{I} or XO sex chromosome constitution has been reported by Sparkes and Motulsky[47] and by Williams *et al.*[70] That the chromosome abnormality is not the primary cause of the autoimmune thyroiditis is suggested by detection of thyroid autoantibodies in unaffected relatives with a normal karyotype. Although the available data are insufficient to draw firm conclusions, it is postulated that the genetic predisposition to develop autoantibodies in a parent is associated either directly or indirectly with an increased occurrence of chromosome errors in their offspring, especially X chromosome abnormalities.[77] That the chromosome error may arise in an early mitotic division of the zygote in these patients as well as during meiosis in a parental germ cell is suggested by the patient with XO/XX/XXX mosaicism.

Gonadal Differentiation in the Syndrome of Gonadal Dysgenesis and Its Variants

The mechanism underlying the ontogeny of the human gonad has been reviewed recently by Grumbach.[35] The primordial bipotential gonad arises along the medial aspects of the mesonephros as a thickening of the celomic epithelium during the fifth week of gestation. Early in its development the indifferent gonad is composed of two unipotential, mesodermal primordia with a disparate physiological, as well as morphological, capacity; an outer cortical component consisting of the "specialized" celomic epithelium of the urogenital ridge and an inner medullary component composed of primary sex cords derived from the downgrowth of celomic epithelium and of mesonephric and gonadal blastemal elements. Even though the primordial gonad is a bipotential structure, each somatic element is unipotential; the cortical component can differentiate only into an ovary and the medulla only into a testis. A third element, the bipotential primordial germ cells, arises from an extra-gonadal site and constitutes the germinal component of the primitive gonad. Contributions by Witschi,[79] Mintz,[80] Hemsworth and Jackson,[81,82] and Ohno *et al.*[83,84] have clarified the origin, migration, and differentiation of these cells. Primordial germ cells that segregate early are first identifiable morphologically and histochemically in the 24-day-old embryo and are located in the dorsal endoderm of the yolk sac, close to the allantoic evagination. From this site the germ cells, increasing in number by mitosis, migrate during the fifth week to the hind gut wall and then through the dorsal mesentery to the primordial gonad in the urogenital ridge seeding the cortex and medulla. In the complete absence of gonocytes, sterile gonadal ridges develop in some lower vertebrates. Although germ cells appear to be essential for ovarian differentiation, apparently this is not true for testicular differentiation. The cortex and medulla seem to induce development of the bipotential primordial germ cells as either oogonia or spermatogonia. In the development of an ovary, the cortex remains associated with the celomic epithelium and continues to increase in size; sex-specific differentiation occurs at a later stage than in the testis. It may be that the more frequent occurrence of true hermophrodism in the chromosomal female is related in part to this delayed differentiation and the incomplete regression of the medullary component. The two X chromosomes in the oogonium and the oocyte are in an isopycnotic state. The isopycnotic appearance of the two X chromosomes suggests that both are genetically active in these cells in contrast to the heterochromatinization of the major portion of one of the two X chromosomes in somatic cells.

Development of rudimentary streak gonads in sex chromatin-negative gonadal dysgenesis seems to be related to the monosomy of the X chromosome. The evidence in humans suggests that at least two normal X chromosomes (without a Y chromosome) are required for the development of normal ovaries, whereas a normal X chromosome and at least one normal Y chromosome are necessary for the development of normal testes. Origin of streak gonads in XO individuals may be explained by loss of the germ cells.[35,36,85,96] Lack of viable germ cells could occur by failure of the primordial germ cells to segregate in the dorsal endoderm, or to survive during or after migration from the extra-gonadal site into the primitive gonad. Recent evidence suggests that in XO individuals the germ cells are lost after they seed the cortex of the primordial gonad.[86] If germ cells fail to survive, cortical or ovarian development of the indifferent gonad cannot take place. If the gonadal blastemal elements do not contain a sufficient number of XY cells, testicular development will not occur. In either situation, gonadal differentiation would be impaired and result in a streak gonad with vestigial medullary elements. It would seem that, in man, a genetically active sex-determining factor(s) on the second sex chromosome (X or Y) is required, in addition to the one euchromatic X chromosome, for the survival of the primordial germ cells.[35,96]

The feminization observed in a few patients, including one fertile case, with an apparent XO sex chromosome constitution, may be explained by a selective nondisjunction which occurs in XO germ cells and gives rise to cells with XX constitution, a phenomenon observed in the creeping vole (*Microtus oregoni*),[40] or by survival of occasional XO germ cells seeded in the ovarian cortex.

However, in our experience, detectable gonadal function in nonmosaic XO

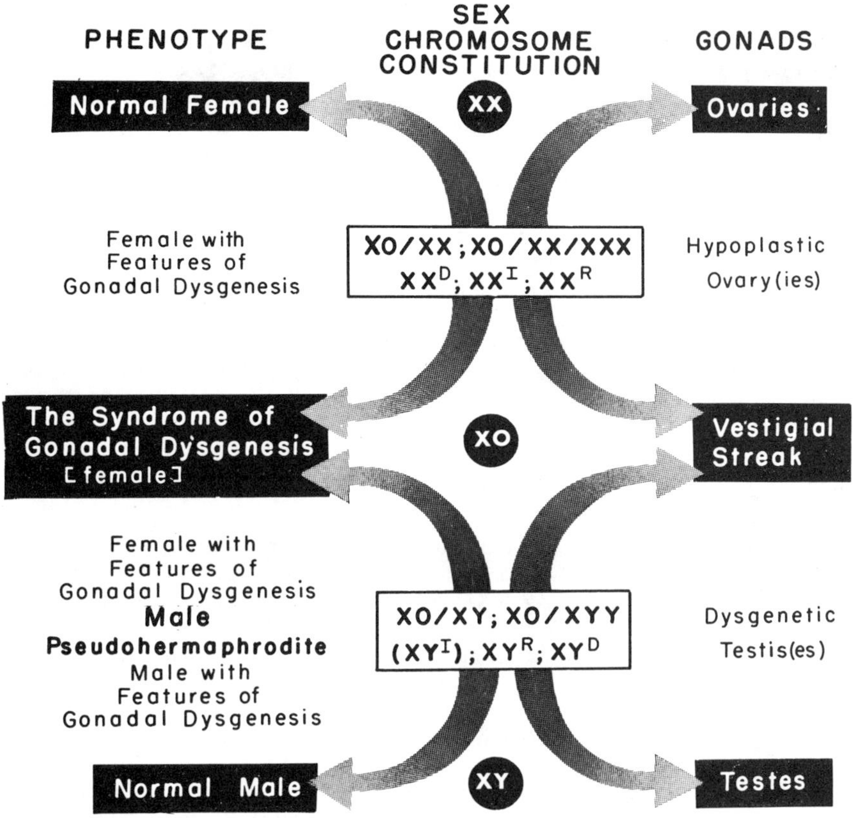

X^D = Deleted X, X^I = Isochromosome X, X^R = Ring X

FIGURE 1. This diagram illustrates the range of phenotypic and gonadal expression which occurs in the variants of the syndrome of gonadal dysgenesis and their relationship to the sex chromosome constitution. The typical phenotypic and gonadal findings in monosomic XO gonadal dysgenesis may be modified by the presence of a mosaic chromosomal constitution or by the presence of a second sex chromosome—a structurally abnormal X or Y chromosome. For example, XO/XX, XO/XXX mosaicis may be associated on the one hand with normal stature, minimal somatic features of Turner's syndrome, and some degree of ovarian differentiation and on the other hand with a clinical picture indistinguishable from classic gonadal dysgenesis. When XO/XY mosaicism or a structurally abnormal Y chromosome is present, varying degrees of testicular differentiation are frequently found which may lead to a spectrum extending from that of a phenotypic male through pseudohermaphrodism to a phenotypic female, depending upon the degree of fetal testicular insufficiency. In addition, the beneficial effects of the normal XY cell line or the presence of some part of a Y chromosome may lead to normal stature and a modification of somatic defects associated with XO monosomy.[35]

individuals is exceedingly rare, and the rather high incidence of menstruation in the reported cases (seven out of 117) is probably due to inherent bias in selection and undiscovered mosaicism. The present study, as well as previous reports,[42,87] amply demonstrates the difficulties of excluding mosaicism.

Variable gonadal development seen in XO/XX, XO/XX/XXX, and XO/XXX mosaicisms, which ranges from nonfunctioning streak gonads to normal ovaries capable of producing regular menses, can be explained by the proportion of primordial germ cells which bear an XO karyotype to those with an XX or XXX constitution. Similarly, in XO/XY and XO/XYY mosaicism, depending on the proportion of XO to XY or XYY bearing germ cells and gonadal blastemal elements, differentiation of the gonad can range from a streak gonad to a normal testis (FIGURE 1). Intermediate differentiation of a gonad between these two extremes would lead to the development of a dysgenetic testis. The spectrum of differentiation of the extragonadal genital structures (genital ducts, urogenital sinus, and external genitalia), which varies from phenotypic female through male pseudohermaphrodite to normal male in these patients, clearly depends on the state of gonadal differentiation.[35,36,85,88,89] Thus, this differentiation spectrum provides an etiological link between the syndrome of gonadal dysgenesis and one type of male pseudohermaphrodism and supports the contention advanced by Grumbach *et al.*[85] that a variant of gonadal dysgenesis may be associated with male pseudohermaphrodism.

Correlative observation of gonadal function in patients with an XO sex chromosome constitution and those with a deletion of a major portion of the short arm of an X chromosome, including XX^{I} and XX^{SD} constitution, suggests that the long arm of an X chromosome may have a modifying effect on the development of streak gonads. This hypothesis is supported by our two patients with an XX^{I} constitution who exhibited a mild degree of feminization as well as the patient with an XX^{SD} who ovulated and menstruated. The effect of the short arm of an X chromosome on gonadogenesis is not entirely clear because of the limited number of patients reported to have either XX^{LD} or XX^{SI} constitution. Only one out of seven such patients was reported to have had uterine bleeding in a recent review.[34] On the other hand, the evidence strongly suggests that a major deletion of either the short or the long arm of an X chromosome leads to impairment in the development of a normal ovary. Thus, it may be concluded that ovary-determining genes are present on both arms of an X chromosome. Although the available data are insufficient to draw a firm conclusion, the findings in patients with a ring X chromosome suggest that the ovary determiners are not located at the terminal ends of an X chromosome. Furthermore, it is postulated that at least some ovary determiners on the short arm of an X chromosome are located in a segment near the centromere. Support for this notion is provided by our well-feminized patient with an XX^{SD} constitution whose X^{SD} chromosome had a minute but recognizable short arm; an observation in sharp contrast to patients with an XX^{I} karyotype in whom, presumably, there is virtually complete deletion of the short arm. Such positional arrangement of ovary-determining genes may also explain the mechanism by which complete segregation of the female determiners is maintained in spermatogenesis, where end-to-end association between the short arm of the X chromosome and one arm of the Y chromosome is observed during meiosis.[90–92] If one assumes that exchange of genetic material occurs by crossing over in such a paired segment, it becomes imperative to suppose that ovary determiners are not located at the terminal end of the short arm. The precocious condensation of both the X and the Y chromosomes observed in meiosis of the XY cell[91] may also contribute to the isolation of the sex-determining genes during spermatogenesis.

The invariable development of testicular tissue in nonmosaic individuals with a Y chromosome points to the presence of potent testis determiner(s) on the Y chromosome. The finding of bilateral streak gonads in a patient with a suspected XX^{I} constitution[32] suggests that testis-determining gene(s) may be on the short arm of the Y chromosome, if we assume that the interpretation of the abnormal chromosome is correct. This notion was advanced by Jacobs and Ross on the basis of their observations of a presumptive XY^{I} constitution in another sexually infantile phenotypic female and of a structurally abnormal chromosome interpreted as a pericentric inversion of the Y in two phenotypical males.[68a] Although the meager data prevent one from drawing firm conclusions, we may speculate from the finding of testicular tissue in patients with a Y^{D} or a y chromosome, that male determiners are not located at the ends of the Y chromosome.

Interrelationship of Sex Chromosome Constitution and Somatic Anomalies of the Syndrome of Gonadal Dysgenesis and Its Variants

Sex chromatin-positive patients with the syndrome of gonadal dysgenesis, whether associated with X chromosome mosaicism or with a structurally abnormal X chromosome, generally have fewer and milder manifestations of somatic anomalies than those with an XO constitution. In particular, incidence of marked congenital lymphedema, webbed neck, and coarctation of the aorta is much lower among sex chromatin-positive patients and all three abnormalities are rarely present in one individual.

Variable phenotypic expression, including shortness of stature and the lesser prevalence of somatic anomalies, in patients with XO/XX, XO/XX/XXX, and XO/XXX mosaicism, can be explained by the proportion of XO cells to XX and/or XXX cells harbored in different tissues and organs during the critical period of embryogenesis (FIGURE 1). The modifying effect on somatic defects of a cell population with either XX or XXX karyotype observed in these mosaic individuals seems to account for some XO/XX mosaics reported as "pure gonadal dysgenesis" whose clinical manifestations were limited to sexual infantilism.

A structurally abnormal X chromosome often has a mitigating effect on the XO phenotype. The observation in patients with an XX^{I} or an XX^{SD} constitution suggests that presence of the long arm of an X chromosome may not abolish the manifestation of short stature and may modify only a few of the associated somatic defects of XO gonadal dysgenesis. Conversely, expression of most of the somatic defects including shortness of stature, are suppressed when a short arm of an X chromosome is present in addition to a normal X, as evidenced by patients with an XX^{LD} or an XX^{SI} sex chromosome constitution. Thus, loss of the short arm of an X chromosome appears to be related to short stature and most of the somatic defects of the XO phenotype in these patients.

There are two possible mechanisms to explain the normalizing effect of the heterochromatinized second X, whether it be a normal X as in normal females or a structurally abnormal X chromosome. First, the entire chromosome is not heterochromatinized and, therefore, some genes are not inactivated. In this model it is assumed that a number of genes on the heterochromatinized X chromosome, particularly those on the short arm, escape heterochromatinization and thus account for the suppression of the Turner's phenotype. Support for this mechanism is provided by the observation of scattered incorporation of tritiated thymidine in the structurally abnormal X chromosomes during an early synthetic period of interphase.[9,23–25] A second possibility is that all X chromosomes are genetically active during early embryogenesis and confer lasting properties upon the cell to express the phenotype dictated by the genotype active at that time. Sole support for this view is derived from the failure to observe sex chromatin masses in normal female embryos before the late blastocyst stage.[93] It is difficult to explain by this mechanism the absence of severe phenotypic abnormality, except for mental retardation, in patients with XXX, XXXX, or XXXXX sex chromosome constitution, since the extra X chromosomes should have exerted their genetic influence during early embryogenesis.

That a Y chromosome has beneficial effects similar to an X chromosome on the XO phenotype is apparent from studies on patients with an XO/XY mosaicism. The spectrum of intermediate phenotypes between normal female or male and XO gonadal dysgenesis can be correlated with the degree of deficiency of an X chromosome or a Y chromosome (FIGURE 1). This observation leads to the concept that the Y chromosome and the X chromosome bear gene loci, possibly homologous, which are responsible for the suppression of the typical phenotype of the syndrome of gonadal dysgenesis, including shortness of stature. This hypothesis has also been advanced by Ferguson-Smith.[34] Evidence adduced from two patients with little or no somatic features of Turner's syndrome in whom presumptive XY^{I} constitution was present, led Jacobs and Ross to suggest that most of the homologous loci may be linked on the long arm of the Y chromosome.[68a] The end-to-end association between the X and Y chromosomes during meiosis of an XY cell may be an expression of crossing over which would indicate the presence of an homologous segment in these two chromosomes with morphological imparity. Some investigators have suggested that the long arm of the Y chromosome and the short arm of the X are terminally associated in spermatogenesis.[92,94] Thus, short stature and most somatic defects of the syndrome of gonadal dysgenesis may be attributed to the loss of either the short arm of an X chromosome or a homologous segment of a Y chromosome.

A Distinct Clinical Entity with Somatic Defects Resembling Turner's Syndrome in Males and Females

The phenotype similar to that seen in the syndrome of gonadal dysgenesis has been reported in females with an XX sex chromosome constitution and in males with an XY constitution (Turner's syndrome in phenotypic males). Recent studies by Grumbach and associates[35,95,96] suggest that these individuals are distinct from the syndrome of gonadal dysgenesis and they were excluded from consideration in the attempt to correlate the phenotype and the karyotype of gonadal dysgenesis. A brief description of this observation, which led to the identification of a distinct entity among the clinically confounding group of boys classified as "male Turner's syndrome" and to the recognition of its counterpart in females, is presented here for the purpose of clarification. In two males and 14 females, some features resembling the syndrome of gonadal dysgenesis were found, including short stature, webbed neck, short neck wtih low hairline, high-arched palate, low-set malformed ears, broad chest, and varying degrees of cubitus valgus. Differentiating features were: (1) a characteristic triangular facies with a broad, beaked apex nasi, ptosis, and antimongoloid palpebral slant; (2) congenital heart disease, commonly pulmonic stenosis and/or atrial septal defect, but not coarctation of the aorta; (3) pectus excavatum; (4) impaired mental development; (5) in males, undescended testes with germinal cell aplasia or hypoplasia; in females, functioning ovaries; and (6) normal karyotype including a sex chromosome constitution and sex chromatin pattern concordant with the phenotype.

Relationship of Heteromorphic X Chromosomes to Sex Chromatin and DNA Replication

When a normal and a structurally abnormal X chromosome are present in a cell, the heteromorphic X is preferentally heterochromatinized. The sex chromatin body in the interphase nuclei of patients with an XO/XX^{R} mosaicism and an XX^{SD} constitution (X^{R} and X^{SD} are structurally smaller than the normal X) was distinctly smaller than in normal females. Conversely, an unusually large sex chromatin mass was present in the interphase and prophase cells of the patients with an XX^{I} constitution (X^{I} is structurally larger than the normal X). The heteromorphic X chromosomes were invariably late in completion of DNA synthesis.[17,77] In experiments designed to study the early stages of chromosomal DNA synthesis, the structurally abnormal X chromosome was unlabeled or lightly labeled but all other complements, including the normal X, were heavily labeled, suggesting asynchronous initiation as well as completion of DNA replication between the normal and the abnormal X chromosomes. Correlation between the size of the sex chromatin mass, morphology of the aberrant X chromosome, and late completion pattern of DNA replication was consistent with previously reported preferential heterochromatinization of the abnormal X chromosome and with the "fixed differentiation" hypothesis of X chromosome behavior.[8–10,17]

Summary

A systematic study of the sex chromosome constitution in over 80 patients with the syndrome of gonadal dysgenesis and its variants combined with a brief review of pertinent literature suggests that: (1) the spectrum of intermediate phenotypes between normal female or male and XO gonadal dysgenesis can be correlated with the degree and type of sex chromosome deficiency; (2) short stature and most somatic defects are attributable to loss either of the short arm of an X chromosome or a small segment of a Y chromosome; (3) failed or impaired ovarian differentiation results from the loss of either arm of an X chromosome and suggests that loci on both the short and long arms are required for development of normal ovaries; (4) streak gonads result from a deficiency of the testis determiners on the Y chromosome or of the ovary determiners on the X chromosome, probably through the loss of primordial germ cells; (5) the late-replicating X chromosome of females is not entirely heterochromatinized and exerts some genic effect on somatic cells, as previously proposed in the "fixed differentiation" hypothesis of X chromosome behavior in man; (6) XO sex chromosome constitution may arise as a consequence not only of meiotic error in the parental gamete, but also as the result of a sex chromosome loss between fertilization and completion of the first cleavage division; (1) a structurally abnormal sex chromosome is predisposed to mitotic errors of segregation for reasons which still remain obscure.

Acknowledgments

The authors gratefully acknowledge the technical assistance of Miss Daisy Breuer and Miss Nancy Carmichael in the preparation of this paper.

References

1. WELSHONS, W. J. & L. B. RUSSELL. 1959. The Y-chromosome as the bearer of male determining factors in the mouse. Proc. Nat. Acad. Sci. U.S.A. **45:** 560.
2. FRACCARO, M. & J. LINDSTEN. 1960. A child with 49 chromosomes. Lancet **ii:** 1303.
3. MILLER, O. J., W. R. BREG, R. D. SCHMICKEL & W. TRETTER. 1961. A family with an XXXXY male, a leukaemic male, and two 21-trisomic mongoloid females. Lancet **ii:** 78.
4. BARR, M. L., D. H. CARR, J. POZSONYI, R. A. WILSON, H. G. DUNN, T. S. JACOBSON, J. R. MILLER, M. LEWIS & B. CHOWN. 1962. The XXXXY sex chromosome abnormality. Canad. Med. Ass. J. **87:** 891.
5. LINDSTEN, J. 1963. The nature and origin of X chromosome aberrations in Turner's syndrome–A cytogenetical and clinical study of 57 patients. Almqvist and Wiksell. Uppsala, Sweden.
6. BAHNER, F., G. SCHWARZ, D. G. HARNDEN, P. A. JACOBS, H. A. HIENZ & K. WALTER. 1960. A fertile female with XO sex chromosome constitution. Lancet **ii:** 100.
7. BAHNER, F., G. SCHWARZ, H. A. HIENZ & K. WALTER. 1960. Turner-Syndrom mit voll ausgebildeten sekundären Geschlechtsmerkmalen und Fertilität. Acta Endocrinol. (Kobenhavn) **35:** 397.
8. GRUMBACH, M. M. & A. MORISHIMA. 1962. Sex chromatin and the sex chromosomes: On the origin of sex chromatin from a single X chromosome. Acta Cytologica **6:** 46.
9. MORISHIMA, A., M. M. GRUMBACH & J. H. TAYLOR. 1962. Asynchronous duplication of human chromosomes and the origin of sex chromatin. Proc. Nat. Acad. Sci. **48:** 756.
10. GRUMBACH, M. M., P. A. MARKS & A. MORISHIMA. 1962. Erythrocyte glucose-6-phosphate dehydrogenase activity and X-chromosome polysomy. Lancet **i:** 1330.
11. LYON, M. F. 1961. Gene action in the X-chromosome of the mouse (*Mus muculus L*). Nature **190:** 372.
12. RUSSELL, L. B. 1961. Genetics of mammalian sex chromosomes. Science **133:** 1795.
13. LYON, M. F. 1962. Sex chromatin and gene action in the mammalian X-chromosome. Amer. J. Human Genet. **14:** 135.
14. DAVIDSON, R. G., H. M. NITOWSKY & B. CHILDS. 1963. Demonstration of two populations of cells in the human female heterozygous for glucose-6-phosphate dehydrogenase variants. Proc. Nat. Acad. Sci. **50:** 481.
15. BEUTLER, E., M. YEH & V. F. FAIRBANKS. 1962. The normal human female as a mosaic of X-chromosome activity: studies using the gene for G-6-PD-deficiency as a marker. Proc. Nat. Acad. Sci. **48:** 9.
16. BEUTLER, E. & M. C. BALUDA. 1964. The separation of glucose-6-phosphate-dehydrogenase-deficient erythrocytes from the blood of heterozygotes for glucose-6-phosphate-deficiency. Lancet **i:** 189.
17. GRUMBACH, M. M., A. MORISHIMA & J. H. TAYLOR. 1963. Human sex chromosome abnormalities in relation to DNA replication and heterochromatinization. Proc. Nat. Acad. Sci. **49:** 581.
18. GRUMBACH, M. M. 1963. Discussion. *In* Second International Conference on Congenital Malformations. New York. The International Medical Congress, Ltd.
19. GORMAN, J. G., J. DI RE, A. M. TREACY & A. CAHAN. 1963. The application of $-Xg^a$ antiserum to the question of red cell mosaicism in female heterozygotes. J. Lab. Clin. Med. **61:** 642.
20. LINDSTEN, J., M. FRACCARO, P. E. POLANI, J. L. HAMERTON, R. SANGER & R. R. RACE. 1963. Evidence that the Xg blood group genes are on the short arm of the X chromosome. Nature **197:** 648.
21. FERGUSON-SMITH, M. A., D. S. ALEXANDER, P. BOWEN, R. M. GOODMAN, B. N. KAUFMANN, H. W. JONES, JR. & R. H. HELLER. 1964. Clinical and cytogenetical studies in female gonadal dysgenesis and their bearing on the cause of Turner's syndrome. Cytogenet. **3:** 355.
22. MACDIARMID, W. D., G. R. LEE, G. E. CARTWRIGHT & M. M. WINTROBE. 1967. X-inactivation in an unusual X-linked anemia and the Xg^a blood group. Clin. Res. **15:** 132 (Abstr.).
23. SCHMID, W. 1963. DNA replication patterns of human chromosomes. Cytogenet. **2:** 175.
24. GERMAN, J. 1964. The pattern of DNA synthesis in the chromosomes of human blood cells. J. Cell Biol. **20:** 37.

25. PETERSEN, A. J. 1964. DNA synthesis and chromosomal asynchrony. Induced parasynchronous DNA synthesis in human leukocyte cultures and chromosomal asynchrony in the early S phase. J. Cell Biol. **23:** 651.
26. MACLEAN, N., D. G. HARNDEN, W. M. COURT-BROWN, J. BOND & D. J. MANTLE. 1964. Sex-chromosome abnormalities in newborn babies. Lancet **i:** 286.
27. CARR, D. H. 1965. Chromosome studies in spontaneous abortions. Obs. Gyn. **26:** 308.
28. HANNAH, A. 1951. Localization and function of heterochromatin in *Drosophila melanogaster*. Adv. Genetics **4:** 87.
29. TRAUT, H. 1964. The dose-dependence of X-chromosome loss and non-disjunction induced by X-rays in oocytes of *Drosophila melanogaster*. Mutation Res. (Amsterdam) **1:** 157.
30. DE LA CHAPELLE, A. 1962. Cytogenetical and clinical observations in female gonadal dysgenesis. Acta Endocrinol. (Kobenhavn). Suppl. 65.
31. SOHVAL, A. R. 1963. Chromosomes and sex chromatin in normal and anomalous sexual development. Physiol. Rev. **43:** 306.
32. COURT-BROWN, W. M., D. G. HARNDEN, P. A. JACOBS, N. MACLEAN & D. J. MANTLE. 1964. Abnormalities of the sex chromosome complement in man. Med. Res. Council, Spec. Rept. (London) **305:** 1.
33. MILLER, O. J. 1964. The sex chromosome anomalies. Am. J. Obs. Gyn. **90:** 1078.
34. FERGUSON-SMITH, M. A. 1965. Karyotype-phenotype correlations in gonadal dysgenesis and their bearing on the pathogenesis of malformations. J. Med. Genet. **2:** 142.
35. GRUMBACH, M. M. 1968. The Reproductive System. *In* Biologic Basis of Pediatric Practice. R. E. Cooke, Ed. Chap. 108, 110. McGraw-Hill Publications, New York, N. Y.
36. GRUMBACH, M. M. & M. L. BARR. 1958. Cytologic tests of chromosomal sex in relation to sexual anomalies in man. *In* Recent Progress in Hormone Research. G. Pincus, Ed. **14:** 255. Academic Press. New York, N. Y.
37. FORD, C. E., K. W. JONES, P. E. POLANI, J. C. C. DE ALMEIDA & J. H. BRIGGS. 1959. A sex chromosome anomaly in a case of gonadal dysgenesis (Turner's syndrome). Lancet **i:** 711.
38. TURNER, H. H. 1938. A syndrome of infantilism, congenital webbed neck and cubitus valgus. Endocrinol. **23:** 566.
39. GRUMBACH, M. M. 1960. Some considerations of the pathogenesis and classification of anomalies of sex in man. *In* Clinical Endocrinology. I. E. B. Astwood, Ed. : 407. Grune & Stratton. New York, N. Y.
40. OHNO, S., J. JAINCHILL & C. STENIUS. 1963. The creeping vole (*Microtus oregoni*) as a gonosomic mosaic. I. The OY/XY constitution of the male. Cytogenet. **2:** 232.
41. GRUMBACH, M. M. 1962. Sex chromatin, sex chromosomes and abnormalities of sex. *In* Laboratory Tests in Diagnosis and Investigation of Endocrine Functions. R. R. Escamilla, Ed. : 463. F. A. Davis Co. Philadelphia, Pa.
42. GRUMBACH, M. M. & A. MORISHIMA. 1961. An XXX/XX/XO sex chromosome constitution in gonadal dysgenesis and other examples of sex chromosome mosaicisms in man (abstr.). Proc. 2nd Internat. Cong. Hum. Genet. Series No. 32. : 99. Excerpta Medica Foundation. Amsterdam, The Netherlands.
43. CARR, D. H., A. MORISHIMA, M. L. BARR, M. M. GRUMBACH, T. LUERS & H. W. BOSCHANN. 1962. An XO/XX/XXX mosaicism in relationship to gonadal dysgenesis in females. J. Clin. Endocrinol. Metab. **22:** 671.
44. DE LA CHAPELLE, A., J. WENNSTRÖM, H. HORTLING & C. H. OCKEY. 1966. Isochromosome-X in man. Part I. Hereditas **54:** 260.
45. ENGEL, E. & A. P. FORBES. 1961. An abnormal medium-sized metacentric chromosome in a woman with primary gonadal failure. Lancet **ii:** 1004.
46. HAMERTON, J. L., G. M. JAGIELLO & B. H. KIRMAN. 1962. Sex-chromosome abnormalities in a population of mentally defective children. Brit. Med. J. **1:** 220.
47. SPARKES, R. S. & A. G. MOTULSKY. 1963. Hashimoto's disease in Turner's syndrome with isochromosome X. Lancet **i:** 947.
48. ULLRICH, O. 1949. Turner's syndrome and status Bonnevie-Ullrich. A synthesis of animal phenogenetics and clinical observations on a typical complex of developmental anomalies. Amer. J. Hum. Genet. **1:** 179.
49. BLANK, C. E., R. R. GORDON & A. BISHOP. 1961. Atypical Turner syndrome. Lancet **i:** 947.
50. LINDSTEN, J., M. FRACCARO, D. IKKOS, K. KAIJSER, H. P. KLINGER & R. LUFT. 1963. Presumptive iso-chromosomes for the long arm of X in man. Analysis of five families. Ann. Hum. Genet. **26:** 383.
51. JACOBS, P. A., D. G. HARNDEN, K. E. BUCKTON, W. M. COURT BROWN, M. J. KING, J. A.

McBride, T. N. MacGregor, N. Maclean, A. Fotheringham & M. Isdale. 1961. Cytogenetic studies in primary amenorrhoea. Lancet **i**: 1183.

52. Tveteras, E. 1965. Gonadal dysgenesis with deleted X chromosome. Acta Paediat. Scand. (Uppsala). Suppl. **159**: 131.
53. London, D. R., N. H. Kemp, J. R. Ellis & U. Mittwoch. 1964. Turner's syndrome with secondary amenorrhoea and sex chromosome mosaicism. Acta Endocrinol. (Kobenhavn) **46**: 341.
54. de Grouchy, J., M. Lamy, H. Yaneva, Y. Salomon & A. Netter. 1961. Further abnormalities of the X chromosome in primary amenorrhoea or in severe oligomenorrhoea. Lancet **ii**: 777.
55. Becker, K. L., J. Paris & A. Albert. 1963. Ovarian dysgenesis due to deletion of the X chromosome. Proc. Mayo Clin. **38**: 389.
56. Conen, P. E., J. D. Bailey, W. H. Allemang, D. W. Thompson & C. Ezrin. 1961. A probable partial deletion of the Y chromosome in an intersex patient. Lancet **ii**: 294.
57. Vaharu, T., R. G. Patton, M. L. Voorhess & L. I. Gardner. 1961. Gonadal dysplasia and enlarged phallus in a girl with 45 chromosomes plus "fragment". Lancet **i**: 1351.
58. Ferrier, P., S. M. Gartler, S. H. Waxman & T. H. Shepard. 1962. Abnormal sexual development associated with sex chromosome mosaicism. II. Ped. **29**: 703.
59. Hustinx, T. W. J. & G. B. A. Stoelinga. 1964. A ring-X-chromosome in part of the somatic cells of a patient with some characteristics of the Turner syndrome. Genet. **35**: 1.
60. Lüers, T., E. Struck & J. Nevinny-Stickel. 1963. Self-perpetuating ring chromosome in gonadal dysgenesis. Lancet **ii**: 887.
61. Lindsten, J. & K. G. Tillinger. 1962. Self-perpetuating ring chromosome in a patient with gonadal dysgenesis. Lancet **i**: 593.
62. Swanson, C. P. 1957. Cytology and cytogenetics. Prentice Hall. Englewood Cliffs, N. J.
63. Morishima, A. & M. M. Grumbach. 1964. The variable clinical pattern of XO/XY mosaicism (abstr.). Proc. Endocr. Soc. Forty-sixth Meeting. : 40. June.
64. Judge, D. L. C., J. S. Thompson, D. R. Wilson, M. W. Thompson. 1962. XY/XO mosaicism. Lancet **ii**: 407.
65. Sohval, A. R. 1963. "Mixed" gonadal dysgenesis: a variety of hermaphroditism. Amer. J. Hum. Genet. **15**: 155.
66. Mellman, W. J., H. D. Klevitt, W. C. Yakovac, P. S. Moorhead & E. Saksela. 1963. 1963. XO/XY chromosome mosaicism. J. Clin. Endocrinol. & Metab. **23**: 1090.
67. Ross, G. T., J. M. Holland, W. S. Kiser & G. W. Douglas. 1965. XO/XY chromosomal mosaicism and extragenital stigmata of Turner's syndrome in a phenotypic male. J. Clin. Endocrinol. Metab. **25**: 141.
68. Cooper, H. L., H. S. Kupperman, O. R. Rendon & K. Hirschhorn. 1962. Sex-chromosome mosaicism of type XXY/XO. New Eng. J. Med. **266**: 699.

68a. Jacobs, P. A. & A. Ross. 1966. Structural abnormalities of the Y-chromosome in man. Nature **210**: 352.

69. Klevit, H. D., W. J. Mellman & W. R. Eberlein. 1963. Triple mosaicism with an isochromosome derived from a partially deleted Y in a male pseudohermaphrodite. Ped. **32**: 56.
70. Solomon, I. L., C. W. Hamm, O. C. Green. 1964. Chromosome studies on testicular tissue cultures and blood leukocytes of a male previously reported to have no Y chromosome. New Eng. J. Med. **271**: 586.
71. Fraccaro, M., M. G. Bott, F. M. Salzano, R. W. R. Russell & W. I. Cranston. 1962. Triple chromosomal mosaic in a woman with clinical evidence of masculinisation. Lancet **i**: 1379.
72. Grumbach, M. M. & A. Morishima. 1961. An XXX/XX/XO sex chromosome constitution in gonadal dysgenesis and other examples of sex chromosome mosaicism in man. Amer. J. Dis. Child. **102**: 691 (abstr.).
73. Boyer, S. H., M. A. Ferguson-Smith & M. M. Grumbach. 1961. The lack of influence of parental age and birth order in the aetiology of nuclear sex chromatin-negative Turner's syndrome. Ann. Hum. Genet. **25**: 215.
74. Nance, W. E. & I. Uchida. 1964. Turner's syndrome, twinning, and an unusual variant of glucose-6-phosphate dehydrogenase. Amer. J. Hum. Genet. **16**: 380.
75. Russell, L. B. 1962. Chromosome aberrations in experimental mammals. *In* Progress in Medical Genetics. Vol. II. A. G. Steinberg & A. G. Bearn, Eds. : 230. Grune & Stratton, New York, N. Y.

76. TURPIN, R., J. LEJEUNE, J. LAFOURCADE, P. L. CHIGOT & C. SALMON. 1961. Présomption de monozygotisme en dépit d'un dimorphisme sexuel; sujet masculin XY et sujet neutre Haplo X. Compt. rend. Acad. Sci. (Paris). **252:** 2945.
77. GRUMBACH, M. M. & A. MORISHIMA. 1964. X-chromosome abnormalities in gonadal dysgenesis: DNA replication of structuarlly abnormal X-chromosomes; relation to thyroid disease. J. Ped. **65:** 1087. (abstr.).
78. WILLIAMS, E. D., E. ENGEL & A. P. FORBES. 1964. Thyroiditis and gonadal dysgenesis. New Eng. J. Med. **270:** 805.
79. WITSCHI, E. 1948. Migration of the germ cells of human embryos from the yolk sac to the primitive gonadal folds. Embryol. **32:** 67.
80. MINTZ, B. 1957. Embryological development of primordial germ-cell in the mouse: Influence of a new mutation, Wj^1. J. Embryol. Exp. Morph. **5:** 396.
81. HEMSWORTH, B. N. & H. JACKSON. 1963. Effect of Busulphan on the developing gonad of the male rat. J. Reprod. Fertil. **5:** 187.
82. HEMSWORTH, B. N. & H. JACKSON. 1963. Effect of Busulphan on the developing ovary in the rat. J. Reprod. Fertil. **6:** 229.
83. OHNO, S., W. D. KAPLAN & R. KINOSITA. 1960. On isopycnotic behavior of the XX-bivalent in oocytes of *Rattus norvegicus.* Exp. Cell Res. **19:** 637.
84. OHNO, S., W. D. KAPLAN & R. KINOSITA. 1961. X-chromosome behavior in germ and somatic cells of *Rattus norvegicus.* Exp. Cell Res. **22:** 535.
85. GRUMBACH, M. M., J. J. VAN WYK & L. WILKINS. 1955. Chromosomal sex in gonadal dysgenesis (ovarian agenesis): Relationship to male pseudohermaphrodism and theories of human sex differentiation. J. Clin. Endocrinol. Metab. **15:** 1161.
86. SINGH, R. P. & D. H. CARR. 1966. The anatomy and histology of XO human embryos and fetuses. Anat. Rec. **155:** 369.
87. BARR, M. L., D. H. CARR, A. MORISHIMA & M. M. GRUMBACH. 1962. An XY/XXXY sex chromosome mosaicism in a mentally defective male patient. J. Mental Defic. Res. **6:** 65.
88. JOST, A. 1953. Problem of fetal endocrinology: the gonadal and hypophyseal hormones. *In* Recent Progress in Hormone Research. G. Pincus, Ed. **8:** 379. Academic Press. New York, N. Y.
89. JOST, A. 1958. Embryonic sexual differentiation. *In* Hermaphroditism, Genital Anomalies, and Related Endocrine Disorders. H. W. Jones & W. W. Scott, Eds. : 15. William & Wilkins Co. Baltimore, Md.
90. FORD, C. E. & J. L. HAMERTON. 1956. The chromosomes of man. Nature **178:** 1020.
91. OHNO, S., W. D. KAPLAN & R. KINOSITA. 1959. On the end-to-end association of the X and Y chromosomes of *Mus musculus.* Exp. Cell Res. **18:** 282.
92. HULTÉN, M., J. LINDSTEN, P. L. MING & M. FRACCARO. 1966. The XY bivalent in human male meiosis. Ann. Hum. Genet. **30:** 119.
93. PARK, W. W. 1957. The occurrence of sex chromatin in early human and macâque embryos. J. Anat. **91:** 369.
94. FORD, C. E. 1963. The cytogenetics of human intersexuality. *In* Intersexuality. C. Overzier, Ed. : 86. Academic Press. New York, N. Y.
95. GRUMBACH, M. M., A. MORISHIMA & N. LIU. 1965. A distinct clinical entity simulating Turner's syndrome in boys and girls associated with congenital heart disease, appropriate gonadal differentiation and a normal sex chromosome constitution (abstr.). J. Pediat. **67:** 966.
96. VAN WYK, J. J. & M. M. GRUMBACH. 1968. Disorders of sex differentiation. *In* Textbook of Endocrinology. 4th edit. R. H. Williams, Ed. : 537–613. W. B. Saunders Co. Philadelphia, Pa.

BIOCHEMICAL CHANGES IN CHROMOSOMAL ABNORMALITIES*

David Yi-Yung Hsia, Henry L. Nadler,
and Ling-yu Shih

Genetic Clinic, Children's Memorial Hospital and
Department of Pediatrics, Northwestern University Medical School
Chicago, Ill.

In 1959, Lejeune and colleagues[1] reported the finding of 47 chromosomes in the cells of children with Down's syndrome. The extra chromosome, a small acrocentric, is believed to be either number 21 or 22. The following year, Nowell and Hungerford[2] showed that patients with chronic myelogenous leukemia carried an abnormally small acrocentric chromosome, the Philadelphia chromosome, which presumably represents a partial deletion of a "G" group chromosome. The finding of elevated levels of alkaline phosphatase in the leukocytes of patients with Down's syndrome[3–5] and the reduction of leukocyte alkaline phosphatase levels in patients with chronic myelogenous leukemia has led to the suggestion that the genetic loci controlling alkaline phosphatase were located on this small chromosome.[6]

The present paper represents a critical review of all data that have been gathered on the enzymatic changes in autosomal trisomy syndromes.

Studies With Peripheral Blood

Whole Blood

In these discussions, whole blood may be defined as material which has been taken out of the vein and directly used for assay without further processing, and includes the combined enzyme activities of red blood cells, white blood cells, platelets, and plasma.

In TABLE 1, we have summarized the data in whole blood of two enzymes from normal controls and patients with Down's syndrome. With galactokinase, there is a 39 percent increase in activity using the galactose-1-^{14}C incubation method.[7] With galactose-1-phosphate uridyl transferase, there is a 40–73 percent increase in activity using the UDPG consumption test in three different studies[8–10] and a 41 percent increase using the galactose-1-phosphate-^{14}C incubation method.[7] There appears to be general agreement that there is an increase in activity of these two enzymes among patients with Down's syndrome.

Red Blood Cells

The red blood cell fraction is usually prepared by removing the plasma and buffy coat, and washing the red blood cells with cold isotonic saline two or three times.

Down's Syndrome. In TABLE 2a, we have summarized the data in red blood cells, of 15 enzymes from normal controls and patients with Down's syndrome. Of these, only four enzymes have been reported to have increased activities. Donnell *et al.*[11] have confirmed the initial observations of Krone *et al.*[7] by finding

* Some of the data reported here were obtained with the aid of research grants from the Chicago Community Trust, the Otho S. A. Sprague Memorial Institute, the Illinois Mental Health Fund, and USPHS grants nos. 1-SO1-FR 5475, 1-SO1-FR 5370, T1-AM-5186, T1-HD-36, and IF-3HD-2984.

TABLE 1

ACTIVITY OF ENZYMES IN WHOLE BLOOD FROM CONTROLS AND DOWN'S SYNDROME

Enzyme	Author	Method of Enzyme Assay	Control No.	Control Mean ± SD	Down's Syndrome No.	Down's Syndrome Mean ± SD	Ratio D/C
Galactokinase	Krone[7]	Gal-1-^{14}C → Gal-1-P-^{14}C (ratio)	18	2.39 ± 0.52	34	3.34 ± 1.02	1.39*
Galactose-1-phosphate uridyl transferase	Brandt[8]	UDPG Consumption (μM/hr/g)	432	26.4 ± 3.6	27	36.9 ± 3.5	1.40*
	Hsia[9]	UDPG Consumption (μM/hr/g)	10	29.8 ± 9.3	10	41.8 ± 7.5	1.40*
	Rosner[10]	UDPG Consumption (μM/hr/g)	12	33.1	10	57.2	1.73*
	Krone[7]	Gal-1-^{14}C → UDP gal-^{14}C (ratio)	18	3.05 ± 0.73	34	4.30 ± 0.87	1.41*

* $p < .01$

TABLE 2

ACTIVITY OF ENZYMES IN RED BLOOD CELLS IN CONTROLS, DOWN'S SYNDROME, AND TRISOMY 18 SYNDROME

Enzyme	Author	Method of Enzyme Assay	No.	Control Mean ± SD	No.	Trisomics Mean ± SD	Ratio T/C
(a) Down's syndrome							
Galactokinase	Donnell[11]	Gal-1-^{14}C → Gal-1-P-^{14}C (μM/hr/ml)	34	0.30 ± 0.065	34	0.36 ± 0.069	1.20*
Galactose-1-phosphate uridyl transferase	Hsia[9]	UDPG Consumption (μM/hr/g)	8	33.3 ± 2.3	10	35.6 ± 7.5	1.07
	Rosner[10]	UDPG Consumption (μM/hr/g)	12	26.3	12	41.7	1.59*
	Hsia[9]	Gal-1-^{14}C → $^{14}CO_2$ (cpm/1.5 hr/g)	20	50,980 ± 12,610	20	49,030 ± 10,690	0.98
	Ng[12]	Gal-1-P-^{14}C → UDP gal-^{14}C (μM/hr/ml)	24	1.89 ± 1.25	20	1.98 ± 1.03	1.05
Glucose-6-phosphate dehydrogenase	Shih[13]	NADPH formation (μM/hr/g)	21	423 ± 85	23	476 ± 40	1.12
	Rosner[10]	NADPH formation (units)	12	336	12	820	2.44*
	Baikie[14]						N.D.
Phosphohexokinase	Baikie[14]	DPNH reduction (μM/min/3.2 g)	20	20.5 ± 2.6	21	29.9 ± 3.0	1.45*
Lactic acid dehydrogenase	Shih[13]	NADH → NAD (μM/hr/10^9 RBC)	12	3.4 ± 1.0	11	3.8 ± 2.0	1.11
		NADH → NAD (μM/hr/mg)	12	195 ± 97	11	155 ± 35	0.79
		NADH → NAD (μM/hr/10^9 RBC)	12	0.53 ± 0.21	11	0.61 ± 0.24	1.15
	Hsia[9]						N.D.
	Baikie[14]						N.D.
Others†	Hsia[9]						N.D.
	Baikie[14]						N.D.
(b) Trisomy 18 syndrome							
Galactose-1-phosphate uridyl transferase	Nadler[15]	Gal-1-P-^{14}C → UDP gal-^{14}C (μM/hr/g Hb)	9	18.4 ± 6.6	9	19.3 ± 3.0	1.04

* $p < .01$ N.D. = No difference

† Hexokinase[14]
Phosphohexose isomerase[9,14]
Aldolase[9,14]
Triose phosphate isomerase[14]
Glyceraldehyde phosphate dehydrogenase[14]
Phosphoglycerate kinase[14]
Phosphoglycerate mutase[14]
Enolase[14]
Pyruvate kinase[9,14]
Glutathione reductase[9,14]

a 20 percent increase in activity of galactokinase in the red blood cells. These studies were carried out by incubating the hemolysate with galactose-1-^{14}C and separating the residual galactose by chromatography on diethyl-aminoethyl-cellulose paper. Baikie *et al.*[13] have presented convincing evidence of a 45 percent increase of phosphohexokinase activity in the red blood cells. As can be seen in FIGURE 1, there is no overlap between the values for controls and mongoloids and the one patient who had a value in the normal range turned out to be a mosaic. Alterations in the other two enzymes are not as definite. Rosner *et al.*[10] have reported an increase of galactose-1-phosphate uridyl transferase activity in the red blood cells, but this has not been confirmed by other studies[9,12] using both similar and different methods for the enzyme assays. Similarly, their report[10] of an increase of glucose-6-phosphate dehydrogenase activity has not been confirmed.[13,14] Thus, it would appear that an increase of enzyme activity in the red

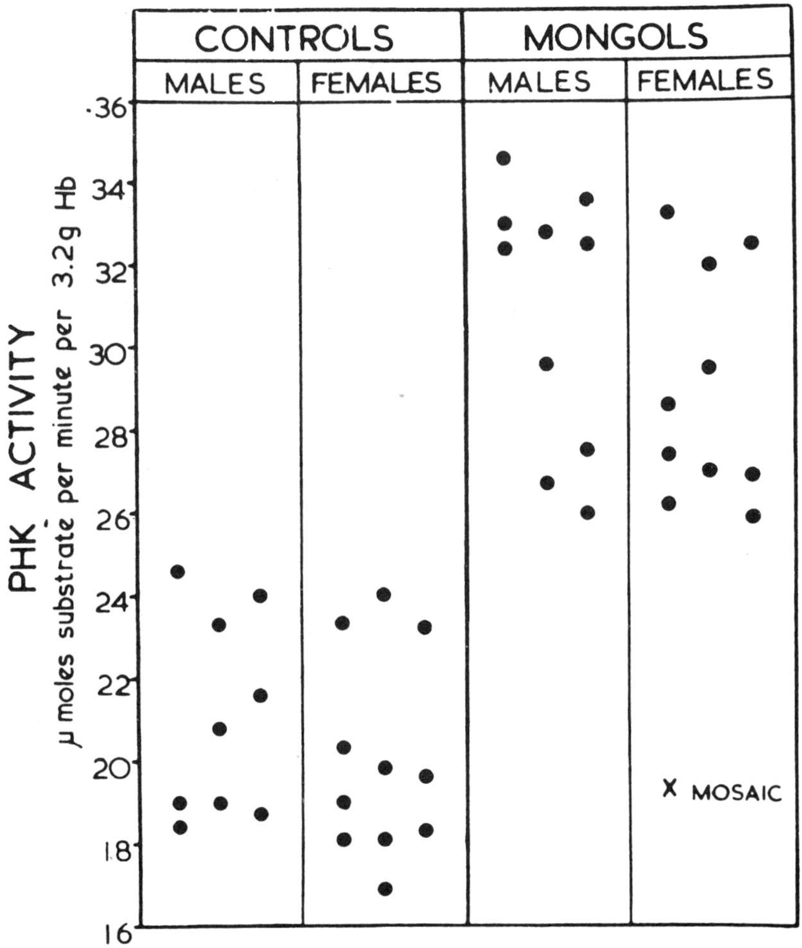

FIGURE 1. Activity of phosphohexokinase in red blood cells from controls and Down's syndrome patients. (Reproduced by permission of Baikie *et al.*[14] and Lancet.)

Table 3

Activity of Enzymes in White Blood Cells in Controls, Down's Syndrome, Chronic Myelogenous Leukemia, Trisomy 18 Syndrome, and Klinefelter's Syndrome

Enzyme	Author	Method of Enzyme		Control		Trisomics or Leukemics		Ratio
		Separation	Assay	No.	Mean ± SD	No.	Mean ± SD	T or L/c
(a) Down's syndrome								
Galactose-1-phosphate uridyl transferase	Hsia[9]	Fibronogen	Gal-1-^{14}C → $^{14}CO_2$ (cpm/1.5 x 2 x 10^7)	20	2,490 ± 1,320	20	4,510 ± 1,780	1.80*
	Mellman[16]	Dextran	UDPG Consumption (μM/hr/10^9)	14	15.5 ± 4.9	14	26.4 ± 12.4	1.70*
	Rosner[10]	Fibronogen	UDPG Consumption (μM/hr/gm RNA)	12	10.0	12	25.5	2.55*
Glucose-6-phosphate dehydrogenase	Mellman[16]	Dextran	NADPH (μM/hr/10^6)	14	9.4 ± 2.6	14	14.4 ± 3.5	1.53*
	Shih[13]	Fibrinogen	NADPH (μM/hr/10^6)	19	1.24 ± 0.13	17	1.72 ± 0.28	1.39*
Acid phosphatase	Mellman[16]	Dextran	Phenylphosphate (μg/hr/10^6)	14	16.6 ± 4.0	14	23.6 ± 7.8	1.42*
	Rosner[10]		*p*-nitrophenol (unitsμmg protein)	12	0.44	12	0.82	1.86*
Alkaline phosphatase	Alter[5]	Dextran	Phenylphosphate (mg/hr/10^{10})	41	66	41	89	1.34*
	Trubowitz[3]		β-glycerophosphate (mg P/hr/10^{10})	22	40 ± 17	22	60.8 ± 27	1.50*
		Histochemical	(scores)	22	40 ± 16	22	70 ± 38	1.75*
	King[4]	Histochemical	(scores)	32	90.7 ± 42.3	32	119.9 ± 41.1	1.32*
	O'Sullivan[17]	Histochemical	(scores)	200	32 ± 16.6	200	78 ± 25.8	2.38*
	Rosner[10]	Fibrinogen	*p*-nitrophenol (units/mg protein)	12	1.34	12	3.18	2.37*
5-Nucleotidase	Rosner[10]	Fibrinogen	ADP (mg P/15 min/mg protein)	12	20.2	12	62.3	3.40*
Lactic Acid dehydrogenase	Shih[13]	Fibrinogen	NADH → NAD (μM/hr/10^6)	16	3.2 ± 2.10	15	3.0 ± 1.70	0.93
			NAD → NADH (μM/hr/10^6)	12	0.87 ± 0.40	11	0.77 ± 0.33	0.89

			(b) Chronic myelogenous leukemia					
Alkaline phosphatase	Valentine[6]	Fibrinogen	β-glycerophosphate (mg P/hr/10^{10})	25	25.8 ± 9.0	14	4.0 ± 1.8	0.15*
	Hsia[19]	Fibrinogen	β-glycerophosphate (mM/hr/10^{10})	6	0.90 ± 0.30	10	0.41 ± 0.58	0.45*
	Frei[18]		PNP (μM/hr/10^{9})	–	17	22	10	0.58*
Galactose-1-phosphate uridyl transferase	Hsia[19]	Fibrinogen	Gal-1-$^{14}C \rightarrow {}^{14}CO_2$ (cpm/1.5 hr/2 x 10^{7})	6	1,255 ± 550	10	310 ± 105	0.24*
			(c) Trisomy 18 syndrome					
Glucose-6-phosphate dehydrogenase	Nadler[15]	Fibrinogen	NADPH (μM/hr/10^{6})	9	1.36 ± 0.41	9	0.95 ± 0.36	0.70
Acid phosphatase	Nadler[15]	Fibrinogen	*p*-nitrophenol (μM/hr/10^{10})	9	5.0 ± 2.1	9	3.1 ± 1.5	0.62*
Alkaline phosphatase	Nadler[15]	Fibrinogen	*p*-nitrophenol (μM/hr/10^{10})	9	0.39 ± 0.11	9	0.72 ± 0.20	1.84*
			(d) Klinefelter's syndrome					
Alkaline phosphatase	Weber[20]	Histochemical	α-napthyl phosphate (LAP/100 cells)	12	48	12	85	1.77*

* $p < .05$

blood cells of patients with Down's syndrome occurs rarely and is not a universal finding.

Trisomy 18 Syndrome. In TABLE 2b, we have summarized the data of Nadler *et al.*[15] with galactose-1-phosphate uridyl transferase in the red blood cells of normal controls and of patients with the trisomy 18 syndrome. Again, no significant differences could be found.

White Blood Cells

The white cell fraction is usually prepared by taking the upper layer of a suspension of whole blood which has been sedimented with either dextran or fibrinogen. The white blood cells are then washed with cold isotonic saline and sometimes with hypotonic saline to hemolyze the remaining red blood cells.

Down's Syndrome. In TABLE 3a, we have summarized the data in white blood cells of six enzymes from normal controls and patients with Down's syndrome. It can be seen that despite the use of a variety of different laboratory methods, there is general agreement that there is an increase in activities of leukocyte galactose-1-phosphate uridyl transferase,[9,10,16] glucose-6-phosphate dehydrogenase,[13,16] acid phosphatase,[10,16] alkaline phosphatase,[3-5,10,17] and 5-nucleotidase.[10] On the other hand, leukocyte lactic acid dehydrogenase does not appear to be altered in Down's syndrome.[13]

Chronic Myelogenous Leukemia with Philadelphia Chromosome. In TABLE 3b,

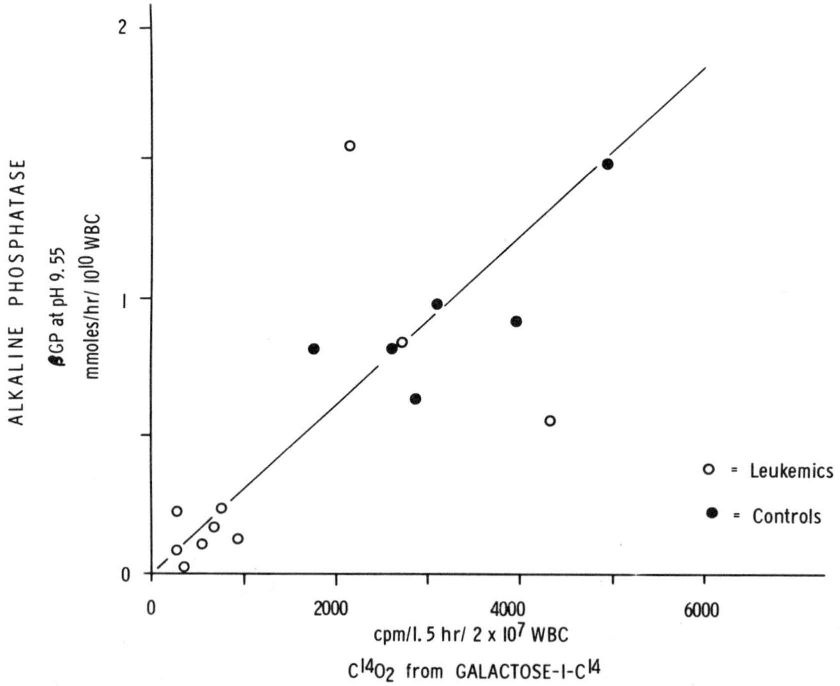

FIGURE 2. Comparison of alkaline phosphatase and galactose-1-phosphate uridyl transferase activities in white blood cells from patients with chronic myelogenous leukemia.

we have summarized the data in white blood cells of two enzymes from normal controls and patients with chronic myelogenous leukemia having the Philadelphia chromosome (Ph^1) during relapse. In 1951, Valentine and Beck[6] called attention to the fact that the activity of alkaline phosphatase in the white blood cells of such patients is lower than that of normal controls and those with leukocytosis. Frei *et al.*[18] have noted that this leukocyte alkaline phosphatase activity increased to normal in two out of 10 patients who achieved a partial remission, and that the majority of patients who achieved complete clinical and hematological remissions had normalization of their leukocyte alkaline phosphatase activity Hsia *et al.*[19] have confirmed these observations with both leukocyte alkaline phosphatase and galactose-1-phosphate uridyl transferase. As shown in FIGURE 2 there was a good correlation in the levels of these two enzymes among patients with chronic myelogenous leukemia both in relapse and in remission.

Trisomy 18 Syndrome. In TABLE 3c, we have summarized the data in white blood cells of three enzymes from normal controls and patients with the trisomy 18 syndrome. It can be seen that there is a significant increase of leukocyte alkaline phosphatase activity,[15] a significant decrease of acid phosphatase activity,[15] and no alteration in glucose-6-phosphate dehydrogenase activity.

Klinefelter's Syndrome. In TABLE 3d, the data of alkaline phosphatase in white blood cells of Klinefelter's syndrome is tabulated. As with Down's syndrome and trisomy 18 syndrome, there is a nonspecific increase of leukocyte alkaline phosphatase activity.

Problems With Peripheral Blood

These data from peripheral blood have to be interpreted with caution because of the problems associated with separation of whole blood, stabilization of enzymes, factors leading to induction, existence of isoenzymes, and the effect of translocations. We shall consider each of these factors individually.

Separation Procedures

There is general agreement that it is difficult to get reliable quantitative data on peripheral blood because there are serious technical difficulties in preparing white blood cells free of red blood cells. Even greater problems occur when one

TABLE 4

COMPARISON OF GALACTOSE-1-PHOSPHATE URIDYL TRANSFERASE ACTIVITY IN WHOLE BLOOD, RED BLOOD CELLS, AND WHITE BLOOD CELLS BETWEEN NORMAL CONTROLS AND DOWN'S SYNDROME

Author	Method of Enzyme Assay	Ratio D/C		
		Whole Blood	Red Blood Cells	White Blood Cells
Brandt[8]	UDPG Consumption	1.40*		
Hsia[9]	UDPG Consumption	1.40*	1.07	
Rosner[10]	UDPG Consumption	1.73*	1.59*	2.55*
Mellman[16]	UDPG Consumption			1.70*
Hsia[9]	Gal-1-^{14}C → $^{14}CO_2$		0.98	1.80*
Krone[7]	Gal-1-^{14}C → UDP gal-^{14}C	1.41*		
Ng[12]	Gal-1-P-^{14}C → UDP gal-^{14}C		1.05	

* $p < .01$

TABLE 5

HEMATOLOGICAL SURVEY OF RED BLOOD CELL ENZYME IN CONTROLS AND DOWN'S SYNDROME

Enzyme	Author		12 Controls	12 Mongoloides	P
Glutamic-oxaloacetic transaminase	Naiman[21]	Units per gm Hemoglobin	3.3	3.4	–
		Units per million RBC	1,150 ± 172	945 ± 158	< .01

tries to prepare red blood cells free of white blood cells. This presents problems as illustrated in TABLE 4, which compares the galactose-1-phosphate uridyl transferase activity in whole blood, red blood cells, and white blood cells. From these data, it is difficult to determine whether the increase in enzymes activity in the red blood cell reported by one study[10] and not by the three other studies[9,12] represents a real difference between controls and Down's syndrome, or whether this is caused by the techniques used for preparing the red blood cell fraction.

Naiman *et al.*[21] have also pointed out that differences can be caused by the expression of enzyme activity in relation to red cell count, particularly in younger cells. As can be seen in TABLE 5, if the red blood cell glutamic oxaloacetic transaminase is expressed as units per million red blood cells, there is a significant difference between mongoloids and controls, whereas if it is expressed as units per gram hemoglobin, no difference can be detected.

Separation of white blood cells is not without problems. We have found that if sedimentation is carried out with fresh three percent fibrinogen, mainly lymphocytes are recovered in the upper white blood cell layer, whereas the polymorphonuclear leukocytes fall to the lower red blood cell layer. If sedimentation is carried out without the addition of Dextran or fibrinogen at 37° C, or with the upper layer of a fibrinogen solution which has been left standing, the differential count of the upper white blood cell layer is the same as that of whole blood. Since Rabinowitz[22] has shown that there may be a ten-to-twentyfold difference in the enzyme activity of different forms of white blood cells as shown in FIGURE 3, the technique used for sedimentation could greatly alter the final result. This emphasizes the importance of expressing future data in terms of pure lymphocytes or pure polymorphonuclear leukocytes. Finally, there appears to be no general agreement on a procedure for the lysis of leukocytes that would give similar results in various laboratories.

Enzyme Stabilization

In our laboratory, earlier studies[1] with glucose-6-phosphate dehydrogenase in white blood cells failed to show a difference between controls and Down's syndrome while later studies[13] showed a 39 percent increase of enzyme activity in the latter group. In its natural state, leukocyte glucose-6-phosphate dehydrogenase is unstable before and after lysis so that over half of its activity is lost within the first four hours. Addition of 25 mM of mercaptoethanol immediately after the blood sample is taken stabilizes the enzyme so that no significant loss of activity takes place in the first eight hours after the blood is withdrawn. The observations without (straight lines) and with (dotted lines) mercaptoethanol in six controls is given in FIGURE 4 and in six mongoloids in FIGURE 5. In FIGURE 6,

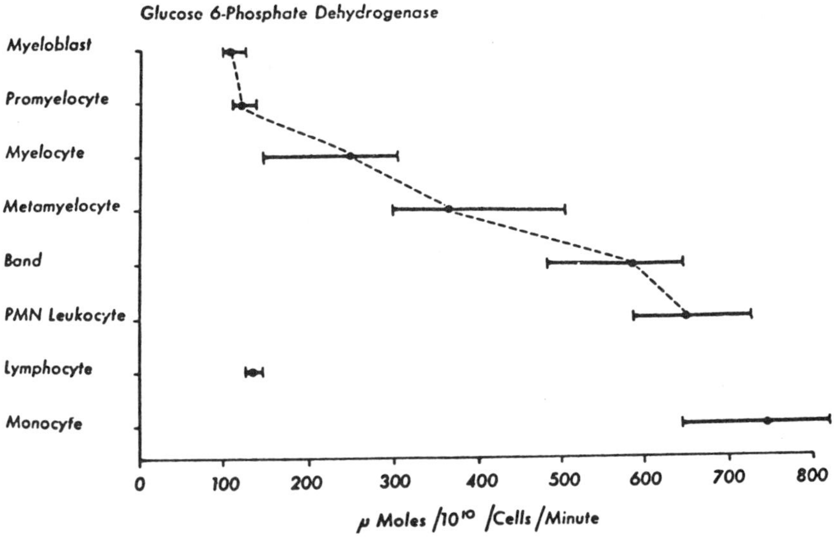

FIGURE 3. Glucose-6-phosphate dehydrogenase activity in different white cells components in granulocytic leukemia. (Reproduced by permission of Rabinowitz[22] and Blood.)

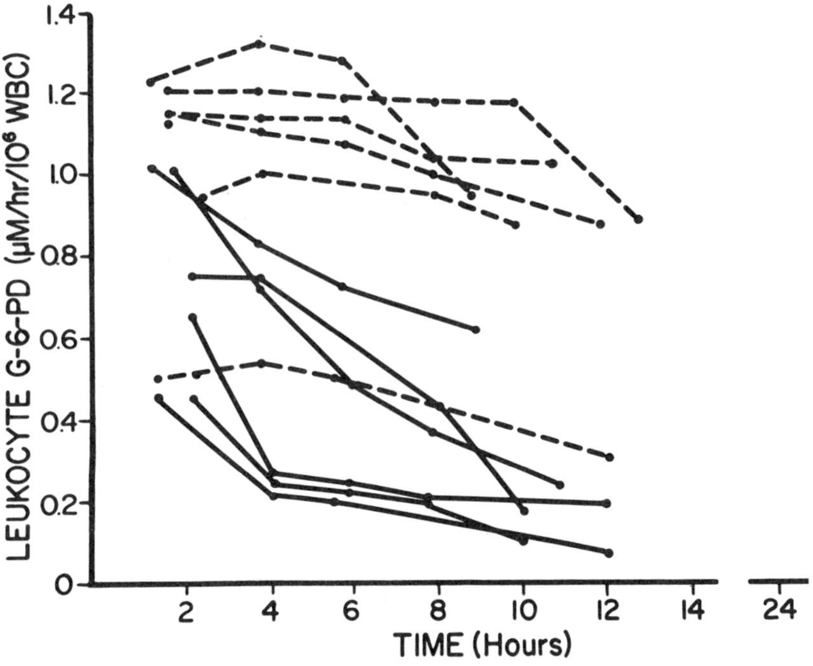

FIGURE 4. Leukocyte glucose-6-phosphate dehydrogenase activity in controls without (solid line) and with (broken line) the addition of 25 mM mercaptoethanol. All values are expressed in terms of time of venipuncture to the time of lysis of leukocytes.

we have made a semi-logarithmic plot of the decay curves of leukocyte glucose-6-phosphate dehydrogenase for the controls (dotted line) and mongoloids (straight line) without mercaptoethanol. It would appear that there is no significant difference in the lability of leukocyte glucose-6-phosphate dehydrogenase between controls and mongoloids.

Enzyme Induction

Although extensive data have been published showing an increase of leukocyte alkaline phosphatase activity in patients with Down's syndrome,[3,5,10,17] and of a decrease in activity in chronic myelogenous leukemia,[6,18,19] these findings remain the least convincing among the biochemical changes in chromosomal abnormalities. In the first place, an increase of leukocyte alkaline phosphatase

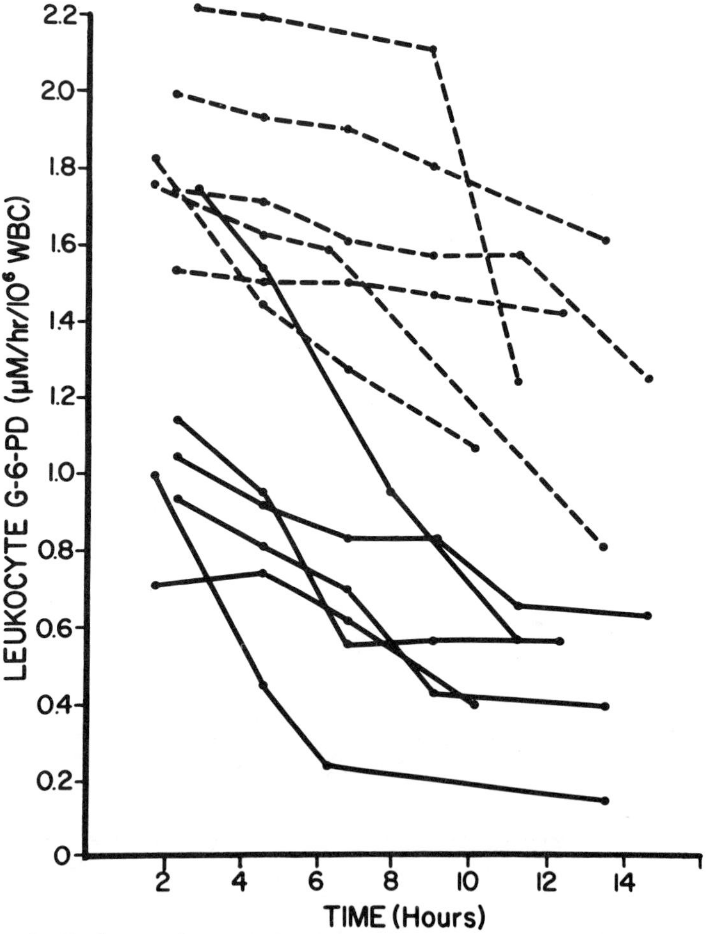

FIGURE 5. Leukocyte glucose-6-phosphate dehydrogenase activity in mongoloid patients without (solid line) and with (broken line) the addition of 25 mM mercaptoethanol. All values are expressed in terms of time of venipuncture to the time of lysis of leukocytes.

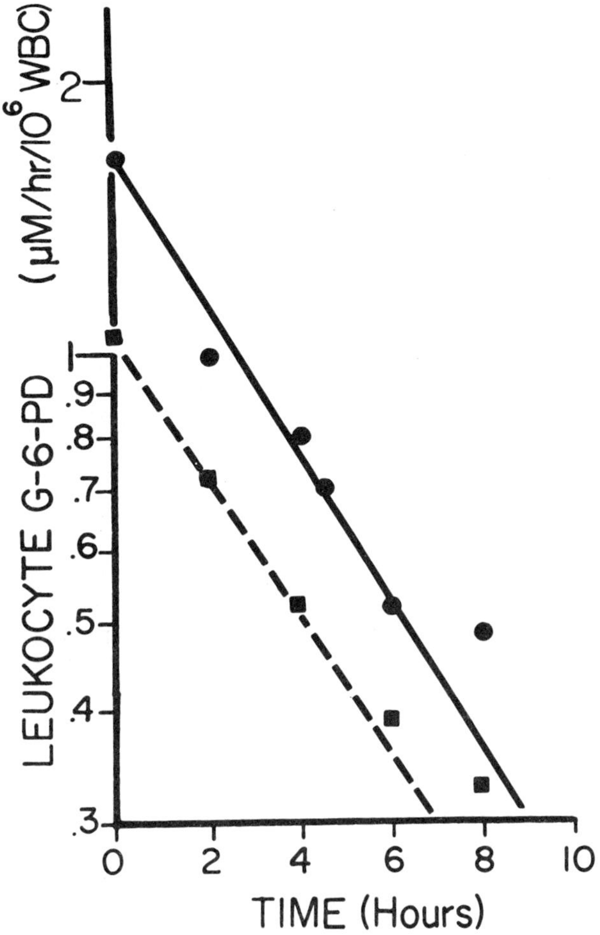

FIGURE 6. Mean rate of fall of leukocyte glucose-6-phosphate dehydrogenase activity for controls (solid line) and mongoloid patients (broken line) without added mercaptoethanol. The data are plotted on a log scale and extrapolated to zero time.

activity has also been noted in trisomy 18 syndrome[15] and in Klinefelter's syndrome.[20] In the second place, an increase of leukocyte alkaline phosphatase activity has been reported in aleukemic patients with refractory anemia, granulocytic hyperplasia of the bone marrow, and a missing chromosome of group 6–12,[23] and an increase of leukocyte alkaline phosphatase activity has been found in a patient with Ph^{1+} chronic granulocytic leukemia.[24] Finally, McCoy and Ebadi[25] have shown that the injection of prednisolone will cause a fivefold increase of leukocyte alkaline phosphatase activity after six hours in Down's syndrome patients as compared with a 3.2-fold increase in controls, a difference which is significant at the $p < 0.25$ level. This induction was actinomycin and puromycin-sensitive and thus dependent upon RNA and protein synthesis.

Role of Isoenzymes

Virtually none of the studies carried out with peripheral blood has examined the possibility of changes in isoenzymes among patients with chromosomal abnormalities. In examining the list of enzymes which have been shown to be abnormal, isoenzymes have been demonstrated with alkaline phosphatase,[26–28] acid phosphatase,[29] and glucose-6-phosphate dehydrogenase.[30]

We have had the opportunity of investigating the isoenzyme characteristics of two enzymes–one abnormal and one normal.[13] Starch gel electrophoresis for glucose-6-phosphate dehydrogenase was performed on white blood cells from 12 controls and 14 mongoloid patients. All were shown to have a single B band (100 percent) and no isoenzymes or variants could be detected in any of the cases. Starch gel electrophoresis for lactic acid dehydrogenase was performed using both red blood cells and white blood cells from ten controls and ten mongoloid patients. As is customary, LDH-1(H type) was much more prominent in erythrocyte hemolysates while LDH-5(M type) was more prominent in leukocyte lysates, but no differences in isoenzyme pattern could be detected between the controls and mongoloid patients. Studies were also carried out with two NAD analogues, namely nicotinamide hypoxanthine dinucleotide (NHXD) and thionicotinamide adenine dinucleotide (TNAD).[31] As shown in TABLE 6, there were no great differences in the ratio of NAD/NHXD between the red blood cells and white blood cells, but there was a marked difference in the ratio of NAD/TNAD with the ratio in the red blood cells below 1.0 and the ratio in the white blood cells above 1.0. Despite these differences, the normal controls and the Down's syndrome patients were similar in terms of the NAD/NHXD and the NAD/TNAD ratios.

Translocation Mongoloid Patients

Recently, Rosner *et al.*[10] have reported that patients with translocation Down's syndrome do not show the characteristic biochemical changes found in trisomic Down's syndrome patients. As shown in TABLE 7, levels of galactose-1-phosphate uridyl transferase, glucose-6-phosphate dehydrogenase, acid phosphatase, alkaline phosphatase, and 5-nucleotidase are not elevated in the 12 translocation patients, but they are markedly elevated in the 12 trisomic patients. These data are difficult to interpret. Rosner has suggested that the translocated position of the chromosome might interfere with normal gene action (position effect) or that the deletion occurring in the process of translocation might be one site on

TABLE 6

SUBSTRATE SPECIFICITY USING NAD ANALOGUES WITH LACTIC ACID DEHYDROGENASE IN RED BLOOD CELLS AND WHITE BLOOD CELLS IN CONTROLS AND DOWN'S SYNDROME

	Red Blood Cells		White Blood Cells	
	Controls Mean ± SD	Down's Mean ± SD	Controls Mean ± SD	Down's Mean ± SD
NAD/NHXD	1.50 ± 0.18	1.50 ± 0.27	1.78 ± 0.21	1.91 ± 0.36
NAD/TNAD	0.70 ± 0.12	0.77 ± 0.15	1.15 ± 0.15	1.09 ± 0.15

NXHD = Nicotinamide hypoxanthine dinucleotide
NAD = Nicotinamide adenine dinucleotide
TNAD = Thionicotinamide adenine dinucleotide

TABLE 7

ENZYME ACTIVITY IN CONTROLS, TRANSLOCATIONS, AND TRISOMY 21[11]

Enzyme	Source	Units	12 Controls	12 Trans-locations	12 Trisomy 21
Galactose-1-phosphate uridyl transferase	WB	μM/hr/gm Hb	53.1	34.6	57.2*
	RBC	μM/hr/gm Hb	26.3	26.9	41.7*
	WBC	μM/hr/gm RNA	10.05	13.13	25.46*
Glucose-6-phosphate dehydrogenase	RBC	units	336	266	820*
Acid phosphatase	WBC	units/mg protein	0.442	0.459	0.823*
Alkaline phosphatase	WBC	units/mg protein	1.34	1.28	3.18*
5–Nucleotidase	WBC	mg P/15 min/mg protein	20.2	23.6	62.3*

* $p < .05$

TABLE 8

ACTIVITY OF ENZYMES IN PLATELETS IN CONTROLS AND DOWN'S SYNDROME

Enzyme	Author	Method of Enzyme Assay	Control No.	Control Mean ± SD	Down's No.	Down's Mean ± SD	Ratio D/C
Glucose-6-phosphate dehydrogenase	Shih[33]	NADPH (μM/hr/10^9)	18	365 ± 17	18	357 ± 18	0.98
Alkaline phosphatase	Shih[33]	*p*-nitrophenol phosphate (μg P/hr/10^{10})	12	55 ± 3.9	13	55 ± 4.9	1.00

TABLE 9

ACTIVITY OF ENZYMES IN CULTIVATED FIBROBLASTS FROM CONTROLS AND AUTOSOMAL TRISOMY SYNDROMES

Enzyme	Author	Method	Control No.	Control Mean ± SD	Down's No.	Down's Mean ± SD	Ratio D/C	18 Trisomy No.	18 Trisomy Mean ± SD	Ratio 18/C	D_1 Trisomy No.	D_1 Trisomy Mean ± SD	Ratio D_1/C
Alkaline phosphatase	Cox[35]	PNP (μM/30 m/0.1 mg					ND						
	DeCarli[36]	PNP					*						
	Walker[38]	PNP (μM/hr/mμg)					ND						
	Nadler[37]	PNP (μM/hr/mμg)	10	.79 ± .12	5	.72 ± .12	0.91	11	.80 ± .06	1.00	4	.84 ± .15	1.06
Acid phosphatase	DeMars[34]	PNP					ND			ND			ND
	Nadler[37]	PNP (μM/hr/mμg)	10	4.4 ± 0.7	5	4.2 ± 0.4	0.98	11	4.1 ± 0.8	0.96	4	4.5 ± 0.7	1.02
Glucose-6-phosphate dehydrogenase	Nadler[37]	NADPH (μM/hr/mμg)	10	.87 ± .45	5	.69 ± .38	0.78	1	.83 ± .44	0.97	4	.94 ± .13	1.08
Galactose-1-phosphate uridyl transferase	Nadler[37]	Gal-1-P-^{14}C (μM/hr/μmg)	10	86 ± 29	5	80 ± 15	0.93	11	.85 ± 18	1.00	4	76 ± 27	0.88
β-Glucuronidase	DeMars[34]	PSPG					ND			ND			ND
UDPG-4-epimerase	Krone[39]	UDP gal → UDPG (m units/mg)					ND						

ND = No difference
* = Not a simple additive effect on enzyme activity level

the chromosome which determines the expression of the enzymes. These observations do point out the importance of karyotyping every patient with Down's syndrome before performing enzyme studies.

Studies With Platelets

In TABLE 8, we have summarized the data in platelets of two enzymes from normal controls and patients with Down's syndrome. There was no difference in the activity of alkaline phosphatase and glucose-6-phosphate dehydrogenase in platelets between the two groups.

Studies With Fibroblasts

In TABLE 9, we have summarized the data of several enzymes from cultivated human fibroblasts derived from normal controls and patients with autosomal trisomy syndromes. In 1964, DeMars[34] was unable to detect any difference in levels of acid phosphatase and β-glucuronidase between strains derived from patients with Down's syndrome, trisomy 18 syndrome, and D_1 trisomy syndrome. The following year, Cox[35] reported no difference in alkaline phosphatase activity between two strains of fibroblasts derived from Down's syndrome patients and eight strains from controls. In studies with human heteroploid cells containing different numbers of small acrocentric chromosomes, DeCarli *et al.*[36] showed that the average increase of one chromosome unit does not result in a simple additive effect upon the enzyme activity level.

In an attempt to determine whether the changes found in peripheral blood of patients with autosomal trisomy syndromes were caused by the consistent influence of the genetic material contained in the extra chromosome, Nadler *et al.*[37] cultivated cells derived from skin biopsies of patients with trisomic Down's syndrome, trisomy 18 syndrome, and D_1 trisomy syndrome, and studied the fibroblasts for alkaline phosphatase, acid phosphatase, glucose-6-phosphate dehydrogenase, and galactose-1-phosphate uridyl transferase. A typical exmple of the findings expressed as micromoles substrate utilized per hour for each day of the experiment with glucose-6-phosphate dehydrogenase is given in FIGURE 7. No significant differences in activity could be demonstrated between strains derived from normal controls and autosomal trisomy syndromes for any of the enzymes studied.

Discussion

Several explanations have been offered for the changes in peripheral blood seen in patients with autosomal trisomy syndromes. Alter *et al.*,[5] Brandt *et al.*,[8] and Baikie *et al.*[14] have all suggested that the extra "G" group chromosome seen in patients with Down's syndrome might contain "structural" genes for certain specific enzymes. Mellman *et al.*[16] and Rosner *et al.*[10] have postulated that this extra chromosome might contain "regulator" genes for certain groups of enzymes. The finding of increased activity of leukocyte alkaline phosphatase in patients with Klinefelter's syndrome,[20] a condition characterized by presence of an XXY chromosome constitution, and the increase of leukocyte alkaline phosphatase activity in patients with both Down's syndrome[3–5] and trisomy 18 syndrome[15] suggest that the increase in enzyme activity is nonspecific. Elevated levels of alkaline phosphatase have also been described in infection, stress, nonproliferative disorders, and pernicious anemia. In addition, the increase of leu-

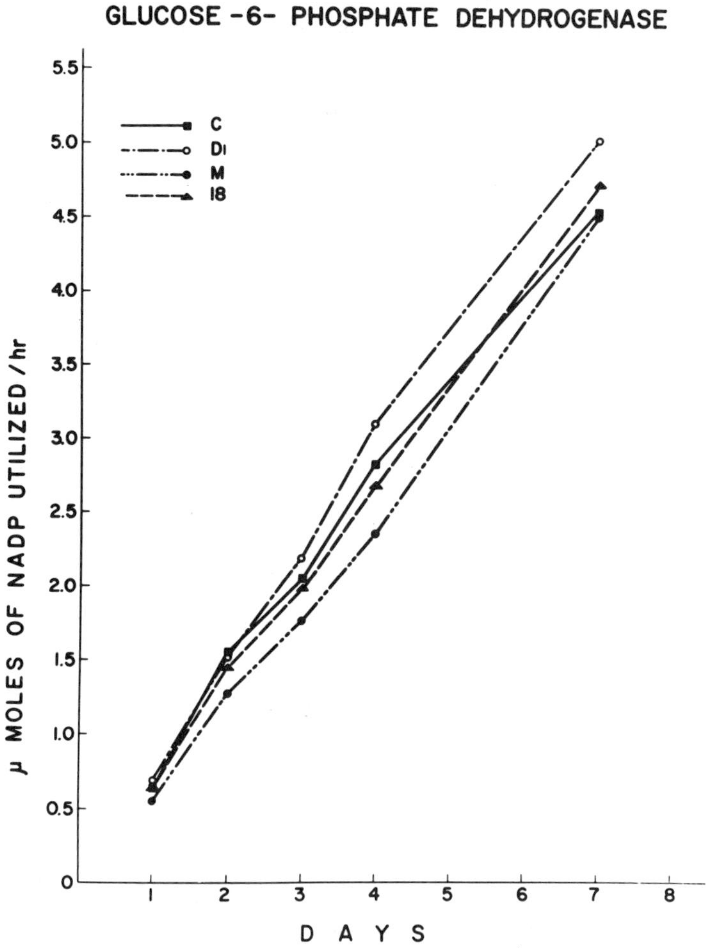

FIGURE 7. The total enzyme activity of glucose-6-phosphate dehydrogenase on each day of experiment for controls (c), D_1 trisomics (D_1), 18 trisomics (18), and mongoloids (M) in cultivated human fibroblasts.

kocyte glucose-6-phosphate dehydrogenase activity in patients with Down's syndrome is difficult to interpret because strong evidence has suggested that the specific genetic locus for this enzyme is present in the X chromosome.

More recently, an alternate hypothesis has been suggested to explain the increase in activity of peripheral blood enzymes in patients with Down's syndrome. Hook and Eagle[40] and others[21,41] have suggested that the enzyme activity is dependent upon cell age and that a shortened life span of the leukocytes in Down's syndrome results in the presence of younger white cells with higher enzyme levels. Two recent studies with conflicting results bear upon this point. Galbraith and Volberg,[42] using the technique of labeling leukocytes *in vitro* with radioactive diisopropyl fluorophosphate (^{32}DFP) to study granulocyte half-life, blood granulocyte mass and granulocyte turnover rate, were unable to demonstrate any difference between normals and four patients with Down's syndrome, but were able to demonstrate a prolonged leukocyte half-life in chronic myelogenous leukemia. On the other hand, Raab *et al.*[43] using comparable techniques involving ^{32}DFP labeling in trisomic mongoloids were able to demonstrate a more rapid granulocyte turnover rate.

The finding of increased enzymatic activity in leukocytes and absence of such changes in fibroblasts derived from patients with autosomal trisomy syndromes would lead us to believe that for the present there is no clear evidence establishing a specific genetic locus for an enzyme, either "structural" or "regulatory" on a specific autosomal chromosome. Studies are currently in progress in our laboratory, first, to define whether any specific component of the leukocyte fraction is responsible for the increase in enzyme activity and second, to determine by starch gel electrophoresis whether there are differences in the form of enzyme present in peripheral blood and tissues.[44,45]

Acknowledgments

The authors wish to express their appreciation to Drs. Herbert Grossman of the Illinois State Pediatric Institute, Paul Tillman of the Dixon State School, and E. Dieterle of the Pflegeanstalt für geistesschwache bildungsunfähige Kinder, Uster, Switzerland for permission to study their patients and to Drs. Tohru Inouye, Michael Makler, and Paul Wong who collaborated in many of these studies.

References

1. Lejeune, J., M. Gautier & R. Turpin. 1959. Etude des chromosomes somatiques de enuf enfants mongoliens. Compt. rend. Acad. Sci. **248:** 1721.
2. Nowell, P. C. & D. A. Hungerford. 1960. Chromosome studies in normal and leukemic human leucocytes. J. Nat. Cancer Inst. **25:** 85.
3. Trubowitz, S., D. Kirman & B. Masek. 1962. The leucocyte alkaline phosphatase in mongolism. Lancet **ii:** 486.
4. King, M. J., E. M. Gillis & A. G. Baikie. 1962. Alkaline-phosphatase activity of polymorphs in mongolism. Lancet **ii:** 1302.
5. Alter, A. A., S. L. Lee, M. Pourfar & G. Dobkin. 1963. Studies of leukocyte alkaline phosphatase in mongolism: a possible chromosome marker. Blood **22:** 165.
6. Valentine, W. N. & W. S. Beck. 1951. Biochemical studies on leucocytes. I. Phosphatase activity in health, leucocytosis, and myelocytic leucemia. J. Lab. Clin. Med. **38:** 39.
7. Krone, W., U. Wolf, H. W. Goedde & H. Baitsch. 1965. Untersuchungen über die Aktivität der Galaktokinase im Blut von Normalpersonen und von Patienten mit G_{Do}–Trisomie. Humangenetik **1:** 279.
8. Brandt, N. J., A. Froland, M. Mikkelsen, A. Nielsen & N. Tolstrup. 1963. Galactosaemia locus and the Down's syndrome chromosome. Lancet **ii:** 700.
9. Hsia, D. Y. Y., T. Inouye, P. Wong & A. South. 1964. Studies on galactose oxidation in Down's syndrome. New Eng. J. Med. **270:** 1085.
10. Rosner, F., B. A. Ong, R. S. Paine & D. Mahanand. 1965a. Biochemical differentiation of trisomic Down's syndrome (mongolism) from that due to translocation. New Eng. J. Med. **273:** 1356.
11. Donnell, G. N., W. G. Ng, W. R. Bergen, J. Melnky & R. Koch. 1965. Enhancement of erythrocyte-galactokinase activity in Langdon-Down Trisomy. Lancet **ii:** 553.
12. Ng, W. G., W. R. Bergen & G. N. Donnell. 1964. Galactase-1-phosphate uridyl transferase assay by use of radioactive galactose-1-phosphate. Clin. Chim. Acta **10:** 337.
13. Shih, L. Y., P. Wong, T. Inouye, M. Makler & D. Y. Y. Hsia. 1965. Enzymes in Down's syndrome. Lancet **ii:** 746.
14. Baikie, A. G., P. B. Loder, G. C. deGruchy & D. B. Pitt. 1965. Phosphohexokinase activity of erythrocytes in mongolism. Another possible marker for chromosome 21. Lancet **:** 412.

15. NADLER, H. L., T. INOUYE & D. Y. Y. HSIA. 1966a. Enzymes in Trisomy-18 syndrome. Lancet **i:** 1270.
16. MELLMAN, W. J., F. A. OSKI, T. A. TEDESCO, A. M. COELHO & H. HARRIS. 1964. Leucocyte enzymes in Down's syndrome. Lancet **ii:** 674.
17. O'SULLIVAN, M. A. & C. V. PRYLES. 1963. Comparison of leukocyte alkaline phosphatase determination in 200 patients with mongolism and in 200 "familial" controls. New Eng. J. Med. **268:** 1168.
18. FREI, E., J. G. TJIO, J. WHANG & P. P. CARBONNE. 1964. Studies of the Philadelphia chromosome in patients with chronic myelogenous leukemia. Ann. N. Y. Acad. Sci. **133:** 1073.
19. HSIA, D. Y. Y., T. INOUYE & P. WONG. 1964. Altered metabolism of leukocytes in Down's syndrome. Clin. Res. **12:** 216.
20. WEBER, W. W., V. MITTWOCH & J. D. A. DELHANTY. 1965. Leucocyte alkaline phosphatase in Klinefelter's syndrome. J. Med. Gen. **2:** 112.
21. NAIMAN, J. L., F. A. OSKI & W. J. MELLMAN. 1965. Phosphokinase activity of erythrocytes in mongolism. Lancet **i:** 821.
22. RABINOWITZ, Y. 1966. DNA polymerase and carbohydrate metabolizing enzyme content of normal and leukemic glass column separated leukocytes. Blood **27:** 470.
23. FREIREICH, E. J., J. WHANG, J. H. TJIO, R. H. LEVIN, G. M. BRITTIN & E. FREI. 1964. Refracting anemia, granulocytic hyperplasia of bone marrow, and a missing chromosome in marrow cells. Clin. Res. **12:** 284.
24. ROSEN, R. B. & R. L. TEPLITZ. 1965. Chronic granulocytic leukemia complicated by ulcerative colitis: elevated leukocyte alkaline phosphatase and possible modifier gene deletion. Blood **26:** 148.
25. MCCOY, E. & M. EBADI. 1966. Induction of leukocyte alkaline phosphatase in Down's syndrome. J. Ped. **68:** 835.
26. BOYER, S. H. 1961. Alkaline phosphatase in human sera and placentae. Science **134:** 1002.
27. ARFORS, K. E., L. BECKMAN & L. G. LUNDIN. 1963. Genetic variations of human serum phosphatases. Acta Genet. **13:** 89.
28. BAMFORD, K. F., H. HARRIS, J. E. LUFFMAN, E. B. ROBSON & T. E. CLEGHORN. 1965. Serum alkaline phosphatase and the ABO blood groups. Lancet **i:** 530.
29. HOPKINSON, D. A., N. SPENCER & H. HARRIS. 1964. Genetical studies on human red cell acid phosphatase. Amer. J. Human Genetics **16:** 141.
30. BOYER, S. H., J. H. PORTER & R. G. WEILBACHER. 1962. Electorphoretic heterogenicity of glucose-6-phosphate dehydrogenase and its relationship to enzyme deficiency in man. Proc. Nat. Acad. Sc. **48:** 1968.
31. KAPLAN, N. O., M. M. CIOTTI & F. E. STOLZENBACH. 1956. Reaction of pyridine nucleotide analogues with dehydrogenases. J. Biol. Chem. **211:** 833.
32. DAWSON, D. M., T. L. GOODFRIEND & N. O. KAPLAN. 1964. Lactic dehydrogenases: Function of the two types. Science **143:** 929.
33. SHIH, L. Y. & D. Y. Y. HSIA. 1966. Enzymes in Down's syndrome. Lancet **i:** 155.
34. DE MARS, R. 1964. Some studies of enzymes in cultivated human cells. Nat. Cancer Institute Monograph **13:** 181.
35. COX, R. P. 1965. Regulation of alkaline phosphatase in skin fibroblast cultures from patients with mongolism. Exp. Cell Res. **37:** 690.
36. DE CARLI, L., J. J. MAIO, F. NUZZO & A. S. BENERCETTI. 1964. Cytogenetic studies with alkaline phosphatase in human heteroploid cells. Cold Spring Harbor Symp. **24:** 223.
37. NADLER, H. L., T. INOUYE, P. JUSTICE & D. Y. Y. HSIA. 1966. Enzymes in cultivated human fibroblasts derived from patients with autosomal trisomy syndromes. (abstr.) III International Congress of Human Genetics. Sept. 1966. : 71.
38. WALKER, F. A. & R. DE MARS. 1966. Enzyme alterations in fibroblasts derived from patients with Down's syndrome. (abstr.) III International Congress of Human Genetics. Sept. 1966. : 103.
39. KRONE, W. & H. BRUNSCHEDE. 1966. UDPG-4-Epimerase in human fibroblast cultures. Humangenetik **2:** 192.
40. HOOK, E. B. & R. R. ENGEL. 1964. Leucocyte life-span, leucocyte alkaline phosphatase, and the 21st chromosome. Lancet **i:** 112.
41. ROSEN, R. B. & H. NISHIYAMA. 1965. Leucocyte life-span and leucocyte alkaline phosphatase. Lancet **i:** 554.
42. GALBRAITH, P. R. & L. S. VALBERG. 1966. Granulopoiesis in Down's syndrome. Pediatrics **37:** 108.

43. RAAB, S. O., N. J. MELLMAN, F. A. OSKI & D. BAKER. 1966. Abnormal leukocyte kinetics—an explanation for the enzyme abnormalities observed in trisomy-21 (Down's syndrome). (abstr.) 36th Annual Meeting Soc. Ped. Res. Atlantic City. May, 1966. : 9.
44. YU, B. P., G. KUMMEROW & T. NISHIDA. 1966. Acid phosphatases of rat polymorphonuclear leucocytes. Proc. Soc. Exp. Biol. Med. **122:** 1045.
45. GRIFFIN, M. J. & R. P. COX. 1966. Studies on the mechanisms of hormone induction of alkaline phosphatase in human cell cultures: II. Rate of enzyme synthesis and properties of base cell and induced enzymes. Proc. Nat. Acad. Sc. **56:** 946.
46. ROBINSON, J. C., J. E. PIERCE, D. P. GOLDSTEIN & W. R. ROSSE. 1966. Leucocyte alkaline phosphatase isoenzymes. Lancet **ii:** 805.

VIRUS-INDUCED CHROMOSOME CHANGES

Pertti Aula,* Warren W. Nichols, and Albert Levan
South Jersey Medical Research Foundation
Camden, N. J.
and
Institute of Genetics, Lund, Sweden

During the last few years the role of viruses as agents capable of producing chromosome changes has been established beyond a reasonable doubt. The group of viruses shown to be able to induce chromosome damage includes DNA as well as RNA viruses and both oncogenic and nononcogenic viruses. The types of chromosome changes also vary from a single gap or break in one chromatid to a total fragmentation of the chromosome set, and from a loss of a specific chromosome to extensive heteroploidization of the cell population.

An exhaustive review of the literature of virus-chromosome relationships is out of the scope of this presentation,[1,2] which is mainly a current review of the work done by our groups.

Interest in the role of viruses among agents causing chromosome changes arose primarily through an attempt to define some of the relationships between the somatic mutation theory and the viral theory of carcinogenesis.

Initially two virus-cell systems were used: Rous sarcoma virus (Schmidt-Ruppin strain) in rat and human cells, and measles virus *in vivo* and *in vitro*. These were subsequently enlarged for various reasons to include other organisms and systems, such as adenovirus-12, with and without a radioactive label, and some human mycoplasma strains such as pleuropneumonia-like organisms (PPLO) in leukocyte cultures. In recent experiments, emphasis has been on attempts to characterize the mechanisms involved in viral-induced chromosome changes. Two distinct types of viral-induced chromosome damage have been observed, single breaks and chromosome pulverization.

Single Breaks

Increased frequency of chromatid breaks was the initial finding in measles,[3] in which measles patients were shown to have 30–70 percent chromatid breaks (percent of cells with one or more breaks) in the leukocyte cultures from the third to fifth day after the onset of rash. A similar, although lower, increase in chromatid breakage was seen later in patients receiving live attenuated measles vaccine.[4] A characteristic feature of chromatid breaks seen in measles patients was the lack of a tendency for reunion of broken chromatids, resulting in a very low number of chromosome rearrangements. This is an important difference when compared with breaks induced by irradiations. Existence of chromosome breaks during measles was confirmed by others,[2,5] but negative results have also been reported.[5,7] The explanation for this difference in observations is not known at the present time, and several possibilities must be considered, such as different or mutant strains of measles virus, other coincident viral infections either enhancing or inhibiting the formation of breaks, or differences in the restitution of the breaks. Chromosome changes identical to those seen in measles have also been seen in chicken pox and possibly in mumps.[2,5]

* Present address: Children's Hospital, University of Helsinki, Helsinki, Finland.

Transformation of cell cultures *in vitro* by oncogenic viruses has often been considered as a model for malignant cellular changes *in vivo*. Chromosome abnormalities have been observed in a majority of the transformation systems studied and consequently are considered as one of the parameters characterizing the transformation process.

Studies of viral-induced malignancies by our groups have utilized a Rous virus system. *In vivo* tumors, tumors carried in tissue culture, and diploid rat embryo cells in tissue culture (to which Schmidt-Ruppin virus was added) exhibited chromosome breaks or evidence that chromosome breaks had occurred previously as shown by rearrangements.[4]

Because the Schmidt-Ruppin strain of Rous virus causes tumors in a large number of animals, including many mammalian species, studies of the effects of the virus on human leukocytes were initiated. These experiments showed inhibition of mitosis when the virus was added at the time the cultures were established. Chromosome breaks occurred when the virus was added at 36 hours, after DNA synthesis had already begun. Chromosome breakage varied from 10–30 percent, and again, the incidence of chromatid rearrangements was very low.[8]

Similar results have been obtained in human leukocyte cultures in recent experiments using the oncogenic adenovirus-12 (FIGURE 1). Interestingly enough, the nononcogenic adenovirus-2 does not seem to have the capacity of producing breaks in leukocyte cultures, as can be seen in TABLE 1. It is important to note that both Rous virus and adenovirus were present in the cells during the synthesis period of cellular DNA.

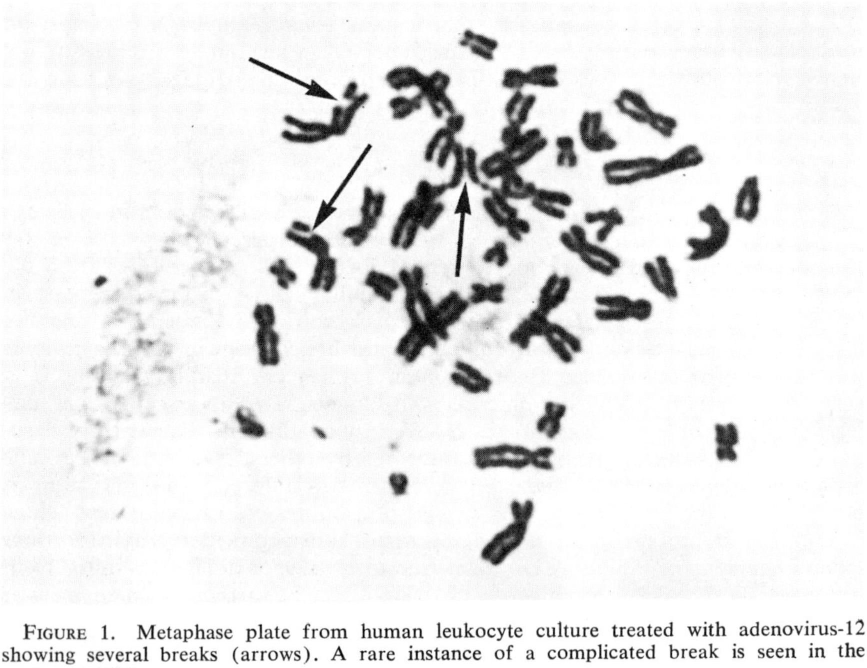

FIGURE 1. Metaphase plate from human leukocyte culture treated with adenovirus-12 showing several breaks (arrows). A rare instance of a complicated break is seen in the center. × 1600.

TABLE 1

PERCENTAGE OF CELLS WITH BREAKS AFTER TREATMENT WITH ADENOVIRUS-12 AND -2 IN HUMAN LEUKOCYTE CULTURES*

Experiment		Percent of Cells with Breaks in 50 Cells		
		Control	Virus at Planting	Virus at 36 hours
Adeno-12	I	6	14	30
Adeno-12	II	3	23	25
Adeno-12	III	6	18	18
Adeno-12	Mean	5	18.3	24.3
Adeno-2	I	6	—	4
Adeno-2	II	6	—	4

* The infectivity titer of both viruses was 2×10^7 PFU/ml as assayed in KB cells. The viruses were kindly supplied and titered by Dr. C. G. Goodheart, Institute for Biomedical Research, Chicago, Ill. Virus treatment was performed by centrifuging the cells for five minutes at 1500 rpm, resuspending in 1cc. of virus suspension for one hour at room temperature and then, after centrifugation, replaced in their own medium.

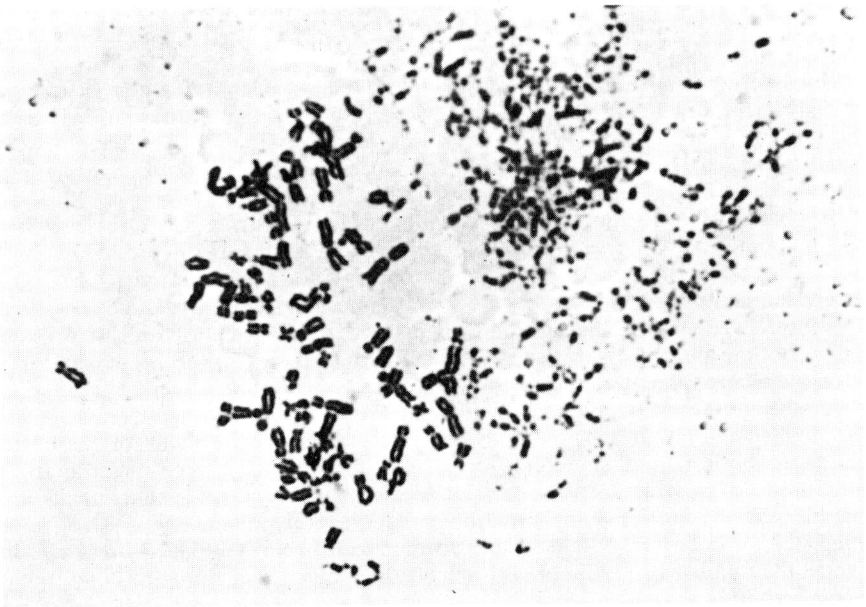

FIGURE 2. A typical pulverization metaphase in HeLa cells treated for six hours with measles virus hemolytic fraction. × 1000.

Chromosome Pulverization

A different type of chromosome damage was seen when measles virus in high multiplicities was added to four different types of human cell cultures.[9] This change consisted of severe fragmentation and scattering of chromatids leading to a picture which prompted us to designate this phenomenon as chromosome pulverization (FIGURE 2). Pulverized chromosomes occurred mainly in large syncytial cells containing different chromosome groups with various degrees of chromosome damage. Pulverization already had occurred after one-hour virus treatment. This phenomenon was seen in human leukocyte cultures, in diploid cell cultures from human embryonic kidneys, and in a heteroploid, continuous human cell line, LU 106, but it was not observed in human diploid cell cultures from embryonic lung tissue. The latter cell cultures, on the other hand, had an increased frequency of single chromatid breaks, if the virus treatment was of 24-hour duration.

Another tissue culture system, presently under investigation from a cytogenetic standpoint, is a strain of the heteroploid line, LU 106, that was converted to a measles carrier line by Norrby.[10] These cells do not go on to cell death and a lytic reaction, as is usual when measles virus is added to LU 106. Instead, they continue to grow and continually support virus growth. In cytogenetic examination, typical chromosome pulverizations are seen in some of the cells. In the cells that appear undamaged on gross examination, the stemline chromosome number has come down to 66–68 in contrast to the usual stemline number of 69–70.

By different chemical treatments, virus fractions could be produced which had a very low infectivity, but showed hemolytic and hemagglutinating activities in one preparation, but only hemagglutinating activity in another preparation. Using these viral fractions in LU 106 cells, it could be demonstrated that pulverization capacity was associated with the hemolytic fraction of the measles virus.[11]

Chromosome pulverization has been observed with several other viruses of the group of myxoviruses including Sendai, NDV and mumps virus.[12,13] The extraordinary rapidity of this process was demonstrated in experiments with Sendai virus in HeLa cells by detecting the first signs of chromosome changes as soon as ten minutes after the virus was added.[14]

In agreement with the observations with measles virus, it was also seen that the noninfective, UV-irradiated Sendai virus was as potent in producing pulverization as the untreated virus, but, in contrast to the measles virus, the pulverization component of the Sendai virus was not associated with any hemolytic capacity. Even though the mechanisms involved in both chromatid breaks and pulverization are unsolved, there is evidence that these two viral-induced chromosome changes are different phenomena. The type of chromosome abnormality that is believed most likely to have mutagenic significance, and therefore of greatest importance in carcinogenesis, is the single break. While many of the chromosome abnormalities, including loss of significant chromosome material from single breaks, would probably be fatal to the cell, it is possible that breaks are an indicator system for point mutations in less severely affected cells. This, then, might be an indicator system similar to that seen in x-ray-induced breakage, in which the number of visible breaks reflects the incidence of mutations and mutagenic activity.

Much of our most recent work has dealt with attempts to evaluate possible mechanisms in viral-induced chromosome changes. Many mechanisms, by which viruses could produce these effects on chromosomes, are possible. These include a combination of viral and cellular genomes or interference with DNA synthesis. Interference is effected either by inhibiting cellular enzymes, competing for nucleic acid building blocks, or by altering a cellular organelle such as the lysosome, which then produces the observed effect through release of DNase or other hydrolytic enzymes. Another possible mechanism is a specific change in the culture medium, either a toxic product or a deficiency of an essential compound. Experiments described below were performed to test some of the listed possible mechanisms of viral-induced chromosome damage.

Observations Made on Radioactively Labeled Adenovirus-12 in Human Leukocyte Cultures

Experiments are being made using adenovirus-12 labeled with tritiated thymidine† in order to get information on the site of viral action in the cells that exhibit chromosome abnormalities. Preliminary results of these experiments seem promising and show a suggestive increase in the number of nuclei exhibiting silver grains in the material exposed to labeled virus compared to cells exposed to tritiated thymidine alone.

Chromosome Breaks Induced by Inhibitors of DNA Synthesis

It was known earlier from work with plant material that some inhibitors of DNA synthesis, such as 5-fluorodeoxyuridine (FUdR)[15] and deoxyadenosine (AdR)[16] were capable of producing chromosome breaks morphologically similar to those seen in virus materials. These substances are thought to produce their chromosomal effects by inhibiting DNA synthesis.

In evaluating inhibitors of DNA synthesis, human leukocyte cultures were treated with the deoxyriboside analogs arabinosylcytosine (AraC),[17] arabinosyladenine (AraA);[18] the deoxyriboside deoxyadenosine (AdR),[17] and the riboside, cytidine triphosphate (CTP).[19]

Morphologically, the breaks produced with these inhibitors of DNA synthesis were identical to those seen in virus experiments–mainly open breaks and gaps and a low tendency for reunion. Whether or not the mechanism of action of viral-induced chromosome breaks and those associated with the inhibition of DNA synthesis are the same, several additional similarities between these two systems are apparent. These include mitotic inhibition, the ability of both to produce chromosome defects shortly after exposure, similar breakage localizations, synergism between Rous virus and CTP, and similarities between long-term base effects and viral-induced transformation.[20] However, these similarities are by no means complete in all cases.

Lysosomal Enzymes in Production of Chromosome Changes

It has been postulated by Allison and Paton[21] that the viral-induced chromosome breaks might be caused by lysosomal enzymes released by the viral attack on the lysosome membranes. This hypothesis was based on the observations of chromosome breaks after cells were treated with vital dyes like acridine orange, which have an affinity for lysosomal membranes. The treated cells are then exposed to visible light illumination of a wave length specific for the dye used in the experiment in order to damage the lysosomal membranes and release the contained enzymes. It is known that the cytopathic effects of several viruses

† Supplied by Dr. C. Goodheart, Institute for Biomedical Research, Chicago, Ill. The radioactive virus contained 2.5×10^{-3} cpm/PFU and a titer of 2.0×10^{7} PFU/ml.

are associated with a release of lysosomal enzymes into the cytoplasm.[22,23] This mechanism could well explain the rapidity and extensiveness of the chromosome pulverization.

This hypothesis has been tested in two types of experiments: (1) an adeno-virus-12-leukocyte system demonstrating single breaks, and (2) a measles virus-

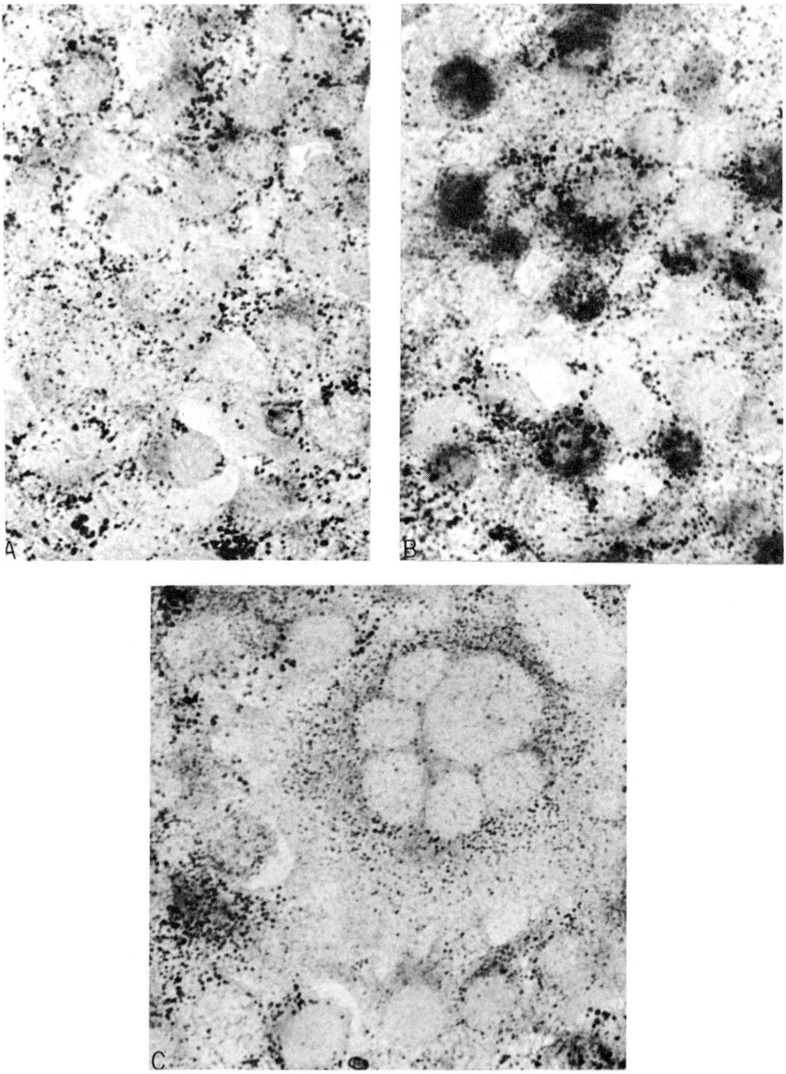

FIGURE 3. Lu 106 cells stained for acid phosphatases with naphtol AS-MX phosphate and fast red violet. × 850.

A. Control cells. Granular staining in cytoplasm.

B. Cells treated with poliovirus for 24 hours showing several cells with diffuse type of acid phosphatase staining.

C. Cells treated with measles virus hemolytic fraction for 24 hours. Large syncytial cell in the center with granular acid phosphatase staining.

HeLa or LU 106 system showing pulverization. In the latter, instead of infective measles virus, the hemolytic fraction showing equal pulverizing capacity was used. In the first type of experiment, acid phosphatases were stained at the time of harvesting of one portion of the cells, while a second portion was used simultaneously for chromosome preparations. The acid phosphatases were stained with 4 percent napthol AS-MX phosphate in acid pH with fast red violet LB in distilled water using two-hour incubation at 37° C.‡ HeLa and LU 106 cells were stained without fixing, but the leukocytes were fixed for one minute before incubation in phosphate solution with cold 10 percent neutral formalin. The results showed no increase of acid phosphatase staining when compared with the uninfected controls in either of the systems studied. HeLa and LU 106 cells, both controls and infected, showed granular staining in the cytoplasm, but only a few cells showed diffuse staining, indicating rupture of lysosomal membranes. Human leukocytes had less granular staining, both infected and controls, than

TABLE 2

ACID PHOSPHATASES AND CHROMOSOME PULVERIZATION IN HELA CELLS TREATED WITH MEASLES VIRUS HEMOLYTIC FRACTION AND POLIOVIRUS (TYPE 3)

Virus	Incubation Time (Hours)	Acid Phosphatases		Chromosomes	
				No. Cells	Percent Pulverization
None	6	+ → ++	granular stain in cytoplasm	50	0
None	24	+ → ++	granular stain in cytoplasm	50	0
Measles	6	+ → ++	granular stain in cytoplasm	80	10
Measles	24	++	granular stain in cytoplasm	60	11
Polio	6	+++	intensified granular stain in cytoplasm	71	0
Polio	24	++++	diffuse cytoplasmic and nuclear staining	No mitosis (cell destruction)	

* Measles virus hemolytic fraction was produced by Dr. Norrby, Karolinska Institute, Stockholm, Sweden, as described earlier.[11] It had a hemolytic activity of 1:320 and it was used in 1:3 dilution. Poliovirus (type 3) had an infectivity titer of $10^{6.5}$ $TCID_{50}$ in HeLa cells.

the cells of the continuous cell lines. An increased and diffuse type of staining was seen in many HeLa and LU 106 cells treated with poliovirus under the same conditions. FIGURE 3 illustrates the difference in acid phosphatase staining in LU 106 cells infected with the hemolytic fraction of measles virus and with poliovirus. The chromosome studies made simultaneously showed pulverization in HeLa cells with measles virus, but no detectable chromosome changes in poliovirus treated cells. Results of a representative experiment are shown in TABLE 2.

The second type of experiment is based on the well established stabilizing effect of cortisone on the lysosomal membranes.[24] It has also been demonstrated

‡ Sigma Chemical Co., St. Louis, Mo.

that treatment of the cells with cortisone decreases the rupture of lysosomes and diminishes the viral cytopathic effect caused by polio[25] and other viral diseases.[26] The same virus cell systems were used as in the previous experiments and the cortisone§ concentrations were from 2.5 μg/ ml to 250 μg/ml. In leukocyte cultures the cortisone treatment slightly decreased the mitotic index. No decrease of break frequency in adenovirus experiments or pulverization frequency in measles experiments could be detected, as can be seen in TABLES 3 and 4.

TABLE 3

ADENOVIRUS-12 INDUCED CHROMOSOME BREAKS IN HUMAN LEUKOCYTES TREATED WITH CORTISONE (POOLED RESULTS FROM TWO EXPERIMENTS)

Cortisone μg/ml	Adeno-12	No. of Cells	Percent Cells with Breaks
—	—	108	4.5
2.5	—	110	6.5
25	—	—	—
—	At planting	110	20.5
2.5	At planting	114	25
25	At planting	(6)	(33.3)
—	At 36 hours	121	21.5
2.5	At 36 hours	121	19
25	At 36 hours	50	20

TABLE 4

MEASLES VIRUS-INDUCED CHROMOSOME PULVERIZATION IN HELA AND LU 106 CELLS TREATED WITH CORTISONE

Cells	Cortisone μg/ml	Measles Virus 6 Hours		Measles Virus 24 Hours	
		No. Cells	Percent Pulverization	No. Cells	Percent Pulverization
LU 106	—	104	8	100	9
LU 106	2.5	100	7	100	12
HeLa	—	60	15		
HeLa	2.5	45	13		
HeLa	—	80	10	60	11
HeLa	25	68	15	50	8
HeLa	250	No mitosis		30	6

These results do not support the hypothesis that viral-induced chromosome changes, either single breaks or pulverization, are caused by hydrolytic enzymes released from the lysosomes after viral attack on the lysosome membranes, at least in these systems. Some recent reports[27] of the effect of acridine orange after illumination with visible light on the DNA of coliphage T7 point to the possibility that chromosome breaks in human cells, after treatment with vital dyes and visible light, could also be due to a direct reaction of the dyes with chromosomal DNA.

§ Cortisone acetate, Merck, Sharp & Dohme, West Point, Pa.

Effect of Human Mycoplasma Strains (PPLO) on the Chromosomes

Two reports have so far been published indicating the possible effect of PPLO's on the chromosomes.[28,29] These findings suggest an extracellular type of mechanism in the chromosome changes, inasmuch as the PPLO's are not thought to have an intracellular phase to their life cycles.

As the first step, human leukocyte cultures were studied after inoculation with three human PPLO strains, *Mycoplasma salivarium, M. hominis* Type II, and *M. fermentans*. Chromosomes were studied after three and five days of culture and the PPLO's were inoculated at the beginning of culturing with approximately 10^6 CFU and 10^3 CFU inoculum size. Preliminary results indicate that *M. salivarium* and *M. hominis II* cause a complete mitotic inhibition when used in the high inoculum of 10^6 CFU. These two PPLO strains are known to be arginine-requiring, and it was therefore interesting to study the effect of arginine on the mitotic inhibition. The mitotic inhibition could be partially reversed by adding arginine in concentrations of 1 mM to 10 mM. This was particularly evident with *M. salivarium*. The effect of *M. fermentans* on the mitotic index was less severe, and the relationship to arginine is still obscure.

Chromosome studies revealed no changes in cells harvested after three days of culture in any of the experiments, but a suggestive increase in the break frequently could be seen in cultures inoculated with 10^3 CFU of *M. salivarium* and harvested after five days. These cultures had break frequencies ranging from 14–22 percent, in contrast to the controls which showed breaks from 3–5.5 percent. The effect of arginine on breaks in cultures with *M. salivarium* was also studied, and in all experiments performed so far, arginine inhibited the breaks; cultures with added arginine had break frequencies equal to those seen in controls. These results are shown in TABLE 5. The blood cultures used, supplemented with 30 percent calf serum, supported the growth of PPLO's well, as indicated by increasing numbers of colonies counted on PPLO agar plates. The increased concentration of arginine did not have any effect on the growth of PPLO's in the blood cultures.

Chromosome breaks in PPLO-inoculated cell cultures pose many interesting questions, particularly when the mechanisms in viral-induced chromosome breakage are taken into consideration. The fact that PPLO's grow extracellularly or in association with the cell membranes, as shown in recent electron microscopic

TABLE 5

CHROMOSOME STUDIES IN BLOOD CULTURES INOCULATED WITH *M. Salivarium**

	Percent of Cells with Breaks in 120 Hours Culture				
Inoculum^{CFU} Experiment	10^6	10^3	10^6 + Arginine	10^3 + Arginine	Control
I	—	17	ND†	ND	4
II	—	22	9	6	4
III	—	14	—	6	6
IV	—	20	6	4	8
Mean	Mitotic inhibition	18.3	7.5	5.3	5.5

* 50 cells analyzed in each culture.
† ND = Not done.

studies,[30] and the effect of arginine on chromosome breaks seen in the present study indicate that environmental and metabolic factors are involved in some of the mechanisms leading to chromosome breaks.

The possibility that contamination with PPLO's is responsible for observed viral-associated chromosome damage seems quite remote, since in the work of our own group and others, PPLO's have been tested for by available methods and were not detected. However, this possibility should be kept in mind. The reverse possibility, that PPLO's might be able to support growth of an undetected virus, is an interesting but remote speculation.

Summary

Results obtained in previous works with measles virus and Schmidt-Ruppin strain of Rous sarcoma virus have shown that there are two types of viral-induced chromosome damage: chromatid breaks and chromosome pulverization. The one which is thought to have mutagenic significance, particularly in carcinogenesis, is the single break.

In recent experiments, emphasis has been on attempts to evaluate some possible mechanisms involved in viral-induced chromosome breakage. Comparison of viral-induced breaks with those produced by some ribosides and deoxyriboside analogs suggests a similar type of mechanism. Breaks in these two systems share several characteristics, such as morphology, time of occurrence, and lack of a tendency for reunion. Experiments are in progress with labeled adenovius-12 in order to detect the site of viral action on the chromosomes.

The possible role of lysosomal enzymes in chromosome breakage has been tested by studying acid phosphatases in cells exhibiting chromosome breaks or pulverization, and by stabilizing the lysosomal membranes with cortisone before virus treatment. The results did not support this hypothesis.

Preliminary results of studies with PPLO-infected human leukocyte cultures indicate that changes, such as depletion of arginine in the growth medium, also can lead to chromosome breaks, suggesting that the mechanism involved in morphologically similar chromosome changes might not be uniform.

References

1. Nichols, W. W. 1966. Studies on the role of viruses in somatic mutation. Hereditas **55:** 1–27.
2. Aula, P. 1965. Virus-associated chromosome breakage. A cytogenetic study of chickenpox, measles, and mumps patients and of cell cultures infected with measles virus. Ann. Acad. Sci. Fenn. A.IV. **89:** 1–78.
3. Nichols, W. W., A. Levan, B. Hall & G. Ostergren. 1962. Measles-associated chromosome breakage. Preliminary communication. Hereditas **48:** 367–370.
4. Nichols, W. W. 1963. Relationships of viruses, chromosomes, and carcinogenesis. Hereditas **50:** 53–80.
5. Gripenberg, U. 1965. Chromosome studies in some virus infections. Hereditas **54:** 1–18.
6. Harnden, D. G. 1964. Cytogenetic studies on patients with virus infections and subjects vaccinated against yellow fever. Amer. J. Hum. Genet. **16:** 201–213.
7. Tanzer, J., Y. Stoitchkov, P. Harel & M. Boiron. 1963. Chromosome abnormalities in measles. Lancet **ii:** 1070–1071.
8. Nichols, W. W., A. Levan, L. L. Coriell, H. Goldner & C. G. Ahlstrom. 1964. *In vitro* chromosome abnormalities in human leukocytes associated with Schmidt-Ruppin Rous sarcoma virus. Science **146:** 248–250.
9. Nichols, W. W., A. Levan, P. Aula & E. Norrby. 1965. Chromosome damage associated with measles virus *in vitro*. Hereditas **54:** 101–118.
10. Norrby, E. A carrier cell line of measles virus in LU 106 cells. In press.

11. NORRBY, E., A. LEVAN & W. W. NICHOLS. 1966. The correlation between the chromosome pulverization effect and other biologic activities of measles virus preparation. Exp. Cell Res. **41:** 241–249.
12. SAKSELA, E., P. AULA & K. CANTELL. 1965. Chromosomal damage of human cells induced by Sendai virus. Ann. Med. Exp. Fenn. **43:** 132–136.
13. CANTELL, K. E. SAKSELA & P. AULA. 1966. Virological studies on chromosome damage of HeLa cells induced by Myxoviruses. Ann. Med. Exp. Fenn. **44:** 255–259.
14. AULA, P. & E. SAKSELA. 1966. Early morphology of the chromosome damage induced by Sendai virus. Hereditas **55:** 362–366.
15. TAYLOR, J. H., W. F. HAUT & J. Tung. 1962. Effects of fluorodeoxyuridine on DNA replication, chromosome breakage and reunion. Proc. Nat. Acad. Sci. **48:** 190–198.
16. KIHLMAN, B. 1963. Deoxyadenosine as an inducer of chromosomal aberrations in *Vicia faba*. J. Cell Comp. Physiol. **62:** 267–272.
17. KIHLMAN, B. A., W. W. NICHOLS & A. LEVAN. 1963. The effect of deoxyadenosine and cytosine arabinoside on the chromosomes of human leukocytes *in vitro*. Hereditas **50:** 139–143.
18. NICHOLS, W. W. 1964. *In vitro* chromosome breakage induced by arabinosyladenine in human leukocytes. Cancer Res. **24:** 1502–1505.
19. NICHOLS, W. W., A. LEVAN, W. K. HENEEN & M. PELUSE. 1965. Synergism of the Schmidt-Ruppin strain of the Rous sarcoma virus and cytidine triphosphate in the induction of chromosome breaks in human cultured leukocytes. Hereditas **54:** 213–236.
20. NICHOLS, W. W. & W. K. HENEEN. 1965. Chromosomal effects of arabinosylcytosine in a human diploid cell strain. Hereditas **52:** 402–410.
21. ALLISON, A. C. & G. R. PATON. 1965. Chromosome damage in human diploid cells following activation of lysosomal enzymes. Nature **207:** 1170–1173.
22. ALLISON, A. C. & K. SANDELIN. 1963. Activation of lysosomal enzymes in virus-infected cells and its possible relationship to cytopathic effects. J. Exp. Med. **117:** 879.
23. ALLISON, A. C. & L. MALLUCCI. 1965. Histochemical studies of lysosomes and lysosomal enzymes in virus-infected cell cultures. J. Exp. Med. **121:** 463–476.
24. WEISSMAN, G. 1965. Lysosomes. New Eng. J. Med. **273:** 1143–1149.
25. MACIEIRA-COELHO, A., M. V. FERNANDES & W. J. MELLMAN. 1965. Cortisone on *in vitro* viral infection. II. Effect on distribution of cytopathic effect and acid phosphatase arrangement in human cells infected with polio virus. Proc. Soc. Exp. Biol. Med. **119:** 631–635.
26. HOTHAM-IGLEWSKI, B. & E. H. LUDWIG. 1966. Effect of cortisone on activation of lysosomal enzymes resulting from mengovirus infection of L-929 cells. Biochem. Biophys. Res. Comm. **22:** 181–186.
27. FREIFELDER, D. & R. B. URETZ. 1966. Mechanism of photoinactivation of coliphage T7 sensitized by acridine orange. Virology **30:** 97–103.
28. FOGH, J. & FOGH, H. 1965. Chromosome changes in PPLO-infected FL human amnion cells. Proc. Soc. Exp. Biol. Med. **119:** 233–238.
29. PATON, G. R. & J. P. JACOBS & F. T. PERKINS. 1965. Chromosome changes in human diploid cell cultures infected with Mycoplasma. Nature **207:** 43–45.
30. ZUCKER-FRINKLIN, D., M. DIVIDSON & L. THOMIS. 1966. The interaction of mycoplasmas with mammalian cells. II. Monocytes and lymphocytes. J. Exp. Med. **124:** **533–542.**

CHROMOSOME POLYPLOIDIZATION IN HUMAN LEUKOCYTES INDUCED BY RADIATION

Carlos E. Nasjleti and Herbert H. Spencer

The Veterans Administration Hospital and The University of Michigan, Ann Arbor, Mich.

Introduction

A great quantity of literature has accumulated on the effects of radiation and radiomimetic agents upon cells. Much of this work has been performed on mammalian cells both *in vivo* and in tissue cultures. Some of these damaging effects can be seen in dividing cells.

After the development of a technique for tissue culture of human peripheral blood, we were able to demonstrate abnormal patterns and chromosomal polyploidy in cultures from patients who had been treated with A-8103 (a piperazine derivative with antitumor activity),[1] nitrogen mustard, 6-mercaptopurine, and A-649 (another antitumor agent).[2] During treatment and for some time after treatment in these patients, structural changes could be seen in the chromosomes as either chromatid or chromosome deletions and chromosomal breakage. Abnormally shaped chromosomes were also seen, particularly ring forms and dicentrics. Although aneuploidy was observed, the major numerical variation consisted of metaphases showing polyploidy with random distribution of chromosomes and diplochromosomes. When normal human leukocytes were tested *in vitro* with the chemotherapeutic agents already mentioned, as well as with streptonigrin and cyclophosphamide,[3] similar results were obtained. From these studies we postulated that two different types of damage were induced in the cells by the chemicals. One type of damage is apparent in the hereditary material, and it can be characterized by the structural chromosomal changes. The second type of damage is interpreted as damage to the mitotic apparatus of the cells, as evidenced by the induction of polyploidy. Simultaneously, initial studies from patients treated with x-rays and cobalt-60 demonstrated that the same type of chromosomal anomalies were present in their peripheral leukocytes as those induced with chemotherapeutic agents. Generally, these were structural variations and chromosome polyploidization. Certainly, chromosomal changes have been described in association with x-radiation[4,5] and ^{131}I therapy[6,7] and, rarely, following diagnostic x-radiation. However, in most of these reports, the occurrence of polyploidy was overlooked, and when polyploidy was mentioned, it was not characterized.

Since both structural damage as well as polyploidy lead to genetic transformation or to somatic cell death, we thought it of paramount interest to determine whether or not induction of chromosomal polyploidy by radiation was a constant feature in human somatic cells. Such effects may have a bearing on both the induction as well as the treatment of cancer.

For the present study, we determined not only polyploidy, but also the amount of aneuploidy, chromosomal breakage, ring forms, translocations, dicentrics, and tricentrics as well as other rearrangements appearing in patients exposed to radiation therapy. In addition, normal human leukocytes were exposed to x-rays in cultures, and information of induced damage was obtained.

Materials and Methods

In Vivo Studies

Samples of blood for culture were taken from 12 patients who had received radiation therapy: Five treated with oral radioactive iodine (^{131}I), three treated with x-rays, and four with γ-rays from a cobalt-60 source. The dose of radiation was from 800–6,085 r given over 8–45 days. Most of these patients were suffering from cancer but four were treated for hyperthyroidism.[9] These men were from 33–74 years of age. The blood samples (10–15 ml) were taken before, during, and sometimes after irradiation. Blood from normal controls were cultured along with that from treated patients. The culture method used was slightly modified from the original technique of Moorhead *et al.*[8] described previously.[9] Briefly, heparinized blood, after drawing, was left in a vacuum tube at room temperature (27° C) for one hour to let erythrocytes sediment. Then 2 ml of leukocyte ladden plasma were added to 8 ml of culture medium 199 (Difco, Co.) containing penicillin and streptomycin, so that the seeding had a concentration of approximately 1×10^5 cells/ml. Final volume per culture was 10 ml and the ratio of supernate to medium was 1:4. To each bottle, 0.5 ml of Phytohemagglutinin M (Difco, Co.) was added. Culture bottles were incubated at 37° C in an atmosphere of 5 percent carbon dioxide and 95 percent air. Bottles were shaken twice daily during incubation. Between 65–67 hours after culture initiation, 0.1 ml of Colcemid® (Ciba Lab.) in a concentration of 10^{-6} M was added. At 72 hours these cells were hypotonically treated with distilled water and fixed with methanol-glacial acetic acid (3:1) mixture. Chromosomal spreading was accomplished by fanning and flaming. For staining, a solution of 2 percent aceto-orcein was used. Plates were scanned for mitotic metaphases under the microscope and metaphases that appeared intact were photographed. The transparencies (2 × 2 inches) obtained were projected on a screen for study. When possible, a minimum of 100 mitosis per culture was analyzed for chromosome number as well as for structural aberrations. Final analysis and karyotypes were prepared following the Denver nomenclature.[10]

In Vitro Studies

For these series the same technique was used except that blood from healthy individuals (one woman and four men) was used, half of the cultures were irradiated, and the total incubation time was 100 hours.

After obtaining blood from the five normal donors, ten cultures were set up and incubated. After 48 hours of incubation, the ten aliquots were taken from the incubator. To five aliquots a 200 r dose of x-radiation was given, using a conventional Westinghouse therapy machine operated at 250 KVP, 15 MA with ½ mm Cu and 1 mm A1 filters. For the radiation procedure, each bottle was placed on a 2-inch board of masonite and received a dose rate of 30.2 r/min for six minutes and 37 seconds. The remaining five aliquots were handled identically but did not receive actual irradiation. Following both the true and sham radiation, all ten aliquots were returned to the incubator for an additional 48 hours, after which Colcemid was added. After 100 hours, cells were taken from the incubator and thereafter handled as in the *in vivo* work.

Results

Cytogenetic studies from normal controls and from patients before radiation therapy were similar and showed a small percentage of breaks and aneuploidy as shown in TABLE 1. Most cells were characterized by a normal chromosomal complement (FIGURE 1).

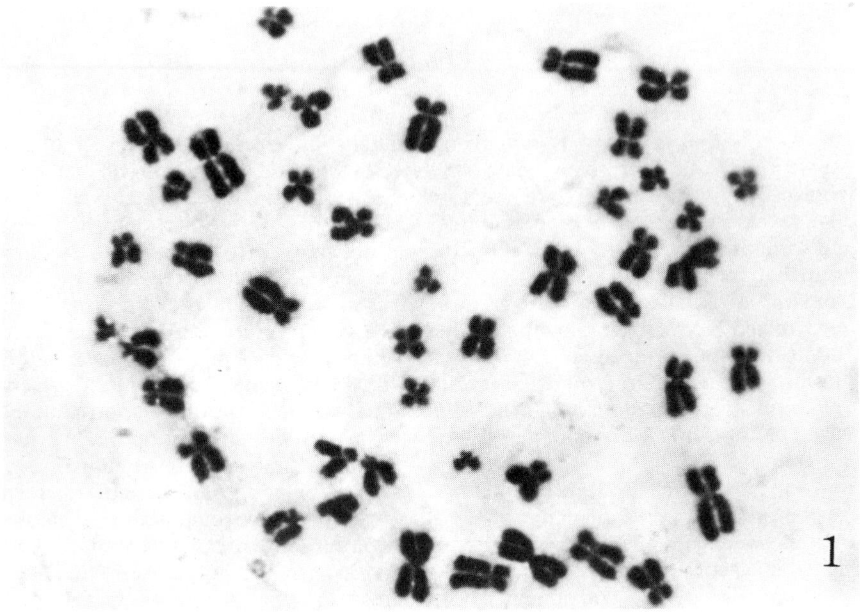

FIGURE 1. Normal female diploid metaphase obtained in a control culture. Aceto-orcein stain. × 1,400; orig. mag. × 2,000.

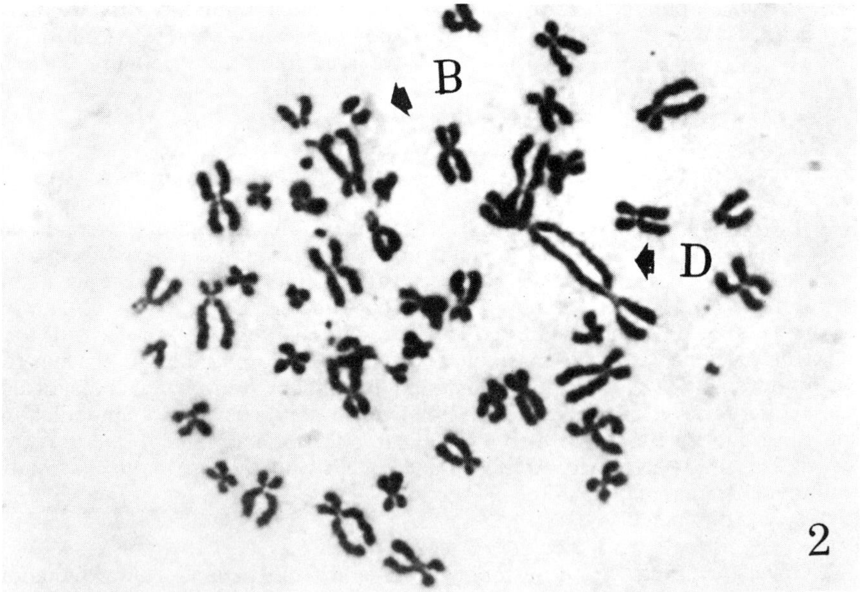

FIGURE 2. Hypoploid metaphase with chromosomal breakage (B) and dicentric chromosome (D) in a 72-hour culture of peripheral leukocytes from a patient treated with ^{131}I. Aceto-orcein stain. × 1,400; orig. mag. × 2,000.

When chromosomal analyses were obtained one week following ^{131}I therapy, an increase in structural chromosome aberrations was evident. For the most part these aberrations consisted of unstable chromosomal type damage, such as acentric fragments, rings, and dicentrics. FIGURE 2 shows a hypoploid cell demonstrating this type of damage. In addition, an increase in polyploid metaphases was

TABLE 1

CHROMOSOME PATTERNS BEFORE RADIATION THERAPY

	Total Cells Counted	Percent Cells with Structural Changes*	Aneuploidy† Percent	Tetraploidy Percent
Normal controls	1200	4	5	0.5
Patients before treatment	1200	3	5	0.5

* Only chromosome breaks were seen.
† Aneuploid cells having one or two chromosomes missing or in excess.

TABLE 2

CHROMOSOME COUNT DISTRIBUTION AFTER ONE TREATMENT WITH ^{131}I*

Diagnosis	Dose (mC)	Diploidy Percent	Aneuploidy Percent	Tetraploidy Percent
Thyrotoxicosis† (four patients)	5.5–9	86	5	9 (4)‡
Thyroid cancer† (one patient)	150	83	5	12 (3)‡

* Cultures established within one week after therapy.
† 100 metaphases were analyzed from each patient.
‡ Numbers in parenthesis indicate number of tetraploid cells that showed endoreduplication.

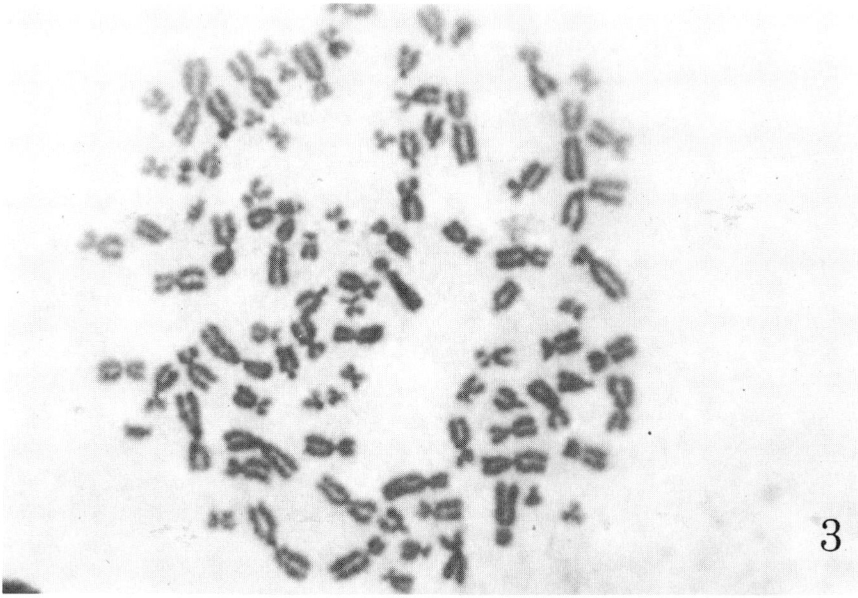

3

FIGURE 3. Tetraploid metaphase with random chromosome distribution in a 72-hour culture of peripheral leukocytes from a patient treated with ^{131}I. Aceto-orcein stain. × 1,120; orig. mag. × 1,600.

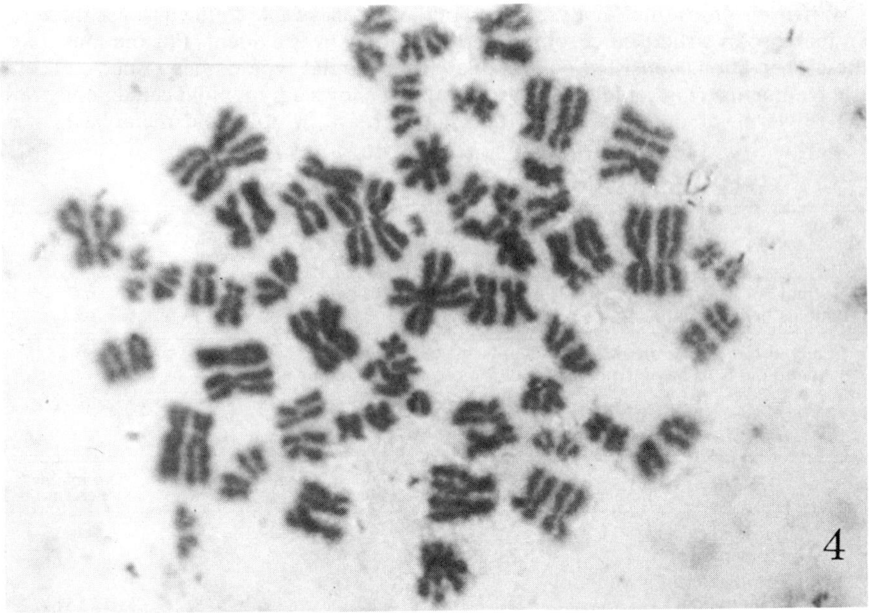

FIGURE 4. Tetraploid endoreduplicated metaphase with typical diplochromosomes in a 72-hour culture of peripheral leukocytes from a patient treated with ^{131}I. Aceto-orcein stain. × 1,120; orig. mag. × 1,600.

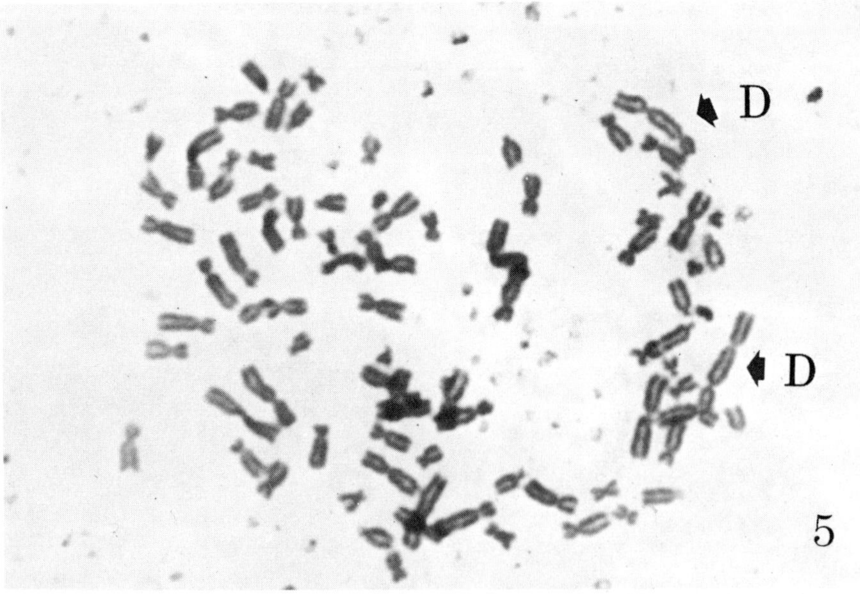

FIGURE 5. Heteroploid metaphase with dicentric chromosomes (D) in a 72-hour culture of peripheral leukocytes from a patient treated with ^{131}I. Aceto-orcein stain. × 1,120; orig. mag. × 1,600.

noted. Tetraploid mitoses constituted the major part of the polyploidy population. However, octoploids and a few cells at the 16-ploidy level were also observed from these patients. Polyploidy was seen with chromosomes distributed at random (FIGURE 3) and in diplochromosomes (FIGURE 4). Furthermore, it was noted that many of the structural aberrations seen in diploids were also seen in tetraploid cells (FIGURE 5).

The one patient, who received a large dose of radioiodine for thyroid carcinoma, did not show any more damage than those patients receiving smaller doses. It seems unlikely that the amount of structural or numerical chromosomal variation will provide an accurate method of biological radiation dosimetry in man. One patient had received radioiodine therapy nine months before our study and showed no chromosome abnormalities in baseline culture. These data are presented in TABLES 2 and 3.

Analyzing 2,200 cells from 22 cultures in patients receiving external radiation (including x-ray and cobalt-60) the prompt appearance of numerical changes and structural abnormalities were documented (FIGURE 6). Approximately two-thirds of the nonmodal metaphases were polyploid and one-third were aneuploid. The patients developed polyploidy that persisted throughout the course of therapy. The structural abnormalities noted were similar to those which have been de-

TABLE 3

CHROMOSOME STRUCTURAL ABERRATIONS AND TOTAL DAMAGE AFTER ONE TREATMENT WITH ^{131}I*

Diagnosis	Acentric Fragments Percent	Dicentrics Percent	Translocations and Other Aberrations Percent	Total Damage Percent
Thyrotoxicosis† (four patients)	10 (6)‡	9 (7)	1	20 (13)
Thyroid cancer† (one patient)	13 (10)	12 (10)	1	26 (20)

* Cultures established one week after therapy .
† 100 metaphases were analyzed from each patient.
‡ Numbers in parenthesis indicate amount of damage found in tetraploid metaphases out of the total number found.

TABLE 4

TETRAPLOID CELLS INCLUDING ENDOREDUPLICATION ANALYZED FOR DICENTRICS AND OTHER STRUCTURAL ABERRATIONS

Therapy	Number of Cells Analyzed	Number of Cells with Dicentrics	Percent
^{131}I	*R – 25	*R – 17	72
	†E – 25	†E – 19	
	50	36	
X-ray	R – 25	R – 17	74
	E – 25	E – 20	
	50	37	
Cobalt-60	R – 25	R – 18	72
	E – 25	E – 18	
	50	36	
Total	150‡	109	73

* R = Tetraploid cells with random distribution of chromosomes.
† E = Tetraploid endoreduplication.
‡ = In these tetraploid cells only 44 percent showed acentric fragments.

scribed many times, with the most frequent abnormalities being the formation of dicentric chromosomes and acentric fragments. It was again noted that the structural aberrations were frequently present in the tetraploid cell.

In our material, when fifty tetraploid cells were selected from each group of patients (treated with ^{131}I, x-ray, and cobalt-60), and these 150 cells analyzed for chromosome structural damage, it was noted that 73 percent of these cells contained dicentrics and 44 percent contained chromosomal fragments (TABLE 4).

In addition, fragmented cells were common in these preparations in which the fragmented chromosome segments underwent pycnotic condensation in the cytoplasm. At other times, cells showed various degrees of superfragmentation of the chromosomes with hyperchromatic micronuclei adjacent to it (FIGURE 7). Similar results were obtained by Koller[11] working with alkylating agents on cells of the Walker rat carcinoma 256.

When human leukocyte cultures were irradiated with 200 r and control cultures were not irradiated, marked differences were seen. A high degree of polyploidy

TABLE 5

SUMMARY OF CHROMOSOMAL ABERRATIONS SEEN FOLLOWING *in Vitro* X-RADIATION WITH 200 R

	Cells Counted	Structural Changes* Percent	Aneuploidy Percent	Tetraploidy Percent
Control	500	3.8	5.4	0
Irradiated cultures	500	52	3.2	12.2†

* Fragments, dicentrics, and translocations.
† Approximately half of the tetraploid cells showed endoreduplication.

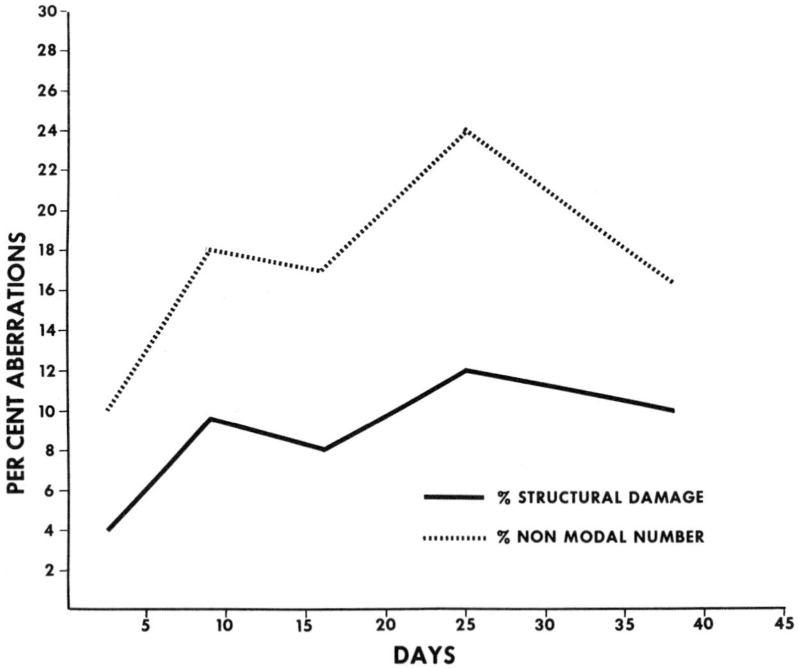

FIGURE 6. Relationship of damage to time during treatment in patients receiving external radiation.

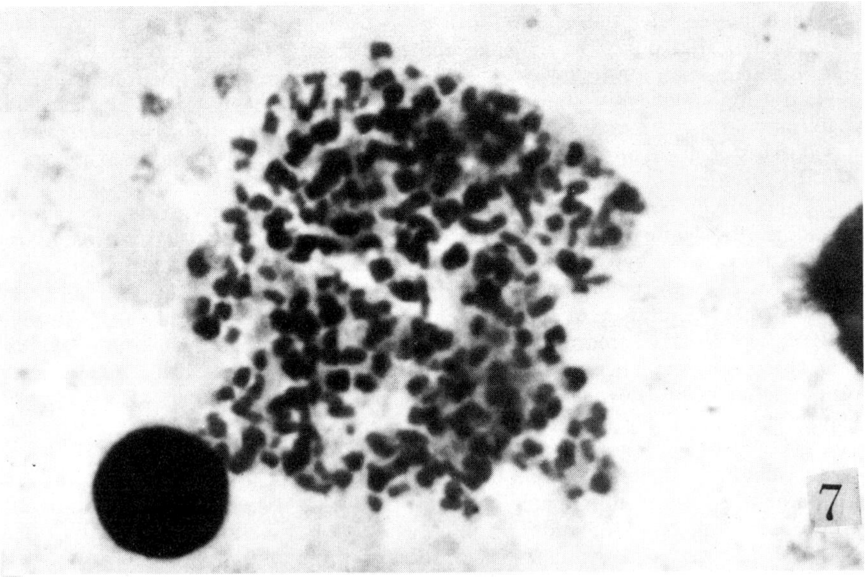

FIGURE 7. Damaged cell showing superfragmentation of chromosomes in a 72-hour culture of peripheral leukocytes from a patient treated with x-rays. Aceto-orcein stain. × 1,400; orig. mag. × 2,000.

and endoreduplication was noted as well as a high percentage of structural abnormalities reaching over 50 percent in some instances (TABLE 5).

DISCUSSION

It has long been known that radiation from x-rays and radioisotopes are capable of inducing mutations, as well as mitotic and chromosomal anomalies in human leukocytes.[12] However, relatively few of these studies characterized the chromosomal polyploidization, and thus failed to estimate the total extent of cytogenetic damage.

We have recently studied polyploidy induced by x-rays in human leukocyte cultures.[9] We observed polyploidy with random distribution of chromosomes and diplochromosomes. Levan and Hauschka[13] have considered the configuration of diplochromosomes at metaphase to be the result of endoreduplication. The fact that an endoreduplicated cell with diplochromosomes is a form of polyploidy was demonstrated by Bell,[14] who used two-wavelength microspectrophotometry to show that tetraploid endoreduplicated cells in an x-irradiated culture of human leukocytes contained about twice as much DNA as diploid cells from the same culture. An earlier review by Geitler[15] showed that endoreduplication has been described in different plant and animal tissues. Diplochromosomes have also been reported in human tumor cells.[16–19]

This investigation was undertaken to provide more needed information on polyploidy induction from ionizing radiation *in vivo*. Unfortunately, many of our patients died in the course of the study leaving us with only a small amount of material for evaluation. Furthermore, an unusually high percentage of cultures established from these patients during treatment failed to grow. Previous experience with patients treated with chemotherapeutic agents for cancer did not produce such a high number of failures. Perhaps, this failure rate could be related to an additional cellular damage induced by radiation in these cases.

It appears that polyploidy is an important change following irradiation, and that this aberration seems to be a fairly constant feature. The time interval, however, during which this abnormality persists cannot be ascertained from our material, and further studies will be needed to settle this question. However, it was noted that structural chromosomal changes and polyploidy persisted during radiation therapy in these patients. In several patients, the cells that contained chromosome abnormalities seemed to lose their proliferative capacity. This was evident from the observation of cytogenetic studies in three patients (two treated for cancer and one for hyperthyroidism), performed three to five months after irradiation, when the large majority of their leukocyte metaphases were characterized by a normal chromosomal complement without evidence of damage. Another patient, who received treatment 11 and nine months prior to our baseline evaluation, showed no evidence of damage before the third therapy with ^{131}I. However, other studies have shown that damage may persist for many years after radiation exposure. Particularly pertinent is the report of Bender and Gooch,[20] who observed chromosomal abnormalities 29 months after radiation in leukocyte cultures of a number of subjects who had been accidentally exposed to mixed gamma and fission neutron irradiation. Calculated absorbed doses received by these individuals varied from 22.8–365 rads. Buckton *et al.*[4] reported that abnormalities persisted for as long as 18 years after x-irradiation in patients treated for ankylosing spondylitis. Recently, Nofal and Beierwaltes[6] noted a statistically significant increased incidence of chromosomal aberrations in count and morphology both acutely and to a lesser extent chronically after radioiodine therapy for hyperthyroidism. These abnormalities were detected as early as one-half hour after the therapy dose, and were found in certain patients 14 years after treatment. These observations on the persistence of chromosomal damage after radiation therapy, lead us to a related consideration that would appear to be of much interest to the present audience.

It is now generally accepted that the metaphases we are analyzing are from transformed lymphocytes in the cultures,[21] but we are uncertain as yet about the life-span of these circulating cells. The persistence of chromosomal aberrations in peripheral lymphocytes for one year or longer after radiation, suggests a possibility that the life-span of lymphocytes may be considerable longer than two- or three-hundred days, as has been recently suggested by Yoffey.[22] However, in our material we observed octoploid and sometimes 16-ploid metaphases from patients during radiation. This seems to indicate that a certain number of lymphocytes in the circulating blood are actively dividing. Present evidence indicates that circulating lymphocytes are in G_0 stage and that in short term or 72 hour cultures, lymphocytes undergo a single division as has been demonstrated by MacKinney *et al.*[23] Those octoploid and 16-ploid cells clearly must have undergone more than one division in the donor's blood, otherwise it would be difficult to explain the finding of cells with such high polyploidy. In addition, although a high degree of polyploidy is good evidence to suggest that these dividing lymphocytes exist, the information gained from radiation-induced tetraploidy from these patients also provides evidence of this. Moreover, in our irradiated cultures using ^3H-thymidine we have seen tetraploids originate from two successive chromosome duplications. The cycle leading to tetraploid cells has approximately the same duration as two cycles of a diploid cell. Certainly this is true for tetraploid metaphases bearing diplochromosomes as well.

Another of our observations is of particular interest. When 150 tetraploid mitoses (75 showing random distribution of chromosomes and 75 showing diplochromosomes) were studied from our patients and were analyzed for the incidence of structural chromosomal aberrations, the following were observed: (1) The only damage seen in these cells were acentric fragments and dicentric chromosomes (three cells showed tricentrics). Ring forms, triradials, quadriradials, or rearrangements were not observed. (2) Dicentrics in numbers of two, four, and sometimes six were detected in 73 percent of tetraploid cells analyzed. (3) Chromosomal breakage was observed only in cells with dicentrics, whereas fragments alone were not seen in these tetraploid cells.

We think that there may be an important point here. Since 27 percent of the cells showed no dicentrics or other noticeable damage, one possibility is that polyploidy could be an independent consequence of the radiation injury to the mitotic apparatus. The possibility that dicentrics and polyploid cells are induced by radiation in different ways is understandable because many target areas may be involved simultaneously. One always sees an increase in the number of acentric fragments, dicentrics, ring forms, and many types of translocations and rearrangements, as well as polyploids in irradiated material. It is evident from this analysis that polyploidy may be related to damage to the mitotic mechanism, and that it may occur without apparent additional chromosomal damage.

On the other hand, we found 73 percent of polyploid cells showing dicentrics, usually accompanied by fragments but no other chromosome-type damage. One also can understand the appearance of dicentrics and fragments together, since these two events are related, and breakage is necessary for dicentrics to be formed. But why is there so high a number of dicentrics and no other type of unstable chromosome anomalies in polyploid cells? Are these two aberrations related to one another? Could dicentrics induce polyploidy independently of the polyploidy induced by radiation alone? This is a possibility that is suggested by our data, although we have no evidence or information as to how this kinetic event may occur. However, it is possible that dicentrics may become a permanent bridge interfering with cleavage, thus giving rise to giant cells or polypolar figures. In this regard, Muller[24] demonstrated that this process appears to be the principal cause of death in early fruit fly (*Drosophila melanogaster*) zygotes derived from irradiated spermatozoa. The association of this polyploidy and dicentric chromosomes is interesting. However, it is evident that further work exploring this hypothesis will have to be done to gain more definite information concerning the basis for this phenomenon.

Summary

1. In our patients following radiation therapy, induction of polyploidy was a prominent feature in addition to the usual chromosomal type abnormalities.

2. In most of our patients we were unable to continue long-term investigation following radiation therapy, but in four patients, studied three to nine months following therapy, no increase in chromosomal aberrations were seen.

3. Seventy three percent of 150 tetraploid cells selected following radiation therapy showed dicentric chromosomes and 44 percent contained acentric fragments. No fragments were seen in tetraploid cells unless a dicentric chromosome was present.

4. Similar chromosomal changes were seen following irradiation to human leukocyte cultures.

Acknowledgments

We are grateful to Dr. Claire J. Shellabarger, Chief, Kresge Radioisotope Laboratory, University of Michigan Medical Center, and Dr. Robert Rapp, Chief, Radiology Department, Veterans Administration Hospital, for making available the facilities used and for advice in some phases of this work. The technical assistance of Mrs. Jean Simons, Mrs. Virginia Hartog, and Mr. Richard Shaw is acknowledged. We are indebted to Mr. Robert McKnight and Mr. Stanley Nance for excellent photographic work, and to Mrs. Doris Watkins for aid with the manuscript.

References

1. Nasjleti, C. E., J. M. Walden & H. H. Spencer. 1965. Polyploidy and endoreduplication induced *in vivo* and *in vitro* in human leukocytes with n,n′-bis-(3-bromopropionyl) piperazine (A-8103). Cancer Res. **25**(3): 275–285.
2. Nasjleti, C. E. & H. H. Spencer. 1966. Chromosome damage and polyploidization induced in human peripheral leukocytes *in vivo* and *in vitro* with: nitrogen mustard, 6-mercaptopurine, and A-649. Cancer Res. **26**(1): 2437–2443.
3. Nasjleti, C. E. & H. H. Spencer. 1967. Chromosome polyploidization in human leukocyte cultures treated with streptonigrin and cyclophosphamide. Cancer **20**(1): 31–35.
4. Buckton, K. E., P. A. Jacobs, W. M. Court-Brown & R. Doll. 1962. A study of the chromosome damage persisting after x-ray therapy for ankylosing spondylitis. Lancet **ii**: 676–682.
5. Warren, S. & L. Meisner. 1965. Chromosomal changes in leukocytes of patients receiving irradiation therapy. J.A.M.A. **193**(5): 351–358.
6. Nofal, M. M. & W. H. Beierwaltes. 1964. Persistent chromosomal aberrations following radioiodine therapy. J. Nucl. Med. **5**: 840–850.
7. Boyd, E., W. Watson-Buchanan & B. Lennox. 1961. Damage to chromosomes by therapeutic doses of radio-iodine therapy. Lancet **i**: 977–978.
8. Moorhead, P. S., P. C. Nowell, W. J. Mellman, D. M. Battips & D. A. Hungerford. 1960. Chromosome preparations of leukocytes cultured from human peripheral blood. Expt. Cell Res. **20**: 613–616.
9. Nasjleti, C. E., J. M. Walden & H. H. Spencer. 1966. Polyploidization and aberration of human chromosomes induced *in vitro* and *in vivo* with ionizing radations. J. Nucl. Med. **7**: 157–176.
10. Human Chromosome Study Group. 1960. A proposed standard system of nomenclature of human mitotic chromosomes. J. Heredity **51**: 213–221.
11. Koller, P. C. 1958. Comparative effects of alkylating agents on cellular morphology. Ann. N. Y. Acad. Sci. **68**: 783–801.
12. Wald, N., G. E. Thoma, Jr. & G. Broun, Jr. 1962. Hematologic manifestations of radiation exposure in man. In Progress in Hematology. L. M. Tocantins, Ed. Vol. 3. : 1. Grune & Stratton. New York, N. Y.
13. Levan, A. & T. S. Hauschka. 1953. Endomitotic replication mechanisms in ascites tumors of the mouse. J. Nat. Cancer Inst. **14**: 1–43.
14. Bell, A. G. 1964. Diploid and endoreduplicated cells: measurements of DNA. Science **143**: 139–140.
15. Geitler, L. 1953. Endomitose und endomitotische Polyploidisierung. Protoplasmatologia *VI/C*. Spring. Vienna, Austria.
16. Levan, A. 1956. Chromosome studies on some human tumors and tissues of normal origin, grown *in vivo* and *in vitro* at the Sloan-Kettering Institute. Cancer **9**: 648–663.
17. Ising, U. & A. Levan. 1957. The chromosomes of two highly malignant human tumours. Acta Path. Microbiol. Scand. **40**: 13–24.
18. Sasaki, M., T. Fukuschima & S. Makino. 1962. Some aspects of the chromosome constitution of hydatidiform moles and normal chorionic villi. Gann **53**: 101–106.
19. Hsu, T. C. & P. S. Moorhead. 1956. Chromosome anomalies in human neoplasms with special reference to the mechanisms of polyploidization and aneuploidization in the HeLa strain. Ann. N. Y. Acad. Sci. **63**: 1083–1095.
20. Bender, M. A. & P. C. Gooch. 1962. Persistent chromosomes aberrations in irradiated human subjects. Radiat. Res. **16**: 44–53.
21. Robbins, J. H. 1964. Tissue culture studies of the human lymphocyte. Science **146**: 1648–1654.
22. Yoffey, J. M. 1964. Further problems of lymphocyte production. Ann. N. Y. Acad. Sci. **113**: 867–886.
23. MacKinney, A. A., Jr., F. Stohlman, Jr. & G. Brecher. 1962. Kinetics of cell proliferation in cultures of human peripheral blood. Blood **19**: 349–358.
24. Muller, H. J. 1954. Nature of genetic effects produced by radiation. *In* Radiation Biology. A. Hollander, Ed. Vol. 1. part 1. : 351–474. McGraw-Hill Book Co. New York, N. Y.

AUTOANTIBODIES IN DOWN'S SYNDROME AND GONADAL DYSGENESIS*

Philip J. Fialkow
Department of Medicine, Division of Medical Genetics
University of Washington, Seattle, Wash.
and
Irene A. Uchida
Department of Genetics, Children's Hospital
Winnipeg, Manitoba, Canada

Increased frequency of thyroid antibodies has been noted both in patients with Down's syndrome[1-5] and in those with gonadal dysgenesis.[6-8] In general terms, the association could be explained by one of two mechanisms. Aneuploidy in an individual may predispose him to develop thyroid autoantibodies, or alternatively, thyroid antibodies or a related factor may predispose him to aneuploidy. In the latter case, it is necessary to postulate that a factor associated with thyroid antibodies in a parent predisposes to aneuploidy in the child. The increased frequency of maternal thyroid dysfunction, claimed by many, but not all, studies of the mothers of patients with Down's syndrome, would be compatible with this suggestion.[4,9-14] No reports of parental thyroid evaluation in gonadal dysgenesis have yet appeared, but several observers have noted examples of parental thyroid antibodies.[8,15,16] These observations suggested that a large group of parents of children with chromosomal abnormalities should be tested for thyroid antibodies. If the antibodies in patients with chromosomal aberrations are secondary to these aberrations, then one need not expect to find thyroid antibodies in the parents who do not themselves have chromosomal disorders. On the other hand, an increased frequency of thyroid antibodies would be compatible with the suggestion that a factor related to the antibodies predisposes these parents to having a child with a chromosomal abnormality.[17]

Initially we measured thyroid antibodies in the families of children with Down's syndrome,[4,18] primarily because they were more available to us than families of patients with gonadal dysgenesis. In that study of 148 mothers of children with Down's syndrome and 148 controls, a significantly increased frequency of thyroid antibodies was noted in the mothers of children with Down's syndrome. Since that time our study has been expanded to include 242 families of patients with Down's syndrome and the data have been analyzed in relation to maternal age. Antinuclear factors, gastric parietal-cell antibodies, and rheumatoid factors have also been measured. In addition, a smaller group of families with gonadal dysgenesis has been tested.

Study Groups

Down's Syndrome

Two groups of families were studied. One hundred ninety families are from Winnipeg and the surrounding areas. Sera from these families were obtained for linkage studies and were stored frozen. Results in the mothers and fathers of these patients were compared with blood-bank donors from the Winnipeg area

* This work was supported by USPHS research grants nos. HD-01682, HE-3091, HD-527 from the National Institutes of Health, and by a grant from The National Foundation.

matched for sex and age. The remaining 52 families resided in the Seattle area and were ascertained through either the Genetics Clinic at the University of Washington (42 families) or a small private school for mentally retarded children (ten families). Families in which there was prior knowledge of thyroid or related diseases were excluded. These 52 families were compared with an equal number of control families from the Seattle area who were matched for maternal age at the time of study. Control families came from the outpatient clinics of the University of Washington Hospital and the Children's Orthopedic Hospital and Medical Center where they were seen either because of a child receiving well baby care (14 families) or because of a child with hemophilia (nine families), muscular dystropy (three families) or some other single gene mutation. Among the offspring only the propositi in the Winnipeg group were studied, and they were compared with age- and sex-matched children attending the Children's Orthopedic Hospital. Sera from the latter were randomly obtained from surplus specimens in the clinical chemistry laboratory, except that children with chromosomal abnormalities, thyroid disease, and "collagen diseases" were excluded.

Gonadal Dysgenesis

Thirty-nine previously unreported families were studied. Eleven of these are from the Winnipeg area, and 28 reside within a 200-mile radius of Seattle. These 28 families were ascertained through the outpatient clinics at the University of Washington Hospital and the Children's Orthopedic Hospital and Medical Center. Results in these families were compared to those expected in an equal number of age- and sex-matched controls. These expected results were calculated from analysis of the controls utilized in the Down's syndrome study.

Serological Tests

The tanned red blood cell test for thyroglobin antibodies and the indirect immunofluorescent test for antibodies to thyroid microsomal antigen were the same as those reported in the earlier study.[18]

Gastric parietal-cell antibodies and antinuclear factors were measured by indirect immunofluorescent techniques. Goat-antihuman gamma globulin conjugated to fluorescein isothiocyanate (Sylvana Company, Milburn, N.J.) was the antiserum and unfixed fresh-frozen sections of surgically removed human gastric mucosa served as the antigen for the parietal-cell antibody test. For the assay of antinuclear factors, goat-antihuman globulin conjugated to fluorescein isothiocyanate (Sylvana Company), unfixed fresh-frozen sections of rat liver, and 1:10 dilutions of the patients' sera were used.

Only a screening latex slide test (Hyland Laboratories, Los Angeles, Calif.) was used to test for rheumatoid factors.

Results

Families with Down's Syndrome

Thyroid Antibodies in Propositi

One hundred twenty-six patients with Down's syndrome between the ages of one year and 24 years were tested and compared with 126 controls. Twenty-five percent of the propositi were seropositive as compared to three percent of the controls ($p<0.005$). Two out of three propositi over 24 years old were seropositive. These results are in general agreement with the four other relevant reports in the literature (TABLE 1).[1-3,5] The data strongly suggest that the frequency of thyroid antibodies is significantly increased in children with Down's syndrome.

Thyroid Antibodies in Parents

Since there was no significant heterogeneity between the results obtained from the two groups (Seattle and Winnipeg), the data were pooled for analysis. No significant difference in thyroid antibodies between fathers and male controls was observed (TABLE 2).

TABLE 1

FREQUENCY OF THYROID ANTIBODIES IN PATIENTS WITH DOWN'S SYNDROME AND CONTROLS

Investigators	Down's Syndrome		Controls		χ^2*	p
	No. Tested	No. Positive	No. Tested	No. Positive		
Mellon *et al.*[1]	35	7 (20%)	35	0	5.7	<0.05
Burgio *et al.*[2]	65	21 (32%)	101	9 (9%)	13.2	<0.001
Saxena & Pryles[3]	50	14 (28%)	30	2 (7%)	4.1	<0.05
Richards *et al.*[5]	174	8 (5%)	90	0	2.9	<0.1
This report	126	32 (25%)	126	4 (3%)	23.6	<0.001

* The chi squares in this and the subsequent tables were calculated using Yates's correction for continuity.

TABLE 2

THYROID ANTIBODIES IN FATHERS OF PATIENTS WITH DOWN'S SYNDROME AND IN CONTROL MALES

	Fathers	Controls	χ^2	p
No. tested	228	228	0.23	>0.5
No. positive	24 (11%)	20(9%)		

TABLE 3

THYROID ANTIBODIES IN MOTHERS OF PATIENTS WITH DOWN'S SYNDROME AND IN CONTROL FEMALES

Investigators	Mothers of Patients with Down's Syndrome		Control Females		p
	No. Tested	No. Positive	No. Tested	No. Positive	
Burgio *et al.*[2]	50	22 (44%)	80	11 (14%)	<0.001
Dallaire & Flynn[19]	44	12 (27%)	101	12 (12%)	<0.05
This report	242	69 (29%)	242	39 (16%)	<0.005

Considering all the mothers, 69 or 29 percent of 242 mothers of patients with Down's syndrome were seropositive in contrast to 39 or 16 percent of an equal number of control females ($p<0.005$). Similar results have been obtained in the two other serological studies of mothers of patients with Down's syndrome known to us (TABLE 3).[2,19]

Age-specific prevalence of seropositivity in the 242 mothers of patients with Down's syndrome did not vary significantly throughout the age range tested (FIGURE 1). Thus, about 30 percent in any age range were seropositive. However, prevalence of thyroid antibodies in our control group, as in other studies,[20,21] increased notably with age, reaching a frequency similar to that seen in the Down's syndrome group (FIGURE 1). The most significant differences were observed in the youngest age group (TABLE 4).

Penrose, from analysis of maternal age and other factors, concluded that children with Down's syndrome can be subdivided into at least two general groups.[22] In one group the frequency of births of children with Down's syndrome increases notably with advancing maternal age, while cases in the other group seem to occur with a frequency independent of maternal age. Inherited translocations fit into the latter group, but they contribute only a small portion to the total, since Penrose now calculates that about 33 percent of all cases may belong in the maternal age independent group. To investigate whether maternal seropositivity is correlated with one or the other of these groups, we have analyzed our data in relation to maternal age at the time of birth of the propositus.[23] Thirty-five years of age was arbitrarily chosen as the dividing line. Thirty-four out of 120 mothers who had their children with Down's syndrome when they were less than 35 years of age were observed to be seropositive, whereas from analysis

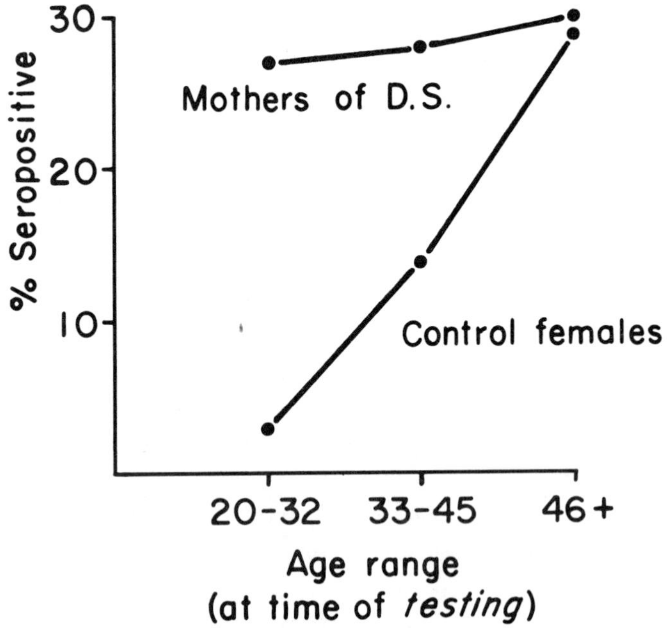

FIGURE 1. Age-specific prevalence of thyroid antibodies in mothers of patients with Down's syndrome and control females.

TABLE 4

THYROID ANTIBODIES IN MOTHERS OF PATIENTS WITH DOWN'S SYNDROME COMPARED WITH CONTROL FEMALES IN RELATION TO AGE AT THE TIME OF TESTING

Age Range at Time of Testing (Years)	Mothers of Patients with Down's Snydrome		Control Females		χ^2	p
	No. Tested	No. Positive	No. Tested	No. Positive		
20–32	66	18 (27%)	66	2(3%)	13.3	<0.001
33–45	97	27 (28%)	97	14 (14%)	4.5	<0.05
45+	79	24 (30%)	79	23 (29%)	–	–
Total	242	69 (29%)	242	39 (16%)	10.0	<0.005

TABLE 5

MATERNAL THYROID ANTIBODIES IN RELATION TO AGE AT TIME OF BIRTH OF CHILD WITH DOWN'S SYNDROME

Maternal Age at Birth of Down's Child (Years)	No. Tested	No. Positive		χ^2	p
		Observed	Expected		
18–34	120	34	11.5	12.5	<0.001
35+	122	35	27.5	0.91	>0.3

of an equal number of age- and sex-matched controls only 11.5 were expected to be seropositive (TABLE 5). This difference is significant at the 0.1 percent level. In marked distinction, there is no significant difference between the observed and expected frequencies of thyroid antibodies in mothers who had their affected children when they were 35 years of age or older.

Parietal-Cell Antibodies

Two out of 108 propositi and none of the 108 controls had gastric antibodies (TABLE 6). Similarly, 17 mothers and 13 controls were seropositive (TABLE 6). These differences are not statistically significant. No difference between fathers and male controls was noted.

Antinuclear Factors

Six out of 122 propositi had antinuclear factors as compared with two controls (TABLE 7). Six out of 158 mothers and two out of 158 control females were seropositive. These differences are not statistically significant.

Rheumatoid Factors

No differences in the frequencies of rheumatoid factors were noted.

Families with Gonadal Dysgenesis

Only thyroid antibody tests have been completed in this group. Fifteen of 37 propositi were seropositive, whereas only 1.5 were expected ($p<0.001$) (TABLE 8). Thirteen of 39 mothers were seropositive compared to 5.5 expected. This difference is at least equal in magnitude to that observed in mothers of patients with Down's syndrome, but it is not statistically significant. This may be because only a relatively small number of families has been studied. Five of 31 fathers were observed to be seropositive and 2.8 were expected to be seropositive. For further analysis the families were divided into two groups: those in which propositi had an XO karyotype and those in which propositi had either mosaicism or an isochromosome X.

XO Group

Seven of 22 propositi were observed to be seropositive, and 0.9 were expected to be seropositive. This difference is significant at the 5 percent level (TABLE 9). The observed and expected numbers of seropositive mothers were 4 and 2.8, respectively (TABLE 9).

Mosaic and Isochromosome X Group

Eight of 15 propositi were observed to be seropositive, and 0.5 were expected ($p<0.01$). Fifteen mothers were tested, and the observed and expected numbers of seropositive mothers were nine and three, respectively ($p<0.1$) (TABLE 9).

Discussion

The data indicate that there is an increased frequency of thyroid antibodies in patients with Down's syndrome and their mothers. There is also an increased frequency in patients with gonadal dysgenesis, and possibly also in their mothers. One may next inquire whether presence of these antibodies is characteristic of any particular type of chromosomal abnormality.

TABLE 6

GASTRIC PARIETAL-CELL ANTIBODIES IN DOWN'S SYNDROME

	Propositi	Mothers	Fathers
No. Tested	108	143	125
No. positive Down's syndrome	2	17	9
No. positive controls	0	13	10

TABLE 7

ANTINUCLEAR FACTORS IN DOWN'S SYNDROME

	Propositi	Mothers	Fathers
No. Tested	122	158	156
No positive Down's syndrome	6	6	5
No. positive controls	2	2	3
χ^2	1.2	1.1	0.12
p	>0.2	>0.2	>0.7

TABLE 8

THYROID ANTIBODIES IN GONADAL DYSGENESIS

	Propositi	Mothers	Fathers
No. Tested	37	39	31
No. positive observed	15 (41%)	13 (33%)	5 (16%)
No. positive expected	1.5 (4%)	5.5 (14%)	2.8 (%9)
χ^2	12.2	3.0	0.21
p	<0.001	<0.1	>0.6

TABLE 9

THYROID ANTIBODIES IN PATIENTS WITH XO AND OTHER TYPES OF GONADAL DYSGENESIS AND IN THEIR MOTHERS

Group	Type	No. Tested	No. Positive		χ^2	p
			Observed	Expected		
Patients	XO	22	7 (32%)	0.9 (4%)	4.01	<0.05
	Mosaics and isochromosomes X	15	8 (53%)	0.5 (4%)	6.94	<0.01
Mothers	XO	23	4 (17%)	2.8 (12%)	–	–
	Mosaics and isochromosomes X	16	9 (56%)	2.8 (18%)	3.63	<0.1

When the data are analyzed in relation to maternal age at the time of birth of the child with Down's syndrome, contrary to what we had initially anticipated, the increased frequency of thyroid antibodies in mothers seems to be almost confined to the maternal age-independent group. Since this group has a relatively high frequency of mosaicism, familial trisomy 21, and translocations, this suggests that the effect may be more important in the more unusual chromosomal abnormalities. Karyotypic studies, as yet incomplete, tend to support this. Thus far, four mosaics have been identified in the Seattle group.[24] Two have mothers with Hashimoto's thyroiditis, one has a seropositive mother without overt thyroid disease, and the fourth has a paternal grandmother with a firm goiter who is seropositive. Furthermore, in the original study of 35 patients with Down's syndrome by Mellon *et al.*,[1] four of the seven seropositive patients had the more unusual karyotypes seen in Down's syndrome, such as mosaicism and translocations. Moreover, in gonadal dysgenesis the frequency of thyroid antibodies is more striking in patients with mosaicism or an isochromosome X and in their mothers than in the XO group.

Several mechanisms might explain the association between maternal thyroid antibodies and chromosomal aberrations. The chromosomal abnormality could initiate the production of thyroid antibodies. This implies that approximately 30 percent of the younger mothers of children with Down's syndrome have significant chromosomal abnormalities. Thus far we have studied five seropositive mothers, two of whom have had detailed study, including counts of 150 cells. To date we have not found significant chromosomal abnormalities in these five subjects, but we are evaluating a larger sample. Alternatively, the birth of a child with Down's syndrome may initiate maternal thyroid autoimmunity. This question, which has been discussed elsewhere,[4,18] could best be resolved by prospective study of a large group of child-bearing women. Unfortunately, this requires obtaining blood specimens from at least 100,000 women. Preliminarily, it seems more likely to us that maternal thyroid antibodies precede abnormal chromosome division.[4,17,18]

One hypothesis is that the maternal thyroid antibodies themselves predispose to the chromosomal aberrations. Since circulating thyroid antibodies are felt to have little, if any, pathogenetic significance, the possibility was explored that these factors indicate a more generalized immunologic disturbance, one manifestation of which might be the birth of a child with a chromosomal aberration. Gastric parietal-cell antibodies and rheumatoid factors were not found significantly more frequently in the families of children with Down's syndrome. Similarly, the propositi and their mothers tended to have more antinuclear factors than did controls, but the differences were not statistically significant. Although it is possible that when a larger number of families of patients with Down's syndrome is studied, a significantly increased frequency of these factors may be observed, this certainly cannot be a very striking phenomenon. Thus, within the limitations of our test systems, there is no evidence to indicate that the mothers of children with Down's syndrome have a generalized immunologic disturbance. Nevertheless, it should be noted that circulating antibodies to rabbit ova have been reported in some mothers of subjects with chromosomal abnormalities.[25]

In view of lack of evidence for a pathogenetic action of circulating antibodies, we have attempted to study the effect of cell-bound factors on cell division *in vitro*. Experiments have been reported which show that extracts prepared from human circulating lymphocytes cause significant increases in the number of hyperploid mitoses of fibroblasts *in vitro*.[26] Since that time it has been shown that these extracts also induce significant increases in chromosomal breaks and rearrangements.[27] These effects are seen only when the extracts are tested on genetically foreign fibroblasts. When the same normal subject donates both the lymphocyte extract and the fibroblasts, these effects are not observed. Thus, self-recognizing mechanisms are involved, but whether or not these effects are related to the *in vivo* chromosomal abnormalities remains a matter of conjecture.

Thus far only the possibility that thyroid antibodies or a related immunologic phenomenon predispose to the chromosomal aberration has been considered. However, the relationship between maternal thyroid antibodies and a child's aneuploidy need not be direct, since thyroid antibodies may reflect another factor which leads to the chromosomal aberration. For example, a virus could induce the formation of thyroid antibodies. It could also possibly induce chromosomal aberrations *in vivo* resulting in, for example, Down's syndrome.[28,29] Evidence currently available does not allow either the rejection or acceptance of this hypothesis. Alternatively, structural or functional abnormalities of the thyroid could lead to "autoimmunity" and perhaps also to chromosomal aberrations.[30,31]

Summary

Thyroid antibodies have been detected in the sera of 25 percent of 126 patients with Down's syndrome as compared to three percent of an equal number of age-

and sex-matched controls ($p<0.001$). They were not detected significantly more frequently in the fathers of such patients than in male controls, but 29 percent of 242 mothers were seropositive compared to 16 percent of an equal number of controls ($p<0.005$). The increased frequency is almost confined to those mothers who had their children when they were younger than 35 years of age, i.e., in the maternal age-independent group. Frequencies of gastric parietal-cell antibodies, antinuclear factors, and rheumatoid factors were not significantly increased in these families.

Thyroid antibodies were observed in 41 percent of 37 propositi with gonadal dysgenesis whereas only four percent were expected ($p<0.001$). They were also detected in 33 percent of 39 mothers of patients with gonadal dysgenesis, whereas 14 percent were expected. This difference is not statistically significant, but only a relatively small number of families was studied. As in the case of Down's syndrome, occurrence of thyroid antibodies seemed to be more striking in one subgroup, those patients who have mosaicism or an isochromosome X.

Presence of thyroid antibodies in women appears to be associated with a higher risk of Down's syndrome and possibly also of gonadal dysgenesis in the offspring. The hypothesis that a factor related to the maternal thyroid antibodies antedates and predisposes to the aneuploidy is favored. The seemingly more striking occurrence of this phenomenon in mothers of children with the more unusual chromosomal abnormalities such as mosaicism may offer some insight into the unknown pathogenetic mechanism.

ACKNOWLEDGMENTS

The studies described herein could not have been accomplished without the collaboration of numerous colleagues including Drs. A. G. Motulsky, P. E. Ferrier, F. Hecht, and G. Martin, and Mrs. Jean Bryant. Carolyn McKinney provided skilled technical assistance. Control samples were obtained from the Manitoba Depot of the Canadian Red Cross Blood Transfusion Service through the courtesy of Miss Catherine Anderson and staff. The kind cooperation of the many families and subjects who participated in this study is gratefully acknowledged.

[NOTE ADDED IN PROOF: Since this paper was submitted for publication, our studies have been expanded and several relevant reports have appeared in the literature.

We have now studied a total of 320 mothers of patients with Down's syndrome, ascertained as described in the text. Ninety-seven or 30 percent are seropositive compared with 54 or 17 percent of an equal number of control females ($p<0.001$). In addition, a fourth report of increased frequency of thyroid antibodies in mothers of subjects with Down's syndrome has been published (Engelberth, O. *et al.*, 1967. Sborn. lék. **69:** 232–238). In a fifth study, an apparent increase of significant clinical thyroid disease was found in such mothers, but the authors were nonetheless unable to confirm an increased prevalence of thyroid antibodies in these women or in their affected offspring (Wren, P. *et al.*, 1967. Lancet **i:** 186-188). An exceptional feature of this study is that a relationship between advancing age and increasing prevalence of thyroid antibodies in control females, almost universally noted by numerous other investigators, was not found.

The observation that the increased frequency of thyroid antibodies in mothers of children with Down's syndrome compared with age-matched female controls is more striking in younger than in older mothers has also been made by other investigators (Dallaire, L. & D. Kingsmill-Flynn. 1967. L'Union Méd du Canada **96:** 1371-1375; Engleberth, O. Personal communication).

The study of thyroid antibodies in families of patients with gonadal dysgenesis has also been expanded and includes 69 propositi, 77 mothers, and 64 fathers. The results will be reported in more detail elsewhere, but they are essentially similar to those reported in the text, i.e., increased prevalence of thyroid antibodies in propositi and in mothers of subjects with either mosaicism or an isochromosome X. Two other groups have found increased frequency of thyroid antibodies in parents of patients with gonadal dysgenesis (Vallotton, O. & A. Forbes. 1967. Lancet **i:** 648–651; Engelberth, O. Sborn. lék. In press), but a third group found this only in propositi and not in their parents (Doniach, D. *et al.,* 1968. Proc. Roy. Soc. Med. **61:** 278–280). Vallotton and Forbes also found increased frequency of antibodies to the ovarian cytoplasm in their subjects' families (Vallotton, O. & Forbes. 1967. Lancet **i:** 648–651). Engel has reported a high frequency of thyroid antibodies in patients with gonadal dysgenesis with both XO and other types of chromosomal aberrations (Engel, E. 1967. Lancet **i:** 1271–1272).]

References

1. Mellon, J. P., B. Y. Pay & D. M. Green. 1963. Mongolism and thyroid antibodies. J. Ment. Defic. Res. **7:** 31–37.
2. Burgio, G. R., F. Severi, R. Rossoni & R. Vaccaro. 1966. Autoantibodies in Down's syndrome. Lancet **i:** 497–498.
3. Saxena, K. M. & C. V. Pryles. 1965. Thyroid function in mongolism. J. Pediat. **67:** 363–370.
4. Fialkow, P. J. 1966. Autoimmunity and chromosomal aberrations. Amer. J. Hum. Genet. **18:** 93–108.
5. Richards, B. W., A. Stewart, P. E. Sylvester & V. Jasiewicz. 1965. J. Ment. Defic. Res. **9:** 245–259.
6. Sparkes, R. S. & A. G. Motulsky. 1963. Hashimoto's disease in Turner's syndrome with isochromosome X. Lancet **i:** 947.
7. Grumbach, M. & A. Morishima. 1964. X-chromosome abnormalities in gonadal dysgenesis: DNA replication of structurally abnormal X-chromosome: relation to thyroid disease. J. Pediat. **65:** 1087.
8. Williams, E. D., E. Engel & A. P. Forbes. 1964. Thyroiditis and gonadal dysgenesis. New England J. Med. **270:** 805–810.
9. Myers, C. R. 1938. An application of the control group method to the problem of etiology of mongolism. Proc. Amer. Assoc. Ment. Defic. **62:** 142–150.
10. Benda, C. E. 1949. Prenatal maternal factors in pregnancy. J. A. M. A. **139:** 979–985.
11. Ek, J. I. 1959. Thyroid function in mothers of mongoloid infants. Acta Pediat. (Uppsala) **48:** 33–42.
12. Coppen, A. & V. Cowie. 1960. Maternal health and mongolism. Brit. Med. J. **1:** 1843–1847.
13. Fialkow, P. J., F. Hecht, J. Bryant & A. G. Motulsky. 1965. Familial predisposition to chromosomal aberrations. Clin. Res. **13:** 124.
14. Zsako, S. & A. R. Kaplan. 1966. The trisomy-21 syndrome and protein-bound iodine in the mothers. Amer. J. Ment. Defic. **70:** 512–514.
15. Sparkes, R. S. & A. G. Motulsky. 1967. The Turner syndrome with isochromosome X and Hashimoto's thyroiditis. Ann. Intern. Med. **67:** 132–134.
16. Grumbach, M. & A. Morishima. Personal communication.
17. Fialkow, P. J. 1964. Autoimmunity: a predisposing factor to chromosomal aberration? Lancet **i:** 474–475.
18. Fialkow, P. J., I. A. Uchida, F. Hecht & A. G. Motulsky. 1965. Increased frequency of thyroid autoantibodies in mothers of patients with Down's syndrome. Lancet **ii:** 868–870.
19. Dallaire, R. & D. Flynn. 1967. Frequency of antibodies to thyroglobulin in relation to gravidity and to Down's syndrome. Canad. Med. Ass. J. **97:** 209–212

20. Hill, O. W. 1961. Thyroglobulin antibodies in 1,297 patients without thyroid disease. Brit. Med. J. **1**: 1793–1796.
21. Doniach, D. & I. M. Roitt. 1964. An evaluation of gastric and thyroid autoimmunity in relation to hematologic disorders. Seminars Hemat. **1**: 313–343.
22. Penrose, L. S. 1961. Mongolism. Brit. Med. Bull. **17**: 184–189.
23. Fialkow, P. J. 1967. Thyroid antibodies, Down's syndrome, and maternal age. Nature **214**: 1253–1254.
24. Fialkow, P. J., J. Bryant & F. Hecht. Unpublished observations.
25. Vallotton, M. B. & A. Forbes. 1966. Antibodies to cytoplasma of ova. Lancet **ii**: 264–265.
26. Fialkow, P. J. & S. M. Gartler. 1966. Hyperploidy effect of lymphocyte extract of fibroblasts *in vitro*. Nature **211**: 713–715.
27. Fialkow, P. J. 1967. Chromosome breakage induced by extracts of human allogeneic lymphocytes. Science **155**: 1676–1677.
28. Robinson, A. & T. T. Puck. 1965. Sex chromatin in newborns: Presumptive evidence for external factors in human nondisjunction. Science **148**: 83–85.
29. Stoller, A. & R. D. Collmann. 1965. Virus aetiology for Down's syndrome (mongolism). Nature **208**: 903–904.
30. Bishun, N. P., W. R. Morton & M. N. Rashad. 1964. Chromosome endoreduplication. Lancet **i**: 1452.
31. Merz, T., T. Pempree & B. R. Migeon. 1966. Thyroxin, satellite association and trisomy. Nature **209**: 1198–1200.

CHROMOSOME ABNORMALITIES IN ANEMIAS*

Gerald E. Bloom and Louis K. Diamond

Divisions of Hematology and Genetics, Medical Service
Children's Hospital Medical Center and the Department of Pediatrics
Harvard Medical School, Boston, Mass.

Cytogenetic techniques were first applied to the study of human disease in 1956.[1] With few exceptions, chromosomal abnormalities have been found only in certain conditions where involvement of multiple organ systems occurs, as in the D1, 17–18, and 21 trisomies. In most diseases due to single gene-determined defects, however, the chromosomal lesion is beyond the resolution of presently available techniques. Several congenital hematologic disorders that occur in childhood, such as some of the congenital neutropenias, appear to be due to a single genetic defect involving only the hematopoietic system,[2] whereas others are associated with involvement of multiple organs. For example, minor congenital abnormalities, including pterygium coli and polydactyly, are occasionally seen in patients with congenital hypoplastic anemia,[3] and aplasia of the radius is present in one form of congenital amegakaryocytic thrombocytopenic purpura.[4] The most prominent congenital malformations occur in patients with constitutional aplastic anemia (CAA), in whom the skeleton, kidneys, heart, and other organs may be affected.[5]

In order to explore the possibility that some of these conditions are associated with chromosomal abnormalities, a systematic cytogenetic investigation of a number of congenital and acquired hematologic diseases was carried out.

Patient Material

Thirty-five children, with a variety of hematologic disorders, both acquired and congenital, made up the study group (TABLE 1). Because of the unusual nature of the findings in the patients with CAA, 1,068 patients without hematologic disease were studied for comparison. These controls were derived from a retrospective analysis of the records of 1,000 consecutive chromosome studies performed prior to December, 1964, as well as a prospective study of 68 nonanemic patients investigated concurrently.

Constitutional aplastic anemia refers to a syndrome of chronic pancytopenia due to bone-marrow aplasia in which there is evidence of a constitutional origin. The 16 patients with this disorder were divided into two groups on the basis of their clinical and hematologic manifestations. Type I (Fanconi's aplastic anemia) is characterized by pancytopenia associated with a variety of well-defined congenital malformations such as aplasia of the radius, polydactyly, and renal ectopy and hypoplasia. Less striking abnormalities including hyperpigmentation, microphthalmia, and brachydactyly may be seen in conjunction with major deformities or are themselves the main features of the disorder along with the pancytopenia. Also included in this group are multiply affected children with aplastic anemia in a family which may have associated congenital deformities. Type II CAA, affecting only males thus far, includes patients without congenital deformities, in whom amegarkaryocytic thrombocytopenic purpura occurs at birth or early infancy, followed by pancytopenia later in childhood.

* Supported by grants from the National Institutes of Health (nos. HE 5255, HE 02405, and GM 09107) and from the John A. Hartford Foundation.

TABLE 1

Hematologic Disorders Studied	Number	Results of Chromosome Studies
Constitutional aplastic anemia		
Type I	14	Abnormal in 12
Type II	2	Normal
Acquired aplastic anemia	7	Normal
Congenital aregenerative anemia	6	Normal
Congenital thrombocytopenia	2	Normal
Congenital thrombocytopenia with aplasia of the radius	1	Normal
Paroxysmal nocturnal hemoglobinuria	1	Normal
Congenital chronic neutropenia	2	Normal

Methods

Chromosome studies on peripheral blood were done according to a modified technique of Moorhead *et al.*[6] Phytohemagglutinin P (Difco) was added at the beginning of the 72-hour culture period to medium 199 enriched with 15 percent fetal bovine serum containing the white-blood-cell-rich plasma. Cells were exposed to Colcemide® two hours prior to harvesting. Bone marrow preparations were performed according to the technique of Tjio and Whang.[7] No culture period was involved other than a one-hour exposure to Colcemide®.

Cells from both peripheral blood and bone-marrow preparations were harvested by exposure to a hypotonic solution for ten minutes followed by fixation in an acetic acid-alcohol solution. Slides were prepared by an air-drying method.

Only in those patients with Type I (Fanconi's variety) CAA were any chromosomal abnormalities found (TABLE 1). No abnormality of chromosome number was encountered in these patients except for a specific type of polyploidy known as endoreduplication in some cells. The most common abnormalities found were a variety of structural aberrations known as chromatid exchanges, and chromatid and isochromatid breaks.

Endoreduplications represent chromosomal duplication with incomplete separation of the partners, so that at metaphase a cell characterized by 46 four-stranded figures results (FIGURE 1). The most frequent abnormalities found in the CAA patients were breaks of one or both chromatids of a chromosome, with angulation, displacement, or loss of chromosomal material distal to the break (FIGURE 2). There was no apparent predilection for one particular chromosome or one group of chromosomes to be involved in the breakage phenomenon. Chromatid gaps consisted of achromatic segments without any change in the orientation of the chromosomal material distal to the gap. In contrast to chromosomal breakage, there was no increase in the frequency of gaps in patients with CAA.

Chromatid exchanges are abnormal arrangements of homologous or non-homologous chromosomes presumably arising as a result of chromatid breakage in two adjacent chromosomes followed by an anomalous reunion of the broken ends (FIGURE 3). A variety of conformations of chromatid exchanges

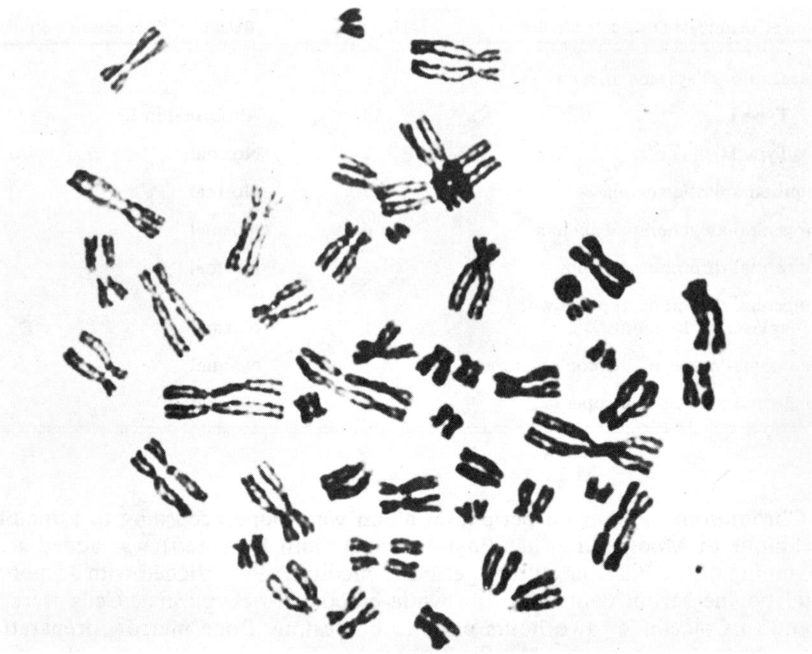

FIGURE 1. Endoreduplicated metaphase figure.

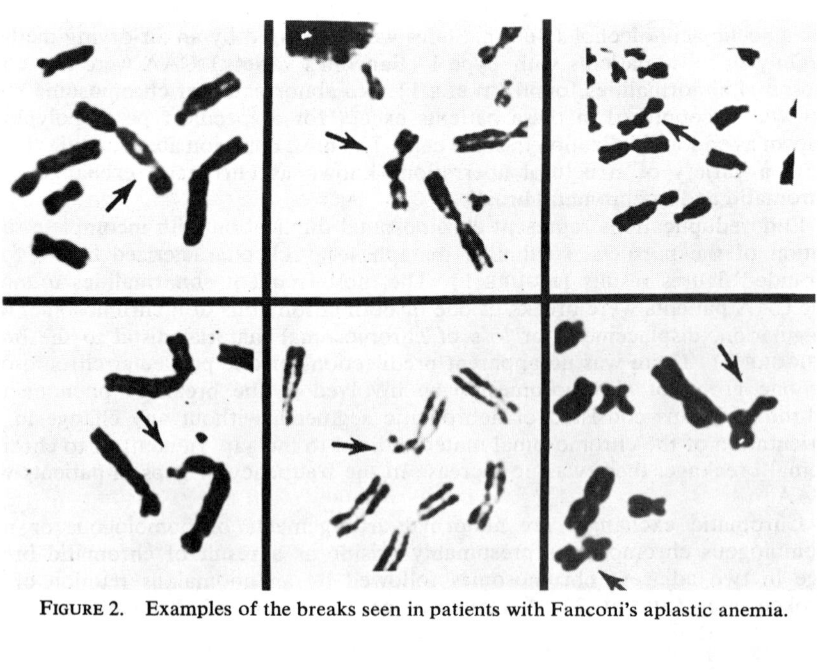

FIGURE 2. Examples of the breaks seen in patients with Fanconi's aplastic anemia.

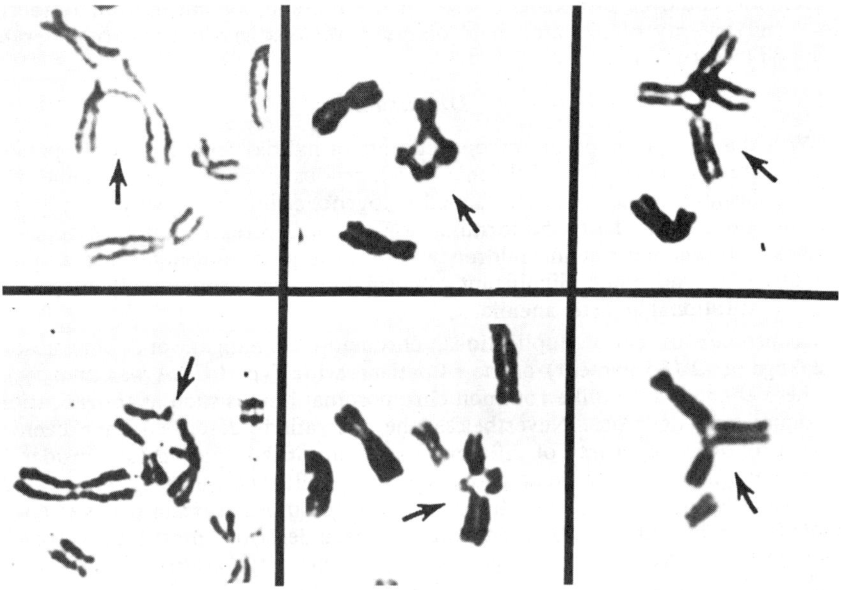

FIGURE 3. Examples of the variety of chromatid exchanges found in Fanconi's aplastic anemia.

was seen. In some, homologous chromosomes participated so that symmetrical figures resulted; in others, broken ends were unattached; and in still others, more than four arms were present indicating that more than two chromosomes were involved.

Because of the unusual nature of these findings, a large number of controls was examined both retrospectively and concurrently with the patients with CAA. A minimum of 15 cells was microscopically karyotyped from each control patient and many more were at least superficially scanned in the process of looking for the best cells (endoreduplications and chromatid exchanges are often easily spotted even under low magnification). From these studies, it was concluded that occurrences in a single chromosomal preparation of more than two chromatid exchanges or two endoreduplications was abnormal. Similarly, when 50 cells were examined, presence of more than one cell with a break was abnormal.

In children with Type I CAA, 12 out of 14 patients had one or more chromosomal abnormalities as described above, whereas both Type II patients were normal. Out of the 12 abnormal Type I patients, an increased incidence of chromosomal breakage was found in 11 and was observed in 4–42 percent of cells examined, 3–17 chromatid exchanges were found in nine patients, and endoreduplications were seen in three patients.

Direct bone-marrow preparations were successful in only one out of seven patients in whom this study was carried out. No chromosomal abnormalities were found in the bone marrow of this patient at a time when the peripheral blood was abnormal.

There was no correlation between incidence of cytogenetic abnormalities and number or type of congenital malformations, except that the chromosomes in Type II patients, who had no congenital anomalies, were normal. Similarly, no correlation could be established between the presence of chromosomal aberrations and severity of hematological disease, previous irradiation, drug therapy, or blood transfusions.

Discussion

With the exception of the cytogenetic abnormalities found in some patients with leukemia, particularly chronic myelogenous leukemia,[8] and some with megaloblastic anemia,[9] no well-defined cytogenetic findings have been reported in other diseases of the blood-forming organs. In the present report, cytogenetic studies were carried out in children with a variety of congenital and acquired hematologic syndromes. Significant abnormalities were found only in patients with constitutional aplastic anemia.

Occurrence of endoreduplications, chromatid exchanges, and chromosome breakage in 12 (85 percent) of the 14 patients with Type I CAA was unexpected as these changes are unlike common chromosomal lesions such as translocations, trisomies, and deletions. Nevertheless, the aberrations described have been reported following a variety of different insults and it is important to consider the possibility that they are related to exogenous influences. For example: endoreduplications occur following irradiation,[10] exposure to certain drugs,[11] and in acute leukemia;[12] chromosome breakage has been described most frequently after radiation exposure[13] but breakage may occur during the course of certain viral illnesses[14] and therapy with cytotoxic drugs;[15] chromatid exchanges have been reported in normal persons, in relatives of mongoloid patients, in Waldenström's macroglobulinemia,[16] and after exposure of human leukocytes to mitomycin C.[17] Nevertheless, occurrence of these chromosomal abnormalities in patients with CAA does not appear to be related to exogenous causes as they occurred in children who had received no radiation, drug therapy, or blood transfusions. Seven patients with acquired aplastic anemia, investigated and treated in a similar manner, showed no such changes. In addition, apparently identical chromosomal changes have now been reported independently by several groups of observers in other patients with Fanconi's aplastic anemia.[18–21]

There are two disease states in which the reported chromosomal findings bear a resemblance to the changes found in our patients with CAA. Kiossoglou and Mitus described chromosomal breakage and endoreduplication in 18 patients with megaloblastosis due to several causes.[9] These patients, however, also had dicentric forms and giant chromosomes which were not found in our patients. Of greater interest is a syndrome described by Bloom,[22] characterized by low birth weight, stunted growth, and a peculiar skin eruption. Like CAA, this disorder is considered to be a recessively determined familial disease associated with an increased incidence of leukemia. In our series of patients with CAA, two developed acute monocytic leukemia. Cytogenetic studies in patients with Bloom's syndrome have shown abnormal numbers of chromatid exchanges and broken chromosomes.[19,23] These changes appear to be very similar to findings in the CAA patients.

The increased incidence of leukemia in CAA and in Bloom's syndrome raises the question of whether the cytogenetic abnormalities in these disorders predispose cells to undergo malignant transformation. It is possible that the hypersusceptibility to chromosomal breakage in both conditions could result in cells whose genome was sufficiently altered so that they were now capable of autonomous proliferation. In this regard, it is of interest that in one of our patients

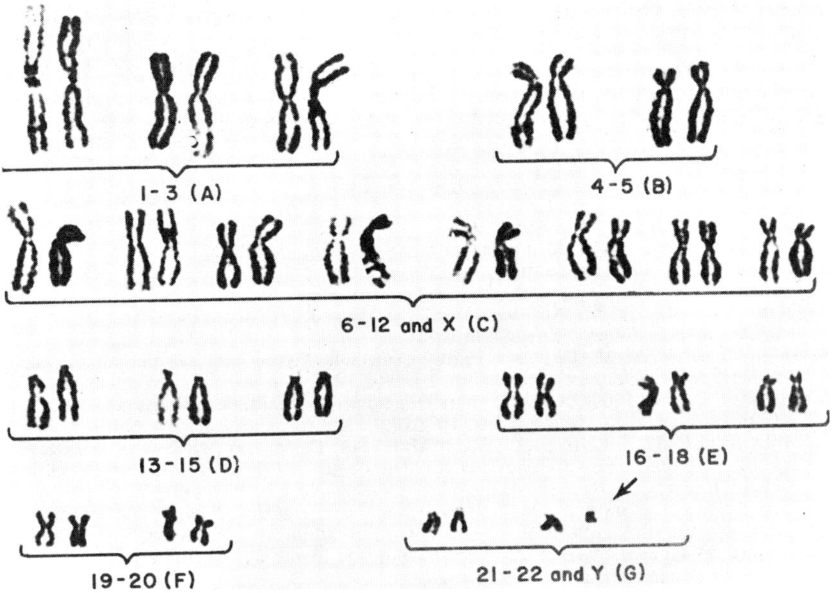

FIGURE 4. Karyotype of a cell appearing to contain a Philadelphia chromosome from a patient with Fanconi's aplastic anemia.

with CAA, a cell was found that appeared to contain a Philadelphia chromosome (FIGURE 4).

The relationship of the chromosomal findings in patients with CAA to the basic disease process in this disorder is unclear. They may be only secondary phenomena and of no etiologic importance. Löhr *et al.*[24] felt that the chromosomal breakage might be due to altered glucose metabolism. They investigated two brothers with Fanconi's aplastic anemia and found low levels of the enzyme hexokinase. However, we studied two unrelated patients with Fanconi's aplastic anemia and found normal levels of this enzyme. Others have suggested that some peripheral lymphocytes serve as a pool that the stem-cell component of the bone marrow draws upon to replenish itself.[25] If these lymphocytes are sufficiently altered by the chromosomal changes described so that their proliferation and maturation is interfered with, then a deficiency of stem cells could occur and aplastic anemia might result.

Whatever the significance of the chromosomal findings in Type I CAA proves to be, it is clear that the changes are specific for this type of aplastic anemia. As a result, they have proved helpful in the diagnosis of CAA where the congenital malformations are minor. It is hoped that further research directed toward a better understanding of the genesis of these cytogenetic abnormalities will eventually lead to more effective forms of treatment for Fanconi's aplastic anemia.

Summary

Chromsomal analyses were carried out in 35 children with various hematologic disorders other than leukemia. These included congenital "pure" red-cell aregenerative anemia, chronic neutropenia, paroxysmal nocturnal hemoglobinuria, congenital thrombocytopenia, acquired aplastic anemia, and constitutional aplastic anemia. Only in the Fanconi type of CAA were any significant findings encountered. The abnormalities included a specific type of polyploidy and increased numbers of chromosomal breaks and chromatid exchanges. These findings do not appear to be related to therapy, irradiation or other apparent exogenous factors but rather to the basic pathologic process in CAA.

References

1. LEVAN, A. 1956. Chromosome studies on some human tumors and tissues of normal origin, grown in vivo and in vitro at Sloan-Kettering Institute. Cancer **9:** 648.
2. KOSTMAN, R. 1956. Infantile genetic agranulocytosis. Acta Paediat. (Suppl. 105) **45:** 1.
3. DIAMOND, L. K., D. M. ALLEN & F. B. MAGILL. 1961. Congenital (erythroid) hypoplastic anemia. Amer. J. Dis. Child. **102:** 403.
4. SHAIN, S. & R. A. M. OLIVER. 1959. Congenital hypoplastic thrombocytopenia with skeletal deformities in siblings. Blood **14:** 374.
5. NILSSON, L. R. 1960. Chronic pancytopenia with multiple congenital abnormalities (Fanconi's anemia). Acta Paediat. **49:** 518.
6. MOORHEAD, P. S., P. C. NOWELL, W. J. MELLMAN, D. M. BATTIPS & D. A. HUNGERFORD. 1960. Chromosome preparations of leukocytes cultured from human peripheral blood. Exper. Cell. Res. **20:** 613.
7. TJIO, J. H. & J. WHANG. 1962. Chromosome preparations of bone marrow cells without prior in vitro culture or in vivo colchicine administration. Stain Techn. **37:** 17.
8. NOWELL, P. C. & D. A. HUNGERFORD. 1960. A minute chromosome in human chronic granulocytic leukemia. Science **132:** 1497.
9. KIOSSOGLOU, K. A. & W. J. MITUS. 1964. Cytogenetic studies in pernicious anemia, megaloblastosis and Di Guglielmo syndrome. Clin. Research **12:** 217.
10. FRIEDMAN, B. I., E. L. SAENGER & M. S. KREINDLER. 1964. Endoreduplication in leukocyte chromosomes: preliminary report of its relation to cancer and whole body irradiation. Lancet **2:** 494.
11. NASJLETI, C. E., J. M. WALDEN & H. H. SPENCER. 1965. Polyploidy and endoreduplication in non-leukemic patients. New Eng. J. Med. **272:** 250.
12. HOUSTON, E. W., W. C. LEVIN & S. E. RITZMANN. 1964. Endoreduplication in untreated early leukemia. Lancet **2:** 496.
13. CONEN, P. E., A. G. BELL & N. ASPIN. 1963. Chromosomal aberrations in infant following use of diagnostic x-rays. Pediatrics **31:** 72.
14. AULA, P. 1964. Chromosomes and viral infections. Lancet **i:** 720.
15. ARRIGHI, F. E., T. C. HSU & E. BERGSAGEL. 1962. Chromosome damage in murine and human cells following Cytoxan therapy. Texas Rep. Biol. Med. **20:** 545.
16. GERMAN, J. 1964. Cytologic evidence for crossing-over in vitro in human lymphoid cells. Science **144:** 298.
17. SHAW, M. W. & M. M. COHEN. 1965. Chromosome exchanges in human leukocytes induced by mitomycin C. Genetics **51:** 181.
18. SCHROEDER, T. M., F. ANSCHÜTZ & A. KNOPP. 1964. Spontaneous aberration of chrosomes in familial panmyelopathy. Humangenetik **1:** 194.
19. GERMAN, J. & R. ARCHIBALD. 1965. Chromosomal breakage in a rare and probably genetically determined syndrome of man. Science **148:** 506.
20. SCHMID, W., R. SCHÄRER, T. BAUMANN & G. FANCONI. 1965. Chromsomenbrüchigkeit bei der familiären Panmyelopathie (typus Fanconi). Schweiz. Med. Wschr. **95:** 1461.
21. SWIFT, M. R. & K. HIRSCHORM. 1966. Fanconi's anemia: inherited susceptibility to chromosome breakage in various tissues. Ann. Intern. Med. **65:** 496.
22. BLOOM, D. 1954. Congenital telangiectatic erythema resembling lupus erythematosis in dwarfs. Amer. J. Dis. Child. **88:** 754.
23. SAWITSKY, A., D. BLOOM & J. GERMAN. 1966. Chromosomal breakage and acute leukemia in congenital telangiectatic erythema and stunted growth. Ann. Intern. Med. **65:** 487.
24. LÖHR, G. W., H. D. WALLER, F. ANSCHÜTZ & A. KNOPP. 1965. Biochemische Defekte in den Blutzellen bei familiaren Panmyelopathie (typus Fanconi). Humangenetik **1:** 383.
25. YOFFEY, J. M. 1962. Present status of lymphocyte problem. Lancet **i:** 206.

GENETICS IN ACUTE LYMPHATIC LEUKEMIA IN CHILDHOOD*

J. Jeffrey McCullough† and Melvyn T. Korobkin

United States Public Health Service, Minnesota Department of Health
Minneapolis, Minn.

and

William Krivit

University of Minnesota Medical School
Minneapolis, Minn.

The genetic influence on cancer development in retinoblastoma, multiple polyposis of the colon, neurofibromatosis, xeroderma pigmentosum, and acanthosis nigricans is quite clear. Nevertheless, the genetic role in the majority of cancers remains unproved. A predisposition for leukemia in childhood, however, has been noted in several specific population groups. These have included concordancy for leukemia in monozygotic twins,[1–3] and patients with Down's syndrome,[4–6] immunological deficiencies,[7–8] and Bloom's syndrome.[9] One of the underlying mechanisms for this increased incidence could be a definite genetic predisposition.[10,11] Isolated instances of familial leukemia other than in concordant monozygotic twins have increased the likelihood of a possible genetic influence. Indeed, Videbaek[12,13] reported that cancer and leukemia were more common in relatives of leukemic patients than in those of controls, but several subsequent studies have not substantiated these findings.[14–16]

The present study attempts to clarify the problem by investigating occurrence of cancer and leukemia in relatives of children with acute lymphatic leukemia treated at the University of Minnesota Hospital. Results are compared with hospital controls and with estimates of the number of cancers expected. We did not find an excess of cancer or leukemia in relatives of leukemic children.

Methods

From July, 1963 to July, 1965, 36 patients under 15 years of age with the diagnosis of acute leukemia were admitted to the University of Minnesota Hospital. The diagnosis was substantiated in all cases by examination of the bone marrow. Five of the patients were dead at the time this study was performed. The parents of all of these children were contacted either personally or by mail and were requested to participate in the study. Twenty-four (67 percent) families agreed to participate.

A questionnaire was given to each set of parents, and they were asked to record information about themselves and the patient's siblings, aunts, uncles, cousins, grandparents, and grandparents' siblings. The following information was obtained: name, present age if living, age at death if deceased, year of death, place of death, cause of death, whether the relative was ever known to have had cancer, hospitalizations, reasons for hospitalization, and name and location of the hospital. Parents were asked to contact members of their family to obtain this information. Finally, one of the authors met with each set of parents to review the information they had obtained. In a few cases the final interview was by telephone.

* Supported by grants from the USPHS, no. CA 08832, and the Graduate School of the University of Minnesota.

† Present address: Department of Laboratory Medicine, University of Minnesota Hospital, Minneapolis, Minn.

Controls were selected in two ways. The first was a random selection of patients admitted to the same pediatric station during the same period of time as the leukemic patients. The only criteria applied were that they not have a malignant disease and that the parents be willing to participate in the study. Final diagnoses of these 17 hospital controls are shown in TABLE 1. The second control group consisted of neighbors of the leukemic families whose only qualification was a willingness to participate in the study. These eight control families were selected by a random method but were not matched for age and sex.

We also calculated for control and leukemia relatives the expected number of cancers based on cancer mortality data for Minnesota.[17]

TABLE 1

DIAGNOSES OF CONTROL PATIENTS ADMITTED TO THE UNIVERSITY OF MINNESOTA HOSPITAL

Case	Diagnosis
1	Bilateral vesicoureteral reflux, chronic cystitis and pyelonephritis
2	Hydrocephalus and meningomyelocele
3	Bladder outlet obstruction with bilateral vesicoureteral reflux, hydroureter, and hydronephrosis
4	Encephalopathy–cause unknown
5	Congenital scoliosis
6	Congenital urethral stricture
7	Congenital mitral stenosis
8	Nephrotic syndrome secondary to Henoch-Schoenlein syndrome
9	Myasthenia gravis, postthymectomy (no thymoma)
10	Penile hypospadias
11	Contractures of burn scar
12	Congenital scoliosis
13	Fractured humerus
14	Interventricular septal defect
15	Tetralogy of Fallot
16	Scoliosis
17	Postrenal transplantation

TABLE 2

RELATIVES FOR WHICH INFORMATION WAS OBTAINED

Relatives	Total Number Relatives of Probands	Total Number Relatives of Controls
Parents	48	50
Siblings	61	76
Maternal aunts and uncles	121	88
Paternal aunts and uncles	61	116
Cousins	358	444
Grandparents	94	100
Grandparents' siblings	531	466
Total	1,274	1,340

Results

A total of 1,274 relatives of 24 leukemia patients and 1,340 relatives of 25 controls compose the basis of this report. The average number of relatives in each family was 53.1 for the leukemic families and 53.6 for the control families. The largest single category of relatives was grandparents' siblings (TABLE 2), which accounted for almost 40 percent of all relatives.

Present age of living relatives and age at death of dead relatives is shown in TABLE 3. There were 217 deaths among leukemic relatives (17 percent) and 204 deaths among control relatives (15.2 percent). No significant difference between the proportion of relatives who were dead in leukemic and control groups was found. As shown in TABLE 4, twenty-nine (13.4 percent) relatives of leukemic children died of cancer, whereas 23 (11.3 percent) deaths in the relatives of controls were due to cancer ($p > .05$).

The number of cancer deaths expected in both groups of relatives was calculated according to the following formula:

$$\text{Expected number of deaths over a five-year interval} = D\left[5\left(\frac{A}{2} + \frac{B}{2} + C\right)\right]$$

where A = number of relatives dead during the given interval, B = number of relatives living in the given interval, C = number of relatives living through the given interval, and D = age specific death rate for the five-year interval. Thirty-seven cancer deaths were expected among the relatives of the patients with leukemia, whereas only 29 were found (TABLE 5). Thirty-five cancer deaths were expected among the relatives of controls, whereas 23 were found.

TABLE 3
AGE DISTRIBUTION OF RELATIVES

Age in Years	Relatives of Probands		Relatives of Controls	
	Living	Dead	Living	Dead
0–4	125	27	107	14
5–9	137	2	148	10
10–14	93	3	121	3
15–19	51	8	78	4
20–24	29	5	56	5
25–29	48	8	40	5
30–34	48	4	45	4
35–39	44	7	40	3
40–44	40	10	76	9
45–49	40	7	57	12
50–54	48	8	63	8
55–59	56	13	54	8
60–64	62	21	62	12
65–69	59	17	46	12
70–74	45	13	44	11
75–79	31	17	23	15
80–84	10	9	11	14
85 and over	5	4	6	7
Unknown	86	34	59	48
Total	1,057	217	1,136	204

TABLE 4

RELATIVES REPORTED TO HAVE DIED OF CANCER AND LEUKEMIA

	Probands				Controls			
Relatives	Total	Dead	Cancer Deaths*	Leukemia Deaths	Total	Dead	Cancer Deaths*	Leukemia Deaths
Parents	48				50	1	1	
Siblings	61	1			76	4		
Aunts and uncles	182	13	1		204	18	3	
Cousins	358	7			444	2		
Grandparents	94	23	7		100	31	7	1
Grandparents' siblings	531	173	21	2	466	148	12	
Total	1,274	217	29	2	1,340	204	23	1

* Includes leukemia.

TABLE 5

NUMBER OF CANCER DEATHS FOUND COMPARED WITH NUMBER EXPECTED

	Relatives of Probands Cancer Deaths		Relatives of Controls Cancer Deaths	
Relatives	Found	Expected	Found	Expected
Parents			1	
Siblings				
Aunts and uncles	1		3	
Cousins				
Grandparents	7	5.8	7	7.6
Grandparents' siblings	21	29.1	12	26.3
All relatives	29	37.3	23	35.7

TABLE 6

CANCERS IN LIVING AND DEAD RELATIVES

	Patients	Controls
Breast	2	5
Female genital	5	1
Colon	2	2
Stomach	6	5
Lung	6	3
Unknown	5	4
Prostate	2	1
Skin	2	3
Oral	1	1
Bladder		1
Lymphoma	1	
Hodgkin's disease		2
Leukemia	2	1
CNS		2
Bone	1	
Pancreas	1	1
Liver	1	
Total	37	32

There were some differences in the types of cancer reported in the leukemia and control groups (TABLE 6); however, the number of cases involved is too small to allow any generalizations. Two cases of leukemia were found in 1,274 relatives of leukemics compared with one case of leukemia in 1,340 relatives of controls. All three cases were in grandparents or grandparents' siblings.

Cancer deaths were more common in the siblings of grandparents of leukemic patients (21, 12.1 percent) than of controls (12, 8.1 percent). However, the 21 cancer deaths reported in the siblings of grandparents of leukemic patients is still less than the 29 cases expected in this group (TABLE 5).

We found no difference between the leukemic and control groups in the proportion of living relatives who were known to have cancer (TABLE 7). When all cancers known to have occurred in all relatives (living and dead) were considered (TABLE 8), there were 37 cancers in 1,274 relatives of leukemia patients as opposed to 32 cancers in 1,340 relatives of controls, which again does not represent a significant difference.

TABLE 7

LIVING RELATIVES REPORTED TO HAVE CANCER

	Probands		Controls	
Relatives	Total Living	Living with Cancer	Total Living	Living with Cancer
Parents	48		49	
Siblings	60		72	
Aunts and uncles	169		186	
Cousins	351		442	
Grandparents	71	4	69	7
Grandparents' siblings	358	4	318	2
Total	1,057	8	1,136	9

TABLE 8

TOTAL NUMBER OF CANCERS REPORTED IN ALL RELATIVES

	Probands		Controls	
Relatives	Total	All Cancers	Total	All Cancers
Parents	48		50	1
Siblings	61		76	
Aunts and uncles	182	1	204	3
Cousins	358		444	
Grandparents	94	11	100	14
Grandparents' siblings	531	25	466	14
Total	1,274	37	1,340	32

Discussion

In the present study the cancer history of 1,274 relatives of 24 children with leukemia was compared with that of 1,340 relatives of 25 controls. We did not find the number of cases of either leukemia or cancer in the patients' relatives to be more than in the controls' relatives or more than expected in the population studied.

If there is an increased incidence of malignant disease in the relatives of children with leukemia, it is a small one. Studies which intend to reveal any difference must be carefully designed so that each type of leukemia is individually analyzed and age ranges are well-defined and well-separated. Because of the length of survival periods and the comparatively low incidence of leukemia in any one area, Miller[11] has estimated that 1,000 siblings of leukemic children must be studied before any excessive occurrence of cancer could be demonstrated in an investigation of this type.

Results from various studies indicate that the genetic influence in leukemia is weak indeed (TABLE 9). The lack of consanguinity in this relatively rare condition is evidence against a recessive gene mechanism. Rare instances of familial occurrence of leukemia[18–22] may indicate that this is a dominant characteristic with extremely low penetrance.

The strongest evidence to date for a genetic influence in leukemia is the concordance ratio of 1:4 for like-sex (presumably monozygotic) twins[1] opposed to the negligible concordance for dizygotic twins. And, the increased incidence of leukemia in Down's and other chromosomal syndromes interests us. Nevertheless, the failure of the overwhelming majority of such affected individuals to manifest leukemia implies important nongenetic determinants.

Yet, the excess risk of leukemia in these specific population groups provokes

TABLE 9

FAMILIAL OCCURRENCE OF LEUKEMIA

Author	Parent's Consanguinity	Number of Leukemic Children	Total Number of Children in Family
Steinberg (1960)	First cousins	3	7
	Second cousins	4	12
Stewart (1961)	Maternal grandparents, first cousins	2	2
	None	2	4
	None	2	5
	None	2	3
Anderson (1951)	None	5	8
Campbell (1962)	None	2	6
Baikie (1961)	None	2	4
Gunz (1966)	None	4	9
Videbaek (1958)	None	2	unknown
Miller (1963)	None	2	4
	None	2	5
	None	2	4
	None	2	7
	None	2*	4

* Identical twins.

certain questions. What, if not genetic, are the determinants of the leukemic process? Future extensive serial analyses of the leukemic child's chromosomal, immunological, and biochemical changes over an extended period should provide fundamental clues. Possible secondary environmental factors, such as the severity of childhood illnesses, immunizations, or dietary patterns predisposing to leukemia should also be ascertained in future studies.

References

1. MacMahon, B. & M. A. Levy. 1964. Prenatal origin of childhood leukemia: Evidence from twins. New Eng. J. Med. **270**: 1082–1085.
2. Anderson, R. C. & H. W. Hermann. 1955. Leukemia in twin children. J.A.M.A. **158**: 652–654.
3. Pearson, H. A., F .W. Grello & T. E. Cone, Jr. 1963. Leukemia in identical twins. New Eng. J. Med. **268**: 1151–1156.
4. Krivit, W. & R. A. Good. 1957. Simultaneous occurrence of mongolism and leukemia: Report of a nationwide survey. Amer. J. Dis. Child. **94**: 289–293.
5. Stewart, A., J. Webb & D. Hewitt. 1958. A survey of childhood malignancies. Brit. Med. J. **1**(5086): 1495–1508.
6. Stewart, A. 1961. Aetiology of childhood malignancies: Congenitally determined leukemias. Brit. Med. J. **1**(5224): 452–460.
7. Peterson, R. D. A., M. D. Cooper & R. A. Good. 1965. Disorders of thymus. Prog. in Medical Genetics **4**: 1–31.
8. ten Bensel, R. W., E. M. Stadlan & W. Krivit. 1966. The development of malignancy in the course of the Aldrich syndrome. J. Pediat. **68**: 761–767.
9. German, J., R. Archibald & D. Bloom. 1965. Chromosomal breakage in a rare and probably genetically determined syndrome of man. Science **148**: 506–507.
10. Miller, R. W. 1964. Radiation, chromosomes, and viruses in the etiology of leukemia: Evidence from epidemiologic research. New Eng. J. Med. **271**: 30–36.
11. Miller, R. W. 1966. Relation between cancer and congenital defects in man. New Eng. J. Med. **275**: 87–93.
12. Videbaek, A. 1947. Heredity in Human Leukemia and Its Relation to Cancer. Opera ex Domo Biologiae Hereditariae Humanae. Universitatis Hafniensis. Copenhagen, Denmark.
13. Videbaek, A. 1958. Familial leukemia. Acta Path. Microbiol. Scand. **44**: 372–377.
14. Busk, T. 1948. Some observations on heredity in breast cancer and leukemia. Ann. Eugen. **14**: 213–229.
15. Busk, T. 1954. Genetical studies in leukemia. *In* Proceedings of the Second National Cancer Conference. 1952. Vol. **2**: 1087–1101. American Cancer Society. New York, N. Y.
16. Steinberg, A. G. 1960. The genetics of acute leukemia in children. Cancer **13**: 985–999.
17. Age-Adjusted and Age-Specific Death Rates for Malignant Neoplasms. 1960. Washington, D. C. Government Printing Office. 1963. (U. S. Public Health Service Publication no. 1113).
18. Anderson, R. C. 1951. Familial leukemia: A report of leukemia in five siblings, with a brief review of the genetic aspects of this disease. Amer. J. Dis. Child. **81**: 313–322.
19. Campbell, W. A. B., A. L. Macafee & W. G. Wade. 1962. Familial neonatal leukemia. Arch. Dis. Childhood **37**: 93–98.
20. Baikie, A. G., W. M. Court-Brown, K. E. Buckton & D. G. Harnden. 1961. Two cases of leukemia and a case of sex-chromosome abnormality in the same sibship. Lancet **ii**: 1003–1004.
21. Miller, R. W. 1963. Down's syndrome (mongolism), other congenital malformations and cancers among the sibs of leukemic children. New Eng. J. Med. **268**: 393–401.
22. Gunz, F. W., P. H. Fitzgerald, P. E. Crossen, I. S. Mackenzie, C. P. Powles & G. R. Jensen. 1966. Multiple cases of leukemia in a sibship. Blood **27**: 482–489.

FAMILIAL AGGREGATES OF THE 21-TRISOMY SYNDROME*

Hans Zellweger
Department of Pediatrics, University of Iowa
Iowa City, Iowa

Mongolism is usually a sporadic event afflicting not more than one individual in a family or kindred. This time-honored experience was one of the few reassuring statements the counselling physician of yore could make when confronted by parents of a mongoloid child. Familial occurrence of mongolism was (and still is) considered as being exceptional. Nevertheless, already some ten years ago, Penrose[1] collected 250 instances of familial mongolism, some fraternal, some nonfraternal cases. The cause of mongolism in general and of familial mongolism in particular remained a widely disputed, but essentially unknown topic until a few years ago, when chromosomal aneuploidy was found to produce disease in man. Mongolism or Down's syndrome arises when a supernumerary chromosome, or major parts of it, is present in all, or at least in a sizeable number of cells. Three main groups of karyotypic aberrations leading to mongolism can be distinguished: (1) trisomy 21 or G_m which is found in over 90 percent of all cases of mongolism; (2) partial trisomy 21, also called translocation or interchange mongolism; and (3) chromosomal mosaicism with a large clone of 21-trisomic cells (mosaic mongolism). Interchange and mosaic mongolism account for less than ten percent of the cases of mongolism. Familial mongolism has been found in association with trisomy 21 and partial trisomy 21. Familial mosaic mongolism has not been described yet, although chromosomal mosaicism is known to occur in rare instances as a familial trait.

Familial Trisomy 21

Trisomy 21 in Twins

Monozygotic twins are concordant with respect to mongolism; exceptions to this rule are rare.[2] Dizygotic twins are, in most instances discordant, one twin only being mongoloid (Table 1). This was already known in the precytogenetic era and was one of the reasons which led Waardenburg[3] to believe that mongolism could be caused by a chromosomal aberration: Discordance of dizygotic twins speaks against environmental factors causing mongolism, whereas the discrepancy between concordance in monozygotic and persistent discordance in dizygotic twins rules out transmission of the trait by a mutant gene.

Mongolism in both monozygotic twins represents a unique category of familial mongolism, since, obviously, only one aneuploid gamete is involved.

Trisomy 21 in Offspring of Individuals with 21-Trisomic Germ Cells

It is logical to assume that the primitive germ cells of trisomy-21 mongoloids are 21-trisomic as well. Similarly, normal individuals with chromosomal mosaicism and a 21-trisomic clone may have the same aneuploid germ cells. Meiosis of a 21-trisomic germ cell leads to gametes with either one or two chromosomes 21. A 21-trisomic spermatogonium divides into two euploid and two aneuploid

* This study was supported by USPHS grants nos. 3R01 HD01820 06S1 and 3R01 HD01822 06S1.

TABLE 1

MONGOLISM AND TWINS

Type of Offspring	One Twin Mongoloid	Both Twins Mongoloid
Dizygotic Twins	155 (sets)	4 (sets)
Monozygotic Twins	4 (sets)	22 (sets)

sperms, whereas an ovum resulting from meiosis of a 21-trisomic ovogonium has presumably an equal chance to be either euploid or aneuploid (FIGURE 1). Fertilization of the former leads to a normal zygote, whereas fertilization of the latter results in a mongoloid offspring. It may be expected, therefore, that mongoloids and individuals with chromosomal mosaicism and a 21-trisomic clone may produce one or even several mongoloid offspring. In reality, however, it is questionable whether mongoloid males are able to reproduce, their fertility being at least reduced, if not completely abolished. We do not know of any mongoloid male who has fathered a child. On the other hand, 13 mongoloid females have been reported as having borne 16 children.[4] Five of the children were mongoloid, eleven were normal. The ratio, five mongoloid to 11 normal offspring, deviates somewhat from the expected one to one ratio and calls for an explanation. Some of these mongoloid women experienced abortions in addition to their full term pregnancies. Recent reports have disclosed that aneuploid zygotes run a fairly high risk of being eliminated during early pregnancy.[5] There is presumptive evidence that only one out of three zygotes with trisomy 21 reaches the end of gestation. The relatively high number of normal offspring of mongoloid mothers may be explained by the premature elimination of some of the aneuploid zygotes. Nevertheless, it can be stated that mongoloid females carry a risk of at least 25 percent of having a mongoloid offspring. Such a high risk calls for effective birth control. Sterilization of mongoloid girls may be advisable.

A few reports have appeared describing mongoloid offspring of phenotypically normal individuals with chromosomal mosaicism and a 21-trisomic clone. Fer-

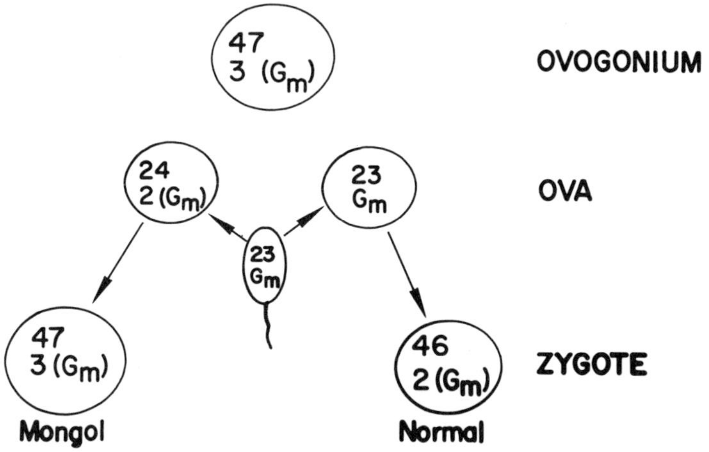

FIGURE 1. Maternal mongolism or mosaicism as a cause of familial trisomy 21.

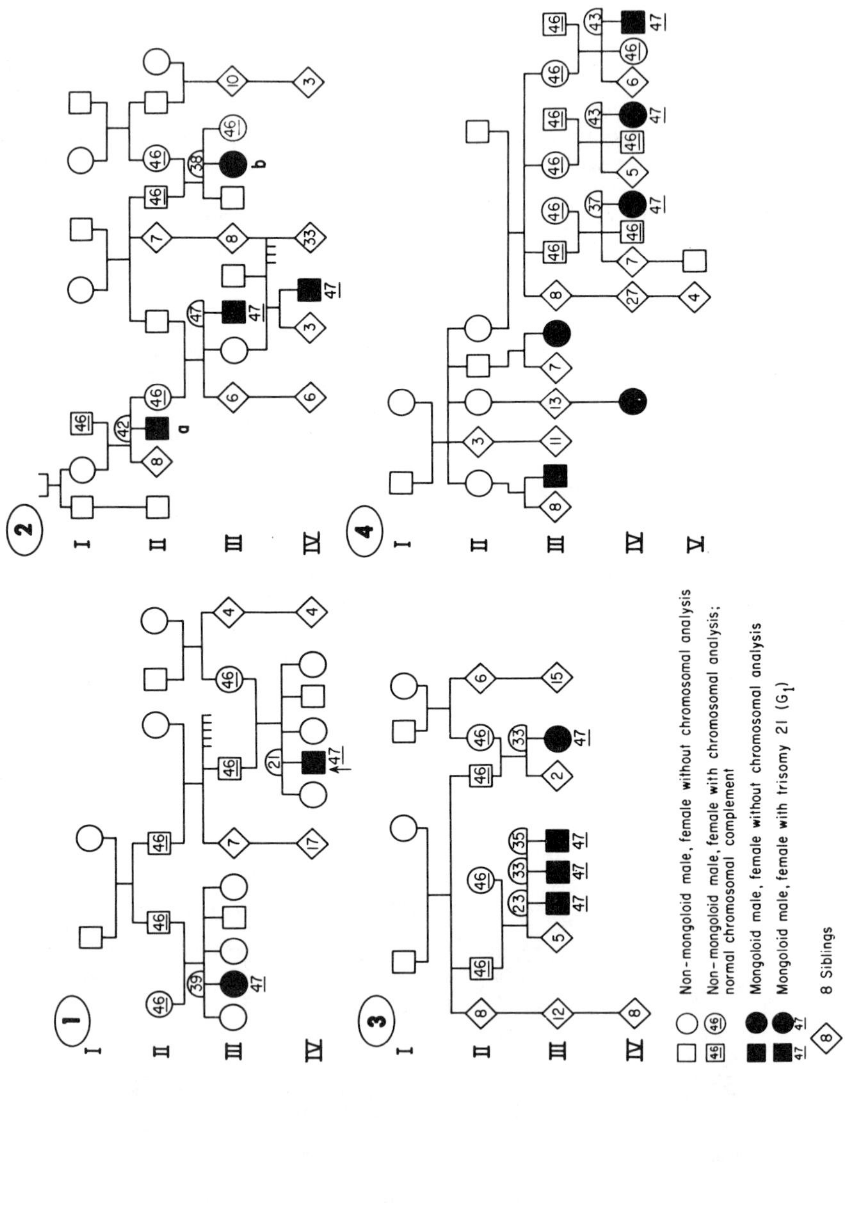
Non-mongoloid male, female without chromosomal analysis
Non-mongoloid male, female with chromosomal analysis; normal chromosomal complement
Mongoloid male, female without chromosomal analysis
Mongoloid male, female with trisomy 21 (G1)
8 Siblings

FIGURE 2.

rier[6] collected four cases from the literature and added two personal observations. Five of the mosaic parents were females, one was a male. We studied, in our laboratory, another mosaic male, who was the father of a mongoloid child.[7] More than one mongoloid child was found in only one of these seven families. Smith *et al.*[8] reported a mosaic mother having two mongoloid children. The same mother has, since then, borne a third mongoloid child.[9] Only a few of the examined white blood cells of this woman were trisomic, most of them were euploid. In spite of that, all her children were mongoloid, i.e., they all were the products of fertilization of aneuploid ova. This, then, would indicate that the ratio of euploid to aneuploid cells in their blood precludes predicting for mosaic individuals, how great is their risk of having aneuploid offspring. At present it is only possible to conclude that a mosaic parent has a high risk of having more than one mongoloid child. This ought to be kept in mind when giving eugenic advice to a mosaic parent.

Trisomy 21 in Siblings and Parents with Normal Karyotypes

A number of instances has been reported in which parents with a normal complement of 46 normal chromosomes had more than one offspring with trisomy 21. We have (excluding monozygotic twins) studied ten such families in our laboratory.[10] Eight sibships had two, and two sibships had three, 21-trisomic siblings; all nonmongoloid individuals of these families who were karyotyped, notably the parents, had a normal chromosomal complement. The cause of fraternal trisomy 21 is presently not known. It has been conjectured that it is caused by a break in a parental chromosome 21, with inversion of the fragment, and reinsertion of it on the same chromosome.[11] Although the light microscopic appearance of this chromosome does not differ from the other chromosome 21, it may no longer act as a homologue. Thus synapsis during the early phases of meiosis may no longer occur, the two chromosomes 21 may segregate independently from each other and may migrate to the same daughter cell, thus giving origin to a 21-disomic gamete. Whether or not this explanation accounts for all instances of fraternal trisomy remains an open question, as is illustrated by the following observation: We studied the kindred of two brothers, both of whom had mongoloid children (FIGURE 2, Pedigree 3). One had three children with trisomy 21, the other, one child with trisomy 21. All nonmongoloid individuals of this kindred who were tested had a normal chromosomal complement. It would be difficult to explain the familial mongolism in this kindred by breakage and inversion of a chromosome 21 unless its occurrence as a familial trait present in several members is presumed.

FIGURE 2. Four pedigrees of familial trisomy 21.

Pedigree 1: Two cases of trisomy 21 in a mongoloid proband and his mongoloid paternal great-uncle (presumptive random association.).

Pedigree 2: Four cases of mongolism (two trisomies 21 and two karyotypically unanalyzed mongoloids) in a wider kindred. Notice that mongoloid (a) and mongoloid (b) are not related to each other. The occurrence of three mongoloids is probably significant, the occurrence of the fourth one is a coincidental finding.

Pedigree 3: Four cases of familial and fraternal trisomy 21.

Pedigree 4: Six cases of mongolism in a wider kindred.

Mongoloids are indicated with black squares and black circles. The number 47 under the black symbol indicates trisomy 21. The white squares and circles indicate nonmongoloid individuals. The number 46 indicates that a normal chromosomal complement was found.

The number in the semicircles above the symbol of the mongoloid patients indicates the age of the mother at the time the respective child was born.

Familial, or rather fraternal, trisomy 21 cannot be predicted. It is presently impossible to predict which karyotypically normal parents of a 21-trisomic child run an increased risk of having a second child with trisomy 21. It is generally agreed that parents of a 21-trisomic child run a risk of having another mongoloid child which is several times higher than that of parents of the same age who do not have a mongoloid child. However, the increase of the risk is not of such magnitude that it should enter as a decisive factor in the family planning. If, however, two siblings are 21-trisomic, the risk of a subsequent child being again 21-trisomic is probably considerable.

Familial Trisomy 21 Occurring in Different Sibships of a Kindred

The overall incidence of trisomy 21 is about one in 600 live births. The probability of two cases of trisomy 21 occurring in aggregates of 50–100 individuals varies between 0.01 and 0.02. It is, therefore, quite possible to find, sometimes, two cases of mongolism in a wider kindred of about 50–100 relatives as a mere consequence of random association. Thus, two cases of mongolism among distant relatives may not be causally related (FIGURE 2, Pedigree 1 and 2). Hanhart[12] considers even mongolism in two first cousins as coincidental.

Since trisomy 21 represents the most frequent form of mongolism, random association of two cases of trisomy 21 will be found more frequently than random association of trisomy 21 with one of the other rarer karyotypic forms of mongolism. Nevertheless, in rare instances, trisomy 21 and translocation mongolism or mosaic mongolism may occur in the same family as shown by two examples studied in our laboratory (FIGURE 3).

In addition to these coincidental instances of familial trisomy 21, kindreds with a more than merely coincidental agglomeration of cases of trisomy 21 have been observed. FIGURE 2, Pedigree 4, represents a family where six cases of mongolism occurred, each in another sibship, yet all closely related to each other (first and second cousins). A familial tendency to nondisjunction of the chromosome pair 21 has to be assumed to understand such observations. Its etiopathogenesis and pattern of transmission is unknown. Minor chromosomal aberrations, such as increased satellite association or small structural alterations of a chromosome, could predispose to nondisjunction. This, however, is at the present time mere speculation and further extensive research is needed to determine the significance of such minor aberrations for the causation of familial nondisjunction.

FAMILIAL INTERCHANGE MONGOLISM (PARTIAL TRISOMY 21)

About a year after trisomy 21 was discovered as a cause of mongolism, a case of sporadic translocation or interchange mongolism with 46 chromosomal elements, including an interchange between two acrocentric chromosomes, was described by Polani *et al.*[13] Shortly thereafter, the first report of familial interchange mongolism appeared: three cases of interchange mongolism and several normal family members with a balanced D/G interchange were described.[14] Since then, numerous cases of balanced interchange and interchange mongolism have been described. They were discussed in a recent review article.[4]

Chromosomal interchange occurs predominantly between acrocentric chromosomes of the groups D and G, rarely between a G chromosome and a nonacrocentric chromosome. A schematic representation of the different interchanges involving a supernumerary chromosome 21 is given in FIGURE 4. The extra

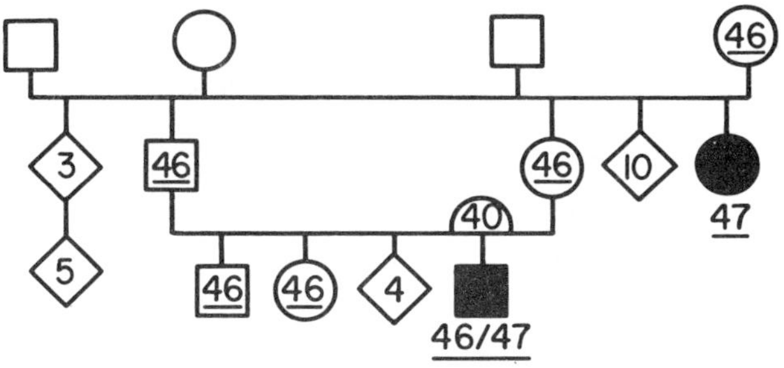

Trisomy 21 and Mosaic Mongolism

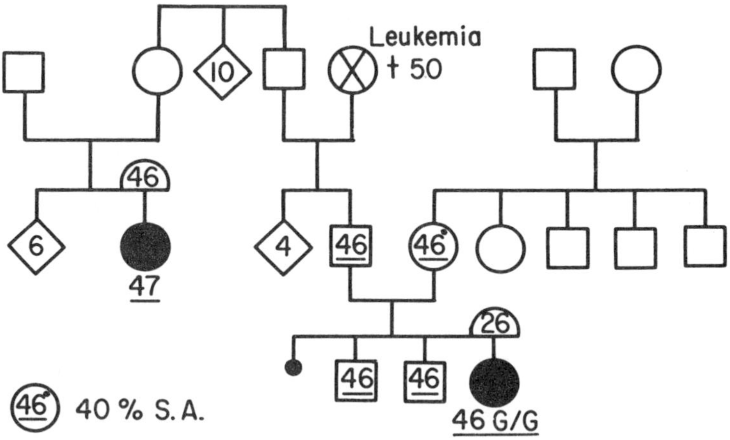

Trisomy 21 and Interchange Mongolism

FIGURE 3. Familial mongolism with two karyotypically different mongoloids in each family.

chromosome 21, or at least major parts of it, can interchange with parts of a large acrocentric chromosome (FIGURE 4, 1), with another chromosome 21 (FIGURE 4, 2), or with a chromosome 22 (FIGURE 4, 3). In rare instances the interchanged chromosome 21 may be hidden in one of the large chromosomes (FIGURE 4, 6). Interchange mongolism is relatively more frequent in offspring of younger mothers. Polani *et al.*[15] found a partial trisomy 21 (interchange) in 8.7 percent of 630 mongoloids borne of mothers below the age of 30 years and only in 1.3 percent of 462 mongoloids borne of mothers above the age of 30 years. Interchange mongolism is often sporadic, yet in about 10 percent of the G/G interchanges and 50 percent of the D/G interchanges, a parent with the respective interchange in balanced form is found. Individuals with a balanced D/G or G/G interchange, respectively, are phenotypically normal. They run an increased risk of having mongoloid offspring because their germ cells have a special segregation pattern during meiosis.

There is good evidence to assume that the three unpaired chromosomal elements, namely the single chromosomes 15 and 21 and the interchanged 15/21 structure, segregate independently from each other and may associate in various combinations forming karyotypically different gametes (TABLE 2). Only three of them, after fertilization with a normal gamete of the other sex, lead to viable zygotes with a normal karyotype, a balanced interchange, or an interchange trisomy.

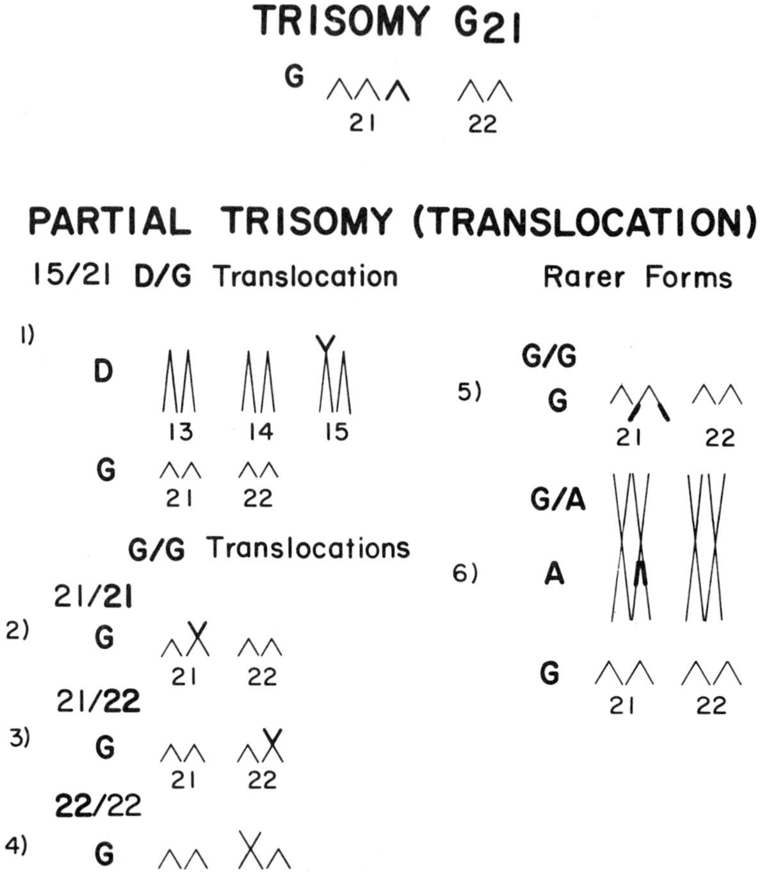

FIGURE 4. Schematic drawing of different types of interchange (translocation) mongolism. The extra chromosome 21 is indicated by the heavy line.

1. 15/21 interchange mongolism.
2. 21/21 interchange mongolism.
3. 21/22 interchange mongolism.
4. 22/22 interchange (nonmongoloid partial trisomy G).
5. Unusual 21/22 interchange (tandem translocation). Very few such cases have been observed.[4,17]
6. Interchange between a 21 chromosome and a larger chromosome. This interchange is microscopically unrecognizable.

TABLE 2

GAMETES AND ZYGOTES IN MATERNAL BALANCED 15/21 INTERCHANGE

Possible Gametes	Possible Zygotes	
1. A,* 15, 21, 15/21	Double partial trisomy 15 & 21	Not yet observed
2. A, 15, 15/21	Partial trisomy 15	Not yet observed
3. A, 15/21, 21	Partial trisomy 21	Interchange mongolism
4. A, 15, 21	Normal karyotype	Normal phenotype
5. A, 15/21	Balanced interchange 15/21	Normal phenotype
6. A, 15	Monosomy 21	Not yet observed (Not viable)
7. A, 21	Monosomy 15	Not yet observed (Not viable)
8. A, –	Double monosomy 15 & 21	Not yet observed (Not viable)

* A = chromosomes 1–14, 16–20, 22, X.
Complete karyotype = A + chromosomes 15, 21, 15/21.

If the mother carries the balanced D/G interchange, the risk of a mongoloid offspring (interchange trisomy) is in the neighborhood of 20 percent. It is less than 20 percent if the father carries the balanced interchange. The same risk figures apply presumably for 21/22 interchanges, yet not for balanced 21/21 interchanges. In the latter case a somewhat different pattern of meiosis is present: here only two gametic karyotypes are possible, one with the 21/21 interchange, and the other without it and with no 21 chromosome at all. Fertilization of the former gamete leads to partial trisomy 21 and interchange mongolism, whereas fertilization of the latter leads to a 21-monosomic zygote, which is not viable. All living offspring of a parent with a balanced 21/21 interchange will be mongoloid, as illustrated by a family[16] where the father had a balanced G/G interchange and whose five children were mongoloid.

Balanced G/G, i.e., 21/22, and D/G interchanges, can be transmitted through several generations. Hence, the respective interchange mongolism can be found in individuals of several sibships and generations of a wider kindred. Balanced 21/21 interchange usually represents a new mutation, because this type of interchange in its balanced form can not be transmitted from generation to generation.

SUMMARY

Familial aggregation of trisomy 21 or partial trisomy 21, respectively, is rare. More than one case of trisomy 21 may occur in the same sibship or in other close or distant relatives. In larger kindreds, familial aggregates of two or three mongoloids may be coincidental, well within the normal expectation for a trait found in one of 600 live births. For other instances of familial trisomy 21, particularly if occurring in siblings or other close relatives, a familial tendency to nondisjunction has to be assumed. Possible causes of such familial tendencies are discussed.

Special karyotypes or configurations comprising familial trisomy-21 mongolism are trisomy 21 in both monozygotic twins and trisomy 21 in offspring of a

21-trisomic woman or of a mosaic parent with a 21-trisomic clone. A parental chromosomal interchange involving a chromosome 21 represents another cause of familial mongolism. In such instances a parent has to be the carrier of the interchange in balanced form.

References

1. Penrose, L. S. 1954. Observations on the aetiology of mongolism. Lancet **ii:** 505.
2. de Wolff, E., K. Schaerer & J. Lejeune. 1962. Contribution á l'étude des jumeaux mongoliens; un cas de monozygotisme hétérocaryote. Helv. Paediat. Acta **17:** 301.
3. Waardenburg, P. J. 1932. Das menschliche Auge und Seine Erbanlagen. Nijhoff, The Hague, Netherlands
4. Zellweger, H. 1966. Familial chromosomal aberrations, Parts I & II. Ann. Paediat. **206:** 317 & 381.
5. Polani, P. E. 1966. Chromosome anomalies and abortions. Develop. Med. Child. Neurol. **8:** 67.
6. Ferrier, S. 1964. Enfant Mongolien–Parent Mosaique. Thése. Genéva, Switzerland.
7. Zellweger, H. Unpublished data.
8. Smith, D. W., E. M. Therman, K. A. Patau & S. L. Inhorn. 1962. Mosaicism in mother of two mongoloids. Amer. J. Dis. Child. **104:** 534.
9. Smith, D. W. Personal communication.
10. Zellweger, H. 1964. Familial mongolism–History and present status. Clin. Pediat. **3:** 291.
11. Zellweger, H. 1965. Mongolismus–Down's Syndrom. Ergebn. Inn. Med. Kinderheilk. **22:** 268.
12. Hanhart, E. 1960. 800 Faelle von Mongoloidismus in konstitutioneller Betrachtung. Arch. Klaus. Stift. Vererbungsforsch **35:** 1.
13. Polani, P. E., J. Briggs, A. Ford, C. Clarke & J. Berg. 1960. A mongol girl with 46 chromosomes. Lancet **i:** 721.
14. Penrose, L. S., J. R. Ellis & J. D. A. Delhanty. 1960. Chromosomal translocation in mongolism and normal relatives. Lancet **ii:** 409.
15. Polani, P. E., J. L. Hamerton, F. Giannelli & C. O. Carter. 1965. Cytogenetics of Down's Syndrome (Mongolism) III. Frequency of interchange trisomies and mutation rate of chromosome interchanges. Cytogenetics (Basel) **4:** 193.
16. Dallaire, L. & F. C. Fraser. 1964. Two unusual cases of familial mongolism. Canad. J. Genet. Cytol. **6:** 540.
17. Soudek, D., R. Laxova & R. Adamek. 1966. Development of translocation 21/22. Lancet **ii:** 536.

HEREDITY AND CARCINOMA

H. T. Lynch,* D. E. Anderson, and A. J. Krush

The University of Texas M. D. Anderson Hospital and Tumor Institute Texas Medical Center, Houston, Tex.

and

A. L. Larsen

The University of Nebraska College of Medicine Omaha, Neb.

Introduction

The concept of a hereditary etiology of malignancy in man has long been a controversial idea in both medicine and genetics. Differences of opinion stem not only from the complexity of the cancer problem itself, but also from the complicated nature of man with his long generation-interval, small number of progeny, marriage customs, natural history of disease, and psychological features, all of which make him an exceedingly poor subject for genetic studies. No small wonder, therefore, that pioneering studies in cancer genetics were initially concentrated on mice,[1-6] birds,[7,8] rabbits,[9,10] cattle,[11,12] and monkeys[13] (TABLE 1).

The systematic study of cancer genetics in man is a relatively recent discipline. Historical reviews on the subject have been compiled by Clemmesen,[14] Jacobsen,[15] Woolf,[16] and Anderson and associates.[17] As early as the beginning of the nineteenth century and probably even earlier, physicians were speculating upon a hereditary etiology for human malignancies.[18] The question, "Is cancer hereditary?" was sent to all English physicians in 1802, but with no apparent results. Bashford[19] in 1908 was one of the first investigators to emphasize the critical role of cultural, geographical, environmental, and ethnic factors in human cancer (TABLE 2). Indeed, he stressed these factors to the extent of detracting from the importance of inherited factors. He believed that more valid information would result from the study of acquired factors. Waaler[20] was one of the first investigators to utilize controls (spouses and their relatives) and mortality statistics in tabulating results from a large population of cancer patients. He also emphasized the importance of endogenous as well as exogenous factors in carcinogenesis. Other pioneering investigators in the cancer field, including Martynova,[21] Wassink,[22] Macklin,[23,24] Penrose,[25] Oliver,[26] Woolf,[16] Videbaek,[27] Busk,[28] Cockayne,[29] Clemmesen,[14] Lockhart-Mummery,[30] Dukes,[31] Griffith and Sorsby,[32] and Gardner,[33] conducted controlled studies in search of a hereditary etiology for malignancies. Emphasis in these studies was primarily on the inheritance of cancer of *specific sites,* most frequently, cancer of the breast.

The first investigation of cancer of *multiple sites* in families ("cancer families") with emphasis on careful pathological correlation was that of Warthin in 1913.[34] He reinvestigated one family (Family G) in 1925.[35] Later this family was updated by his colleagues, Hauser and Weller, in 1936.[36]

This report presents our experience with six "cancer families." Details concerning these families will be presented to serve as prototypes for our concept of a hereditary multiple-cancer syndrome.

* Present address: Department of Preventive Medicine, The Creighton University School of Medicine, Omaha, Neb.

TABLE 1

HISTORY OF CANCER GENETICS IN ANIMALS

Investigator	Year	Contribution
Slye, M.[3]	1914	Cancer in mice
Heston, W. E.[5,6]	1942	Cancer in mice
Bittner, J. J.[1]	1944	Cancer in mice
Rous, P.[7]	1911	Cancer in birds
Sanarelli, G.[9]	1898	Cancer in rabbits
Shope, R. E.[10]	1933	Cancer in rabbits
Bevan, E. W.[12]	1925	Cancer in cattle

TABLE 2

HISTORY OF CANCER GENETICS IN MAN

Investigator	Year	Contribution
Bashford, E. F.[19]	1908	Emphasis on cultural, geographic, environmental, ethnic factors.
Waaler, G. H. M.[20]	1931	Use of controls (spouses) and mortality statistics.
Wassink, W. F.[22]	1935	*Cancer of specific sites*: Breast
Penrose, L. S. *et al.*.[25]	1948	Breast
Macklin, M. T.[23]	1959	Breast
Woolf, C. M.[16]	1955	Stomach
Macklin, M. T.[24]	1960	Stomach
Lockhart-Mummery, P.[30]	1925	Colon (Polyposis coli)
Dukes, C. E.[31]	1930	Colon (Polyposis coli)
Cockayne, E. A.[29]	1933	Xeroderma pigmentosum
Griffith, A. D. & A. Sorsby[32]	1944	Retinoblastoma
Virchow, R.[45]	1947	Neurofibromatosis
Gardner, E.J.[33]	1951	"Gardner's syndrome"
Straith, F. E.[46]	1939	Nevoid basal cell carcinoma syndrome
Binkley, G. W. & H. H. Johnson, Jr.[47]	1951	Nevoid basal cell carcinoma syndrome
Warthin, A. S.[34]	1913	Cancer in families

Material and Methods

Protocol in the study of "cancer families" has been published elsewhere.[37] Major criteria for a "cancer family" consist of the following: (1) a minimum of 25 percent of first-degree relatives of probands must show histological evidence of carcinoma; (2) these patients' lesions must involve multiple anatomic sites; (3) individuals in such families generally experience onset of malignancies at a relatively early age, usually significantly lower than that for the same malignancy in the general population; (4) several generations are frequently affected; (5) segregation ratios may be found; and (6) carcinoma of the endometrium, colon, and multiple primary malignancies are found more frequently in these families than in the general population.

Results

Family 1 consists of 198 individuals, of whom 43 have had malignant neoplasms. Among these affected individuals, ten had carcinoma of the colon and

13 had endometrial carcinoma. Eight individuals had multiple primary malignancies and four showed the combination of endometrial and colon carcinoma. Other anatomic sites were involved in 29 of the 43 affected individuals.

Family 2 consists of 31 individuals, of whom 18 have had malignant neoplasms. Nine individuals had carcinoma of the colon, five had endometrial carcinoma, and six had multiple primary malignant neoplasms. Of the latter, two had the combination of endometrial and colon carcinoma. Other anatomic sites were involved in ten of the 18 affected individuals.

Family 3 consists of 15 individuals, of whom eight have had malignant neoplasms. Four individuals had carcinoma of the colon and three had endometrial carcinoma. Out of two individuals who had multiple primary malignancies, one had the combination of endometrial and colon carcinoma. Other anatomic sites were involved in three of the eight affected individuals.

Family 4 consists of 14 individuals, of whom 12 have had malignant neoplasms. Nine individuals had carcinoma of the colon, one had endometrial carcinoma, and two individuals had multiple primary malignancies. Other anatomic sites were involved in two of the 12 affected individuals.

Family 5 consists of 391 individuals, of whom 74 have had malignant neoplasms. Thirty-five individuals had carcinoma of the colon, 21 had endometrial carcinoma, and ten had multiple primary malignancies .Of those with multiple primary tumors, four had the combination of endometrial and colon carcinoma. Other malignancies were involved in 21 of the 74 affected individuals.

Family 6 (FIGURE 1) consists of 35 individuals, of whom ten have had malig-

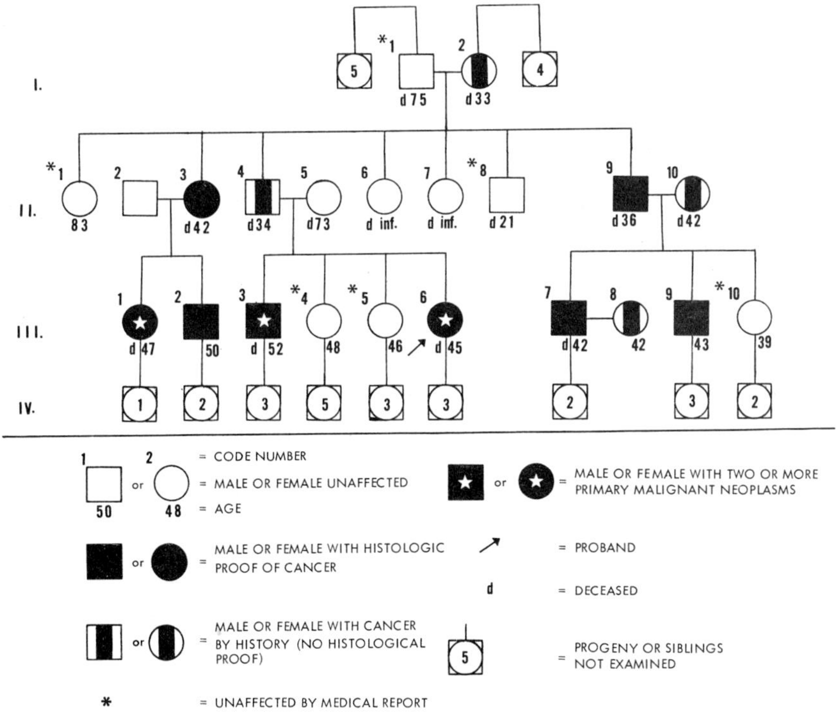

FIGURE 1. Pedigree of cancer family 6.

nant neoplasms. Eight individuals had carcinoma of the colon, two had endometrial carcinoma, and three individuals had multiple primary malignancies, two of whom had the combination of endometrial and colon carcinoma. Other anatomic sites were involved in three of the ten affected individuals. The following paragraphs detail the case history of the proband in Family 6, which is a prototype of a patient with the hereditary multiple-cancer syndrome.

This white female had been in good health until age 42, when she underwent a resection of the transverse colon for a tumor that proved histologically to be a malignant carcinoid. Six months later a diagnosis of adenocarcinoma of the endometrium was established. She underwent radium implantation and external radiation therapy, followed by panhysterectomy approximately two months later. About four months following the diagnosis of endometrial carcinoma, she underwent an anterior resection for a third primary malignancy, adenocarcinoma of the rectosigmoid.

This patient was a nonsmoker and used alcohol infrequently. There were no known unusual environmental exposures. She was gravida 4, para 3, and had experienced one miscarriage. The family history was striking for the presence of malignant neoplasms (TABLE 3 and FIGURE 1).

A physical examination during this latter hospitalization showed the patient to be normotensive. She was 5 feet 6 inches tall and weighed 120 pounds. There were cystic lesions of the breast, pectus excavatum, mild thoracic scoliosis, and a left inguinal mass that subsequently proved to be carcinoma of the rectosigmoid colon. The remainder of the physical examination was within normal limits.

An endocrine evaluation revealed normal thyroid and adrenal function; the latter evaluation included a normal response to metyrapone-suppression studies. A mammogram of the breast revealed bilateral fibrocystic disease.

The remainder of the laboratory work, including liver function studies and blood glucose levels, was within normal limits. The patient did well for several months after her last hospitalization but then began a downhill course and died at age 45. Autopsy revealed generalized carcinomatosis.

TABLE 4 summarizes the occurrence of endometrial carcinoma, carcinoma of the colon, and multiple primary malignant neoplasms in the "cancer families." An overall total of 18.7 percent multiple primary malignancies was found in these six families.

The average age of onset of endometrial carcinoma in the six "cancer families"

TABLE 3

REGISTRY OF MALIGNANT NEOPLASMS IN FAMILY 6

Pedigree No.	Age	Sex	Colon	Endometrium	Lip	Lung	Malignant-Carcinoid Tumor
I 2	d 33	F	33*	–	–	–	–
II 3	d 42	F	42†	–	–	–	–
II 4	d 34	M	34*	–	–	–	–
II 9	43	M	40†	–	–	–	–
III 1	d 47	F	44†	47†	–	–	–
III 2	50	M	48†, 49†	–	–	–	–
III 3	d 52	M	–	–	46†	52†	–
III 6	d 45	F	43†	42†	–	–	42†
III 7	d 42	M	40†	–	–	–	–
III 9	43	M	41†	–	–	–	–

* = malignancy by history.
† = malignancy histologically confirmed.

TABLE 4

REGISTRY OF MALIGNANT NEOPLASMS IN SIX "CANCER FAMILIES"

Family Number	1	2	3	4	5	6
Total number in family	245	64	19	14	517	51
Males	117	33	7	6	258	26
Females	128	31	12	8	259	25
Total over age 20	198	31	15	14	391	35
Total number of individuals with a malignancy	43	18	8	12	74	10
Individuals with carcinoma of colon	10	9	4	9	35	8
Individuals with endometrial carcinoma	13	5	3	1	21	2
Individuals with multiple primary malignancies	8	6	2	2	10	3
Individuals with endometrial and colon carcinoma	4	2	1	0	4	2
Individuals with cancer of other sites	29	10	3	2	21	3

was 45, whereas that for carcinoma of the colon was 43. The average age of onset for endometrial carcinoma in the general population is approximately 62, and is approximately 55 for carcinoma of the colon.

Discussion

Despite the frequency of malignant neoplasms in the population, and the varied and prodigious efforts directed to the problem during the past century, the etiology of carcinoma remains an enigma.

During the past several decades, the role of hereditary factors in the etiology of malignant neoplasms has been a subject of considerable interest. Challenging facts have emerged. Classical Mendelian inheritance patterns have been identified for some site-specific malignancies, and definite, albeit less clear hereditary roles have been indicated for many others. However, in spite of this intense interest, little attention has been focused on so-called "cancer families," wherein cancer of multiple sites is prevalent. Since Warthin's first description, only occasional reports have described this phenomenon in other families. This suggests that the phenomenon is rare. However, our experience belies this, since we have now made the same observation in several families during the past five years.

Our findings in six "cancer families" have shown an exceedingly high incidence of malignant neoplasms, the most frequent being carcinoma of the colon and endometrium. In addition, an unusually high incidence of multiple primary malignant neoplasms has been observed, with the most frequent combination in females being carcinoma of the colon and endometrium. In males, carcinoma of the colon is also frequently observed, but no one lesion has consistently appeared as the second primary malignancy. Age of onset for the malignancies in these "cancer families" is consistently lower than that for the same lesions occurring sporadically in the general population.

Present research in several additional "cancer families," although less thoroughly studied to date, is, nevertheless, revealing a pattern similar to that found in the six families discussed here.

Because of the high frequency of endometrial carcinoma in the "cancer families," we recently studied 154 females with histologically confirmed diagnoses of this malignancy, who were seen during a 20-year period at a university hospital. Details of this work have been published elsewhere.[38] A critical finding relating to the present discussion is that although 11 percent of these patients had multiple primary malignant neoplasms, not a single individual showed the combination of endometrial and colon carcinoma, the most frequent combination in our "cancer families." A further finding was that 16 percent of these probands had first-degree relatives with endometrial carcinoma.

Interestingly, several reports in the literature also show a familial occurrence of endometrial and colon carcinoma, multiple primary malignancies, and an early age of onset for these lesions and these cases presumably pertain also to "cancer families."[39–41] These reports have been concerned primarily with the occurrence of multiple primary malignancies. Unfortunately, in many cases the genetic information has been limited.

In a large series of patients with multiple primary malignancies, Moertel[42] found families with histories of carcinoma significantly exceeding those found in a control group having single malignancies and in a second control group of patients selected for absence of malignancies.

Therefore, it appears that hereditary factors may contribute to the phenomenon of multiple primary malignant neoplasms. Unfortunately, Moertel's data do not provide information as to the variety and patterns of malignancies in his families. Hence, it is not possible to know to what extent he might have been dealing with so-called "cancer families." It is significant, however, that relatives in his multiple primary groups developed malignancies at younger ages than did those in his control groups.

The findings from our study suggest an inherited predisposition to malignancies of multiple anatomic sites, but in particular, to colon and endometrial carcinoma in females, and colon and other carcinomas in males. In addition, an increased incidence of multiple primary malignant neoplasms characterizes these "cancer families." These data, therefore, indicate that carcinoma of the colon, in combination with endometrial carcinoma and other malignancies is not fortuitous, but that these malignancies are etiologically related. We propose, therefore, that these collective findings are compatible with a concept of a hereditary multiple-cancer syndrome.

We further propose that there are at least two genotypes for endometrial carcinoma, one appears to be site-specific as found in the endometrial carcinoma series of 154 patients. Support for this hypothesis has also been provided by Murphy[43] and Brøbeck.[44] The other genotype for endometrial carcinoma is that associated with colon carcinoma and, to a lesser extent, carcinoma of other sites in members of "cancer families" having our newly proposed hereditary multiple-cancer syndrome.

Occurrence of multiple carcinomas in families is of significant practical importance. For example, while an annual proctosigmoidoscopic examination should be a routine cancer detection procedure for all adults past the age of 40, it assumes urgent proportions for members of "cancer families." It should be performed at an early age, since carcinoma of the colon occurs at a significantly younger age than in patients with sporadic colon carcinoma. In like manner, a careful evaluation of the endometrium should be made on all women in "cancer families" as they approach the risk age for this lesion. A conventional Papanicolaou smear of cervical secretions will not be sufficient in most cases; an endometrial suction biopsy is the preferred method for detection of endometrial carcinoma. Should signs or symptoms be present, a dilatation and curettage should then be performed.

Whenever abdominal surgery is necessary, a careful examination of all abdominal viscera, including the ascending, transverse, and descending colon should be performed, to rule out the presence of occult or frankly advanced primary malignancy in these organs.

Unexplained upper-gastrointestinal symptomatology should be carefully evaluated in these patients, and, when indicated, an upper-gastrointestinal series, gastric fluoroscopy, gastric analysis for the presence of total and free HCl, and gastric cytological studies should be carried out.

In addition to specific cancer-screening techniques, it must constantly be remembered that members of such "cancer families" are also a high-risk group for malignancies of *all* anatomic sites.

Summary

Research during the past 50 years has identified hereditary etiologic factors for certain malignant neoplasms of *specific anatomic sites;* indeed, in some cases a classical Mendelian inheritance pattern has been confirmed. However, very little attention has been focused upon families showing cancer of *multiple anatomic sites* ("cancer families"). This report has presented data on six such families. Endometrial and colon carcinoma were the most frequent lesions, multiple primary malignancies occurred frequently, and the age of onset for malignancies was lower than that for the same tumors occurring on a sporadic basis. The most frequent combination was colon and endometrial carcinoma. It is proposed that these data are compatible with the concept of a hereditary multiple-cancer syndrome. Regularity in health maintenance examination is advocated for members of families with the hereditary multiple-cancer syndrome.

References

1. Bittner, J. J. & F. R. Heilman. 1944. Cancer Res. **4:** 779.
2. Little, C. C. 1954. Genetics, Biological Individuality, and Cancer. Stanford University Publications. Stanford, Calif.
3. Slye, M. 1927. J. Cancer Res. **11:** 135.
4. Strong, L. C. 1945. J. Nat. Cancer Inst. **5:** 339.
5. Heston, W. E. 1952. Amer. J. Hum. Genet. **4:** 314.
6. Heston, W. E. 1965. Cancer Res. **25:** 1326.
7. Rous, P. 1911. J. A. M. A. **56:** 198.
8. Rubin, H. & R. K. Vogt. 1962. Virology. **17:** 184.
9. Sanarelli, G. 1898. Centralbl. Bakt. fur Parasitenkunde. **23:** 865.
10. Shope, R. E. & E. W. Hurst. 1933. J. Exp. Med. **58:** 607.
11. Anderson, D. E. 1963. Ann. N. Y. Acad. Sci. **108:** 948.
12. Bevan, E. W. 1925. Trans. Roy. Soc. Trop. Med. Hyg. **19:** 153.
13. Munroe, J. S. & W. F. Windle. 1963. Science. **140:** 1415.
14. Clemmesen, J. 1965. Acta Path. Microbiol. Scand. (Suppl.) **174:** 1.
15. Jacobsen, O. 1946. Op. Dom. Biol. Hered. Hum. (Kobenhavn) **11:** 1.
16. Woolf, C. M. 1955. Univ. Calif. (Berkeley) Publ. Public Health. **2:** 265.
17. Anderson, V. E., H. O. Goodman & S. C. Reed. 1958. Variables Related to Human Breast Cancer. University of Minnesota Press. Minneapolis, Minn.
18. Hoffman, F. L. 1915. The Mortality from Cancer throughout the World. Prudential Press. Newark, N. J.
19. Bashford, E. F. 1908. Lancet. **ii:** 1508.
20. Waaler, G. H. M. 1931. Norske Vidensk. Akad. Skr. Mat. Nat. Kl. **2:** 5.
21. Martynova, R. P. 1937. Amer. J. Cancer. **29:** 530.
22. Wassink, W. F. 1935. Genetica. **17:** 103.
23. Macklin, M. T. 1959. J. Nat. Cancer Inst. **22:** 927.
24. Macklin, M. T. 1960. J. Nat. Cancer Inst. **24:** 551.
25. Penrose, L. S., H. J. Mackenzie & M. N. Karn. 1948. Brit. J. Cancer. **2:** 168.
26. Oliver, C. P. 1958. Ann. N. Y. Acad. Sci. **71:** 1198.
27. Videbaek, A. A. 1947. Nyt. Nordisk Forlag. H. K. Lewis and Co., Ltd. London, England.
28. Busk, T. 1952. Proceedings of the Second National Cancer Conference. **2:** 1087.
29. Cockayne, E. A. 1927. Cancer Review. **2:** 337.

30. Lockhart-Mummery, P. 1925. Lancet. i:427.
31. Dukes, C. E. 1952. Ann. Eugen. **17:** 1.
32. Griffith, A. D. & Sorsby. 1944. J. Ophthal. **28:** 279.
33. Gardner, E. J. 1951. Amer. J. Hum. Genet. **3:** 167.
34. Warthin, A. S. 1913. Arch. Intern. Med. **12:** 546.
35. Warthin, A. S. 1925. J. Cancer Res. **9:** 279.
36. Hauser, I. J. & C. W. Weller. 1936. Amer. J. Cancer. **27:** 434.
37. Lynch, H. T., M. W. Shaw, C. W. Magnuson, A. L. Larsen & A. J. Krush. 1966. Arch. Intern. Med. **117:** 206.
38. Lynch, H. T., A. J. Krush, A. L. Larsen & C. W. Magnuson. 1966. Amer. J. Med. Sci. **252**(4): 381.
39. Heinzelmann, N. F. 1964. Helv. Chir. Acta **31:** 316.
40. Savage, D. 1956. Brit. Med. J. **2:** 341.
41. Stalker, L. K., R. B. Phillips & J. De J. Pemberton. 1939. Surg. Gynec. Obstet. **68:** 595.
42. Moertel, C. G., M. B. Dockerty & A. H. Baggenstoss. 1961. Cancer. **14:** 231.
43. Murphy, D. P. 1952. Heredity in Uterine Cancer. Harvard University Press. Cambridge, Mass.
44. Brøbeck, O. 1949. Heredity in Cancer Uteri: A Genetical and Clinical Study of 200 Patients with Cancer of the Corpus Uteri. Universitetsfarlaget. Aarhus, Denmark.
45. Gates, R. R. 1946. Human Genetics. The MacMillan Co. New York, N. Y.
46. Straith, F. E. 1939. Amer. J. Orthodon. Oral Surg. **25:** 673.
47. Binkley, G. W. & H. H. Johnson, Jr. 1951. Arch. Derm. (Chicago) **63:** 73.

GENETIC STUDIES OF DISEASES ASSOCIATED WITH CHROMOSOMAL ABERRATIONS

Richard H. Osborne
University of Wisconsin, Madison, Wis.

The papers presented in this section have dealt with four quite distinct, but interrelated problem areas: first, the multiple causes of chromosomal changes, both oncogenic and nononcogenic viruses and radiation (Aula *et al.,* 1968 Nasjleti & Spencer, 1968); second, the variety of chromosomal changes which can result from the action of anyone of these agents: polyploidy, endoreplication, fragmentation, ring forms, dicentrics, and rearrangements (Aula *et al.,* 1968 Nasjileti & Spencer, 1968); third, the variety of disease entities which can result from these changes: congenital malformations and benign and malignant neoplastic disease; associated anemias and immunological irregularities were also discussed (Fialkow & Uchida, 1968; Bloom & Diamond, 1968); fourth, the familial incidence, or genetic susceptibility or resistance of the host to chromosomal changes or the disease processes associated with such changes (McCullough *et al.,*1968; Zellweger, 1968; Lynch *et al.,* 1968). It is to this fourth area that I shall primarily address my remarks, and most particularly from the standpoint of cancer etiology. In doing this, however, my intention is to focus attention upon the actual unity of what I have designated as four separate problem areas.

To investigate the possible role of the genetic or host factor in cancer etiology, it is usual to approach the problem as though a specified form of the disease, as listed in the Manual of Tumor Nomenclature (1953), constitutes a unique and completely delineated disease entity. It is also assumed that the disease process is in all probability initiated by the impact of a single environmental agent or event upon a specific, and relatively simple, genetic system. The results of studies based upon these simplifying propositions have been essentially negative, or at best inconclusive (McCullough *et al.,* 1968), as might be anticipated from the multiple causes and effects of chromosomal changes (Aula *et al.,* 1968; Nasjleti & Spencer, 1968; Fialkow & Uchida, 1968; Bloom & Diamond, 1968). Investigations of quite a different type from those reported in this monograph may help to make this point clear.

A major milestone in cancer studies was recognition of the multiplicity of the disease and the variety of its histological types. Evidence has long been mounting, however, which clearly indicates that in studies of cancer etiology, some grouping of types on biological grounds is necessary, and that each form of the disease is not a unique entity, either in respect to the responsible causative agent or a host susceptibility factor. One example is the ABO blood group cancer association. Blood group A, for reasons still unknown, marks a genotype with a statistically increased susceptibility to neoplastic disease of the stomach (Aird *et al.,* 1953), of the ovary (Osborne & DeGeorge, 1963), and of the salivary gland (Cameron, 1958; Osborne & DeGeorge, 1962). Three body sites and several histological types, both benign and malignant, are involved in the blood group association. This may be surprising to the hospital administrator for it cuts across the boundaries of three absolutely different services (Gastric, Gynecology, and Head and Neck), but there is a unifying biological element. The associated types are predominantly of glandular epithelium and all are characterized by atypical cell regeneration or metaplasia.

Similarly, it is quite possible that in lymphatic leukemia, the genetic susceptibility may not be specifically to lymphatic leukemia itself, but to a particular combination of different lymphoid tissue neoplasms. Family studies might be profitably carried out which included some combination of lymphatic leukemia, Hodgkin's disease, lymphosarcoma, reticulum cell sarcoma, and fibrosarcoma. The age of incidence of these lymphatic diseases differ. Age-dependent physiological changes might be one of the factors responsible for the specific form the disease process takes. All involve lymphoid tissue and all are characterized by a marked reduction in antibody formation (Wintrobe, 1956). On the basis of such common elements, it is not likely that only a single genetic mechanism, predisposing to a failure in antibody formation, is the only genetic factor conditioning susceptibility. In fact, it is not necessary to assume that a failure of the immunogenetic capacity of the host is entirely genetic (Osborne & DeGeorge, 1967).

The possibility of the interaction of two or more environmental events or agents in the initiation of malignant disease should also be considered in future genetic studies of human cancers. The accumulative effects of radiation and virus in mouse leukemia are well known. Also to be considered are less obvious physiological alterations that may enhance virulence of an oncogenic agent or depress defense mechanisms. Of great potential value for studies of this nature are twin pairs discordant for malignant disease, or concordant pairs in which marked differences in age of onset or other factors occur. (Osborne & DeGeorge, 1964 & 1967). One example will suffice here.

A pair of five-year-old monozygotic twin boys differed markedly in body weight and stature. The smaller member of the pair, Richard, had his tonsils removed. Following this he experienced a marked growth spurt and increase in weight; he shortly surpassed his previously more robust twin who showed an average growth rate for that age level. Richard developed acute leukemia, but several years later, his twin was still alive and free of leukemic symptoms. If there is a genetic susceptibility to leukemia, as monozygotic twins they were identical in this respect. As twins they had shared the same prenatal environment, and at the time Richard contracted his disease, the same postnatal environment and infectious exposures. The reason his twin had not had a tonsillectomy was that his sore throats had prevented scheduling his operation. Growth rate at ages 4–6 is at a low point. During this period there is also very little increase in lymphoid tissue. Richard experienced a growth spurt abnormal for this developmental stage with, undoubtedly, some alteration or disruption in physiological homeostasis. Is it possible that this constituted "factor X" and led to development of the disease process?

Studies of host susceptibility and resistance to neoplastic disease have been notoriously unsuccessful. Studies of chromosomal abnormalities, viral- and radiologically-induced chromosomal changes, as well as other types of evidence, suggest far more complicated etiologies for most cancers than a "single event-single gene interaction." More sophisticated studies will be needed to further our understanding of susceptibilities to these diseases.

References

Aird, I., H. H. Bentall & J. A. F. Roberts. 1953. Relationship between cancer of the stomach and the ABO groups. Brit. Med. J. 1: 799–801.

American Cancer Society. 1953. Manual of Tumor Nomenclature and Coding. American Cancer Society. New York, N. Y.

Aula, P., W. W. Nichols & A. Levan. 1968. Virus-induced chromosome changes. This monograph.

BLOOM, G. E. & L. K. DIAMOND. 1968. Chromosome abnormalities in anemias. This monograph.
CAMERON, J. M. 1958. Blood groups in tumors of salivary tissue. Lancet **i**: 238–240.
FIALKOW, P. J. & I. A. UCHIDA. 1968. Autoantibodies in Down's syndrome and gonadal dysgenesis. This monograph.
LYNCH, H. T., D. E. ANDERSON, A. J. KRUSH & A. L. LARSEN. 1968. Heredity and carcinoma. This monograph.
MCCULLOUGH, J. J., M. T. KOROBKIN & W. KRIVIT. 1968. Genetics in acute lymphatic leukemia in childhood. This monograph.
NASJLETI, C. E. & H. H. SPENCER. 1968. Chromosome polyploidization in human leukocytes induced by radiation. This monograph.
OSBORNE, R. H. & F. V. DE GEORGE. 1967. The ABO blood groups in parotid and submaxillary gland tumors. Amer. J. Hum. Genet. **14**: 199–209.
OSBORNE, R. H. & F. V. DE GEORGE. 1963. The ABO blood groups in neoplastic disease of the ovary. Amer. J. Hum. Genet. **15**: 380–388.
OSBORNE, R. H. & F. V. DE GEORGE. 1964. Neoplastic diseases in twins: Evidence for pre- or perinatal factors conditioning cancer susceptibility. Cancer **17**: 1149–1154.
OSBORNE, R. H. & F. V. DE GEORGE. Cancer and contagious disease in twins: The Interrelation of host defense mechanisms. Cancer. In press.
ZELLWEGER, H. 1968. Familial aggregates of the 21-trisomy syndrome. This monograph.

Part II. Leukocytes in Genetic Anomalies

NEUTROPHIL NUCLEI AND THE SEX-CHROMOSOME COMPLEMENT

Ursula Mittwoch
Galton Laboratory, University College
London, England

The relationship between leukocytes and disease has been recognized for over a century. In his book on cellular pathology, published in 1858, Rudolph Virchow wrote that in his opinion the leukocyte occupies an established place in pathology. The majority of circulating leukocytes consist of polymorphonuclear leukocytes, or granulocytes. These cells comprise some of the most distinctive cell-types of the body, and their morphology was described by Paul Ehrlich in 1879. Nevertheless, the fact that certain morphological characteristics are a result of the sex-chromosome constitution escaped investigators for another 75 years.

The nuclear appendage of polymorphonuclear leukocytes, which is present in cells from normal females and absent from cells of normal males, was first described by Davidson and Smith (1954), who called this appendage a "drumstick." This finding was soon confirmed by a number of authors (Mittwoch, 1964b).

Drumsticks occur in eosinophilic and basophilic as well as in neutrophilic polymorphonuclear leukocytes (FIGURES 1–3). However, for practical purposes, only those occurring in the neutrophils are usually considered. This is because eosinophils, and particularly basophils, are relatively infrequent, and, in addition, the coarse granules present in these cells often obscure the detailed morphology of the nucleus.

A typical drumstick consists of a piece of condensed nuclear material with a rounded outline and a surface area of about 1.5 μm^2; this forms the head of the drumstick, which is attached to the rest of the nucleus by a thin filament of varying length. Drumsticks are characteristics of neutrophils from normal females and indicate the presence of two X chromosomes in the karyotype. Formation of drumsticks in patients with XXY- and multiple X-chromosome constitution will be discussed later.

One reason for the relatively late discovery of the drumstick is undoubtedly to be found in the presence of many other types of nuclear appendages that may be encountered in neutrophils from different individuals. Considerable care is needed to distinguish true drumsticks from other nuclear appendages, which may be of different sizes and shapes (FIGURES 4 & 5). Although these latter types of appendages are not sex-specific and bear no direct relation to the sex-chromosome complement, some of them may reflect other chromosome constitutions (Huehns *et al.*, 1964).

Even in their original publication, Davidson and Smith (1954) suggested that, like the Barr body of epithelial and other tissue cells, the drumstick may represent condensed X-chromosomal material. At first, however, certain difficulties in the evaluation of drumstick data left the alternative hypothesis open, namely that, unlike the Barr body, the drumstick may be merely a secondary sexual characteristic. Probably the most significant data on this subject have come from studies of drumsticks in patients with structurally abnormal X chromosomes.

Drumsticks are absent in the XO type of Turner's syndrome, but in patients who carry a structurally abnormal X chromosome, drumstick-like structures are

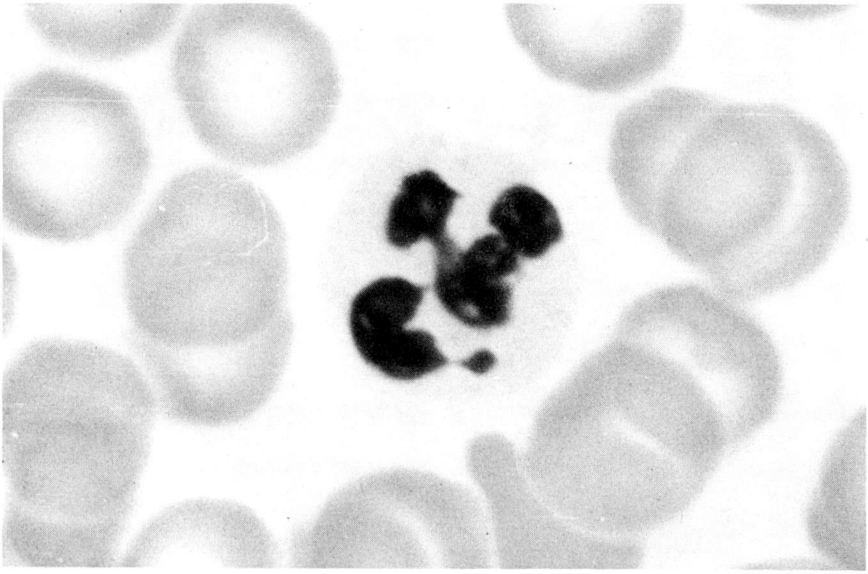

FIGURE 1. Drumstick in neutrophil. ~ × 2,800.

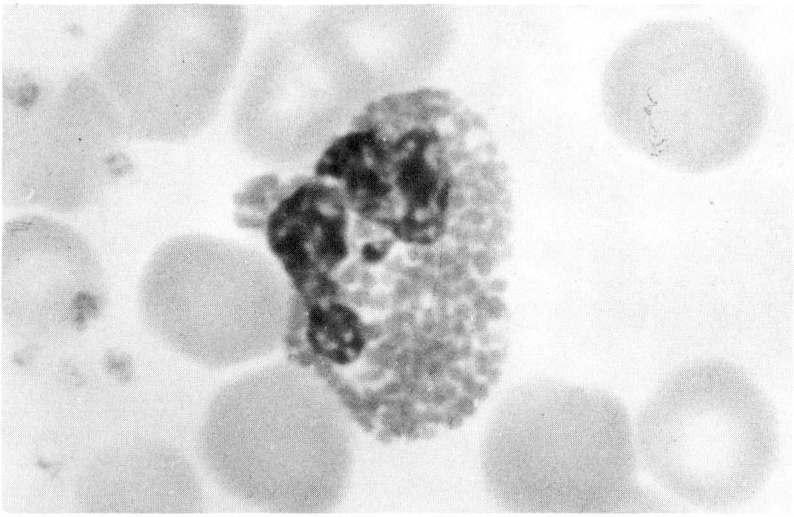

FIGURE 2. Drumstick in eosinophil. ~ × 2,800.

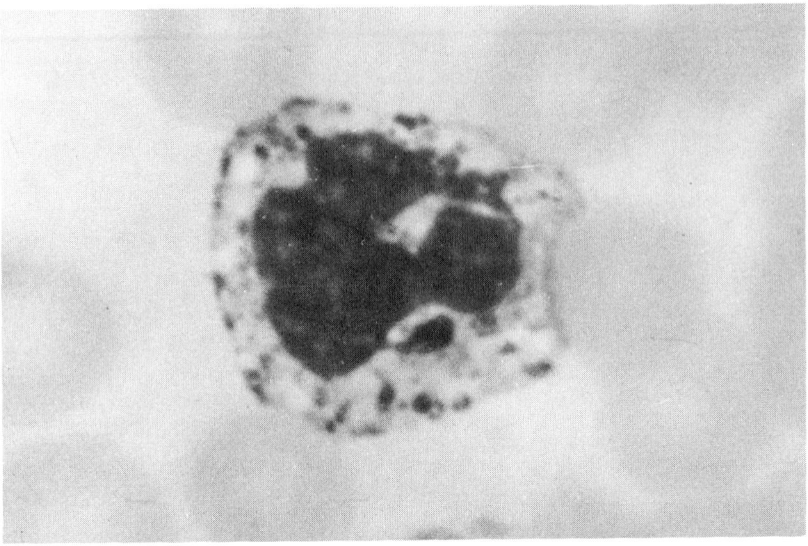

FIGURE 3. Drumstick in basophil. ~ × 2,800.

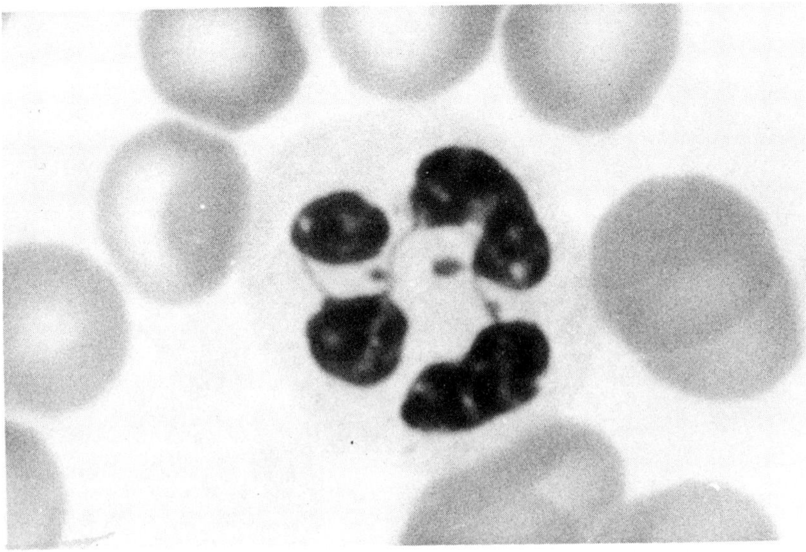

FIGURE 4. Small, nonsex-specific appendages in neutrophil.

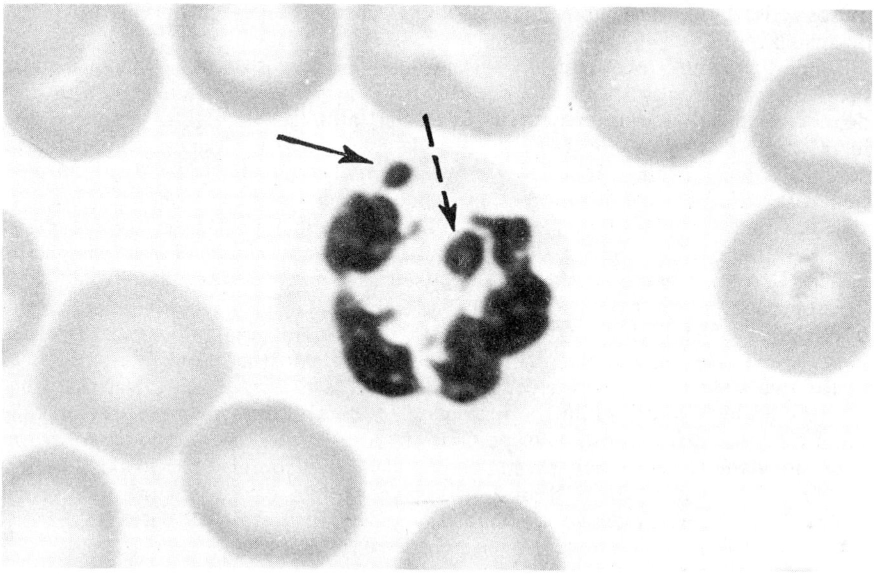

FIGURE 5. Drumstick (solid arrow), minor lobe (broken arrow) and small, nonsex-specific appendages in neutrophil. ~ × 2,800.

usually found. In the most common type of structural abnormality of the X chromosome, the presumed isochromosome of the long arm of the X chromosome (Fraccaro *et al.*, 1960), the neutrophils bear drumstick-like appendages, the heads of which appear to be larger than those of normal drumsticks. The incidence of these apparently large drumsticks is also greater than that of normal drumsticks. The increase in size of these drumsticks has been confirmed by quantitative measurements. MacLean (1962) found that the ratio of the area of the drumstick to that of the rest of the nucleus was greater in two patients with isochromosomes of the long arm of the X compared with the value found in two normal women. Conversely, this ratio was decreased in a patient with a deleted X chromosome. Similar results were reported by Bamford *et al.* (1964).

Fraccaro *et al.* (1964) compared the sizes of drumsticks of six normal women, six patients with isochromosomes of the long arm of the X, and three patients with deleted X chromosomes. The technique employed was to photograph all drumstick-bearing neutrophils and to put the negatives into a photographic enlarger through which the outlines of the nuclei were drawn at a total magnification of 8,000 diameters. The area bounded by the tracings were then measured by means of a planimeter. Mean drumstick areas for the different karyotypes were found to be as follows: normal X chromosomes, 1.54 μm^2; iso-X chromosome, 1.93 μm^2; and deleted X chromosomes, 1.10 μm^2. Although there was considerable variation in the mean drumstick areas from individuals, some of which is likely to reflect the error involved in drawing the outlines of the greatly enlarged images, the differences between the means were significant at the 5 percent level; and the results may be regarded as strong evidence that the drumstick is a direct expression of the X-chromosome constitution. Thus, like Barr bodies (Ohno *et al.*, 1959) drumsticks must be assumed to originate from a single X chromosome, which is present in addition to the first one. If the second X chromosome is structurally abnormal, it is this chromosome which will form the drumstick.

Large drumsticks occurring in patients with isochromosomes will not usually present any difficulty to an experienced observer, since appendages of this size do not normally occur on neutrophil nuclei, and the regular outline and the intense and even staining of the drumstick head make it virtually impossible to confuse it with a minor lobe. Nevertheless, small drumsticks found in conjunction with deleted X chromosomes may be difficult to distinguish from nonsex-specific nuclear appendages, and a deliberate choice must generally be made whether the size of a given structure falls within the range of nonsex-specific appendages, or whether it should be classed as a small drumstick.

If one accepts the proposition that, basically, drumsticks are equivalent to the Barr bodies of epithelial and other tissue cells, a number of differences become apparent. These are mainly quantitative and relate to the respective incidences of the two structures. The incidence of drumsticks is very much lower than that of Barr bodies. Thus, while the incidence of Barr bodies in buccal-smear cells from females varies from 20–70 percent (Moore, 1966), the incidence of drumsticks is of the order of only three percent of all neutrophils (Davidson & Smith, 1954). Mittwoch (1964a) found that in a sample of 12 apparently normal women, the mean incidence of drumstick varied from 1.6–7.2 percent; the differences were highly consistent over eight weekly intervals.

In patients with Klinefelter's syndrome, the presence of a Y chromosome does not appear to influence the incidence of Barr bodies, so that the buccal-smear test constitutes a good screening technique for diagnosing not only patients with XXY sex-chromosome constitution, but also cases with mosaicism of the XY/XXY type (MacLean, 1966). By contrast, the incidence of drumsticks in patients with Klinefelter's syndrome is considerably less than that of normal females (Davidson & Smith, 1958). Again, the frequencies of Barr bodies and drumsticks in patients with three X chromosomes appear to be very different. The Barr bodies of such patients provide a very characteristic picture, since a proportion of cells will contain two Barr bodies, and the incidence of cells with single Barr bodies is also increased (Jacobs *et al.*, 1959; Johnston *et al.*, 1961). By contrast, the incidence of drumsticks in most patients is not increased, but tends to be below normal (Mittwoch, 1964b & c). Double drumsticks, which were first described by Jacobs *et al.* (1959), are so rare that their enumeration is virtually impossible, and they cannot, therefore, be used as an additional test for diagnosing the triple X condition.

One factor which is known to affect the frequency with which drumsticks are formed is the degree of lobulation of the polymorphonuclear nucleus; drumsticks are more likely to be found in nuclei with four or five lobes than in those with only one or two lobes (Davidson & Smith, 1954). It is likely that this may explain some of the apparent divergences of Barr bodies and drumsticks in patients with abnormal sex-chromosome constitutions.

Mittwoch (1961) found that mean lobe counts of neutrophil nuclei from patients with Klinefelter's syndrome were lower than those of normal and mentally retarded controls; this finding was confirmed by Weber *et al.* (1965). It is likely that some other types of abnormal sex-chromosome constitutions, such as XXX and XXXY, may also result in a lowering of the lobe count (Mittwoch, 1964c). By contrast, in patients with Turner's syndrome, either of the XO type or with a structurally abnormal X chromosome, no decrease in nuclear lobing has been observed (Mittwoch, 1966). It appears, therefore, that some sex-chromosome abnormalities, and particularly Klinefelter's syndrome, are associated with decreased lobing of the polymorphonuclear leukocytes, as well as an inhibition in the extrusion of drumsticks. Thus, the low incidence of drumsticks in Klinefelter's syndrome may be explained as reflecting a disturbance in leukocyte maturation.

Both these abnormalities, decreased neutrophil segmentation and low incidence of drumsticks, are also encountered in patients with mongolism (Turpin & Bernyer, 1947; Mittwoch, 1957). These patients also have an increased level of leukocyte alkaline phosphatase (Trubowitz *et al.*, 1962; Lennox *et al.*, 1962; King *et al.*, 1962; Alter *et al.*, 1963; O'Sullivan & Pryles, 1963). Using a cytochemical technique, Weber *et al.* (1965) presented evidence of an elevated leukocyte alkaline phosphatase level in Klinefelter's syndrome. Patients examined for this study comprised 12 patients with Klinefelter's syndrome, 12 mentally retarded males, and 12 mentally retarded females. The leukocyte alkaline phosphatase level of the females was found to be higher than that of the males, although the difference was not statistically significant. The leukocyte alkaline phosphatase level of the Klinefelter patients was found to be slightly higher than that of the females and significantly higher than that of the males.

Weber *et al.* (1965) further attempted to score for alkaline phosphatase and count the number of nuclear lobes in the same cells. This was done by counterstaining the blood films with Mayer's hematoxylin after applying the cytochemical treatment for alkaline phosphatase. The results suggested that there may be a gradual falling off of leukocyte alkaline phosphatase levels in cells with three and four lobes. If these results can be confirmed, they might explain the observed increases in leukocyte alkaline phosphatase in Klinefelter's syndrome as well as in mongolism, for in both conditions, cells within three and more nuclear lobes are in short supply. As there is likely to be some type of correlation between lobe number and the stage of maturity which the cells have reached, it would appear as if there is a shortage of the more mature neutrophils in mongolism as well as in Klinefelter's syndrome. In mongolism, Mellman *et al.* (1967) have provided evidence for a shortened life-span of the polymorphonuclear leukocytes.

Perhaps the most interesting problem that arises from these findings is the question whether trisomy for two quite unrelated chromosomes, i.e., the sex chromosomes and the autosome 21, may result in the same defect at the cellular level. Although merely conjectural at present, this idea is capable of being tested through detailed comparisons of the morphological and chemical characteristics of the cells in Klinefelter's syndrome and in mongolism. It would appear that leukocytes are particularly well-suited for this kind of comparative study.

References

ALTER, A. A., S. L. LEE, M. POURFAR & G. DOBKIN. 1963. Studies in leukocyte alkaline phosphatase in mongolism: a possible chromosome marker. Blood **22:** 165–177.

BAMFORD, S. B., C. M. CASSIN, D. L. DILBA & G. W. MITCHELL. 1964. Neutrophil appendages as indicators of sex chromosome aberrations. Acta Cytol. **8:** 323–331.

DAVIDSON, W. M. & D. R. SMITH. 1954. A morphological sex difference in the polymorphonuclear neutrophil leucocytes. Brit. Med. J. **ii:** 6–7.

DAVIDSON, W. M. & D. R. SMITH. 1958. The neutrophil sex module in Klinefelter's syndrome. *In* Symposium on Nuclear Sex. D. R. Smith & W. M. Davidson, Eds. : 93–101. Heinemann. London, England.

EHRLICH, P. 1879. Ueber die specifischen Granulationen des Blutes. Arch. Anat. Physiol., Phys. Abt. **1879:** 571–579.

FRACCARO, M., D. IKKOS, J. LINDSTEN, R. LUFT & K. KAYSER. 1960. A new type of chromosomal abnormality in gonadal dysgenesis. Lancet **ii:** 1144.

FRACCARO, M., J. LINDTEN, U. MITTWOCH & ZONTA, L. 1964. Size of drumsticks in patients with abnormalities of the X-chromosome. Lancet **ii**: 43–44.

HUEHNS, E. R., M. LUTZNER & F. HECHT. 1964. Nuclear abnormalities of the neutrophils in D_1 (13–15)-trisomy syndrome. Lancet **i**: 589–590.

JACOBS, P. A., A. G. BAIKEE, W. M. COURT-BROWN, T. N. MACGREGOR, N. MACLEAN & D. C. HARNDEN. 1959. Evidence for the existence of the human "superfemale." Lancet **ii**: 423–525.

JOHNSTON, A. W., M. A. FERGUSON-SMITH, S. D. HANDMAKER, H. W. JONES & C. S. JONES. 1961. The triple X syndrome. Brit. Med. J. **ii**: 1046–1052.

KING, M. J., E. M. GILLIS & A. G. BAIKIE. 1962. The polymorph alkaline phosphatase in mongolism. Lancet **ii**: 661.

KLINGER, H. P. 1957. The sex chromatin body in fetal and maternal portions in the human placenta. Acta Anat. (Basel) **30**: 371–397.

LENNOX, B., H. ST. C. WHITE & J. CAMPBELL. 1962. The polymorph alkaline phosphatase in mongolism. Lancet **ii**: 991–992.

MACLEAN, N. 1962. The drumsticks of polymorphonuclear leucocytes in sex-chromosome abnormalities. Lancet **i**: 1154–1158.

MACLEAN, N. 1966. Sex chromatin surveys of newborn babies. *In* The Sex Chromatin. K. L. Moore, Ed. : 202–210. W. B. Saunders. Philadelphia, Pa.

MELLMAN, W. J., S. O. RAAB, F. A. OSKI & T. A. TEDESCO. 1968. Abnormal leukokinetics in 21 trisomy. This monograph.

MITTWOCH, U. 1957. Some observations on the leucocytes in mongolism. J. Ment. Defic. Res. **1**: 26–32.

MITTWOCH, U. 1961. Nuclear sex and chromosome structure in mongolism and the Klinefelter syndrome. *In* Human Chromosomal Abnormalities. W. M. Davidson & D. R. Smith, eds. : 97–105. Staples Press. London, England.

MITTWOCH, U. 1964a. Frequency of drumsticks in normal women and in patients with chromosomal abnormalities. Nature (London) **201**: 317–319.

MITTWOCH, U. 1964b. Sex chromatin. J. Med. Genet. **1**: 50–76.

MITTWOCH, U. 1964c. The incidence of drumsticks in patients with three X chromosomes. Cytogenetics **2**: 24–33.

MITTWOCH, U. 1966. Unpublished observation.

MOORE, K. L. 1966. The development of clinical sex chromatin tests. *In* The Sex Chromatin. K. L. Moore, Ed. : 173–185. W. B. Saunders. Philadelphia, Pa.

OHNO, S., W. D. KAPLAN & R. KINOSITA. 1959. Formation of the sex chromatin by a single X-chromosome in liver cells of *Rattus norvegicus*. Exp. Cell Res. **18**: 415–418.

O'SULLIVAN, M. A. & C. V. PRYLES. 1963. A comparison of leukocyte alkaline phosphatase in 200 patients with mongolism and in 200 "familial" controls. New Eng. J. Med. **268**: 1168–1170.

TRUBOWITZ, S., D. KIRMAN & B. MASEK. 1962. The leucocyte alkaline phosphatase count in mongolism. Lancet **ii**: 486–487.

VIRCHOW, R. 1858. Die Cellularpathologie in ihrer Begründung auf physiologische und pathologische Gewebelehre. Hirschwald. Berlin, Germany.

WEBER, W. W., U. MITTWOCH & J. D. A. DELHANTY. 1965. Leucocyte alkaline phosphatase in Klinefelter's syndrome. J. Med. Genet. **2**: 93–156.

NEUTROPHILS IN THE 13(D_1)-TRISOMY SYNDROME

E. R. Huehns,* M. Lutzner,† and F. Hecht‡
Department of Medicine and Pathology
University of Washington, Seattle, Wash.

The clinical syndrome associated with 13(D_1) trisomy has already been well described (Patau *et al.*, 1960) and includes severe developmental and mental retardation, as well as a number of malformations, including eye anomalies, harelip and cleft palate, polydactyly, congenital heart disease, and arhinencephalia. Anatomical malformations of varying severity are well known in most congenital chromosomal abnormalities. More recent studies have shown that in a number of such conditions, biochemical abnormalities can be detected in certain cells. Examples of this are the persistence of embryonic and fetal hemoglobin in D trisomy (Huehns *et al.*, 1964), or the increase in both leukocyte alkaline phosphatase (Trubowitz *et al.*, 1962) and erythrocyte galactose-1-phosphate uridyl transferase (Brandt *et al.*, 1963) levels in trisomy 21. Occurrence of these biochemical anomalies is discussed elsewhere in this monograph. In addition to the gross anatomical and biochemical abnormalities, abnormalities of cellular organization might be expected, and in this paper an example of this is described.

The finding that the nuclei of the neutrophil leukocytes in a patient with D_1-trisomy syndrome have an abnormal structure led to the examination of blood films from a number of such individuals. We have examined six patients with proved trisomy of one of the chromosomes of the 13–15 group associated with the typical clinical features of the D_1-trisomy syndrome. Their ages ranged from one day to almost five years. In every case, most of the neutrophil leukocytes showed an abnormal number of nuclear projections (FIGURE 1). Since the original observation on six patients (Huehns *et al.*, 1964), several observers have confirmed the presence of this nuclear abnormality, and to date, it has been found in 25 patients (Powars *et al.*, 1964; Fine *et al.*, 1965; Lutzner & Hecht, 1966; Taylor, 1966; Walzer *et al.*, 1966; Méhes, 1966; Mutalik & Borgaonkar, 1966). The nuclear projections range from 1–6 or even more per cell (TABLE 1). Their appearance and size (approximately 0.25–1.5 μ) are extremely variable. Some are small sessile projections, but other appear definitely pedunculated. The appearance of the projections in blood smears made at different times from the same patient is also variable. They are Feulgen-positive, indicating that they are part of the nucleus.

In addition to the nuclear projections, the nuclear lobulation appears abnormal (FIGURE 1). Often the nucleus looks twisted and individual lobes are not clearly separated. In other cells, several lobules appear to grow out from one point. The chromatin patterns of the nuclei are coarse and lumpy, but the cytoplasm and granules of the cells appear normal. The abnormal projections are also found in eosinophils of peripheral blood but are difficult to see, because the prominent cytoplasmic granules may obscure the nuclear outline. Examination of other cells in the blood smear revealed no abnormality. Bone marrow from one of our patients has been examined, and no abnormality could be detected in the mylocytes or more primitive cells. The more mature band-forms show only

* Present address: University College Hospital Medical School, London, England.
† Present address: Dermatology Branch, National Cancer Institute, National Institutes of Health, Bethesda, Md.
‡ Present address: Department of Pediatrics and Division of Experimental Medicine, University of Oregon Medical School, Portland, Ore.

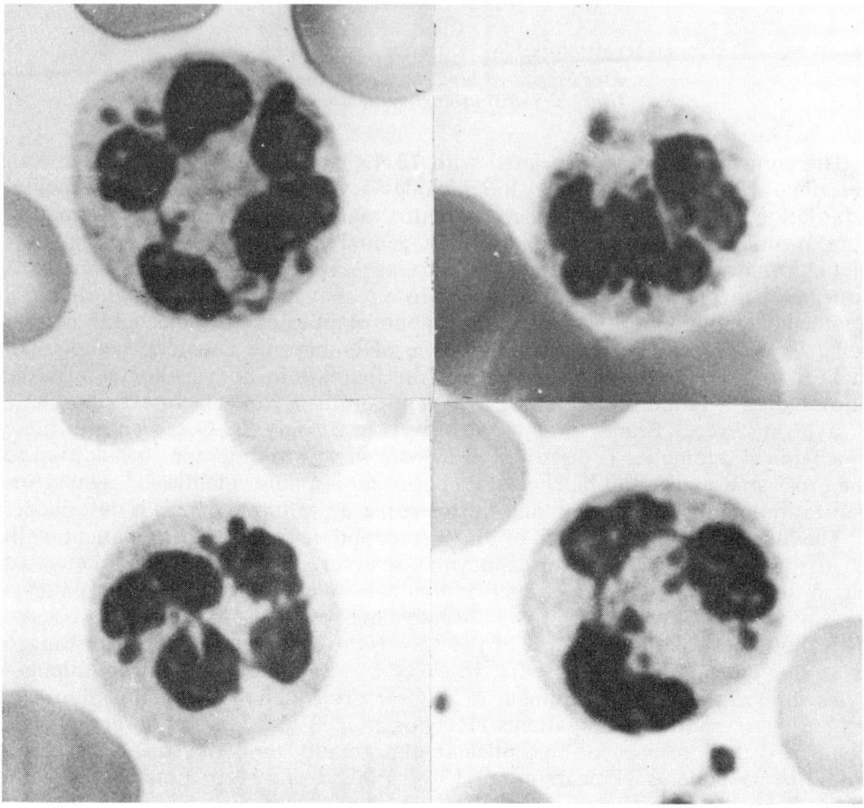

FIGURE 1. Typical peripheral blood neutrophils from D_1 (13–15) trisomy. All cells show the anomalous nuclear projections (Wright's stain; × 3,040; orig. mag. × 3,800; From Huehns *et al.*, 1964).

some anomalous "bumps" along their nuclear borders. The abnormality could only be detected with certainty in the mature polymorphonuclear cells.

The presence of some nuclear projections in normal polymorphonuclear leukocytes has been described, and these are more common in the male (Davidson, 1961). A comparison of the number of projections per cell clearly distinguishes between normal and abnormal cells. Results of such counts by various authors are summarized in TABLE 1. From these data, it can be calculated that in normal individuals the average percentage of polymorphonuclear cells which have one or more nuclear projections is 17 (range 2–40), whereas in D_1-trisomy syndrome it is 62 (range 35–86). The average percentage of cells with two or more projections in normal individuals is 3 (range 0–16), whereas in D_1-trisomy syndrome it is 27 (range 15–52). It can be seen that the cells in this condition are clearly distinguished from normal cells by the proportion of nuclei with two or more projections (Walzer *et al.*, 1966).

There are a few other conditions in which an increased number of nuclear projections is found. Gruner (1915–1916), who was quoted by Davidson (1961), suggested a relationship between a high frequency of leukocyte nuclear projec-

TABLE 1

NUCLEAR PROJECTIONS IN D_1 TRISOMY

	Percentage of Cells with "x" Projections						
x =	0	1	2	3	4+	1 or more	2 or more
Fine *et al.* (1965)							
D-trisomic male (1)	37	22	19	13	9	63	41
Control males (3)	73	18	6	2	1	27	9
Control females* (4)	59	21	13	4	3	41	20
Walzer *et al.* (1966)†							
D trisomy (9)	49	24	15	7	5	51	27
Controls (74)	87	10	2	1	0	13	2
This paper							
D trisomy (2)	27	21	21	15	16	73	52
Controls (5)	66	25	6	2	1	34	9
XO/XX (90:10) mosaic (1)	40	28	18	9	5	60	32

* Presumably including sex chromatin.

† These authors counted only projections 0.5–1.5 μ in size. Using these carefully defined criteria, the differentiation between D_1 trisomy and normals becomes more marked, whereas the count in the patient with XO/XX mosaicism becomes almost normal.

tions and carcinoma or sarcoma but did not comment on this any further. We have seen one patient with leukemia whose leukocytes showed a similar abnormal appearance.

Powars (1964) has carefully screened "many" patients for increased numbers of nuclear projections and has found two such patients without D_1-trisomy syndrome. One of these is an 84-year-old woman and the other a ten-year-old child with lupus erythematosus. An increased number of projections has also been seen in women treated with androgens (Méhes, 1966). This author found that 22 percent of neutrophils (range 10–32) had one or more projections compared with 9 percent (5–16) in controls (see also preceding discussion). Seman (1959) described a family in which an increased number of leukocyte nuclear projections was present in several individuals. This appears to be an autosomal dominant trait. Photographs of affected cells are very similar in appearance to those in the D_1-trisomy syndrome.

Finding this anomaly in D_1 trisomy prompted us to examine blood smears from patients with other chromosomal abnormalities. Two patients with E (17–18) trisomy and several with Down's syndrome (trisomy 21) were studied, but none of the white blood cells had the bizarre appearance found in the neutrophils from the patients with D_1-trisomy syndrome. Recently, Taylor (1966) reported a similar abnormality in patients with the XO condition. She found that the number of cells with one or more nuclear projections was 55.2 ± 5.4 in five such individuals, whereas it was 28.6 ± 4.7 in normal controls, and was 85.7 ± 4.7 in D_1 trisomy (four patients). We recently studied blood smears from a patient with XO/XX mosaicism (kindly referred by Dr. M. d'A. Crawfurd), and these confirmed Taylor's observation, although the picture was not as striking as that seen in D_1 trisomy because the projections were slightly smaller. An increased number of projections has also been seen in a partial C trisomy (Lutzner & Hecht, 1966).

From the preceding results, it would appear that detection of the white cell abnormality together with other clinical findings of D_1 trisomy would be helpful in diagnosing this condition. One group of authors (Kakulas & Rosman, 1965) used this in a retrospective study of the cases of arhinencephalia previously published by Yakovlev (1959). They concluded that in eight out of ten cases the nuclear abnormalities described here were present, suggesting D_1 trisomy. If their interpretation is correct, then, as Becker (1965) points out, there must be a number of patients suffering from D_1 trisomy with arhinencephalia and abnormal white cells without other obvious congenital abnormalities.

The situation in D/D-translocation-trisomy patients and patients with partial trisomy is more complex (Walzer *et al.*, 1966). These authors examined three patients with D/D-translocation trisomy and found an increased nuclear projection count in two (TABLE 2). However, the white cells in the third patient were normal, as was also the case in the patient reported by Erkman *et al.* (1965). Walzer *et al.* (1966) interpret these results in two ways. The first suggestion is that the syndrome has a limited expression because many of the congenital malformations associated with this syndrome are not found in all patients. The second idea and the one favored by these authors is that some of the loci concerned with the occurrence of the increased number of projections are located near the centromere of the D_1 chromosome. In the two patients with the elevated nuclear projection counts, these postulated loci are triplicated, whereas in their patient with the normal count, these loci are lost when the translocation occurs. In support of this hypothesis, they cite two unpublished patients. One, with an elevated nuclear projection count, is probably trisomic for the proximal two-thirds of the D_1 chromosome and eusomic for the remainder, whereas the other has normal white cells and is apparently trisomic for the distal portion of the long arm of the D_1 chromosome but eusomic for the centromeric region.

Electron microscopic studies, of thin sections of white cells obtained from the buffy coat of two of our patients and prepared by the method of Luft (1961), showed that the projections seen by light microscopy have a complex ultrastructure (FIGURES 2 & 3). This has not been described previously and was not present in sections from the white cells of one normal neonate. The pedunculated projections consisted of nucleoplasm in the form of long stalks with terminal swellings. The sessile nodules were also composed of nucleoplasms and were separated from the main part of the nucleus by an electron-light space. In some sections, a narrow link of the nucleoplasm between the two parts could be seen. These findings indicate that there is abnormal separation of some of the nucleoplasm from the main part of the nucleus. A detailed description of the electron microscopic appearances has been published (Lutzner & Hecht, 1966).

Unfortunately, electron microscopic studies are not yet available on the pro-

TABLE 2

NUCLEAR PROJECTIONS IN D/D-TRANSLOCATION TRISOMY*

	Percentage of Cells with "x" Projections						
x =	0	1	2	3	4+	1 or more	2 or more
Case 1	73	21	5	1	0	27	6
Case 2	55	21	16	4	4	45	24
Case 3	53	26	14	6	1	47	21
Controls (74)	87	10	2	1	0	13	2
					Control range	2–37	0–10

* Modified from Walzer *et al.*, 1966.

jections found in other conditions already referred to, and it is possible that these may, in fact, be different.

Lawler *et al.* (1966) described a patient with marrow dysplasia, an extra chromosome in the C group, and an increased number of drumsticks; approximately half the neutrophils showed a drumstick. The proportions of cells with one or more nuclear projections was 31 percent and only one percent had two or more projections, both values being well within the normal range given in TABLE 1. The electron microscopic appearance of the cells differed from that seen in D_1 trisomy. In the one normal we examined by electron microscopy, no structures such as those present in D_1 trisomy were seen. The data, however, do not exclude their occurrence in occasional normal white cells. In this connection, the reports by Davies and Tooze (1964 & 1966) are of interest. These workers found a similar electron microscopic appearance in the mitotic cells from the spleen of the newt, *Triturus cristatus.* They suggest that the appearance of the newt cells and those described here in D_1trisomy, as well as those described by Epstein and Achong (1965) and Epstein *et al.* (1965) in human lymphoblasts in tissue culture are all examples of the same general phenomenon.

The significance and causation of this white cell anomaly is presently unknown. Walzer *et al.* (1966) suggest that it might be due to developmental retardation and quote their finding of a slight increase in the number of nuclear projections in newborn infants as compared with older children. Other workers have also found an increased number of nuclear projections in the white cells of newborn infants (Mutalik & Borgaonkar, 1966). These authors examined some premature infants, but their white cell nuclei did not have a greater number

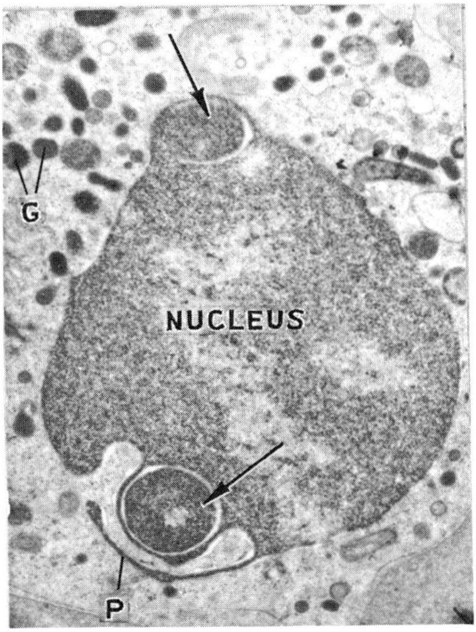

FIGURE 2. Electron micrograph of part of a peripheral blood neutrophil from a two-month-old boy with D_1 (13–15) trisomy. Two sessile nodules are indicated by arrows at the periphery of the nucleus. A pedunculated projection (P) is also shown. Normal specific granules (G) are seen in the cytoplasm (uranyl and lead acetate stain; × 13,000; From Huehns *et al.,* 1964).

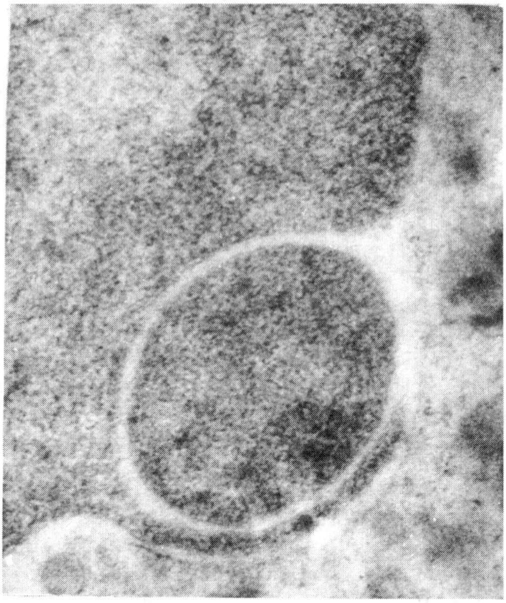

FIGURE 3. Electron micrograph of another sessile nodule at higher magnification (× 50,000; From Huehns *et al.*, 1964).

of projections than were found in the white cells of full-term infants. Further data, such as studies of white cells during fetal life and more detailed electron microscopic studies, are needed before this hypothesis can be accepted. Another group of authors (Snodgrass *et al.*, 1966) has suggested that it may be related to the prominent chromosomal satellites seen in D_1 trisomy, but this explanation appears unlikely.

Acknowledgment

We wish to thank Dr. G. M. Martin for the Feulgen stains.

References

BECKER, A. E. 1965. Lancet **ii:** 911.
BRANDT, N. J., A. FRØLAND, M. MIKKELSEN, A. NIELSEN & N. TOLSTRUP. 1963. Lancet **ii:** 700.
DAVIDSON, W. M. 1961. Brit. Med. Bull. **17:** 190.
DAVIES, H. G. & J. TOOZE. 1964. Nature **203:** 990.
DAVIES, H. G. & J. TOOZE. 1966. J. Cell. Science **1:** 214.
EPSTEIN, M. A. & B. G. ACHONG. 1965. J. Nat. Cancer Inst. **34:** 241.
EPSTEIN, M. A., Y. M. BARR & B. G. ACHONG. 1965. Brit. J. Cancer **19:** 108.
ERKMAN, B., U. BASRUR & P. E. CONEN. 1965. J. Pediat. **67:** 270.
FINE, R. N., M. Y. F. WOO WANG & C. W. HEATH. 1965. Pediatrics **35:** 712.
GRUNER, O. C. 1915–1916. Brit. J. Surg. **3:** 506.
HUEHNS, E. R., F. HECHT, J. V. KEIL & A. G. MOTULSKY. 1964. Proc. Nat. Acad. Sci. USA **51:** 89.
HUEHNS, E. R., F. HECHT & M. LUTZNER. 1964. Lancet **i:** 589.
KAKULAS, B. A. & N. P. ROSMAN. 1965. Lancet **ii:** 717.
LAWLER, S. D., H. E. M. KAY & M. S. C. BIRBECK. 1966. J. Clin. Path. **19:** 214.
LUFT, J. H. 1961. J. Biophys. Biochem. Cytol. **9:** 409.
LUTZNER, M. A. & F. HECHT. 1966. Lab. Invest. **15:** 597.

MÉHES, K. 1966. Blood **28:** 598.
MUTALIK, G. S. & D. S. BORGAONKAR. 1966. Proc. 3rd Int. Congr. Human Genetics. 1966. : 70. Chicago, Ill.
PATAU, K., D. W. SMITH, E. THERMAN, S. L. INHORN & H. P. WAGNER. 1960. Lancet **i:** 790.
POWARS, D. 1964. J. Pediat. **65:** 1089.
POWARS, D., R. ROHDE & D. GRAVES. 1964. Lancet **i:** 1363.
SEMAN, G. 1959. Rev. Hematol. **14:** 409.
SNODGRASS, G. J. A. I., L. J. BUTLER, N. E. FRANCE, L. CROME & A. RUSSEL. 1966. Arch. Dis. Child. **41:** 250.
TAYLOR, A. I. 1966. Lancet **i:** 149.
TRUBOWITZ, S., D. KIRMAN & B. MASEK. 1962. Lancet **ii:** 486.
WALZER, S., P. S. GERALD, G. BREAU, D. O'NEILL & L. K. DIAMOND. 1966. Pediatrics **38:** 419.
YAKOVLEV, P. I. 1959. J. Neuropath. Exp. Neurol. **18:** 22.

THE CHEDIAK-HIGASHI ANOMALY AND THE ALEUTIAN TRAIT IN MINK: HOMOLOGOUS DEFECTS OF LYSOSOMAL STRUCTURE*

D. B. Windhorst,† J. G. White, A. S. Zelickson, C. C. Clawson, P. B. Dent, B. Pollara, and R. A. Good

University of Minnesota Medical School, Minneapolis, Minn.

The Chediak-Higashi syndrome was first described less than 30 years ago and is perhaps one of the most important of genetic diseases for modern cell biology. Beguez-Cesar (1943) and Steinbrinck (1948) published the first case reports, in the Cuban and German literature, respectively, and in 1952 Chediak described the Cuban patients further. Higashi (1954) reported the disease in a Japanese family as well as the results of the first histochemical studies. He appears to have had some inkling of the broad significance of the trait as revealed in his title, "Congenital Gigantism of Peroxidase Granules." Sato (1955), Higashi's mentor, first applied the double eponym by which the trait is most commonly known today.

A mutation producing an unusual blue-gray cast to the coat color of ranch mink was first observed in 1941. Animals manifesting this recessive trait were soon recognized to be highly susceptible to disease and poor breeders, but fortunately, their color rapidly became highly prized enough to justify the increased economic risk to the mink rancher maintaining these animals. It is to this circumstance that we owe the knowledge that the gene acts to dilute all other colors, and that it is probably not an allele at the albino locus (Shackleford, 1950). Alert veterinary scientists related the Aleutian trait to the Chediak-Higashi (CH) trait in 1963 (Leader *et al.*), and this same group has reported detecting the trait in a rare strain of purebred cattle (Padgett *et al.,* 1964).

It has become increasingly certain that the mink trait is homologous to the human anomaly. Both conditions are based on a single autosomal recessive gene. This is clearly demonstrable in the mink, and is a highly reasonable assumption in the human condition. For example, Kritzler *et al.* (1964) found that eight out of 16 sets of phenotypically normal parents were consanguinous, ten out of 19 cases reported were male and 29 out of a total of 69 siblings were affected, including the propositi. Sadan *et al.* (1965) have reported two sibships from consanguinous marriages in a complexly interrelated kinship. They found that assuming the trait to be an autosomal recessive character provided an entirely acceptable pattern of inheritance through six generations involving some 73 persons.

Both the mink and the affected children have similar primary phenotypic manifestations and secondary diseases.

Primary manifestations easily determinable in very young Aleutian mink as well as in infants with the CH trait are the pigmentary dilution and the anomalous "inclusions" in the leukocytes. As seen in peripheral blood smears, the leukocyte cytoplasmic bodies are usually more or less neutrophilic in neutrophils, basophilic in basophils, and eosinophilic in eosinophils. In addition, lymphocytes and monocytes often have one or several large azurophilic

* Aided by grants from the National Foundation, American Cancer Society, and USPHS grants nos. AM-02917, AI-05153, AI-00798, CA-05887, and AE-06314.

† Present address: Department of Medicine, Division of Dermatology, The University of Chicago School of Medicine, Chicago, Ill.

1a

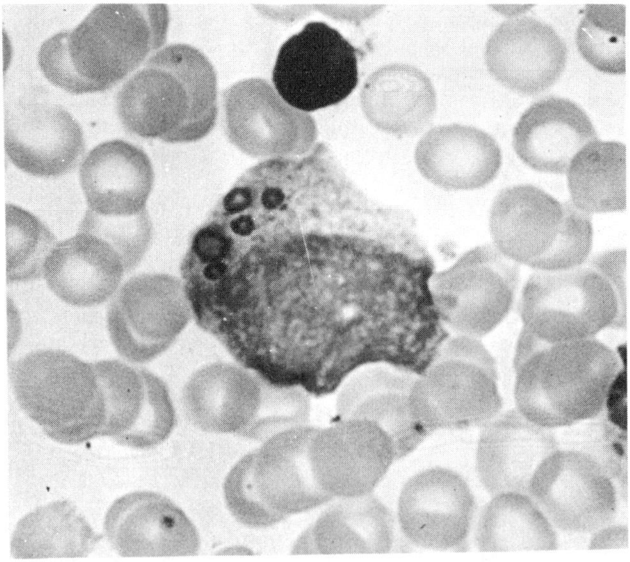

1b

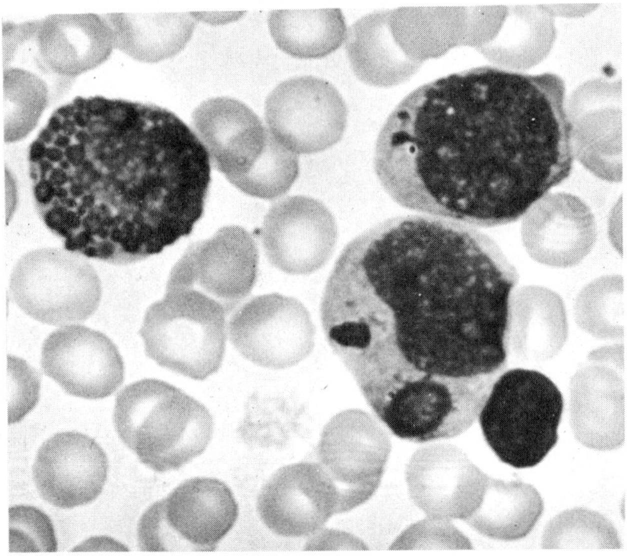

FIGURE 1a. Neutrophil myelocyte from bone marrow of child with the Chediak-Higashi (CH) syndrome. Five massive granulations are apparent in the cell. The small normal sized granules impart a particulate background to the rest of the cell cytoplasm. × 1,466 (orig. mag. × 2,240).

FIGURE 1b. Additional cells from the same sample. The massive size of the particles can be appreciated in the lower of the two myelocytic cells on the right. An eosinophil with giant granules is present on the left side of the illustration. × 1,482 (orig. mag. × 2,280).

granules. The number of cells showing the abnormality may be quite variable, and cells having abnormal granules may also contain many which are normal in size, shape, and staining reactions.

Anomalous granules in the leukocytes and marrow of the affected children have been the subject of extensive investigations. Bessis *et al.* (1961) reported the first electron microscopic studies of leukocytes, and concluded, on the basis of the ultrastructural morphology as well as histochemical examination by light microscopy, that the giant granules result from fusion of substances liberated by the breaking-up of normal granules. They reported similar findings in marrow and emphasized that CH bodies in no way resembled Doehle bodies.

Mauri and Silingardi (1964) reviewed and extended the histochemical observations. Silingardi concluded that the giant granules of the myeloid cells were relatively normal in content, that is, their histochemical properties seem to relate them to the usual granules. The granules in reticulum and lymphoid cells, on the other hand, exhibit staining characteristics unlike those of the myeloid cells, and, according to Mauri, also unlike any normal granulation of the mononuclear cell types. The latter point is difficult to evaluate since

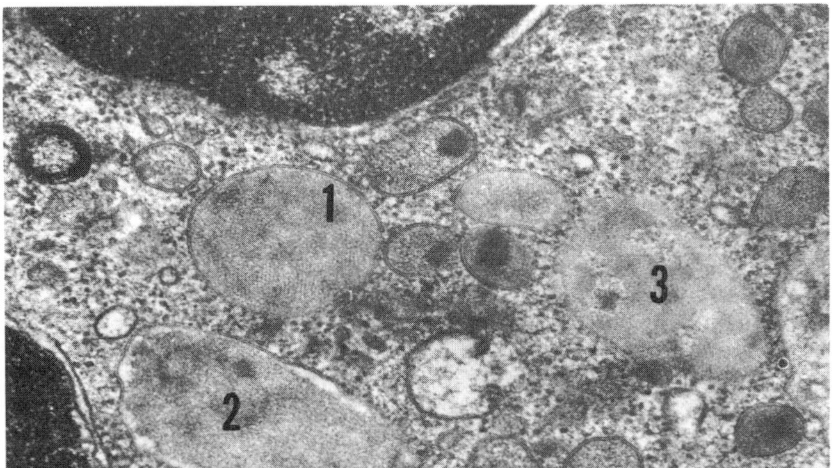

FIGURE 2. Electron micrograph of a CH neutrophil. Four giant granules are marked by numbers. Particle 1 is well preserved, including its laminar internal structure evident in the vertical lines at the lower half of the granule. Particles 2, 3, and 4 are less well preserved, and are probably in early stages of breakdown. The area indicated by arrows is a massive CH granule having a somewhat different internal structure. Normal sized granules are evident between the CH particles. × 46,400 (orig. mag. × 58,000).

"normal" granulations of reticulum and lymphoid cells are not easily seen by light microscopy. In any event, these authors think that the abnormal granules of lymphocytes and monocytes contain ribonucleoproteins, polysaccharides, and lipids in excessive amounts.

Sadan found that even the large granules of the polymorphonuclear cells are histochemically abnormal, since they did not stain for alkaline phosphatase as did the normal granules.

Perhaps the most important finding in the histochemical studies is that the abnormally large granules are variable according to their respective cell lines. This at least suggests that the bulk of the substance of the granules is not a storage material.

Four patients with the CH trait have been studied at the University of Minnesota within the past seven years. Two (JeB and JuB) have been the subject of a previous comprehensive report (Page *et al.*, 1962). They as well as the other two children (L. J. and R. A.) have been the source of information given in various other publications by the authors of this paper (see References). Hematological studies, including ultrastructural examination of peripheral blood and bone marrow (White, 1966a & b; White, 1967) have been compatible with the earlier reports. FIGURE 1 illustrates the appearance of peripheral blood smears and bone marrow in the CH trait, while FIGURES 2–9 are from representative ultrastructural studies.

Leader and his co-workers (1963) studied Aleutian and non-Aleutian mink cells with a battery of histochemical stains. They concluded that there were no

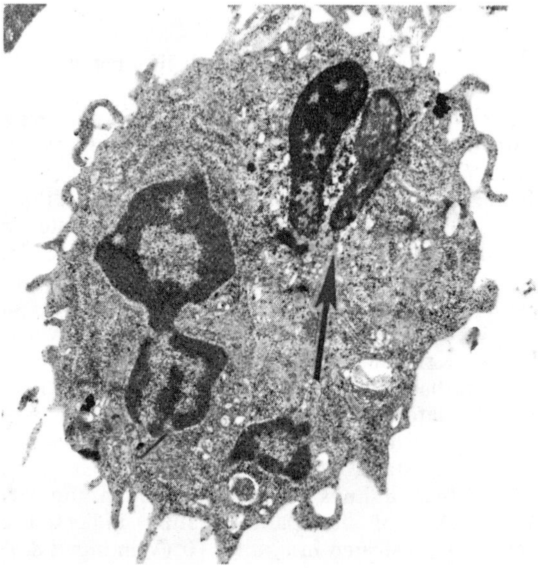

FIGURE 3a. CH neutrophil from peripheral blood sample fixed initially in glutaraldehyde and incubated in modified Gomori media for acid phosphatase activity. Two massive particles (arrows) are specifically stained by the enzyme reaction product, lead phosphate. Note the absence of acid phosphatase activity in normal sized cytoplasmic granules which have been demonstrated histochemically and biochemically to contain this enzyme in previous studies. The giant granules appear to permit penetration of the applied substrate more readily than the normal granules. × 15,800.

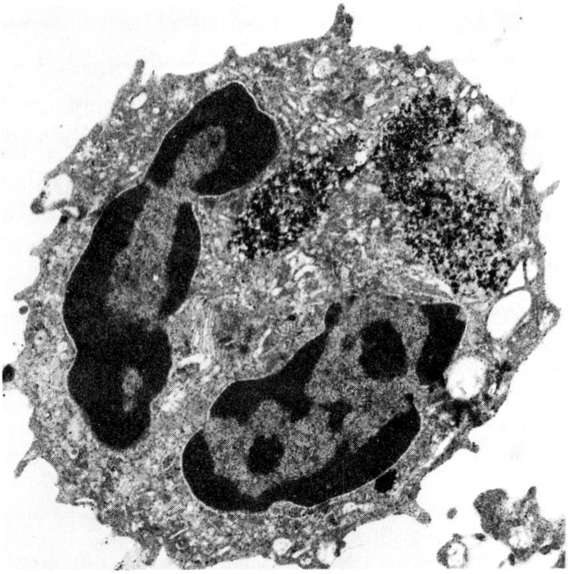

FIGURE 3b. CH neutrophil from the same sample as the cell in 3a. In this example, the enzyme reaction product is deposited in massive CH granules which appear to be in various stages of disintegration. × 13,800.

differences in staining patterns for a given cell line between the giant granules and normal granules from non-Aleutian animals.

Pigmentary findings in mink differing only at Aleutian locus from wild type or "dark" mink include a coat color which is dark gunmetal gray and reduced, but not absent, pigment in the eyes (Shackleford, 1950).

Children with the CH syndrome manifest pigmentary dilution involving the skin, as well as the hair and fundi. There is often associated photophobia and nystagmus. In children born of fair-skinned parents, these findings can easily mimic classical albinism, and thus, the concept of partial albinism has come to be associated with the human CH trait. Darker-skinned parents, however, clearly produce CH children whose pigment is diluted, never absent (Chediak, 1952; Higashi, 1954; Kritzler *et al.,* 1964).

The term albinism has been classically associated with a genetic trait in which the enzymatic defect is expressed as a decreased to absent tyrosinase activity on otherwise normal-appearing melanin granules. This biochemical abnormality is now well established, and the pigment defect it produces has no correlation with the other findings in the CH-Aleutian anomaly. Histochemical examination of the skin of our patient (JuB) indicated the presence of tyrosinase activity, as is illustrated in FIGURE 10 (Windhorst & Zelickson, 1966).

It was the recognition that the CH pigmentary dilution is not albinism which first led us to the hypothesis that the pigmentary change might be related to the leukocyte findings on the basis of abnormally large melanin granules. This proved to be the case (Windhorst *et al.*, 1966). Although many granules which appear normal can be seen, there are numerous giant forms. Melanin, being insoluble and electron-dense, is a "built-in" histochemical marker for tyrosinase activity, and is absent from the granules of melanocytes of classical albinos. Melanin was definitely present in the granules of this child (JuB), although possibly somewhat decreased in amount, considering that her basic coloration was brunette. The presence of the melanin clearly outlines the lamellated substructure of the melanin granules, and it is this feature which provides the strongest evidence that there may be some primary synthesis of giant granules, that is, very large melanin granules are present which appear to have a relatively normally organized substructure (FIGURE 11). As can be seen from the illustrations, there also appears to be some fusion of granules, and further studies in skin and hair of this child have indicated that there may be excessive destruction of melanin granules in structures resembling giant secondary lysosomes (Zelickson *et al.*, 1967) (FIGURE 12). Thus, it seems that the mechanism of formation of giant granules may be quite complex.

The interrelationship of leukocyte granules and melanin granules brought into sharper focus reports of earlier authors (Kritzler *et al.*, 1964; Page *et al.*, 1962) as to the presence of unusual "inclusions" in other cell lines, specifically,

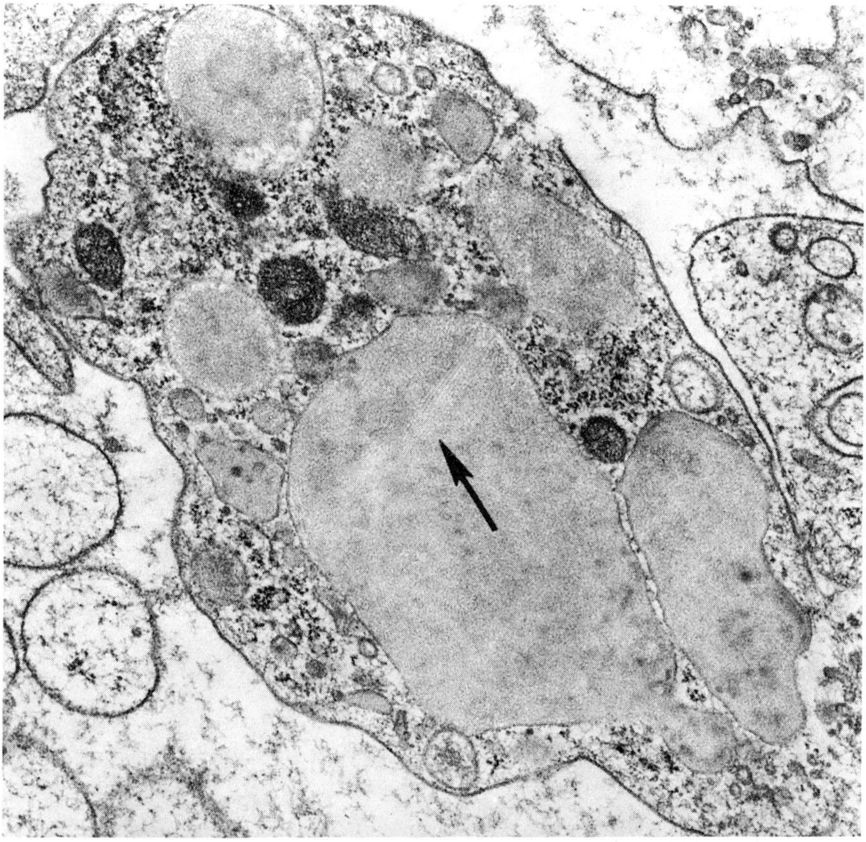

FIGURE 4. Neutrophil myelocyte from CH bone marrow sample. Laminar substructure of one particle is indicated (arrow). × 9,270 (orig. mag. × 10,300).

histiocytes, renal tubular cells, and neurons. The probability that the bodies in the granulocytes were structurally abnormal, but histochemically normal, granules, and the recognition that the melanocyte, a secretory cell, was producing abnormally large melanin granules, gave credence to the possibility that the CH trait is a widespread disease of cytoplasmic organelles of the type that usually have a single limiting membrane.

Independently, in an extensive study, Lutzner and Tierney (1965) and Lutzner *et al.* (1965) produced clear evidence that such is the case for the mink. They found that any tissue which normally produces membrane-limited cytoplasmic organelles may contain abnormally large structures. They examined bone marrow, iris, kidney, spleen, scent gland, pancreas, gastric and duodenal mucosa, pituitary, and liver with the electron microscope (FIGURE 13). Skin and hair were examined by light microscopy. Differences between the melanin granules of the Aleutian and non-Aleutian mink are readily seen with the light microscope and are illustrated here with material from our animals (FIGURE 14).

Various tissues from our patients, when studied with the electron microscope, have contained large cytoplasmic granules. The list of involved cells in human material now includes granulocytes and their precursors, lymphocytes, monocytes, histiocytes, renal tubular cells, neurons, melanocytes, epidermis, Schwann cells (Lockman *et al.*, 1967), and erythroid precursors (FIGURE 7).

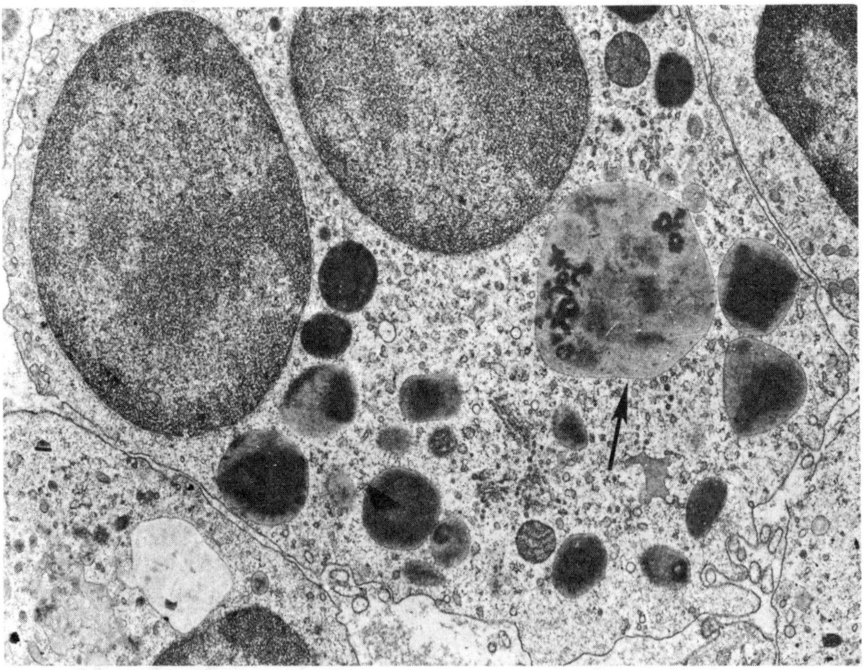

FIGURE 5. Eosinophil from CH bone marrow. The cell contains the usual admixture of normal sized granules and enormous particles characteristic of the CH syndrome. The massive particle indicated contains many peculiar dark structures resembling myelin configuration at high magnification. × 6,525 (orig. mag. × 8,700).

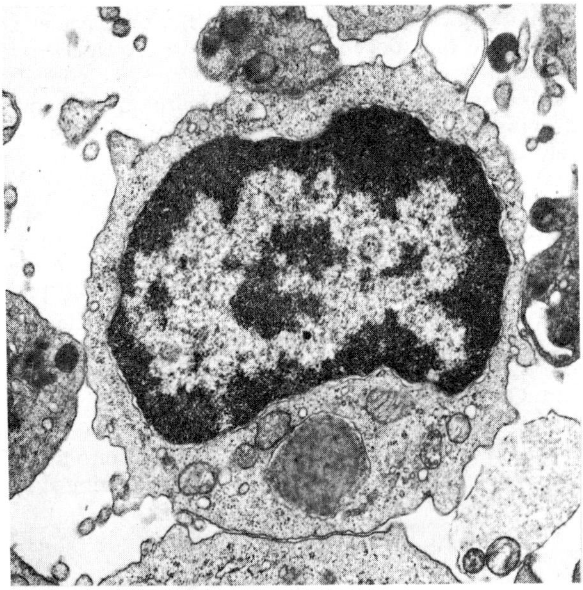

FIGURE 6a. Lymphocyte from CH peripheral blood. A single giant granule is present in its cytoplasm. × 17,750.

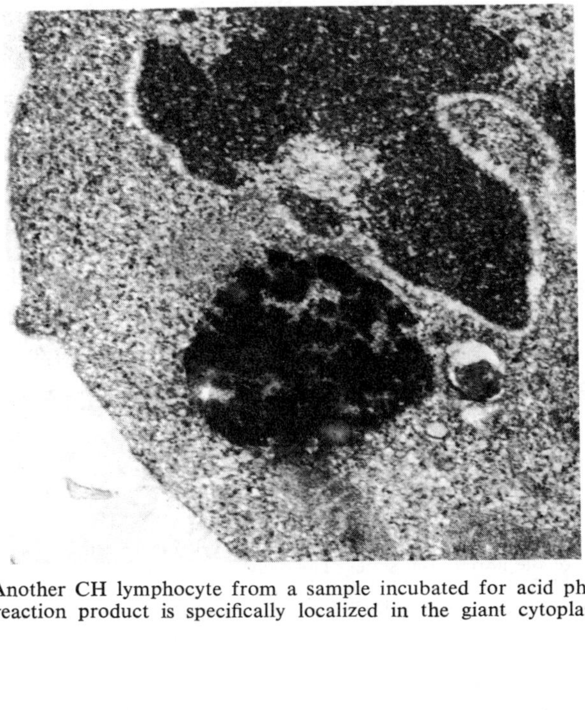

FIGURE 6b. Another CH lymphocyte from a sample incubated for acid phosphatase activity. Enzyme reaction product is specifically localized in the giant cytoplasmic particle. × 34,100.

Thus, the primary phenotypic expression in the two species is not only very similar, but extends to the subcellular level in an extremely extensive manner. The questions posed by this knowledge are indeed exciting: Is this primarily a defect of membrane structure? Is it a failure in a membrane-stabilizing component of cytoplasm? Is the defect genetically coded and operating within each cell—surely it would have to be a very primitive portion of the DNA—or is there a failure of some central control, such as a hormone?

To date, these questions have been examined only in preliminary ways. Most interest has centered around the possibility of defective membrane structure, particularly since several patients have had changes in their serum lipids (Kritzler *et al.*, 1964; Cat *et al.*, 1965; one of our cases). There has been no consistent pattern to these changes, however, and Kritzler found a familial distribution of his patient's abnormal lipid pattern consistent with a separate genetic control.

A. Page and G. A. Padgett (personal communication) have studied the phospholipid metabolism in phagocytizing cells of one patient, mink, and cattle. They found that the cellular incorporation of ^{32}P into the cellular phospholipid fractions was normal in both resting and phagocytizing states.

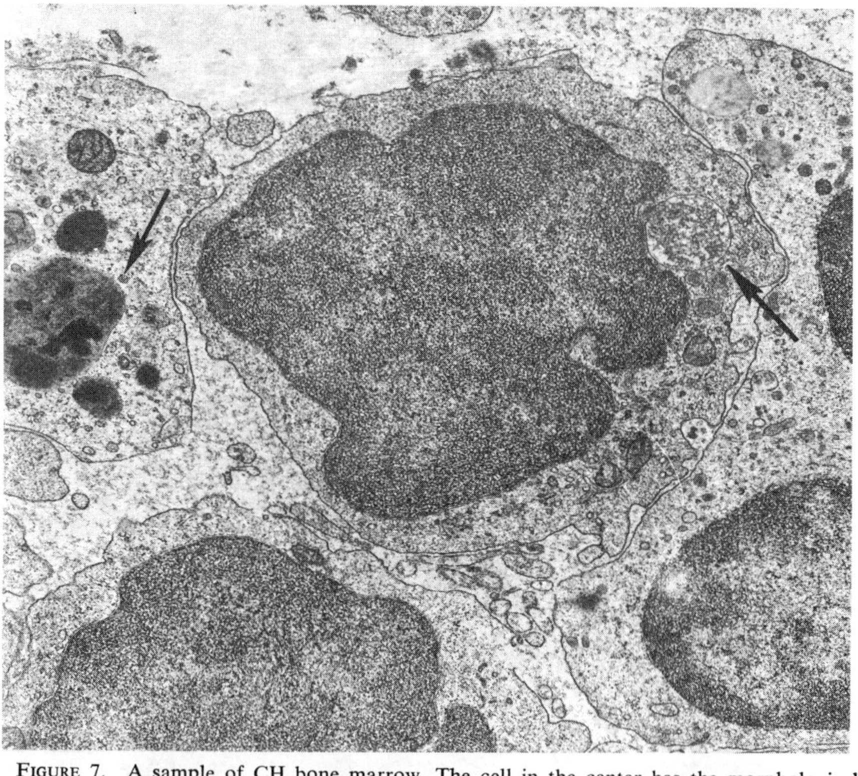

FIGURE 7. A sample of CH bone marrow. The cell in the center has the morphological characteristics of the normoblast series. The arrow indicates a giant granule in its cytoplasm. The cell on the left is an eosinophil with a giant particle (arrow). Anomalous particles have not been previously described in the erythroid series of CH patients. × 8,160 (orig. mag. × 10,200).

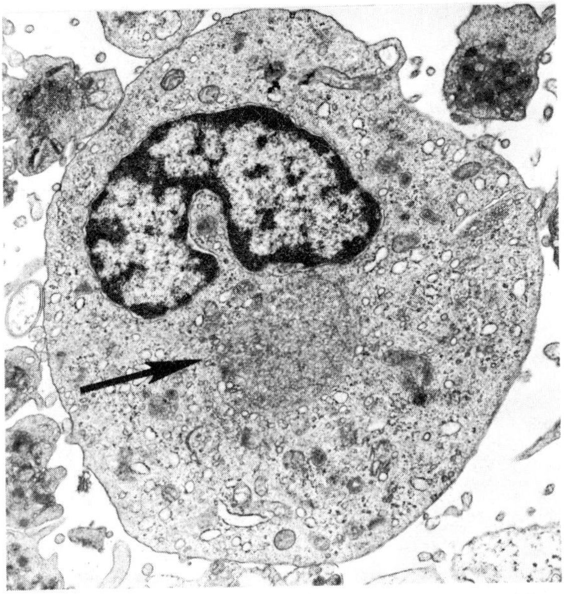

FIGURE 8a. Monocyte from CH peripheral blood. A giant granule forming in the Golgi zone is indicated (arrow). × 21,350.

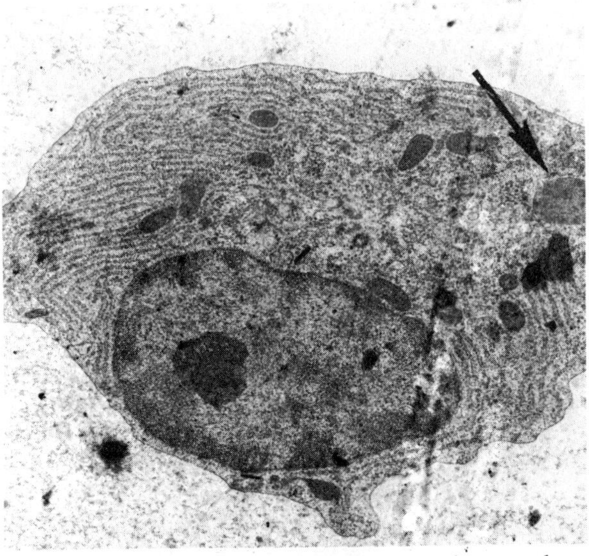

FIGURE 8b. CH plasma cell. The giant particle indicated by the arrow has a laminar substructure when viewed at high magnification. × 38,600.

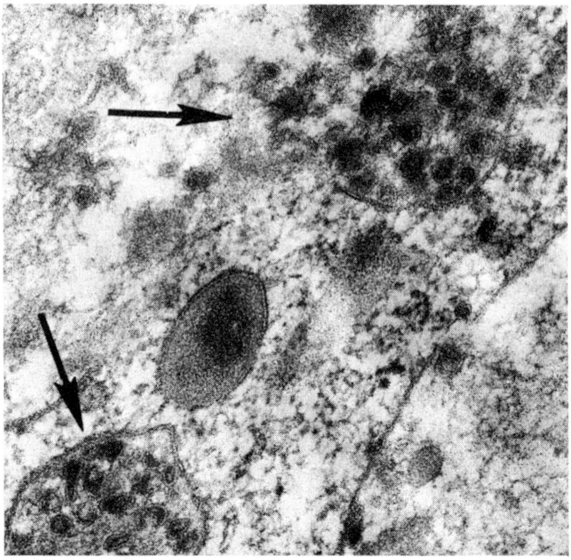

FIGURE 9. Virus-like particles (arrow) in a CH leukocyte. Small particles with dark centers and surrounding pale areas were found in the degenerating CH granules of neutrophils from two patients with the syndrome after development of lymphoreticular malignancy. A normal neutrophilic granule separates the two degenerating pockets containing virus-like particles. × 64,000.

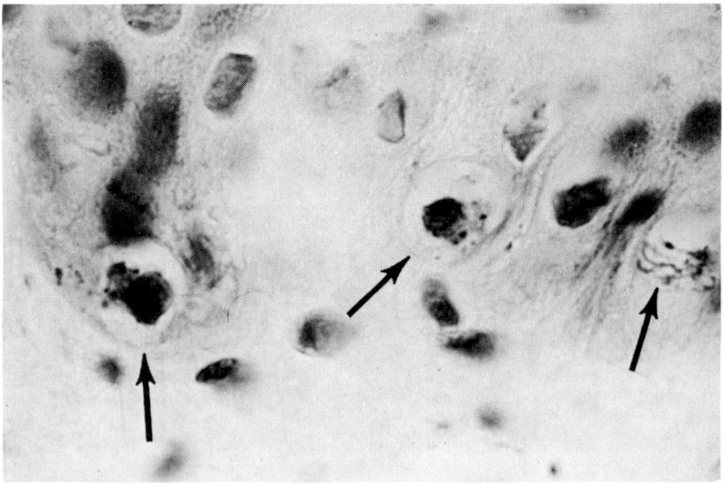

FIGURE 10a. Tyrosinase activity in epidermis of a child with CH syndrome. Several melanocytes (arrows) are seen in which very large melanin granules have formed. The area of skin was exposed to ultraviolet light daily for five days prior to excision of the skin. The tissue was then sectioned in a cryostat and incubated with tyrosine. × 1,000.

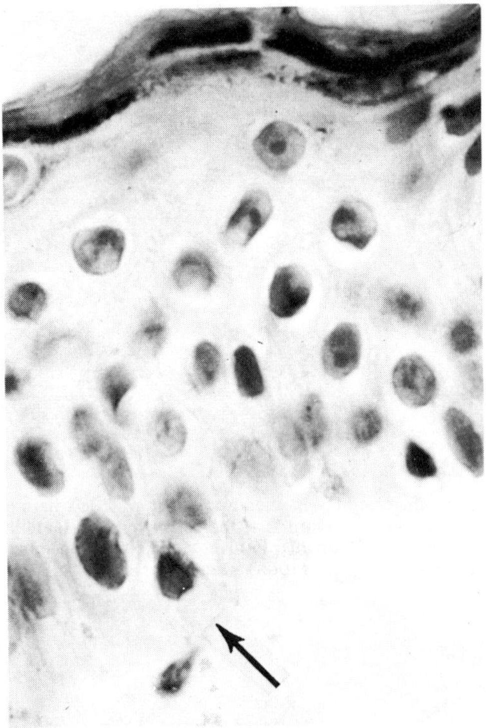

FIGURE 10b. Melanocyte (arrow) and melanin granules from normal skin similarly irradiated and processed. × 1,000.

Page *et al.* (1962) found abnormally low levels of blood 5-hydroxytryptamine in their two patients even after dietary tryptophan loading. Although this seems to be an isolated observation, the interesting suggestion was made that there may be a defective platelet-binding capacity for 5-hydroxytryptamine. This may then come back to membrane structure.

The possibility that the basic defect lies with a central-control mechanism operating to influence cell structure via a humoral factor would appear to have been ruled out by the studies of Dent *et al.* (1966). Cells from one of our patients were maintained in tissue culture for several subcultures extending over a five-month period. These isolated cells continued to show the granular abnormality.

Secondary manifestations of the two traits center around the illnesses to which the CH children and the Aleutian mink are prone. Both are susceptible to infections, and both tend to die at an early age.

The mink are particularly likely to acquire Aleutian mink disease, which has been found to be due to a filterable agent (Henson *et al.*, 1963). This disease, which can affect any strain of mink, produces a hyperglobulinemia associated with a plasma-cell proliferation. Accumulations of plasma cells and lymphocytes occur around vessels, particularly in the liver, spleen, and kidneys. Porter *et al.* (1965) have shown that some chronically infected animals may develop

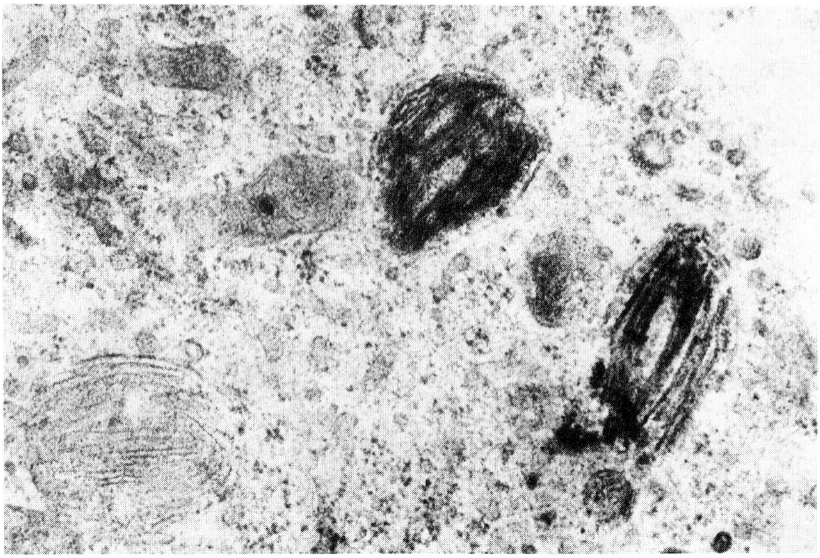

FIGURE 11. Giant melanin granules in melanocyte of plucked hair of child with CH syndrome. Note size relative to the mitochondria, the fairly orderly lamellated substructure, and apparent fusion of two granules at top of picture. × 39,100 (orig. mag. × 46,000). (Reproduced by permission of Windhorst *et al.* (1966) and Science.)

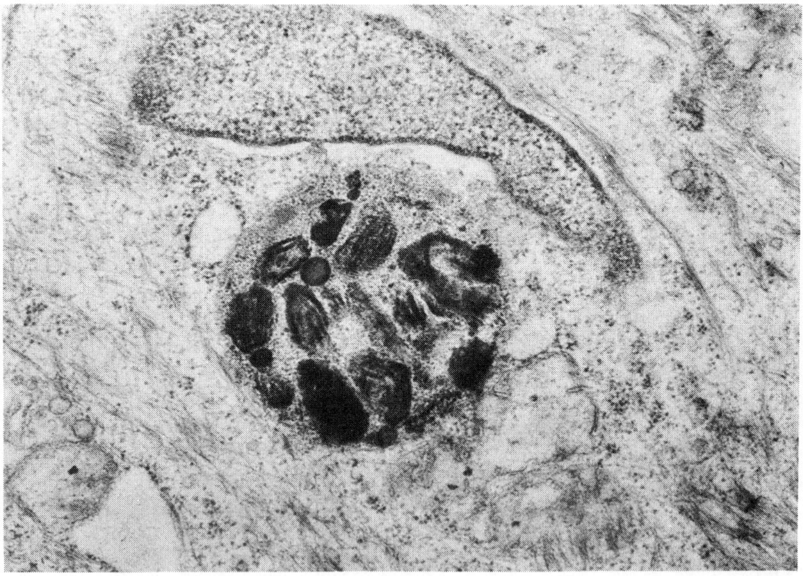

FIGURE 12. Apparent degradation of melanin in epidermal cell of child with CH syndrome. The tonofilaments indicate that this is an epithelial cell rather than a melanocyte. Several mitochondria are present. A very large mass apparently containing many melanin granules in various stages of breakdown is present in the perinuclear area. Similar structures can occasionally be found in normal skin and in phagocytic cells near areas of epidermal disease. × 39,100 (orig. mag. × 46,000).

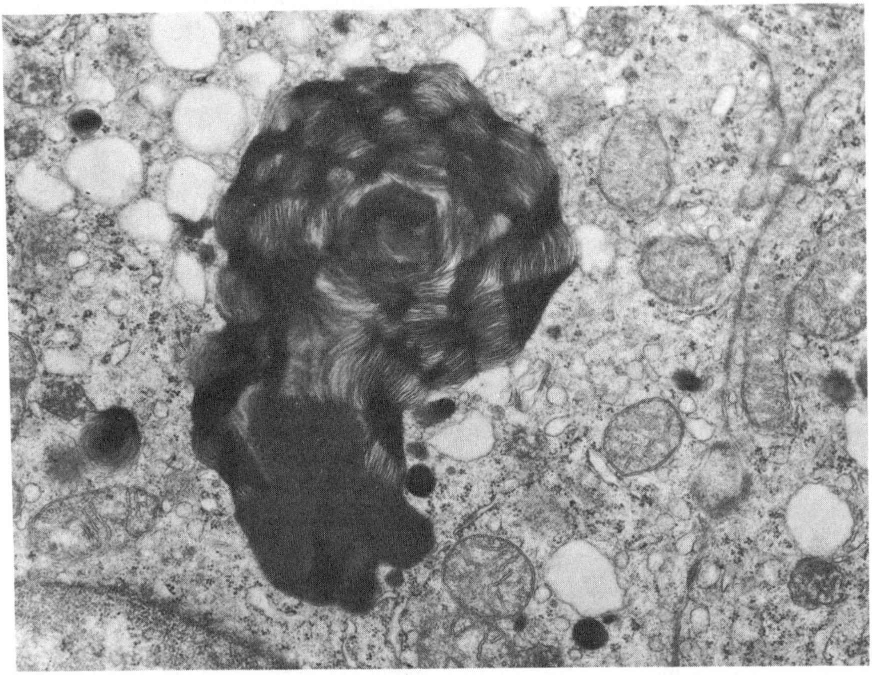

FIGURE 13. Portion of a scent gland cell from an Aleutian mink. Normal-appearing granules are round and composed of concentric membranes. A large inclusion is similarly composed of concentric and lamellar membranes, but has irregular contours and contains homogeneous dense areas. Mitochondria are shown. Approximately × 16,250 (orig. mag. approx. × 25,000). (Reproduced by permission of Lutzner *et al.*, 1966 and Laboratory Investigation.)

a monoclonal hyperglobulinemia reminiscent of that seen in multiple myeloma.

The children may have recurrent ulcerations of the oral mucosa as well as fevers of undetermined origin, pyodermas, and pneumonia (Page *et al.*, 1962; Donahue & Bain, 1957; Efrati & Jonas, 1958), although these latter illnesses are less severe than those in agammaglobulinemic children and children with other forms of immunologic deficiency.

Those children who manage to survive the recurrent infections almost invariably succumb to a fulminant terminal illness that is characterized clinically by fever, anemia, thrombocytopenia, granulocytopenia, hepatosplenomegaly, lymphadenopathy, and in some cases peripheral and central neuropathy. In a number of patients, jaundice is found. Often, the duration of this terminal illness is only a few weeks, and the immediate cause of death is hemorrhage or infection. Temporary remissions have occurred spontaneously (Page *et al.*, 1962) and following splenectomy (Spencer and Hogan, 1960). In one of our cases (Dent *et al.*, 1966), we were able to induce repeated remissions with chemotherapy. The dramatic response (disappearance of jaundice, lymphadenopathy, and peripheral neuropathy), which followed antitumor chemotherapy, has been taken as evidence that death is due to a malignant process rather than to an infectious or allergic phenomenon.

Histological examinations of pre- and postmortem material from these patients have revealed widespread infiltration and destruction of the normal architecture of various tissues by immature lymphoid cells and histiocytes (FIGURE 15). The malignant cell type has been difficult to characterize, a situation analogous to that in Hodgkin's disease. We think, however, that the nature of the infiltrative process is most compatible with a diagnosis of malignant lymphoma.

Recent experimental observations from our laboratory (Dent *et al.,* 1966) have given support to the clinicopathological evidence leading to this conclusion. Spleen cells from a patient dying with the typical lymphoma of CH syndrome were established in tissue culture for five months. During this time they displayed a loss of contact inhibition characteristic of malignant cell growth. These same cells, when transplated to the hamster cheek pouch, produced a transient nodule further reflecting their neoplastic potential.

Electron microscopic studies (White, 1966a) have revealed the presence of virus-like particles (FIGURE 9) within the peripheral leukocytes of two children with the CH lymphoma. One of these children was studied prior to the development of lymphoma and no virus particles were seen at that time. Similarly, no virus particles were present in the leukocytes of a third patient who had not yet developed lymphoma.

It seems, therefore, that in the CH syndrome, the widespread defect in cell granules results in a consistent susceptibility to the development of a viral-associated lymphoma-like condition. In a previous paper (Dent *et al.,* 1966), we have reviewed the relationship of lysosomes, virus infection, and neoplasia, and have attempted to put forward a unified hypothesis explaining the unusual susceptibility to lymphoma in these patients. It is obvious that much remains to be learned about the nature of this malignancy; however, we feel that this genetic abnormality may hold a key to many basic problems in oncogenesis.

These secondary symptoms thus provoke additonal questions: What functional defect or defects lead to the catastrophic events of infectious illnesses, peculiar selective susceptibility to viruses, and malignancy? How does the primary genetic anomaly produce the functional defect?

A number of the children and mink have been examined with various *in vitro* measurements of defense capacity. Saraiva *et al.* (1959), as well as Page and his co-workers (1962), have found a normal capacity to form antibodies in a total of three different patients. Leader *et al.* (1963) reports that mink form neutralizing antibodies against distemper virus in normal amounts and exhibit a normal capacity to become immunized against a challenge of botulism toxin. The children had normal levels of gamma globulins unless afflicted with their fatal illness, in which case hyperglobulinemia was relatively common, a situation reminiscent of the Aleutian disease.

The capacity to develop delayed-type hypersensitivity is apparently adequate in the children. One of our patients had a positive delayed-allergic reaction to mumps antigen. Our patients and Saraiva's patients were clearly able to handle the usual viral diseases of childhood in a normal manner.

Levine *et al.* (1966) have produced experimental allergic encephalomyelitis (EAE) in the Aleutian mink with the same ease as in non-Aleutian strains. Since EAE seems to be primarily based on a cellular hypersensitivity, Levine's work adds additional evidence that delayed hypersensitivity is normal in this trait. Aleutian animals with EAE did not appear more or less severely affected than non-Aleutian mink.

It had naturally been assumed from the earliest studies that the structural

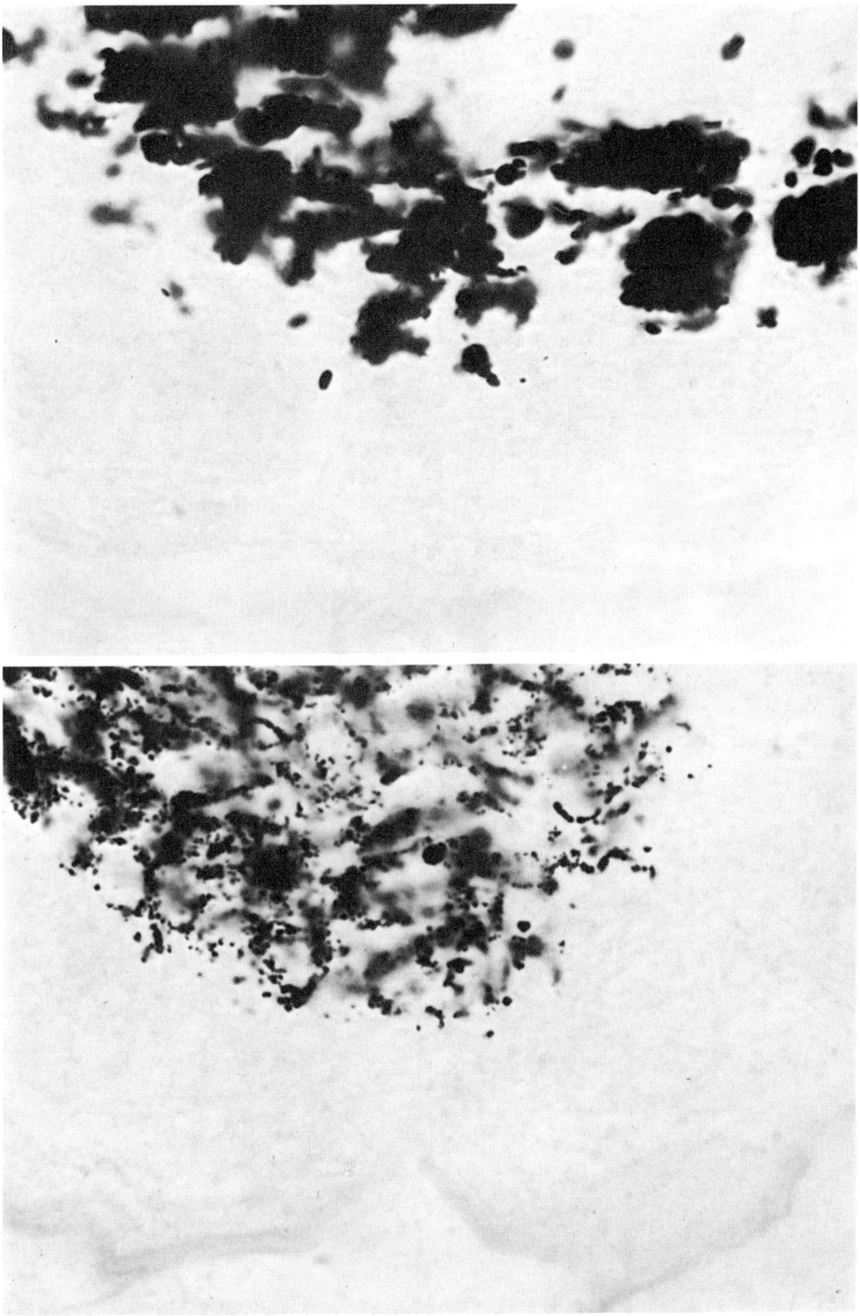

FIGURE 14. Melanin granules in the bulb of mink hair follicles. *Top.* Aleutian mink follicle. *Bottom.* Non-Aleutian mink follicle. The formalin-fixed tissue has been stained by Masson's silver technique. Both approximately × 950 (orig. mag. approx. × 1,000).

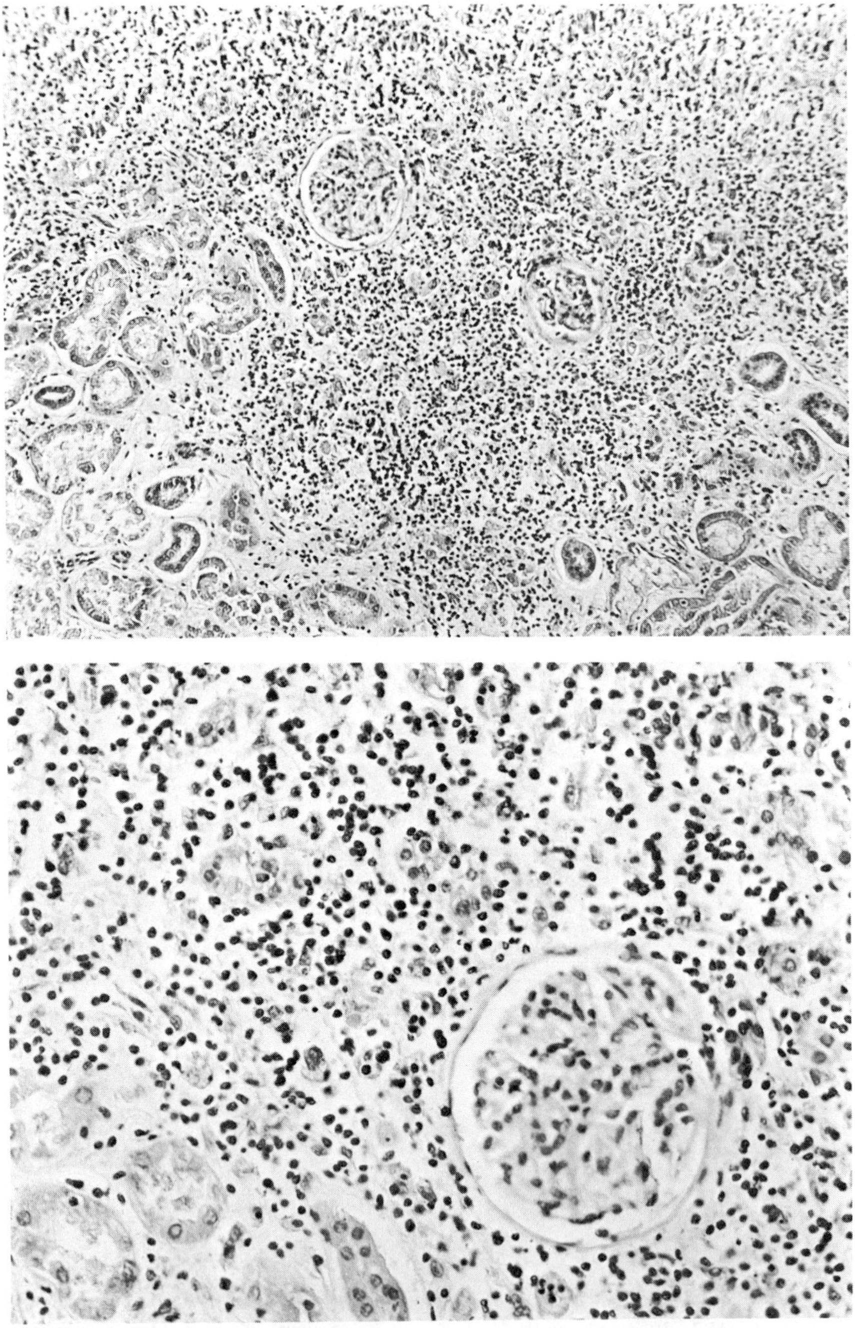

FIGURE 15. Photomicrographs of the kidney of a CH patient (JuB) who died from the associated lymphoma. There is a preponderance of lymphoid cells with scattered large histiocytes. *Top.* × 38 (orig. mag. × 40). *Bottom.* × 327 (orig. mag. × 350).

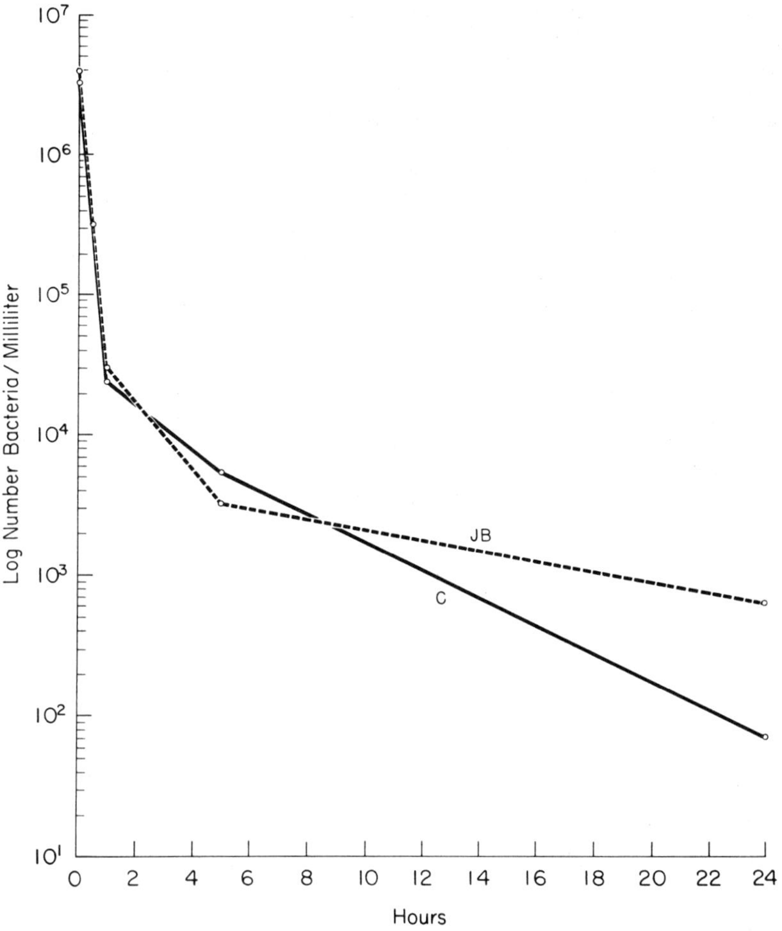

FIGURE 16a. Quantitative measurement of the capacity of isolated leukocytes from a CH patient (JB) to kill bacteria compared with cells from a healthy person (C).

abnormality in the peripheral leukocytes had something to do with the high mortality, and consequently, a number of attempts has been made to demonstrate a functional incapacity of the neutrophils.

Leader *et al.* (1963) states as a preliminary observation that mink exhibit a defective sequence of cell migration in skin-window preparations, and suggests that a "lesser degree of positive chemotaxis is the operating defect in the CH-Aleutian trait." However, normal inflammatory cycles have been repeatedly demonstrated in skin-window preparations of three of our patients (Page *et al.*, 1962 and personal communication).

Page *et al.* (1962) and Saraiva *et al.* (1959) report normal phagocytic capacity in the cells of their patients when measured by observation of uptake of bacteria by neutrophils.

We have compared Aleutian and non-Aleutian mink, as well as Case 2 from the report of Page *et al.* (1962), with a quantitative *in vitro* phagocytosis test.

This test has the demonstrated capacity to measure a defect of neutrophilic function in another hereditary condition (Holmes *et al.*, 1966 and 1968). Although the test not only measures the deficiency of neutrophilic function in patients with fatal granulomatous disease of childhood, but also is sensitive enough to detect the female carriers of this sex-linked trait, we found no abnormality in either the CH child or mink (FIGURES 16 a & b).

To date, established methods of functional examination for defective defense have been unrewarding to the CH trait. We, nonetheless, believe that these patients, with their increased susceptibility to infections and malignancy, lack an important mechanism of bodily defense that must be diligently sought. Of several possible new ways of measuring this particular abnormality of body defense, direct examination of the abnormal granules has offered the most rewarding information.

J. G. White (1966b), using carefully applied ultrastructural histochemical techniques, has clearly shown that the giant granules in the neutrophils of the CH children are positive for acid phosphatase activity. This observation further relates these abnormal granules to the normal neutrophilic granules, which have been shown by Cohn and Hirsch (1960) to be lysosomes in the strictest sense of the word. Further, White's studies indicate that the structure-linked latency of the granules in the abnormal cells is considerably less than that of normal

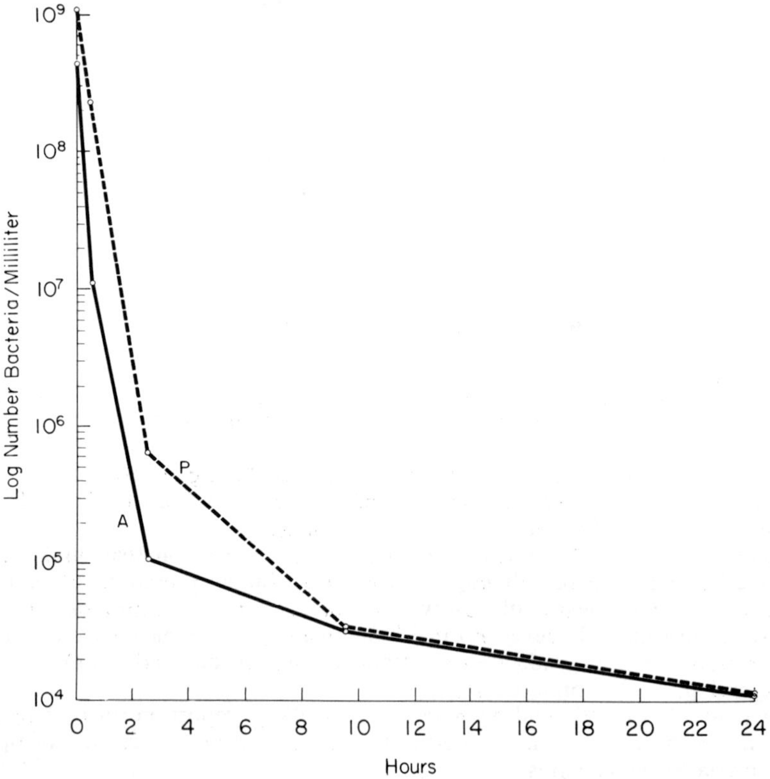

FIGURE 16b. A similar quantitation of Aleutian (A) and non-Aleutian (P) cells. Method of Holmes *et al.* (1966).

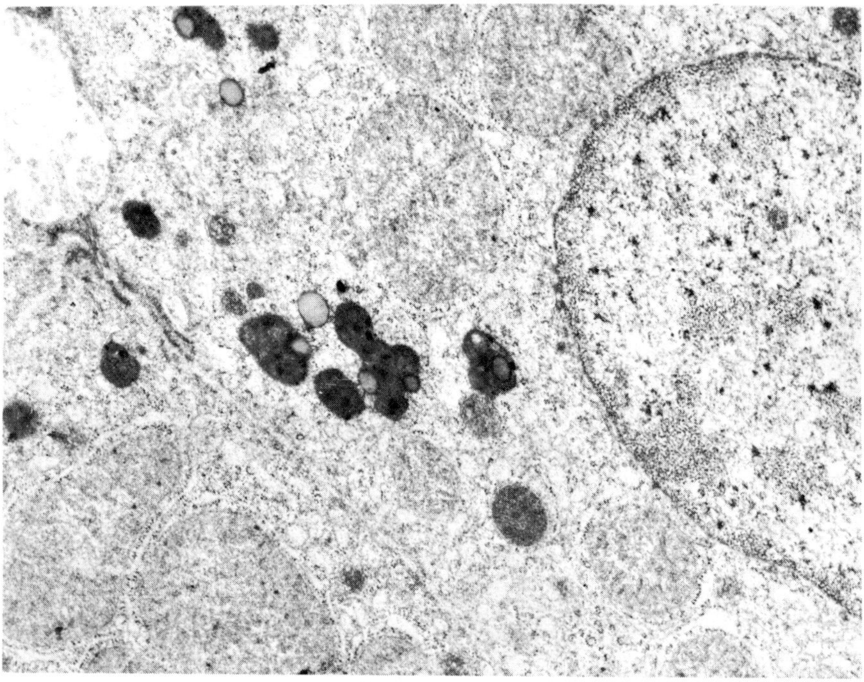

FIGURE 17a. Liver from a normal mink lacking the Aleutian trait. Several densely staining granules are seen within the hepatocyte cytoplasm. These granules are composed of lighter-appearing vesicular areas within a darker matrix of irregular density. The nucleus of the cell lies to the right and a bile canaliculus is in the upper left. Several mitochondria are present which indicate the relative small size of the dense granules. Combined osmic acid and glutaraldehyde fixation. Vestopal® embedding. Uranyl acetate and lead citrate staining. × 14,500.

neutrophils; that is, the enzyme is much more accessible to the applied substrate. The additional finding that numerous leukocytes (mononuclears as well as neutrophils) appear to be demonstrating an excessive amount of tissue sequestering activity has led to the hypothesis that the lysosomal enzymes may, even in the *in vivo* situation, be somehow capable of damaging cytoplasmic structures (White, 1966c). FIGURES 3a & b illustrate the presence of acid phosphatase in the giant neutrophilic granules.

The now classical concept of the lysosome as derived by deDuve has been recently reviewed by him (deDuve and Wattiaux, 1966a). He and his coworkers have demonstrated that the acid hydrolases in the subcellular fractions of liver homogenates can be differentially sedimented in a centrifugal field, separating them from the mitochondrial enzymes. Novikoff's (1963) morphological studies with ultrastructural histochemical methods have correlated and extended the mechanistic understanding of cell function which the lysosome provides.

DeDuve and Baudhuin (1966) have also described still another class of subcellular particles in rat livers. They have termed these newly defined particles "peroxisomes", since they contain primarily peroxidases rather than acid hydrolases. Their work would indicate that, in rat liver at least, peroxisomes are morphologically and functionally distinct from lysosomes. We knew from Higashi's work in 1954 that abnormal leukocyte granules of the CH patients contained peroxidase. We now know that abnormally large CH leukocyte granules also contain an acid hydrolase, acid phosphatase. Normal neutrophilic granules of healthy persons and CH patients also contain these two enzymes. It is unresolved whether, in leukocytes as distinct from rat liver, the two types of enzyme are "packaged" together. Let us say that the possibility that normal neutrophils produce more than one type of cytoplasmic granules is a subject of current interest (Bainton & Farquhar, 1966; Breton-Gorius, 1966).

Although direct biochemical examination of the CH neutrophilic granules would be of great interest, methods for the isolation of neutrophilic lysosomal granules for study of their chemical and physical characteristics are incom-

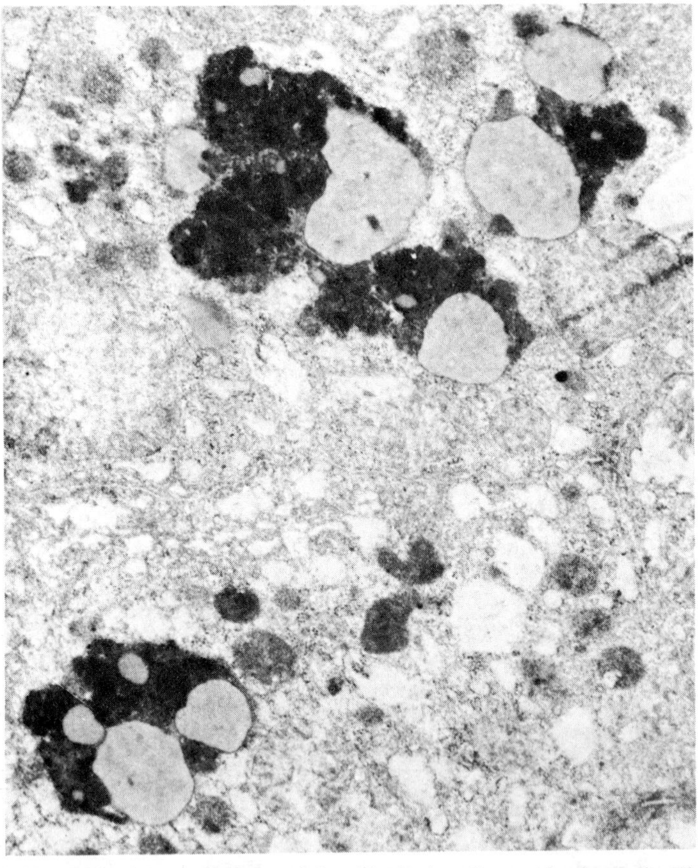

FIGURE 17b. Liver from a healthy mink with the hereditary Aleutian trait. This micrograph, which is the same magnification as FIGURE 17a, shows the large size of the hepatic cytoplasmic granules that are characteristic of the granules found in a variety of cell types in animals homozygous for the Aleutian trait. The visible structural composition of these granules is not essentially different from that seen in the normal non-Aleutian mink liver. Combined osmic acid and glutaraldehyde fixation. Vestopal® embedding. Uranyl acetate and lead citrate staining. × 14,500.

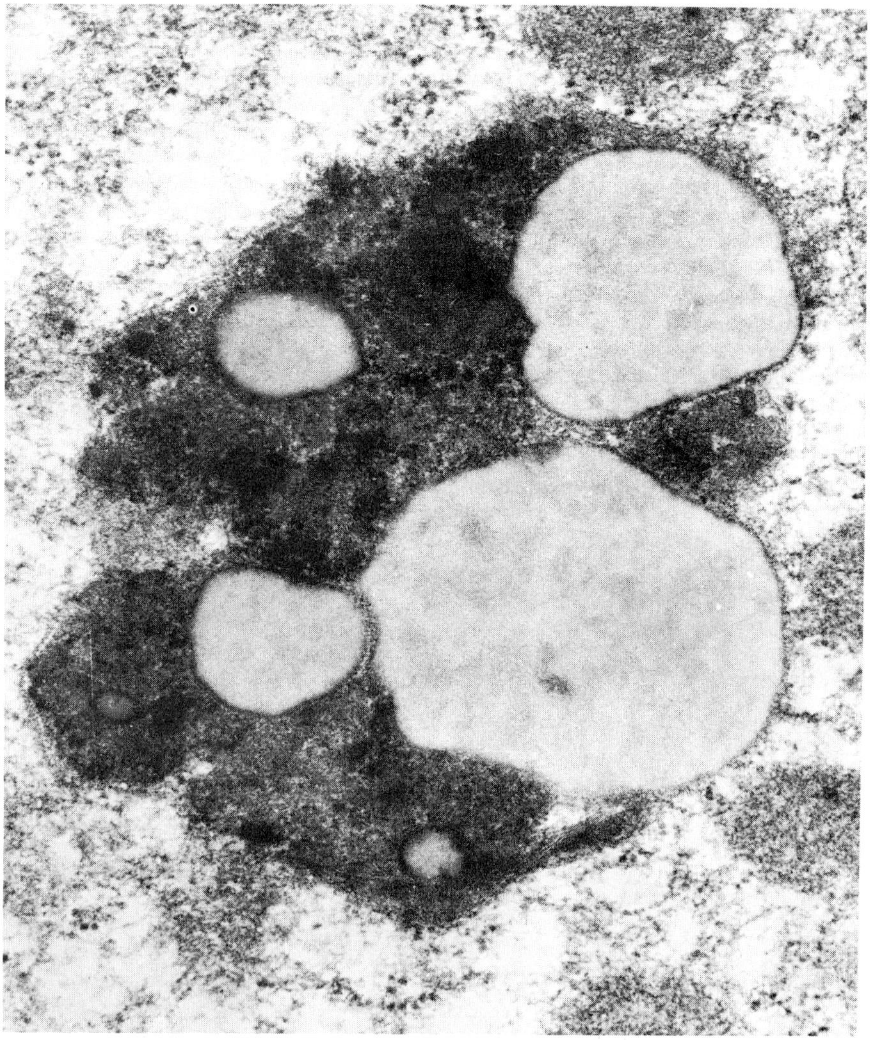

FIGURE 17c. Higher magnification electron micrograph of one of the granules from the hepatocyte of an Aleutian mink. A membrane is visible at several points around the periphery of this large cytoplasmic granule. The granule is composed of several lighter staining regions (which may be individually bound by a membrane) lying in a coarsely granular, densely staining matrix. Combined osmic acid and glutaraldehyde fixation. Vestopal® embedding. Uranyl acetate and lead citrate staining. × 56,000.

pletely developed. Cohn and Hirsch (1960) were able to make their studies in part by using rabbit polymorphonuclear leukocytes which normally have very large stable granules. Meanwhile, it is evident that since the final illness in the children is a lymphocytic and possibly histiocytic process, it is imperative to keep a broad view of the physiological defect. With such considerations in mind, the possibility of examining the defect of lysosomal structure with established techniques of biochemical analysis of subcellular components was explored.

These procedures are best standardized for liver, and livers of Aleutian mink contain abnormally large granules as can be seen in FIGURE 17. Thus, the following studies have been made with Aleutian and non-Aleutian mink livers. Although the complexities of the procedures require that defective and control animals be processed on separate days, each set of animals was kept on the same diet, and all liver homogenizations were performed by the same person (D. W.) in a standardized manner using a motor driven homogenizer of the Potter-Elvejhem type with a Teflon® pestle. All homogenates were subject to 800 x g for ten minutes to remove unbroken cells and nuclei before being used further. The supernatant material from this initial centrifugation (the "postnuclear supernate") was subjected to additional centrifugal procedures and then analyzed for localization of various enzymes characteristic for the cytoplasmic organelles. Because of their particulate nature and density, lysosomes and mitochondria are usually found in that portion of the material which becomes sedimented (the "sedimentable" phase) under certain conditions of centrifugation. The amount of acid phosphatase activity was used to estimate the distribution of lysosomal contents.

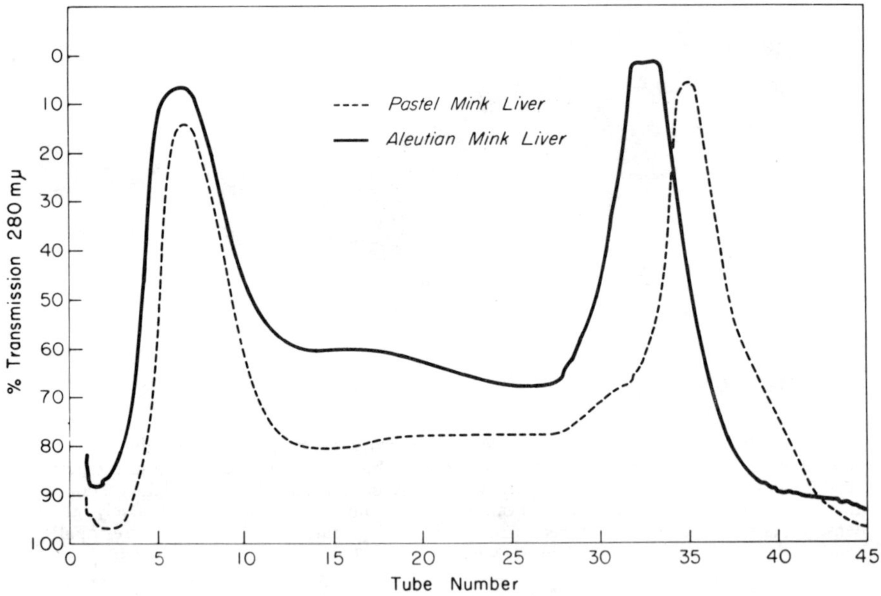

FIGURE 18a. Sucrose density gradient studies (B–IV rotor, zonal ultracentrifuge) of the postnuclear supernate from homogenates of Aleutian and non-Aleutian (Pastel) mink liver. The sucrose gradient was 10–30 percent sucrose linear with volume with a 50 percent cushion. Density increases with tube number. Samples were centrifuged at 20,000 × g for 60 minutes. The graph shows protein distribution as measured by absorption at 280 mμ. The first peak is the soluble phase, and the second peak is known to contain intact particles from the cell cytoplasm such as mitochondria and lysosomes.

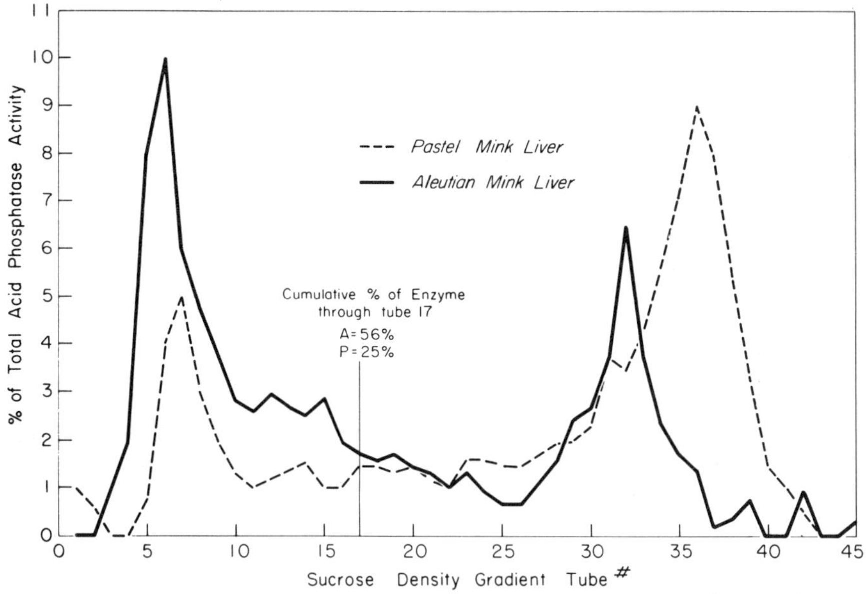

FIGURE 18b. Distribution of acid phosphatase activity (nitrophenyl phosphate technique) expressed as percent of total enzyme activity. Tube 17 was selected to distinguish between a "soluble" vs. "sedimentable" enzyme because of the consistent finding that, under the conditions of the zonal runs, the distribution of the enzyme above and below this area of the gradient was equivalent to the partitioning of enzyme activity when an aliquot of the homogenate was centrifuged in the Sorvall centrifuge at 20,000 × *g* for 20 minutes.

One of the earliest findings was that, compared to control animals, livers of Aleutian mink uniformly yielded less sedimentable acid phosphatase activity (Windhorst, 1966). The actual percent of the enzyme activity in the sedimented phase from the livers of the Aleutian animals was generally less than 40 percent of that total activity of the postnuclear supernatant. Out of five Aleutian animals studied, the range of sedimentable acid phosphatase activity was 15–44 percent. By contrast, the control mink livers had 45–75 percent of the acid phosphatase activity in the sedimented phase. Total acid phosphatase activities per gram of tissue (wet weight) have been widely variable in both types of animals, but generally comparable between the two genotypes.

These findings could indicate that the sedimentation parameters used were inappropriate for the liver lysosomes of mink in general and for Aleutian mink in particular, since we could easily sediment 80–90 percent of the acid phosphatase activity of postnuclear supernates of rat liver, a figure comparable to many others in the literature. It seemed more likely, however, that (1) some factor, possibly the carnivorous diet of mink, affects the capacity of their lysosomal membranes to resist rupture by the homogenization procedure, and that (2) the Aleutian lysosomes were manifesting a profoundly increased susceptibility to the trauma.

Considering the possibility that the abnormal granules might be separable by other centrifugal techniques, we attempted to disperse the cytoplasmic particles in a sucrose density gradient. For this purpose we have used a zonal ultracentrifuge with a B–IV rotor. As described by Anderson (1966), this instrument is designed to separate particulate matter in zone-density gradients set up and withdrawn while the machine is in motion. This instrument offered the opportunity to examine directly the relationship of the solubilization of mink liver lysosomes and their sedimentation properties (FIGURE 18a).

As can be seen on examination of FIGURE 18b, the decrease in Aleutian acid phosphatase activity in the denser area of the gradient is clearly related to a marked increase in enzyme activity in the portion of the gradient which contains cellular components in soluble form. By contrast, the non-Aleutian animal shows considerably less enzyme activity in the soluble area of a comparable gradient.

When the same gradients were examined for uricase activity, similar results were evident, as was true for malic dehydrogenase (FIGURES 18c & d). Uricase is considered to be an enzyme marker for peroxisomes in rat livers, although the presence of peroxisomes in mink liver is unproven. Malic dehydrogenase is principally associated with mitochondria.

An attractive hypothesis to explain the possible involvement of three subcellular structures in the measurable defect would be that they all possess

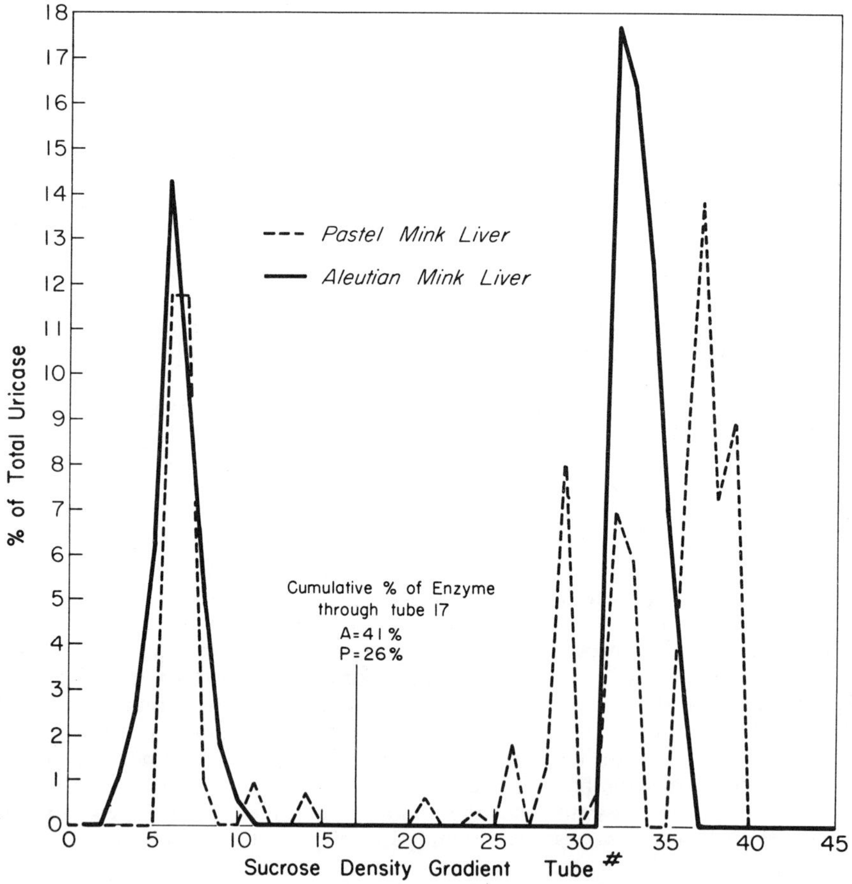

FIGURE 18c. Distribution of uricase activity.

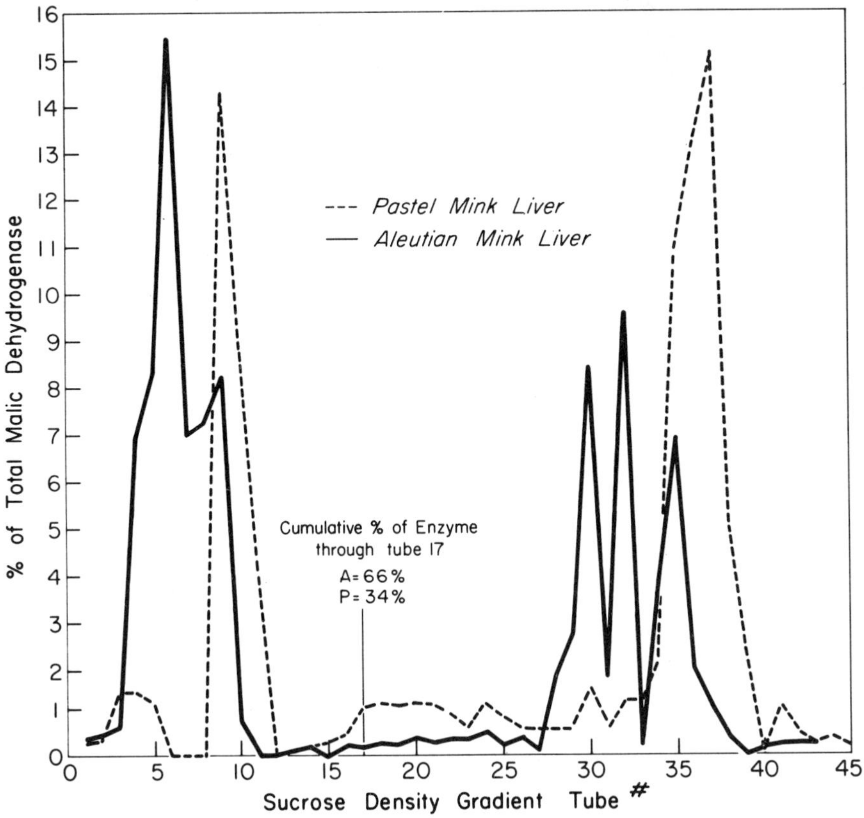

FIGURE 18d. The pattern of malic dehydrogenase activity.

abnormal membranes. This concept has two serious disadvantages, namely, the divergent structure and origin of mitochondria and the lack of morphological evidence of their participation in the CH trait. Possibly, common structural units exist for all membranes or, conjecturally, membranes surrounded by cytoplasm may depend on a stabilizing substance from the cytoplasm for maintenance of their physical integrity.

Such speculation might be more productive if one could relate it to other known features of the CH trait. DeDuve and Wattiaux, in reviewing and discussing the known and hypothetical functions of lysosomes (1966), have developed a concept of dynamic equilibrium for the primary lysosomes, phagocytic vacuoles, and sequestered areas of cytoplasm being digested for reasons of cell differentiation or reconstruction. These structures are regarded as being in constant interaction with each other (the "vacuolar apparatus") with the net result being that most acid-hydrolase-containing structures of liver will, at any one time, be secondary lysosomes. If an animal is manipulated to stimulate its liver to increase uptake of extracellular material or increase autophagic activity, lysosomal enzymes will be found uniformly distributed within all particles except peroxisomes and mitochondria after relatively short periods of time. In addition, such liver will demonstrate an increased fragility of the secondary lysosomes on homogenization. DeDuve and Wattiaux (1966) also suggest that in some situations of increased demand, lysosomal enzymes may not "keep up" with all of the substrates presented to them, and there will be a net accumulation of undigested material occurring in secondary lysosomes and residual bodies.

With these considerations in mind, it would seem feasible to suppose that the apparently increased destruction of melanin granules by epidermal cells (FIGURE 12) and the cytosegregation in the leukocytes of the children with CH disease may also be occurring in the mink livers. One can then suggest that the involvement of peroxisomal and mitochondrial enzymes in the measurable biochemical abnormality is a result of their passive inclusion in excessive autophagic activity and subsequent accumulation in secondary lysosomes.

This hypothesis does not offer an explanation for the presumed excessive autophagy. Theoretically, something is operating to denature cytoplasmic constituents or to produce random cytoplasmic segregation at a greater than usual rate. In searching for the mechanism for this postulated process, it is necessary to remember that the secondary lysosomes are larger than normal, and that the melanin granules are evidently synthesized in their primary form as particles larger than normal. The possibility that the primary membrane structure of lysosomes, melanin granules, and organelles of other cell lines is abnormal thus remains an attractive possibility.

The work reported here is barely begun. In particular, there are a number of approaches that can be made with the mink liver lysosome system–different methods of cell ruptures to try, more enzymes to examine, and different gradients to be used with a view to defining the physical properties of the abnormal granules. In addition, extensive ultrastructural studies of mink livers are in order. In fact, a great deal of morphology remains to be worked out. Further, several vital clinical questions remain unanswered. Is the anemia and thrombocytopenia of CH children a consequence of the malignancy or of primary defects in the erythrocyte and platelet cell lines? And, knowing that secretory granules are involved in mink, what are the secretory capacities of both exocrine and endocrine glands of the children? The primary question seems to be this: What is the molecular basis for this defect which seems to affect cells in the very organelles which express their specific identity?

In summary, the Chediak-Higashi-Aleutian anomaly is an autosomal recessive trait which produces gigantic abnormalities of unit-membrane-limited organelles in every tissue so far examined. The phenotypic manifestations are pigmentary dilution and giant granules in leukocytes. Secondarily, but quite uniformly, the mink and the children demonstrate an unusual defective defense against infections and malignancy which is not measurable by any known parameter of innate or acquired immunity.

Our studies indicate that: (1) there may be a primary failure in a mechanism controlling size in the process of granule synthesis as revealed by the abnormally large melanin granules; (2) there is quite probably abnormal fusion of granules, possibly increased membrane permeability leading to release of damaging enzymes, and increased tissue turnover in relation to excessive production of cytosegresomes or autophagic structures; (3) the defect can be partially quantitated by biochemical study of mink liver homogenates; (4) the findings in the livers are compatible with the concept of an increased distribution of lysosomal enzymes within a hyperactive vacuolar apparatus that appears to be more susceptible to damage from homogenization than lysosomes from livers of normal animals; and (5) enzymes commonly associated with mitochondria and peroxisomes are more easily released in the homogenization of Aleutian liver, as compared to the homogenization of non-Aleutian liver.

Acknowledgments

Most of the mink in this work were graciously donated by mink farmers of the state of Minnesota, to whom we are most grateful.

References

ANDERSON, N. G. 1966. Zonal centrifuges and other separation systems. Science **154:** 103.

BAINTON, D. F. & M. G. FARQUHAR. 1966. Origin of granules in polymorphonuclear leukocytes. J. Cell Biol. **28:** 277.

BEGUEZ-CESAR, A. 1943. Neutropenia cronica maligna familiar con granulaciones atipicas de los leucocitos. Bol. Soc. Cub. Ped. **15:** 900.

BESSIS, M., J. BERNARD & M. SELIGMAN. 1961. Etude Cytologique d'un cas de maladie de Chediak. Nouv. Rev. Franc. Hemat. **1:** 422.

BRETON-GORIUS, J. 1966. Structures périodiques dans les granulations éosinophiles et neutrophiles des leucocytes polynucléaires du sang de l'homme. Nouv. Rev. Franc. Hemat. **6:** **195.**

CAT, I., L. P. MARINONI, D. J. GIRALDI, M. B. ALMEIDA, A. S. NETO, H. BRAGA & A. Q. DA SILVA. 1965. Chediak-Higashi syndrome with familial idiopathic hyperlipemia. Letter to the Editor. Lancet **i:** 1398.

CHEDIAK, M. 1952. Nouvelle anomalie leucocytaire de acracère constitutional et familial. Rev. Hemat. **7:** 362.

COHN, Z. A. & J. G. HIRSCH. 1960. The isolation and properties of the specific cytoplasmic granules of rabbit polymorphonuclear leucocytes. J. Exp. Med. **112:** 983.

DEDUVE, C. & P. BAUDHUIN. 1966. Peroxisomes (microbodies and related particles). Physiol. Rev. **46:** 323.

DEDUVE, C. & R. WATTIAUX. 1966. Functions of lysosomes. Ann. Rev. Physiol. **28:** 435.

DENT, P. B., L. A. FISH, J. G. WHITE & R. A. GOOD. 1966. Chediak-Higashi syndrome: Observations on the nature of the associated malignancy. Lab. Inves. **15:** 1634.

DONAHUE, W. L. & H. W. BAIN. 1957. Chediak-Higashi syndrome–A lethal familial disease with anomalous inclusions in the leucocytes and constitutional stigmata–Report of a case with necropsy. Pediatrics **20:** 416.

EFRATI, P. & W. JONAS. 1958. Chediak's anomaly of leukocytes in maligiant lymphoma associated with leukemic manifestations: Case report with necropsy. Blood **13:** 1063.

HENSEN, J. B., J. R. GORHAM & R. W. LEADER. 1963. The familial occurrence of hypergammaglobulinemia in mink. Texas Rep. Biol. Med. **21:** 37.

HIGASHI, O. 1954. Congenital gigantism of peroxidase granules. Tohoku J. Exp. Med. **59:** 315.

HOLMES, B., A. R. PAGE, D. B. WINDHORST, P. G. QUIE, J. G. WHITE & R. A. GOOD. 1968. The metabolic pattern and phagocytic function of leukocytes from children with chronic granulomatous disease. This monograph.

HOLMES, B., P. G. QUIE, D. B. WINDHORST & A. A. GOOD. 1966. Fatal granulomatous disease of childhood–An inborn abnormality of phagocytic function. Lancet **i:** 1225.

KRITZLER, R. A., J. Y. TERNER, J. LINDENBAUM, J. MAGIDSON, R. WILLIAMS, R. PREISIG & G. B. PHILLIPS. 1964. Chediak-Higashi syndrome–cytologic and serum lipid observations in a case and family. Amer. J. Medicine **36:** 583.

LEADER, R. W., G. A. PADGETT & J. R. GORHAM. 1963. Studies of abnormal leukocyte bodies in the mink. Blood **22:** 477.

LEVINE, S., G. A. PADGETT & R. W. LEADER. 1966. Allergic encephalomyelitis in Chediak-Higashi mink. Arch. Path. **82:** 234.

LOCKMAN, L. A., W. A. KENNEDY & J. G. WHITE. 1967. The Chediak-Higashi syndrome: Electrophysiologic and electron microscopic observations on the peripheral neuropathy. J. of Pediat. **70:** 942.

LUTZNER, M. A. & J. H. TIERNEY. 1965. Electron microscopic study of widespread cytoplasmic inclusions in a genetic syndrome of Aleutian mink. Fed. Proc. **24:** 429.

LUTZNER, M. A., J. H. TIERNEY & E. P. BENDITT. 1965. Giant granules and widespread cytoplasmic inclusions in a genetic syndrome of Aleutian mink. Lab. Invest. **14:** 2063.

MAURI, C. & V. SILINGARDI. 1964. A cytological and cytochemical study of Chediak's leukocytic anomaly. Acta Haemat. **32:** 114.

NOVIKOFF, A. B. 1963. *In* Lysosomes–Ciba foundation symposium. A. V. S. deReuck & M. P. Cameron, Eds. : 36–63. Little, Brown, & Co. Boston, Mass.

PADGETT, G. A., R. W. LEADER, J. R. GORHAM & C. C. O'MARY. 1964. The familial occurrence of the Chediak-Higashi syndrome in mink and cattle. Genetics **49:** 505.

PAGE, A. R., H. BERENDES, J. WARNER, & R. A. GOOD. 1962. The Chediak-Higashi syndrome. Blood **20:** 330.

PORTER, D. D., F. J. DIXON, & A. E. LARSEN. 1965. The development of a myeloma-like condition in mink with Aleutian disease. Blood **25:** 736.

SADAN, N., D. YAFFEE, L. ROZENSZAJN, H. ADAR, B. SOROKER & P. EFRATI. 1965. Cytochemical and genetic studies in four cases of Chediak-Higashi-Steinbrinck syndrome. Acta Haemat. **34:** 20.

SARAIVA, L. G., M. AZEVEDO, J. M. CORREA, G. CARVALHO & J. D. PROSPERO. 1959. Anomalous panleukocytic granulation. Blood **14:** 1112.

SATO, A. 1955. Chediak and Higashi's disease. Tohoku J. Exp. Med. **61:** 201.

SHACKLEFORD, R. M. 1950. Genetics of the ranch mink. Pillsbury publishers. N. Y.

SPENCER, W. H. & M. J. HOGAN. 1960. Ocular manifestations of Chediak-Higashi syndrome. Amer. J. Opthal. **50:** 1197.

STEINBRINCK, W. 1948. Uber eine neue granulations–anomalie der leukocyten. Deutsch. Arch. Klin. Med. **193:** 577.

WHITE, J. G. 1966a. Virus-like particles in the peripheral blood cells of two patients with Chediak-Higashi syndrome. Cancer **19:** 877.

WHITE, J. G. 1966b. The Chediak-Higashi syndrome: A possible lysosomal disease. Blood **28:** 143.

WHITE, J. G. 1967. The Chediak-Higashi syndrome: Cytoplasmic sequestration in circulating leukocytes. Blood **29:** 435.

WINDHORST, D. B. 1966. Studies on a hereditary defect involving lysosomal structure. Fed. Proc. **25:** 358.

WINDHORST, D. B. & A. S. ZELICKSON. 1966. The pigmentary anomaly of the Chediak-Higashi syndrome. Clin. Res. **14:** 276.

WINDHORST, D. B., A. S. ZELICKSON & R. A. GOOD. 1966. Chediak-Higashi syndrome: Hereditary gigantism of cytoplasmic organelles. Science **151:** 81.

ZELICKSON, A. S., D. B. WINDHORST, J. G. WHITE & R. A. GOOD. 1967. The Chediak-Higashi syndrome: Formation of giant melanosomes and the basis of hypopigmentation. J. Invest. Derm. **49:** 575.

MORPHOLOGY OF LEUKOCYTIC HYPERGRANULATION IN BATTEN'S DISEASE*

Sheila Donahue, Itaru Watanabe, and Wolfgang Zeman

Section of Neuropathology, Indiana University Medical Center Indianapolis, Ind.

Introduction

While studying lymphocytic vacuolization in patients with Spielmeyer-Vogt disease, Strouth[1] noticed a peculiar, hitherto undescribed azurophilic granulation of the polymorphonuclear cells. Because some of the patients were in a state of decortication with respiratory and urinary infections, the question of toxic granulations naturally arose. This possibility was quickly eliminated since the granules, unlike toxic granulations, could not be clearly visualized in supravital stains.

Occasional failures in reproducing the findings made standardization of the staining technique mandatory. Moreover, proper evaluation of the preparations seemed to require the blood films to consist of single cell layers with optimal spread of the leukocytes. This is assured by drawing out a few cubic millimeters of blood between two chemically cleaned coverslips. Only the initially discharged blood can be utilized, because later samples contain abundant fibrin and platelets, which interfere with the staining reaction and the spreading of leukocytes. The films are air-dried; fixed in absolute methanol for three minutes; air-dried again; and stained for one hour in a Giemsa solution (Harleco), 1 drop per ml of distilled water adjusted to pH 6.5 with 0.1 M phosphate buffer of pH 7.4. The coverslips are washed in three changes of distilled water, air-dried, and mounted in Permount®. With this technique, the abnormal granules appear as clearly defined azurophilic dots measuring from 0.2 μ to about 0.5 μ in diameter. They are distinguished from normal neutrophilic granulations by larger size, sharper definition, and intense azurophilia. These characteristics are important because the method described here stains neutrophilic granules more clearly and in greater numbers than do ordinary Giemsa or Wright stains.

In order to test the pathognomonic specificity of the finding, a large number of control smears, both from healthy persons and from children with other neurological diseases, were examined, using the standardized technique. This study revealed a small number of hypergranulated leukocytes in many normal individuals. Furthermore, the size and number of granules varied from one cell to another, both in controls and in patients with Spielmeyer-Vogt disease. These observations required a quantitative approach; neutrophils were arbitrarily graded (FIGURE 1), and 200 granulocytes were differentially counted. Only well-spread, undamaged cells were scored. This approach established that normal individuals do not have more than 15 percent hypergranulated neutrophils of grade 2+ and none of grade 3+.[2]

Not having had personal experience with the Alder anomaly,[3] we felt it necessary to examine smears from patients with gargoylism, a condition in which this anomaly has been repeatedly reported. Films from five patients were available, but only one had the Alder anomaly. The Alder granules were distinctly different from the findings described here, since they were frequently

* This study was supported in part by USPHS grant no. NB 4607.

of a size greater by one order of magnitude and also occurred in monocytic elements.

Because of the traditional concept that Spielmeyer-Vogt disease is an age-dependent variant of familial amaurotic idiocy,[4] an effort was made to study the blood of patients with the Tay-Sachs type and with the so-called late infantile form of Bielschowsky-Jansky. These experiments revealed azurophilic hypergranulations to be very frequent in patients with Spielmeyer-Vogt disease and with late infantile amaurotic idiocy. A basophilic hypergranulation with fewer, larger, and focally distributed granules was observed in three out of six patients with Tay-Sachs disease.[2] Only in one patient were the findings so similar to the azurophilic hypergranulation that they defied differentiation.

The apparent specificity of the azurophilic hypergranulation supports our previous concept on the nosology of amaurotic familial idiocy. The traditional classification of this group is entirely at variance not only with genetic data, but also with our histochemical, morphological and ultrastructural observations on 12 brain biopsies.[5] We suggest the classification in TABLE 1.

The Table shows that cases diagnosed as "late infantile amaurotic idiocy" are either instances of Batten's disease or constitute different entities characterized

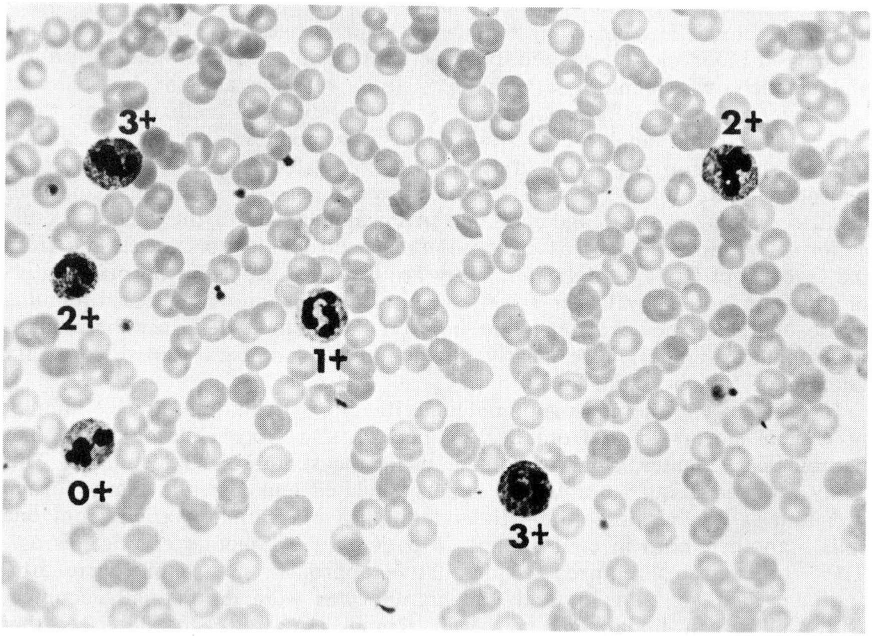

FIGURE 1.
0+ = no abnormal granules
1+ = several dozen weakly stained, definitely abnormal granules seen at about 1,000 times magnification
2+ = several dozen deeply staining granules conspicuous at 400 times magnification
3+ = the cytoplasm is obscured by azurophilic granules

Blood smear from father of patient with Batten's disease. For staining technique see text. The degree of hypergranulation of the leukocytes is given. Note the washed out appearance of neutrophilic granules in cell grading 0+. Granules in the cell of 1+ are slightly out of focus. × 520.

TABLE 1

FAMILIAL AMAUROTIC IDIOCIES*

Traditional Designation of "Subtypes"	Actual or Probable Nosologic Entities	
	Chemically Defined	Chemically Undefined
Congenital F.A.I. (Normann-Wood)	G_{D3} gangliosidosis	no known equivalent
Infantile F.A.I. (Tay-Sachs)	G_{M2} gangliosidosis	no known equivalent
Late Infantile F.A.I. (Bielschowsky-Jansky)	G_{M1} gangliosidosis (G_{M3} gangliosidosis)	
Juvenile Amaurotic Idiocy (Spielmeyer-Vogt, Batten-Mayou, Sjögren)	not reported	Myoclonic variant of cerebral lipidosis or Batten's syndrome or Batten's disease
Adult F.A.I. (Kufs)	not reported	

* Review of the literature indicates that G_{M2} gangliosidosis or Tay-Sachs disease is rarely confused with other entities. On the other hand, the diagnosis of late infantile familial amaurotic idiocy or the Bielschowsky-Jansky type has been applied to cases of G_{M1} gangliosidosis. However, most cases appear to belong to the chemically undefined Batten's syndrome or the myoclonic variant of cerebral lipidosis. A case of G_{M3} gangliosidosis was described under the term Niemann Pick's disease (Jørgensen. 1964. Acta Neuropath. **4**: 90.) It is quite possible that the myoclonic variant of cerebral lipidosis or Batten's syndrome or Batten's disease comprises a number of different genetic entities.

by the pathological accumulation of the monosialogangliosides G_{M1} and G_{M3} and termed generalized gangliosidosis.[6] No blood smears from patients with this condition were available.

The possibility that the azurophilic hypergranulation could indicate the carrier state of Batten's disease was also investigated in a large number of blood relatives. This part of the study forms the subject of the report by Merritt *et al.*[7] immediately following in this monograph.

THE PRESENT STUDY

After the diagnostic significance of leukocytic hypergranulation had been established, the nature of the abnormal granules was investigated. The following possibilities were considered:

1. Azurophilic hypergranulation is an abnormal retention of azurophilic granules in the peripheral leukocytes. In their studies on rabbit bone marrow, Bainton and Farquahr[8] showed that such granules are formed in the Golgi complex of progranulocytes (promyelocytes). As the cells divide and their offspring mature in the bone marrow, the azurophilic granules become progressively less numerous, whereas the specific granules, produced on a different face of the Golgi complex, increase numerically. These authors observed that azurophilic granules do not form in the myelocytes and subsequent cell types.

2. Azurophilic hypergranulation is closely related to toxic granulation. Although there is no *prima facie* evidence in support of this assumption, the fact that the blood smears of many of our patients were interpreted as showing toxic granulations was deemed sufficient reason to explore this possibility.

TABLE 2

COMPARATIVE MORPHOLOGY OF AZUROPHILIC LEUKOCYTIC GRANULES (STANDARDIZED GIEMSA STAIN)

	Batten's Disease	Toxic Granulations	Alder Granulations
Number/cell	20–100	> 50	10–30
Size	0.3–0.5 μ		1–2 μ
Shape	distinct round to ovoid		irregularly round
Activity of alkaline phosphatase	normal	markedly increased	normal
Effect of H_2O at pH 5.4 for ten min	reduction in number of stained granules	none	none
Supravital stain	not visualized	marked granularity	not tested

3. Azurophilic hypergranulation is due to the presence of a hitherto unrecognized organelle. Even though hypergranulation is present in normal individuals, the small number of cells with this change may have escaped observation in electron microscopic preparations.

In order to test these assumptions, a variety of morphological studies were undertaken. Blood films from 16 patients with Batten's disease and of many more relatives with definite azurophilic hypergranulation were available. Control films were obtained from patients with toxic granulations and from healthy individuals whose granulocytes did not display more than 20 percent of leukocytes of grade 1+ and 2+.

As not all neutrophils of patients with Batten's disease are hypergranulated, it is impossible to recognize whether a particular cell contains an abnormally high number of azurophilic granules in blood films subjected to histochemical techniques. Such specimens have to be evaluated by statistical methods. The same difficulty seems to apply to electron microscopic observations. The problem is, however, somewhat mitigated since the hypergranulated neutrophils have a slightly greater density than normally granulated cells. On centrifugation, therefore, they tend to accumulate directly on top of the erythrocytes. Later, proper alignment of the specimen blocks allows sections containing a cell population enriched with hypergranulated elements to be obtained.

HISTOCHEMICAL OBSERVATIONS

Hypergranulated neutrophils did not yield reactions for the demonstration of dehydrogenases, qualitatively and quantitatively different from those seen in normal granulocytes. The granules were not stained by the dichlorodiphenyldichloroethane (DDD) reaction for the demonstration of sulfhydryl groups, nor did they react with the periodic acid-Schiff reaction (PAS), Sudan black B, or Oil red O. This established that the granules do not contain lipofuscin, the material that accumulates in the nerve cells in Batten's disease. Like neutrophils with toxic granulations, the hypergranulated cells were positive for acid phosphatase, but to an extent that was not distinctly different from normal neutrophils. Cells with azurophilic hypergranulation gave a reaction for alkaline phosphatase commensurate with that of normal neutrophils, but markedly less than that seen in cells with toxic granulations.

Digestion with ribonuclease did not alter the azurophilic granules or the toxic granules. However, toxic granules proved resistant to immersion in distilled water, a treatment that rendered the azurophilic granules slightly indistinct and less deeply stained. The distilled water, obtained from a commercial still, had a pH of 5.4. Fresh double-distilled water with a pH of 6.5 did not alter the degree of azurophilic hypergranulation.

Obviously, these studies were not helpful in establishing the nature of the abnormal granules. They did, however, produce differential morphological criteria summarized in TABLE 2.

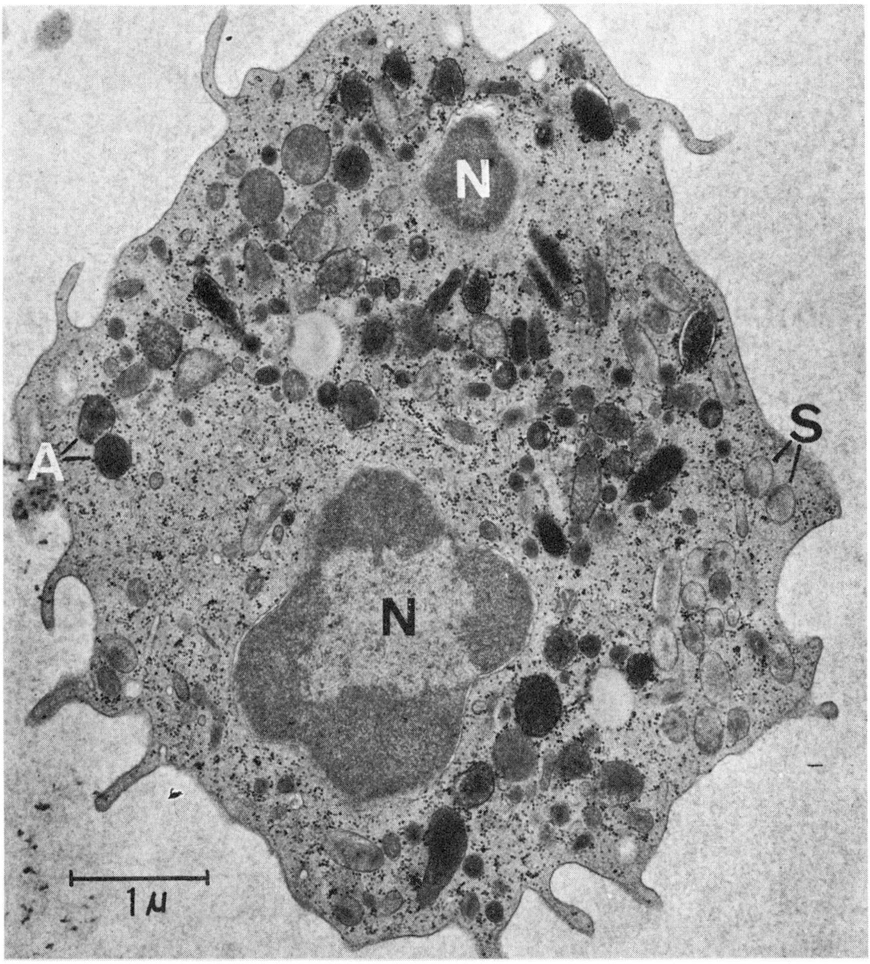

FIGURE 2. Normal neutrophilic leukocyte from peripheral blood. Large dense azurophilic granules (A) and smaller less dense specific granules (S) are easily identified. Dense glycogen particles are distributed more or less evenly through the cytoplasm. Nucleus (N). Uranyl acetate and lead citrate. × 18,000.

Electron Microscope Observations

Preparation of peripheral neutrophils for electron microscopic observation required endless modifications and precautions[9] until we finally arrived at the following technique: Venous blood is mixed with a sufficient amount of EDTA to prevent coagulation, and centrifuged at 1,000 rpm for nine minutes. The plasma is removed with a capillary pipette leaving as little as possible without disturbing the buffy layer. The tube must not be tilted. Cold phosphate buffered

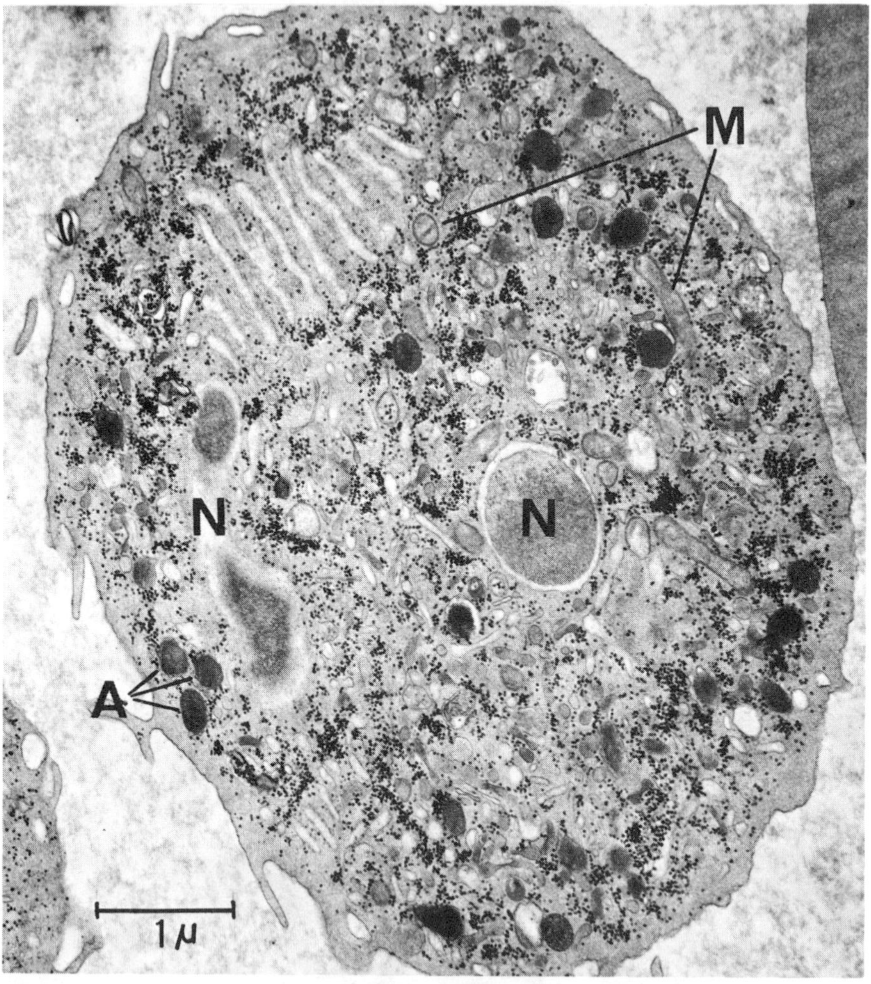

Figure 3. Neutrophilic leukocyte from peripheral blood of patient with toxic granulations. Large dense azurophilic granules (A) are identified. Smaller, less dense, specific granules are intermingled with granules that are intermediate in size and density. Endoplasmic reticulum is prominent and several mitochondria (M) are present. The cell is so filled with organelles that the glycogen particles have been crowded together. Nucleus (N). Uranyl acetate and lead citrate. × 18,000.

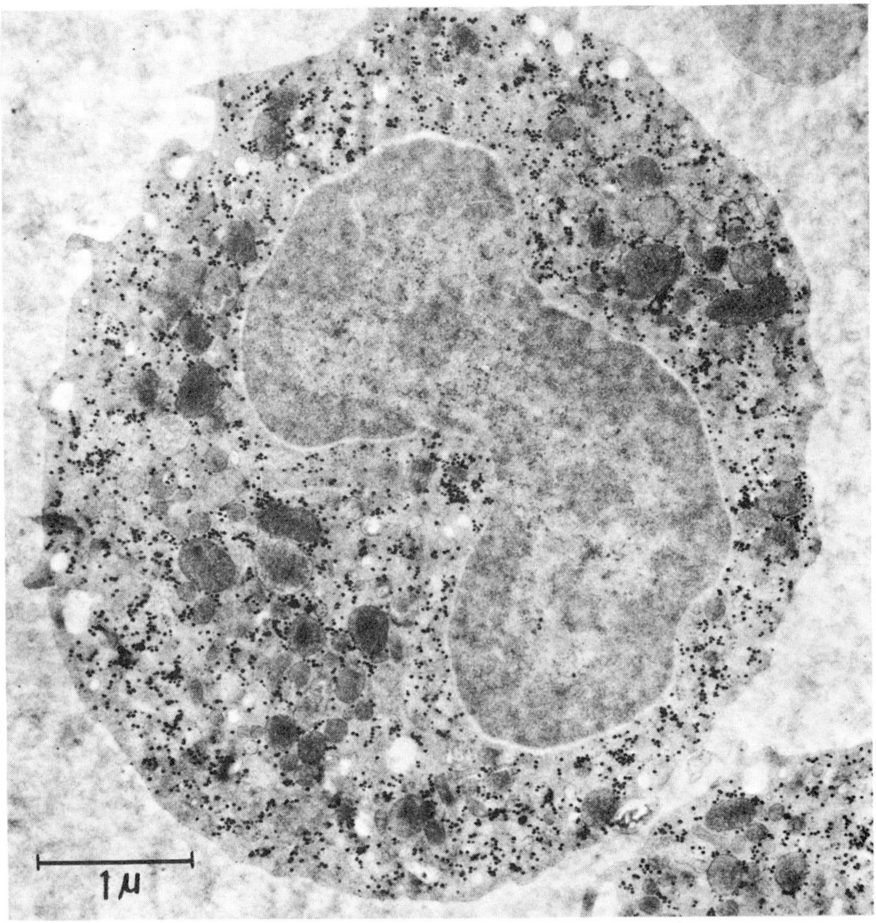

FIGURE 4. Neutrophilic leukocyte from the peripheral blood of patient with Batten's disease. Granules cover a continuous spectrum of sizes and density so that it is difficult to identify the azurophilic and specific granules. The majority are of intermediate size and density. Endoplasmic reticulum is sparse and mitochondria are inconspicuous. Uranyl acetate and lead citrate. × 19,500.

6.25 percent glutaraldehyde is added carefully in approximately the quantity of the plasma that was removed. After one hour at 4° C, the now firm buffy layer is detached from the test tube with a needle and removed as a disk. The disk is fixed at 4° C for another hour in a fresh solution of buffered glutaraldehyde. The disk is washed in buffer and cut into small blocks, oriented relative to the gravity gradient. The blocks are placed in 1 percent buffered osmic acid at 4° C for one hour; dehydrated in graded ethanol solutions; rinsed in two changes of propylene oxide; passed through three changes of Araldite® 502 (Ciba Co., Inc.) and DDSA† in a ratio of 27:23,

† Dodecenyl succinic anhydride.

respectively, leaving them for one hour in the first and second and overnight in the third; and embedded in Araldite®: DDSA: DMP–30‡ in a ratio of 27:23:1.

This procedure permits the reproducible demonstration of azurophilic granules and eliminates extraction of the granules almost completely. FIGURE 2 shows a normal neutrophil with large, dense azurophilic granules and a greater number of smaller, lighter, so-called specific granules. Mitochondria are sparse, there is little endoplasmic reticulum, and the Golgi apparatus is inconspicuous. A neutrophil with toxic granulations is depicted in FIGURE 3. Again, the azurophilic granulations are conspicuous. The endoplasmic reticulum is very well developed and occupies a major portion of the cytoplasm. Somewhat surprisingly, azurophilic granules are not present in increased numbers in the hypergranulated cells from patients with Batten's disease (FIGURE 4).

‡ Dimethyl phthalate.

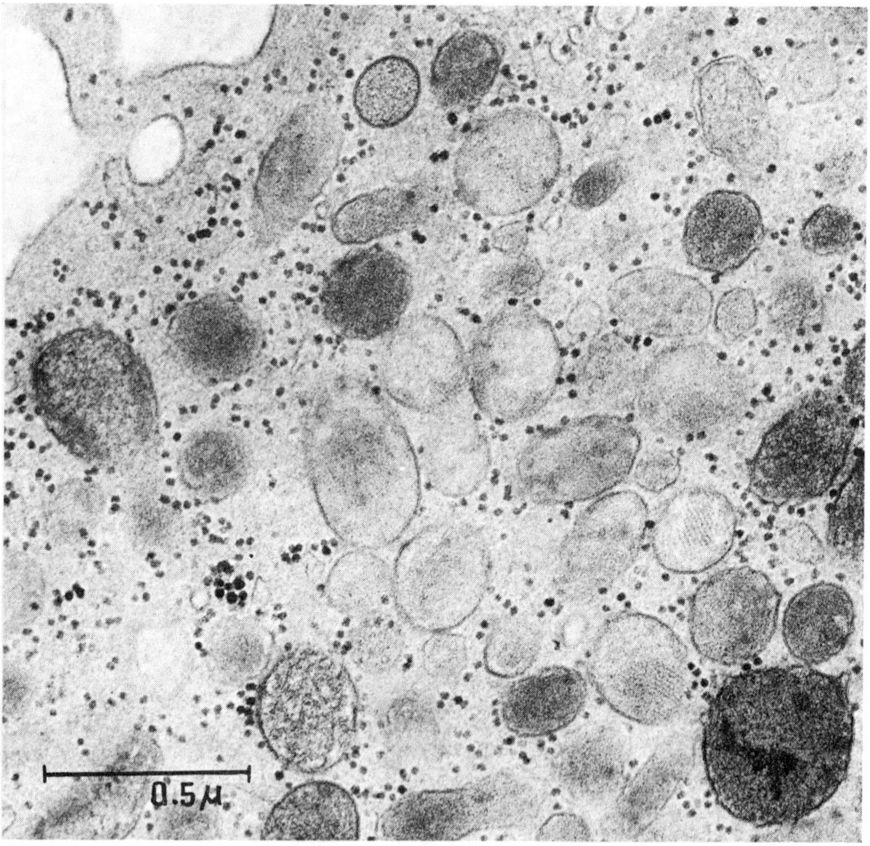

FIGURE 5. Cytoplasm of neutrophilic leukocyte. Large dense azurophilic granules can be distinguished from the more numerous smaller, less dense, specific granules. Structures suggestive of crystalline nature are present in some of the specific granules. The granules are bounded by well-defined membranes. A rare mitochondrion is present in the upper right corner of the micrograph. Uranyl acetate and lead citrate. × 52,500.

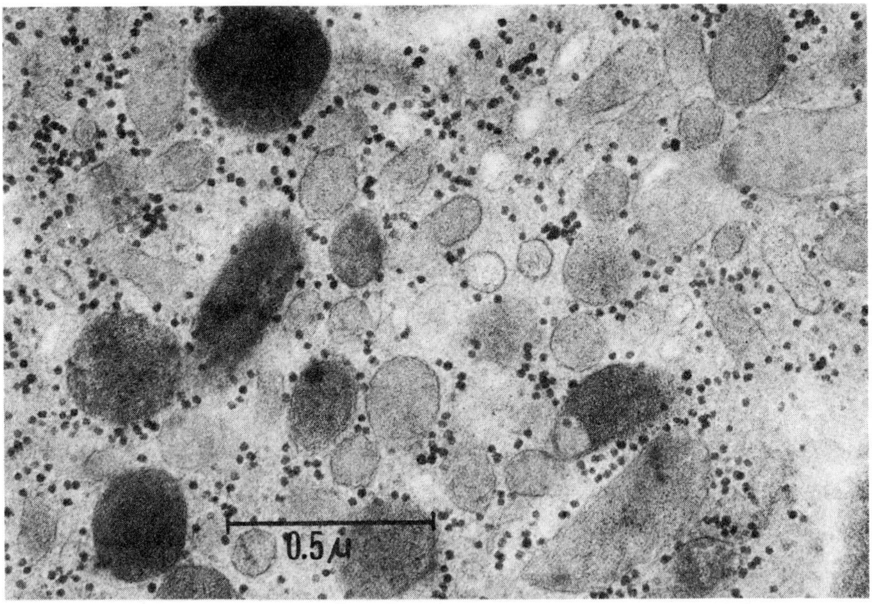

FIGURE 6. A neutrophilic leukocyte from a patient with toxic granulations. The granules vary in size and density. There are intermediate forms, larger and denser than specific granules, but smaller and less dense than azurophilic granules. Uranyl acetate and lead citrate. × 52,500.

The normal neutrophil displays two types of granules, specific and azurophilic (FIGURE 5). Cells with toxic granulations (FIGURE 6) and with hypergranulation (FIGURES 7 & 8) seem to contain a third type of granule with an intermediate density. These granules are larger than the specific granules, approaching the size of the azurophilic granules. Although counts have shown that the number of granules is about the same in the normal, hypergranulated, and toxic granulocytes, the total volume occupied by the granules is greater in the two latter types. In leukocytes with toxic granulation, in which there is also a considerable expansion of the endoplasmic reticulum, one observes, therefore, a crowding of the cytoplasm recognizable by a peculiar bunching of the glycogen granules.

Higher resolution shows still other abnormalities in the hypergranulated neutrophils from patients with Batten's disease. All cytoplasmic granules in these cells, regardless whether they are specific, azurophilic, or intermediate, are bounded by a single-layered membrane (FIGURE 10). In contrast, the granules of normal leukocytes possess a trilaminar limiting membrane (FIGURE 9).

DISCUSSION

We are now convinced that azurophilic hypergranulation is associated with the heterozygous and homozygous genotypes of families with Batten's disease. The nature of this association remains obscure.

Results of the present investigation suggest that the abnormal azurophilic granules seen in Giemsa-stained smears correspond to a type of leukocytic granules hitherto undefined by electron microscopic studies. This organelle has a density and size between the specific and the azurophilic granules, which prompts us to call it an "intermediate granule." It remains to be established whether this is a distinct organelle or whether we are dealing with altered specific or nonspecific granules. The second possibility is suggested by the abnormal limiting membrane which bounds all the granules in the hypergranulated leukocytes. Although the monolayered limiting membrane is conceivably an artifact, attributable to fixation, dehydration, and embedding, it may, nevertheless, indicate a more basic abnormality. This is supported by the fact that the stainability of the granules with the Giemsa technique is easily altered by immersion in acidic water, which presumably causes acid hydrolysis of the membranes. An additional argument is based on observations made during our early attempts to produce electron microscopic preparations of the hypergranulated cells. In specimens not treated according to the technique outlined above, a marked extraction of the granules occurred in the cells of a patient with Batten's disease (FIGURE 11), far more than in the control material.

These observations suggest that the intermediate granules, accounting for the azurophilic hypergranulation in the leukocytes of patients with Batten's disease, result from an abnormality in the membranes of the specific and azurophilic granules. This presumably molecular lesion leads to reproducible

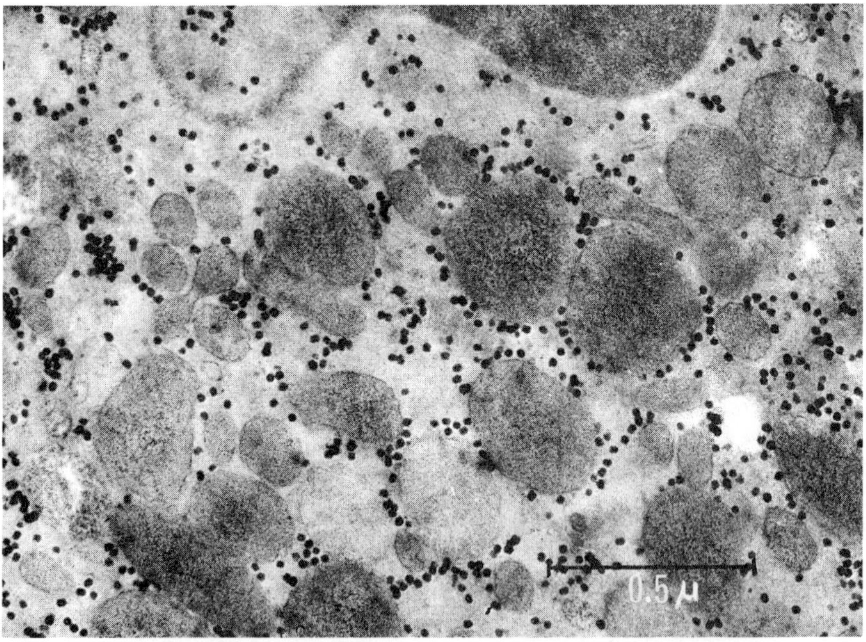

FIGURE 7. Granules in a neutrophilic leukocyte from the peripheral blood of a patient with Batten's disease. There is variation in the size and density of the granules and no specific or azurophilic granules can be identified with certainty. The majority are of the intermediate type. Uranyl acetate and lead citrate. × 52,500.

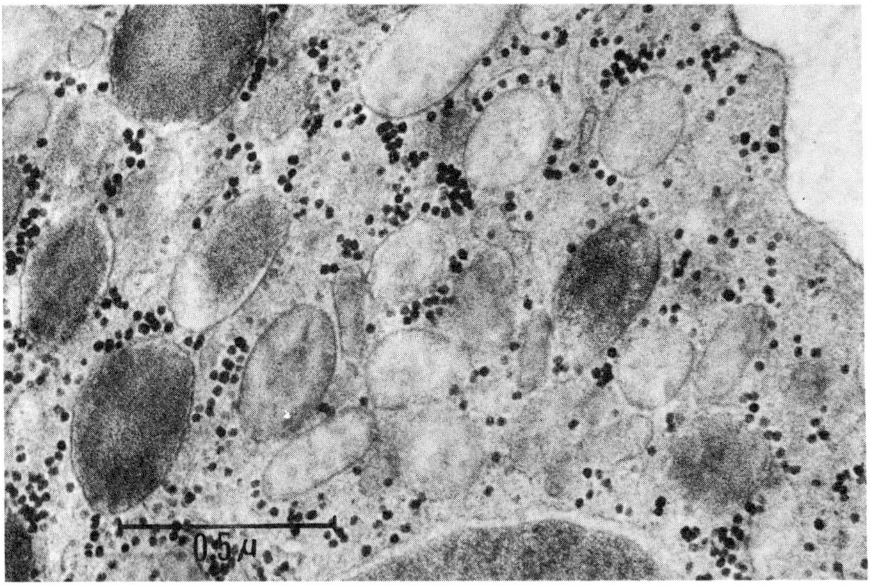

FIGURE 8. Granules in a neutrophilic leukocyte from the peripheral blood of a different patient with Batten's disease. There is similar variation in the size and density of the granules. Thus, the majority are intermediate with only a few identifiable as azurophilic or specific granules. Uranyl acetate and lead citrate. × 52,500.

artifacts in the form of a striking cytochemical staining phenomenon, demonstrable by the Giemsa technique.

SUMMARY

Histochemical and electron microscopic studies on the nature of the azurophilic hypergranulations of leukocytes in Batten's disease are reported. The exact nature of the phenomenon could not be elucidated, but it appears that the abnormal granulation is due to the prevalence of an intermediate granule in the polymorphonuclear cells. In electron microscopic preparations, the leukocyte granules from patients with Batten's disease are bounded by a unilaminar membrane, in contrast to the trilaminar membrane of the granules in controls. The possibility that this finding may represent a molecular lesion is discussed.

ACKNOWLEDGMENTS

We thank the staff of the Department of Neurology for help in obtaining the blood specimens, and Mrs. N. Hoggatt, Mrs. D. Meyer, and Miss C. Alyea for technical assistance.

[NOTE ADDED IN PROOF: Subsequent studies have revealed that both normal and hypergranulated neutrophils from patients with Batten's disease contain three types of granules: azurophilic, specific, and large cylindrical ones with crystalline inclusions. These inclusions are very rare in hypergranulated neutrophils.]

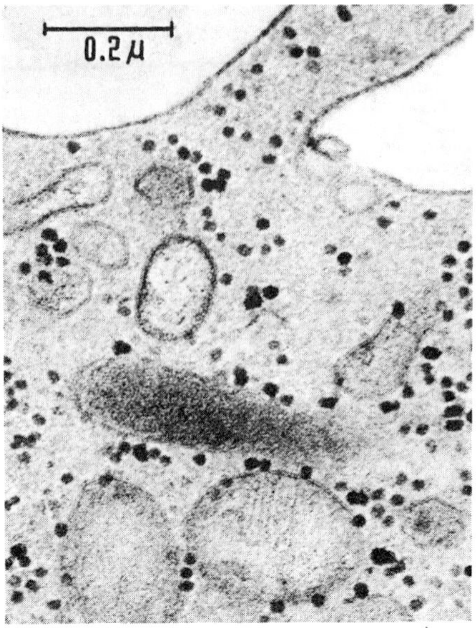

FIGURE 9. Normal neutrophilic leukocyte. The granules are limited by definite trilaminar membranes comparable to the plasma membrane. A specific granule in the lower center shows a lattice suggestive of a crystalline structure. Uranyl acetate and lead citrate. × 75,000.

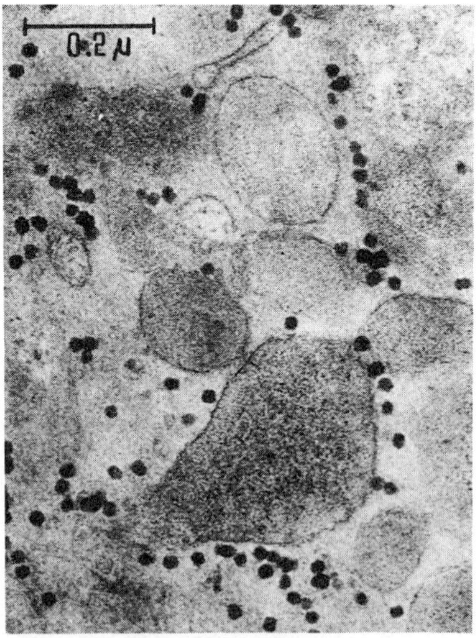

FIGURE 10. Batten's disease. Neutrophilic leukocyte. All granules have a thin single-layered limiting membrane. When compared with the membranes in FIGURE 9, prepared also by the standard technique, the difference is evident. Uranyl acetate and lead citrate. × 75,000.

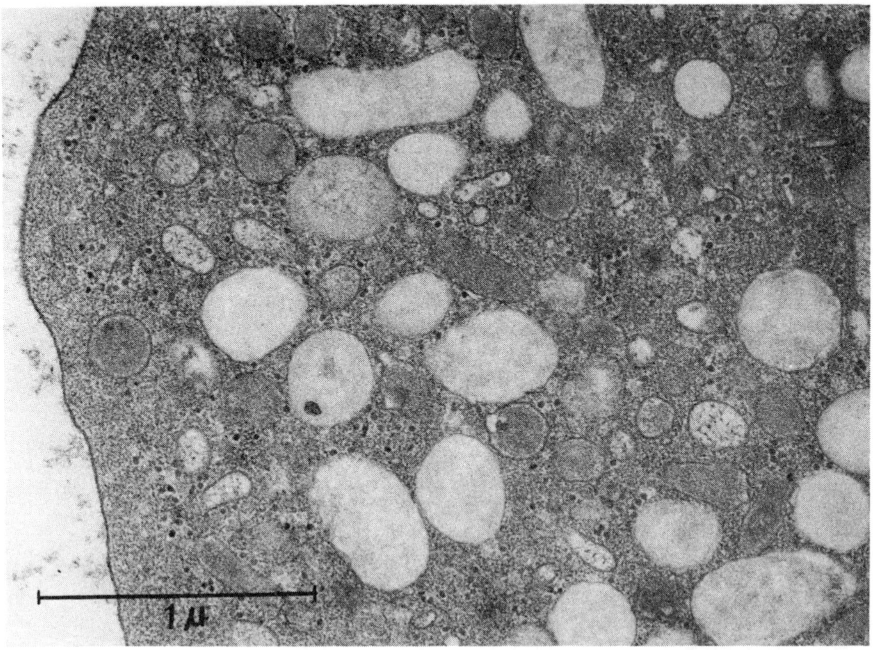

FIGURE 11. Neutrophilic leukocytes of a patient with Batten's disease. Not prepared by standard technique. The various degrees of extraction can be most easily seen in the larger granules. The cytoplasm is dense, and the smaller granules and glycogen particles are distinguished with difficulty. The limiting membranes and plasmalemma are well preserved. Uranyl acetate and lead citrate. × 35,600.

REFERENCES

1. STROUTH, J. C., W. ZEMAN, & A. D. MERRITT. 1966. Leukocyte abnormalities in familial amaurotic idiocy. New Eng. J. Med. **274:** 36.
2. ZEMAN, W. &J. C. STROUTH. 1966. Neutrophil hypergranulations versus lymphocytic vacuolization as markers for hetero- and homozyogtes with Spielmeyer-Vogt disease. *In* Inborn Errors of Sphingolipid Metabolism. S. M. Aronson & B. W. Volk, Eds. : 475–484. Pergamon Press. Oxford, England.
3. ALDER, A. 1957. Die Pelger-Huëtsche Kernanomalie–Die konstitutionell bedingte Granulationsanomalie. *In* Handbuch der gesamten Hämatologie. L. Heilmeyer & A. Hittmair, Eds. : 354–364. Urban & Schwarzenberg. Munich, Berlin, Vienna, Germany.
4. VOLK, B. W. 1964. Tay-Sachs Disease. : 1–16. Grune & Stratton. New York, N. Y.
5. DONAHUE, S., W. ZEMAN, & I. WATANABE. 1966. Electron microscopic observations in Batten's disease. *In* Inborn Errors of Sphingolipid Metabolism. S. M. Aronson & B. W. Volk, Eds. : 3–22. Pergamon Press. Oxford, England.
6. O'BRIEN, J., M. B. STERN, B. H. LANDING, J. K. O'BRIEN, & G. N. DONNELL. 1965. Generalized gangliosidoses: another inborn error of ganglioside metabolism? Amer. J. Dis. Child. **109:** 338.
7. MERRITT, A. D., S. A. SMITH, J. C. STROUTH, & W. ZEMAN. 1968. Detection of heterozyotes in Batten's disease. This monograph.
8. BAINTON, D. F. & M. G. FARQUAHR. 1966. Origin of granules in polymorphonuclear leukocytes. J. Cell Biol. **28:** 277.
9. WATANABE, I., S. DONAHUE, & N. HOGGATT. 1967. Method for electron microscopic studies of circulating human leukocytes and observations on their fine structure. J. Ultrastruct. Res. **20:** 366.

DETECTION OF HETEROZYGOTES IN BATTEN'S DISEASE*

A. D. Merritt, S. A. Smith, J. C. Strouth, and W. Zeman

Department of Medical Genetics and Section of Neuropathology
Indiana University Medical Center, Indianapolis, Ind.

Nosology of the hereditary and degenerative central nervous system disorders in children has been discussed by Donahue *et al.*[1] Familial amaurotic idiocies clearly include several clinical entities. It is our contention that the late infantile, juvenile, and possibly the adult forms (Kufs's disease) represent a single distinct entity (and probable cerebral lipidosis), without, as yet, a specific identifiable biochemical defect. This disorder we will refer to as Batten's disease (Batten-Spielmeyer-Vogt disease).

In 1931, Sjögren[2] demonstrated that Batten's disease was inherited as an autosomal recessive and, further, that the ethnic origin of such children was almost universally non-Jewish in contrast to their Jewish origin in Tay-Sachs disease. Clinical symptoms of Batten's disease were noted to be unique, including a small head, lack of a macular cherry-red spot, and an onset often well beyond the age of one year. Clinical differentiation of the disorder has recently been defined at the ultramicroscopic level.[3,4] Electron microscopic studies of the structure of cerebral lipid bodies in Batten's disease reveal highly characteristic accumulations in the perikarya which are distinctly different from the membranous cytoplasmic bodies of Tay-Sachs disease, as described by Terry and Korey.[5]

The observation by von Bagh and Hortling,[6] followed by the exhaustive study by Rayner,[7] demonstrating lymphocytic vacuolization in amaurotic idiocy provided the impetus for our initial studies of peripheral blood smears from patients with Batten's disease. Morphological studies on the characteristics of granulation found in the cytoplasm of polymorphonuclear leukocytes of patients with Batten's disease are the subject of the preceding paper by Donahue *et al.*[1] Strouth, *et al.*[8] studied leukocytic abnormalities found in children with cerebral disorders and in patients with Batten's disease. These studies were further discussed by Zeman.[9]

Only toxic granulation produces similar azurophilic granulation of neutrophils. Toxic granulation might be expected to be found in patients with Batten's disease in its advanced stages, because such patients are bedfast and vegetative. On the other hand, parents and a proportion of siblings who are in good health manifest neutrophilic granulation that is quantitatively similar to patients with Batten's disease. Usually the general health status and marked affinity of toxic granulation for neutral red in supravital preparations, in contrast to the lack of staining of the leukocytic granules of Batten's disease, provides adequate differentiation. Results of studies on 17 families, including one or more children with Batten's disease, are the subject of this paper.

Materials and Methods

Peripheral blood smears were taken from all probands and, whenever possible, from their parents and normal siblings. All family members were exam-

* Supported in part by USPHS grants nos. GM 1056 and NB 04607, and the James Whitcomb Riley Memorial Association.

ined and pathological examination of affected individuals was performed whenever possible. Giemsa staining at pH 6.5 of fresh air-dried smears after methanol fixation for three minutes provided the best results.

Results

Polymorphonuclear leukocytic granulations are illustrated in FIGURE 1. Those individuals graded negative for the leukocytic hypergranulation trait have few or no granules, whereas those that are positive have 15 percent or more neutrophils containing dozens of azurophilic-staining granules. Fortunately, it is usually easy to decide, without grading of cells, whether a smear is positive or negative. In some instances, a differential count, with grading of cells as 0, 1+, 2+, and 3+, as described in the preceding paper,[1] is necessary to classify the individual, although it has been difficult to discern an exact cutoff point. It is important to note that the degree of leukocytic hypergranulation does not differ quantitatively between individuals with Batten's disease and their positive unaffected relatives.

To date, 17 families have been studied (FIGURES 2–4). The probands in 16 families presented a typical clinical syndrome of progressive psychomotor deterioration, characteristic of Batten's disease. There are 24 affected members in these 16 sibships, 12 of whose diagnoses have been confirmed by pathological examination from brain biopsy or autopsy by one of us (W.Z.). The proband in Family 10 (II-1), however, had Tay-Sachs disease with megalencephaly and typical cherry-red maculae, but lacked electroencephalographic abnormalities at 15 months of age. The early age of onset in this patient, although not usual in Batten's disease, does not in itself exclude the latter diagnosis.[3]

It may have been a good thing that we were not discouraged by Family 1, since the child with Batten's disease, confirmed by brain biopsy, does not have increased granulation, nor does either of his parents.

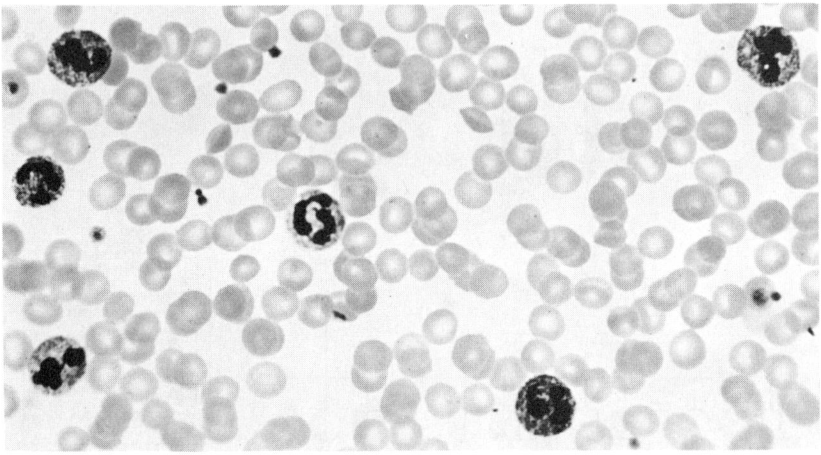

FIGURE 1. A peripheral blood smear, obtained from the father of a child with Batten's disease (Family 8), demonstrating leukocytic hypergranulation of varying degrees. Only the central leukocyte is graded as normal. × 400.

Family 2 is an interesting instance of consanguinity, consisting of an uncle-niece marriage producing three children. Hypergranulation is present in both parents and in their three children.

Family 3 at first appeared to exclude a simple relationship between the neutrophilic granulation and Batten's disease. However, on close questioning, the mother admitted to a long-term extramarital relationship. The biological father is deceased and was not tested. Based on blood group studies, the mother's marriage partner was excluded as the father of the child with Batten's disease and his two alleged full brothers. A single legitimate daughter carries the trait of leukocytic hypergranulation, as does her husband and their one child. A maternal first cousin and his child also carry the trait.

Family 4 has two children with Batten's disease. Two out of the four tested normal siblings demonstrate increased neutrophilic granulation as do both parents. Individual II-3, who died at the age of two months, was stated to have had congenital heart disease.

Family 5 is also consanguineous. In this case the relationship is that of double third cousins with an inbreeding coefficient of 1/128. Both parents carry the leukocytic hypergranulation trait as do two of their three children available for examination. The second child, with a clinical history characteristic of Batten's disease, died at the age of 15 months.

Family 6 expresses the trait in an autosomal dominant fashion, with both

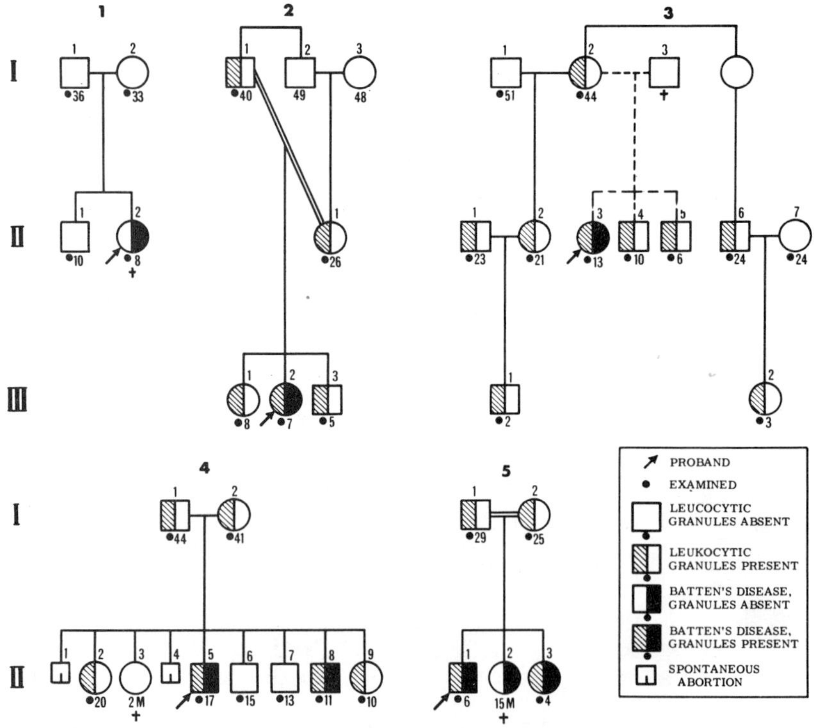

FIGURE 2. Pedigrees of Families 1–5. Dotted lines indicate an extramarital union and double lines consanguinity. Ages at examination are beneath the symbols.

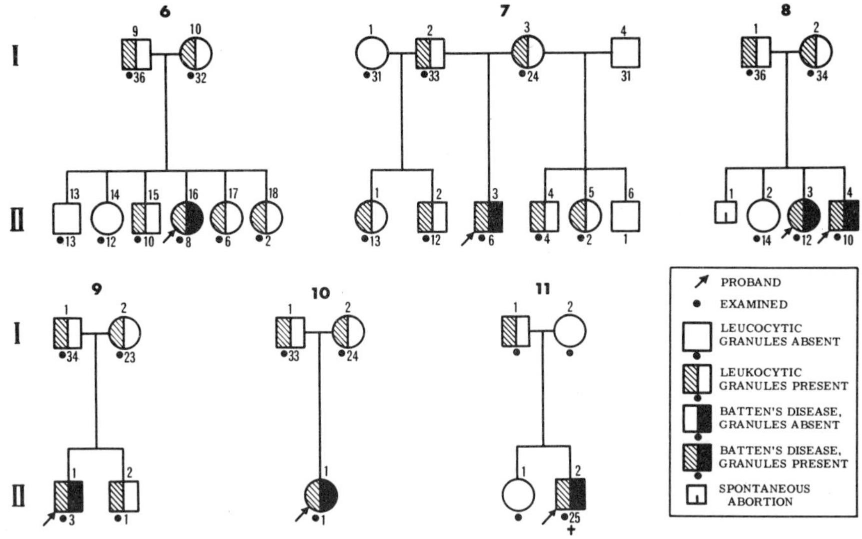

FIGURE 3. Pedigrees of Families 6–11. Dotted lines indicate an extramarital union and double lines consanguinity. Ages at examination are beneath the symbols.

parents and four out of six children (including one child with Batten's disease) having hypergranulated leukocytes.

Family 7 has an only child with Batten's disease. The other marriage partners of both parents do not have increased leukocytic granulation. The children resulting from other parental marriages provide evidence for segregation of the trait.

Family 8 is difficult to interpret. The two children with Batten's disease, not confirmed pathologically, have minimally positive blood smears. Their sister is clearly negative. The mother has easily demonstrable neutrophilic hypergranulation, whereas the father is quantitatively borderline but classified as positive.

Family 9 has two children, one with Batten's disease and one manifesting the hypergranulation trait only. Both parents have leukocytic hypergranulation.

The proband in Family 10 is the child mentioned earlier, whose clinical manifestations are quite suggestive of Tay-Sachs disease. No brain biopsy has been performed. In total, we have examined six patients with Tay-Sachs disease in five families. Two of these demonstrated some increased granularity in their neutrophils. However, it is our feeling that the color of the granules was blue rather than the reddish-blue usually encountered in our patients with Batten's disease.

The mother in Family 11 is an exception, since she demonstrates no increase in leukocytic granularity. The father and proband have the trait.

Two out of six daughters in Family 12 have Batten's disease, and three out of four normal sisters carry the hypergranulation trait, as do their parents.

Family 13 has two children with Batten's disease, one with neutrophilic hypergranulation; the other was not tested. Five normal siblings are without evidence of increased leukocytic granulation. Because the father was an exception, and did not demonstrate the hypergranulation trait, polymorphic blood-group, se-

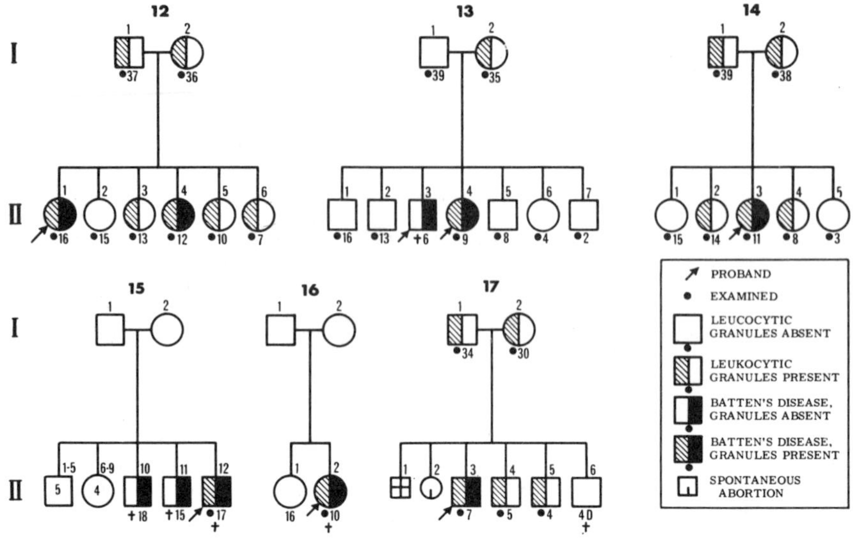

FIGURE 4. Pedigrees of Families 12–17. Dotted lines indicate an extramarital union and double lines consanguinity. Ages at examination are beneath the symbols.

rum protein, and erythrocytic enzyme studies were performed, but no paternal exclusion for the affected girl (II-4) was obtained.

Family 14 is consistent with an autosomal dominant transmission of the hypergranulation trait. Clinically the proband had only psychomotor retardation without fundoscopic abnormalities. On the basis of leukocytic hypergranulation in this family, the presumptive diagnosis of Batten's disease was made. Two years later a brain biopsy was performed, confirming the diagnosis in the proband.

Family 15 is incompletely evaluated. However, the proband demonstrates increased neutrophilic granulation. There were three children with Batten's disease in this large sibship of 12.

Only the proband in Family 16 has been evaluated. The child as yet is only mildly affected and pathological confirmation has not been obtained.

In Family 17, the child with Batten's disease and two brothers have increased azurophilic granulation in their neutrophils.

Sibships containing individuals with Batten's disease are summarized in FIGURE 5. By observation, the trait of increased leukocytic granulation segregates as an autosomal dominant and Batten's disease occurs as an autosomal recessive disorder. If leukocytic hypergranulation identifies the gene responsible for Batten's disease, then affected individuals are presumably homozygous for the trait.

In TABLE 1, segregation analysis of the disease by the a priori method of Bernstein[10] demonstrates a good fit for autosomal recessive inheritance of Batten's disease. The expected number of affected individuals in our 17 sibships was 25.65, the observed 25.

Results of studies of the neutrophilic leukocytes in these families are summarized in TABLE 2. A total of 82 individuals was tested. Two out of 17 parental sets were not tested; only one of the remaining 30 parents, a deceased father, was not tested. Exceptions to an autosomal dominant inheritance pattern with heterozygosity of parents of children with Batten's disease include a father in Family 13; a mother in Family 11; and both parents in Family 1, and their child, our only exception in tested children with Batten's disease. Males and females with Batten's disease were 12 and 13, respectively. The total number of normal male and female siblings, 21 and 23, respectively, was approximately equal, and out of those tested for leukocytic hypergranulation, seven males and ten females were positive, whereas eight males and seven females were negative for the trait.

Discussion

Although Batten's disease is considered quite rare, we have been able to accumulate considerable experience with the disorder during the last few years. Consanguinity was present in two families, a characteristic of rare recessive disorders. Out of the 25 patients in 17 families, 12 cases have been confirmed by biopsy or autopsy and 12 cases have demonstrated a rather typical clinical course. One patient has the clinical expression of Tay-Sachs disease, as yet unconfirmed by pathological studies.

The general problem of leukocytic granulation is still far from clarified. In particular, we do not know what the granules seen in our patients may represent at a biochemical level.

We think that we have demonstrated a definite relationship between Batten's disease and the marked azurophilic granulation as seen in the neutrophils of these patients, even though there is one exception. Further, examination of peripheral blood smears has been useful clinically as in Family 3. Since most parents (25 out of 29 tested), and 17 of their 32 normal children, demonstrate a quantitatively similar degree of hypergranularity of their leukocytes, it would

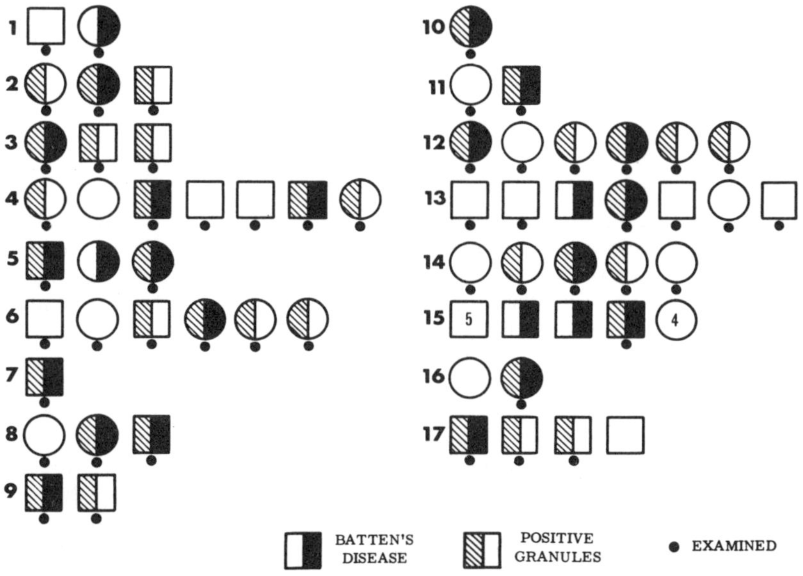

FIGURE 5. Sibship summary of live-born children in 17 families with Batten's disease.

TABLE 1

SEGREGATION ANALYSIS OF BATTEN'S DISEASE (A PRIORI METHOD OF BERNSTEIN)

Sibship Size	No. of Sibships	Affected	
		Expected	Observed
1	2	2.00	2
2	4	4.57	4
3	4	5.19	7
4	1	1.46	1
5	1	1.64	1
6	2	3.65	3
7	2	4.04	4
12	1	3.10	3
Total	17	25.65	25

TABLE 2

SUMMARY OF NEUTROPHILIC HYPERGRANULATION IN 17 FAMILIES WITH BATTEN'S DISEASE

	Positive	Negative	Not Tested	Total
Father	12	2*	3	17
Mother	13	2*	2	17
Affected males	8	1*	3	12
Affected females	12	0	1	13
Normal male sibs	7	8	6	21
Normal female sibs	10	7	6	23
Total	62	20	21	103

* Exceptions.

appear that leukocytic hypergranulation may be inherited as an autosomal dominant. This is, therefore, presumptive evidence that this trait may be the heterozygous expression of the gene causing Batten's disease. With both parents positive, i.e., having hypergranulation, the expected number of siblings having the trait would be two-thirds. Although the number of those having hypergranulation is somewhat smaller, it does not differ significantly from the expected segregation ($p > 0.1$ for males, females, and both sexes taken together). Although there is variation in the amount of leukocytic granulation, there is no evidence for dosage compensation, as patients with Batten's disease and their positive siblings and parents show quantitatively similar degrees of hypergranulation.

There are the exceptions: Family 1 in whom both parents and their child with Batten's disease did not demonstrate the trait, and the two other parents from different families, who also did not manifest leukocytic hypergranulation. In addition, the presence of typical leukocytic azurophilic hypergranulation in a patient clinically manifesting Tay-Sachs disease indicates that we must be cautious in stating that there is an exclusive direct relationship between azurophilic hypergranulation and Batten's disease. It is conceivable that either the clinical picture is leading us astray and that in truth we are dealing with Batten's disease, or that patients with Tay-Sachs disease may occasionally manifest granulation indistinguishable from that seen in our patients with pathologically confirmed Batten's disease. If the association of leukocytic hypergranulation with Batten's disease can be confirmed by other investigators in patients whose pathological diagnosis is established, this simply tested marker will attain additional scientific substantiation and subsequent diagnostic stature.

Summary

1. Leukocytic hypergranulation in Batten's disease has been evaluated in 82 individuals in 17 families.

2. With one exception, all tested patients affected with this autosomal recessive disease have increased granulation of their neutrophils, as well as one patient clinically presenting as Tay-Sachs disease.

3. Further, with four exceptions, all tested parents demonstrate the trait, and normal siblings have leukocytic hypergranulation as frequently as would be expected for an autosomal dominant trait transmitted from heterozygous parents.

4. There is no evidence of dosage compensation for the trait of leukocytic hypergranulation.

5. With the noted reservations, it is hypothesized that leukocytic hypergranulation identifies the carrier state of Batten's disease, and that affected patients are homozygous for this trait.

Acknowledgments

We appreciate the help of Mrs. J. Hamon and Mrs. M. LeStourgeon in obtaining family information and blood specimens, and the technical assistance of Mrs. D. Meyer and Miss C. Alyer.

References

1. DONAHUE, S., I. WATANABE & W. ZEMAN. 1968. Morphology of leukocytic hypergranulation in Batten's disease. This monograph.
2. SJÖGREN, T. 1931. Die juvenile amaurotische idiotie (Klinsche und Erblichkeitsmedizinische Untersuchungen). Hereditas (Lund) **14**: 197–426.
3. ZEMAN, W. & S. DONAHUE. 1963. Fine structure of the lipid bodies in juvenile amaurotic idiocy. Acta Neuropath. **3**: 144–149.
4. DONAHUE, S., W. ZEMAN & I. WATANABE. 1966. Electron microscopic observations on different forms of juvenile amaurotic idiocy. Proc. 3rd Int. Sym. Sphingolipidosis and Allied Diseases. Pergamon Press. New York, N. Y.
5. TERRY, R. D., J. R. KOREY & M. WEISS. 1962. Electron microscopy of the cerebrum in Tay-Sachs disease. *In* Cerebral Sphingolipidoses : 49–56. Academic Press, Inc. New York, N. Y.
6. V. BAGH, K. & H. HORTLING. 1948. Blodfynd vid juvenil amaurotisk idioti. Nord. Med. **37–38**: 1073–1076.
7. RAYNER, S. 1962. Juvenile amaurotic idiocy in Sweden. Institute for Medical Genetics. Uppsala, Sweden.
8. STROUTH, J. C., W. ZEMAN & A. D. MERRITT. 1966. Leukocyte abnormalities in familial amaurotic idiocy. New Eng. J. of Med. **274**: 36–38.
9. ZEMAN, W. & J. C. STROUTH. 1966. Leukocytic hypergranulation versus lymphocytic vacuolization as markers for heterozygotes and homozygotes with Batten-Spielmeyer-Vogt Disease. Pergamon Press. New York, N. Y.
10. BERNSTEIN, F. 1929. Variations und Erblichkeitsstatistik. Hdbch. Vererbgswiss. Gebruder Borntrager. Berlin, Germany.

BIOCHEMICAL GENETICS OF GLUCOSE-6-PHOSPHATE DEHYDROGENASE VARIATION*

Akira Yoshida, George Stamatoyannopoulos, and Arno G. Motulsky
Department of Medicine (Division of Medical Genetics) and Department of Genetics University of Washington, Seattle, Wash.

The study of enzymes with identical function in different tissues is of considerable genetic interest. Generally, it might be expected that an enzyme catalyzing a given reaction has an identical structure regardless of the tissue of origin. However, there is evidence that pyruvate kinase from red blood cells differs structurally from white cell pyruvate kinase. In keeping with this finding, genetically determined pyruvate kinase deficiency in red blood cells is not associated with pyruvate kinase deficiency in white blood cells. The exact structural relationship of white cell and red cell pyruvate kinase is unknown, although peptide analysis suggests that the white cell and red cell enzymes may share common polypetide chains.[1] In the case of lactic dehydrogenase, there are considerable differences in the isozyme patterns from different tissues; these differences, however, are related to the occurrence of various proportions of the two types of lactic dehydrogenase subunits, the H type and the M type[2,3] in different tissues.

Glucose-6-phosphate dehydrogenase (G-6-PD), the first enzyme in the shunt pathway of carbohydrate metabolism, has attracted much attention because a genetically determined deficiency of this enzyme in red blood cells is associated with a variety of hemolytic reactions, such as hemolytic anemia precipitated by drugs, by fava beans, or by infections. Furthermore, many different mutations affecting red cell G-6-PD have been discovered.[4,5] Most studies on G-6-PD have been performed with red blood cells. White cell G-6-PD has been studied less intensively, but in general it appears to have the same characteristics as red cell G-6-PD. Recently it has been claimed, however, that significant structural differences exist between red cell and white cell G-6-PD.[6] Such differences would imply separate genetic control of red cell and white cell G-6-PD. A body of genetic, enzymic and serologic evidence will be presented pointing to the identity of the erythrocyte and leukocyte G-6-PD.

Evidence for the Identity of Red Cell and White Cell G-6-PD

Genetic Evidence

Extensive genetic studies have indicated that the most common variants of G-6-PD, such as the Negro variant associated with normal enzyme activity (A+), and the two variants associated with enzyme deficiency, i.e., the Negro (A−) and the Mediterranean (B−), are X-linked traits. Less extensive studies with other, less common G-6-PD variants suggest that all these mutants are X-linked. It is likely, therefore, that all G-6-PD variants are alleles at the same locus on the X chromosome.† Many G-6-PD variants have been detected because of altered electrophoretic behavior of the red cell enzyme. When white cell G-6-PD from such mutant individuals is subjected to electrophoresis, the electrophoretic mobility of the white cell G-6-PD is identical to that of red cell

* This study was supported by USPHS grants nos. HD-02497-01 and H-3901.

† In an earlier report, Shaw[7] claimed the existence of an autosomal locus for G-6-PD in the liver of *Peromyscus*. More recent studies[8,9] suggest that the principal substrate for the liver enzyme is galactose-6-phosphate and not glucose-6-phosphate.

G-6-PD. For example, the two common Negro types of G-6-PD, A+ and A–, show the identical fast component on electrophoresis, regardless whether the enzyme is derived from red cells or white cells.[10] Similarly, mutant G-6-PD from other tissues, such as fibroblasts from skin or uterine muscles, show electrophoretic patterns identical to those obtained with red cell G-6-PD[11,12] The finding that a given mutation of G-6-PD occurs with identical electrophoretic mobility in different tissues, suggests that the normal enzyme is structurally identical in the various tissues and, therefore, when a mutation occurs, the enzyme is altered in all tissues in an identical manner.

Enzymic Evidence

Bonsignore *et al.*[6] suggested that white cell G-6-PD differed from red cell G-6-PD on the basis of the following findings: (1) white cell G-6-PD was more labile than the red cell enzyme, (2) the electrophoretic mobility of white cell enzyme was slower than that of red cell enzyme at pH 8.3, (3) the Michaelis constant for nicotinamide adenine dinucleotide (NAD) and G-6-P in white cell and red cell G-6-PD was found to differ, and (4) the two enzymes differed in optimum pH. Since the genetic evidence pointing to the identity of red cell and white cell G-6-PD is strong, we considered that the findings of Bonsignore *et al.* were caused by various impurities contaminating the white cell enzyme preparations, rather than by real structural differences. In order to elucidate this problem, the following experiments were performed.

1) Crude white cell G-6-PD was prepared according to the methodology used by Bonsignore *et al.* We confirmed that the crude white cell enzyme was labile and inactivated by more than 50 percent of its initial activity after storage for 24 hours at 0–4° C. When crude white cell G-6-PD preparations were purified through DEAE-cellulose columns, the enzyme stabilized and exhibited no inactivation after storage for more than one month. It is likely, therefore, that the instability of the crude leucocyte enzyme is caused by some contaminating material in the white cells which is removed by purification through the DEAE-cellulose column. The most likely sources of contamination are pepsin or cathepsin types of proteolytic enzymes, since di-isopropyl-fluorophosphate did not protect against instability.

2) Electrophoresis was performed on both crude and partially purified G-6-PD from red cells and white cells using TEB-buffer system, pH 8.6.[13] No difference in electrophoretic mobility could be observed by this method, or when the electrophoresis was performed under the conditions employed by Bonsignore *et al.*

3) Michaelis constants for G-6-P and nicotinamide adenine dinucleotide phosphate (NADP), and the optimum pH were determined on normal red cell and white cell G-6-PD. No significant differences could be demonstrated (TABLE 1). It is known that even normal red cell enzyme may show two different

TABLE 1
COMPARISON OF ERYTHROCYTE AND LEUCOCYTE G-6-PD (B+)

Enzyme	Michaelis Constant		Optimal pH
	for G-6-P	for NADP	
Erythrocyte enzyme	$3.9–5.2 \times 10^{-5}$	$4.4–5.7 \times 10^{-6}$	8.0
Leukocyte enzyme	$3.5–4.1 \times 10^{-5}$	$4.6–5.3 \times 10^{-6}$	8.0

K_m values for G-6-P and four different K_m values for NADP under certain conditions.[14] Justice *et al.*[15] also could not find any differences in K_m for G-6-P and NADP, or in the optimal pH between red cell and white cell enzyme.

Serologic Evidence

For the serologic experiments, rabbit anti-normal G-6-PD serum was prepared using crystalline red cell normal (B+) enzyme.[16] The antigen neutralized the white cell enzyme exactly as it did the red cell enzyme. Quantitative neutralization tests showed no difference in neutralization levels between the erythrocyte and leukocyte enzymes: 1 ml of anti-normal G-6-PD serum neutralized about 9 units of leukocyte G-6-PD as well as 9 units of erythrocyte G-6-PD. In the agar-gel diffusion precipitation test, a single and continuous precipitation line was found between the anti-normal G-6-PD serum and the enzyme, regardless of whether red cell or white cell G-6-PD was placed in the well. No spur suggesting structural dissimilarities was discovered (FIGURE 1). Accordingly, leukocyte enzyme is serologically both qualitatively and quantitatively indistinguishable from erythrocyte enzyme.

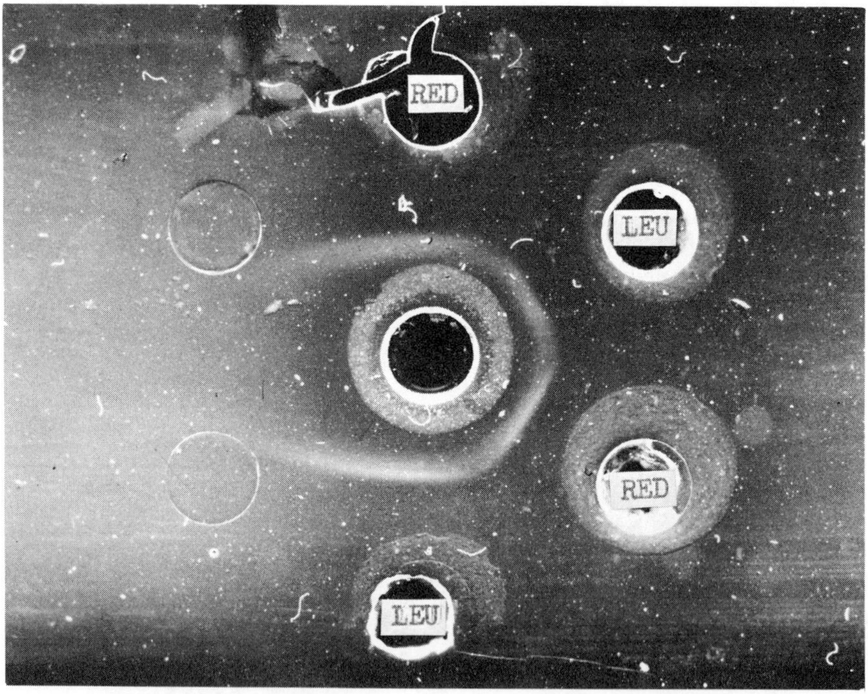

FIGURE 1. Precipitation pattern of double-diffusion test in an agar plate (Ouchtelony plate). Partially purified red cell enzyme and leucocyte enzyme were dissolved in 0.05 M phosphate buffer (pH 6.8) containing 10^{-3} M EDTA, 10^{-3} M mercaptoethanol and 2×10^{-5} M NADP to give a concentration of about 4 units per ml, and placed in a well. Anti-serum was placed in a center well. The anti-serum was obtained by immunizing a rabbit with crystalline red cell glucose-6-phosphate dehydrogenase. RED = red cell enzyme, LEU = leucocyte enzyme.

Considering the genetic, enzymic and serologic evidence presented above, it can be concluded that red cell and white cell G-6-PD are identical.

Characteristics of Normal and Mutant G-6-PD

Detailed knowledge regarding the structure of normal and mutant G-6-PD is still lacking. A series of investigations was undertaken to elucidate the biochemical genetics of G-6-PD and some of its variants.

Normal Enzyme[17]

Normal human G-6-PD was purified from 10 liters of blood by column chromatography using DEAE-cellulose, calcium phosphate gel, CM-cellulose, DEAE-Sephadex, and CM-Sephadex in the column. The crystalline preparation was obtained in an overall yield of 50 percent. This yield and a specific activity of 750 were significantly greater than those previously reported for purification of this enzyme. The sedimentation pattern for analytical centrifugation and interference pattern of sedimentation equilibrium indicated a homogeneous preparation. The sedimentation constant $S_{w,20}$ was 10.0 S at a protein concentration of 0.3 percent. The molecular weight of the enzyme was estimated as about

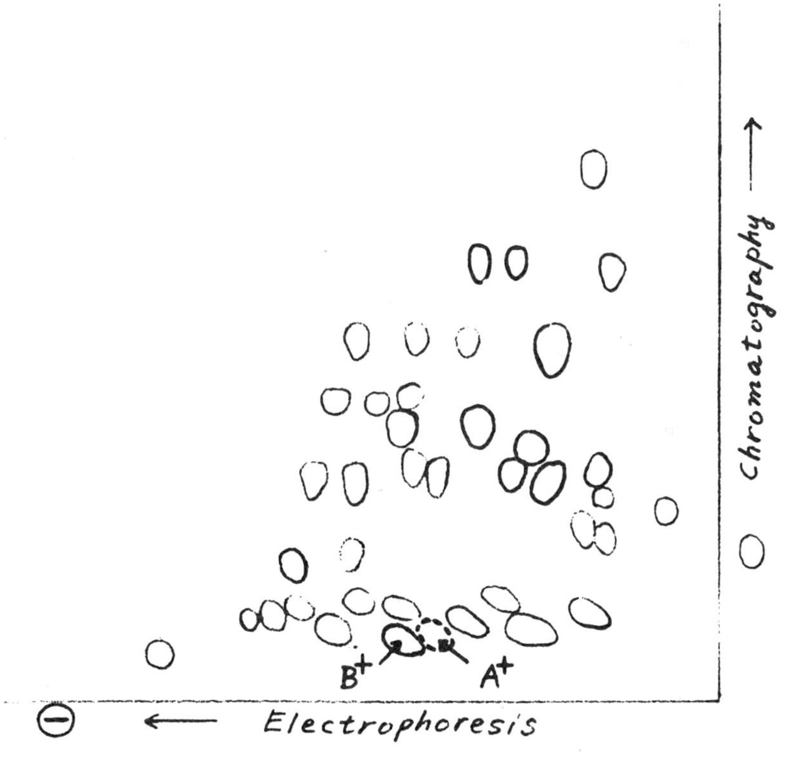

FIGURE 2. Fingerprint of tryptic hydrolysates of reduced, S-carboxymethylated normal glucose-6-phosphate deyhdrogenase (B+). The common Negro variant (A+) showed an identical fingerprint pattern, except that spot marked (B+) was replaced by spot marked (A+) in the variant.

TABLE 2

CHARACTERISTICS OF GLUCOSE-6-PHOSPHATE DEHYDROGENASE VARIANTS

Group	Variant and References	Population Origin	Enzyme Activity in RBC (% of Normal)	Electro-phoretic Mobility (% of Normal)	Column Behavior	K_m for G-6-P	K_m for NADP	Second G-6-P Utilization	Heat Lability	pH Optima	Population Frequency	Remarks
Normal	Normal (B+)[4,10,17]	Various	100	Normal 100	Normal	50–78	2.9–4.4	<4	Normal	Truncate	Usual	
Severe enzyme deficiency associated with chronic nonsphero-cytic hemo-lytic anemia	Oklahoma[4,18]	West European	4–10	Normal 100	?	127–200	20	<4	Low	Narrow peak	Rare	
	Chicago[19]	West European	9–26	Normal 100	?	58–76	3.1–3.7	<4	Very low	Truncate	Rare	
	Eyssen[10]	West European?	0	Slow 90	?	?	?	?	Labile (in cold)	?	Rare	
	Type IV[14]	Italian	2–16	Fast 110	?	Slightly increased	Slightly increased	Normal	Very labile	?	Rare	
Severe enzyme deficiency	Mediterranean (B–)[20]	Greek, Sardinian, Sephardic Jew, Asiatic Indian	0–7	Normal 100	Different from normal (B+) on $CaPO_4$ gel (this paper)	19–26	1.2–1.6	23–37	Low	Biphasic	Common	Serologically distinguishable from normal (B+) (this paper) Normal heat lability reported in Jewish type[21] Greek type may be hetero-geneous[22]
Moderate enzyme deficiency	Negro (A–)[4,10,16]	Negro	8–20	Fast 110	Different from B+ and A+ in DEAE-Sephadex[23] and CM-Sephadex[16]	Normal	Normal	<4	Normal	Truncate	Common	Serologically indistinguishable from B+ and A+[16] Young cells have almost normal enzyme activity[16]
	Seattle[24]	Welsh-Scottish, Greek	8–21	Slow 90	?	15–25	2.4–2.8	7–11	Normal	Slightly biphasic	Rare	Young cells have normal enzyme activity[25]

	(D−)[26]	Irish, German	15	Slow 90	?	?	?	?	?	?	Rare	Identical to G-6-PD (Seattle?)
	Canton[27]	South Chinese	4–24	Fast 105	?	20–36	2.0–2.4	4–15	Slightly reduced	Biphasic	Common	
	West Bengal[28]	Asiatic Indian	9	Slow 90 (TEB) 94 (TRIS)	?	31	6.6	<4	Normal	Truncate	Rare	
Mild enzyme deficiency	Type I[14]	Negro	35	Normal 100	?	Normal	Normal	Normal	?	?	Rare	
	Telhashomer[29]	Sephardic (Tunisian) Jew	25–40	Slow 60–70	?	30–40	?	Normal	Normal	Slightly biphasic	Rare	
	Barbieri[30]	Italian	40–60	Fast 135	?	Increased	Increased	?	Normal	?	Rare	
	Mild Greek Type (B−)[31,32]	Greek	12–45	Normal 100	?	?	?	?	Labile	?	Common	
	Kerala[28]	Asiatic Southeast Indian	50	Slow 75 (TEB) 90 (TRIS)	?	23	1.5	7.4	Normal	Biphasic	Rare	
Very mild or no enzyme deficiency	Negro (A+)[4,10,33,34]	Negro	88	Fast 110	Different from B+ and A− in DEAE- and CM-Sephadex[13,16]	Normal	Normal	<4	Normal	Truncate	Very common	Serologically indistinguishable from B+ or A−[16]
	Austin I[35]	Negro	72	Slow 80	Separable on CM-Sephadex from B+, A+, A−[25]	62–72	3.3	<4	Normal	Truncate	Rare	Probably identical to G-6-PD Ibadan[13]
	Austin II[35]	Negro	75	Slow 90	?	68	3.1	<4	Normal	?	Rare	Probably identical to G-6-PD C[10] or Baltimore[13]
	Madison[36,24]	Norwegian	100	Slow 70 (TEB) 90 (TRIS)	?	?	?	?	?	?	Rare	
	Andrha Porodesh[37]	Asiatic Indian	100	Fast 110 (pH 7.5) 120 (pH 9.0)	?	?	?	?	?	?	?	

240,000. Treatment with 4N Guanidine-HCl and mercaptoethanol dissociated the enzyme into subunits of a molecular weight of approximately 40,000 each, suggesting 6 subunits. Digestion with trypsin yielded 40 peptide spots (FIGURE 2). Amino acid analysis indicated 6.2 percent lysine and 8.04 percent arginine residues. From the number of peptide spots it could be concluded that G-6-PD consisted of 6 identical subunits, each with a molecular weight of 40,000, since the expected number of tryptic peptides in a protein of a molecular weight of 40,000 is about 40 (about 19 lysine residues and about 22 arginine residues per subunit). Removal of NADP from the enzyme caused dissociation into inactive or weakly active subunits of a molecular weight about one-half that of the native protein. The enzyme could be partially inactivated (specific activity 180–200) by dilution, without dissociation into the subunits. Analogs of glucose-6-phosphate accepted as substrate were 2-desoxy-glucose-6-phosphate and galactose-6-phosphate. NAD was a weak substrate.

Mutant Enzymes

A total of at least 20 different glucose-6-phosphate dehydrogenase variants have been recognized so far. Their characteristics are outlined in TABLE 2. Initial classification was best accomplished by noting the severity of the enzyme deficiency, the presence of chronic hemolytic anemia without drug administration, the altered electrophoretic mobility, and the population frequencies (i.e., whether rare mutations or frequent polymorphisms). Some of the more frequently occurring G-6-PD variants have been recently studied in greater detail in our laboratory.

Negro Variant of G-6-PD Associated with Normal Activity (A+)[33,34]

About 18 percent of American Negroes have an electrophoretically rapid G-6-PD not associated with enzyme deficiency in red cells. This variant is inherited as an X-linked trait,[10,38] and the enzyme is usually referred to as the A+ enzyme. A+ enzyme was purified from 10 liters of human blood by methods similar to those used for the normal (B+) enzyme. Detailed enzymic and structural studies were performed. The A+ enzyme, like the normal (B+) enzyme, was found to be an hexamer with a molecular weight of 240,000. A sedimentation constant ($S_{w,20}$) of 9.0 S was found as compared with that of 10.0 S for the normal enzyme, suggesting that the A+ molecules are more asymmetric than the B+ molecules. The Stokes radius was calculated at 5.5 mμ for the normal enzyme and 6.2 mμ for the A+ enzyme. The optimal pH for the A+ enzyme was found to be at pH 8.8 rather than at pH 8.0 as for the normal enzyme. When NAD instead of NADP was used as substrate, A+ enzyme was 25 percent more active in the presence of 7×10^{-3} M $MgCl_2$ than in the absence of $MgCl_2$, whereas the B+ enzyme showed reduced activity in the presence of $MgCl_2$. Michaelis constants for major substrates and for substrate analogues were not essentially different from the normal (B+) enzyme (TABLE 3). No serologic differences between the normal (B+) and the A+ enzymes could be demonstrated by double-diffusion precipitation tests in agar-gel (Ouchterlony method) or by quantitative neutralization tests using anti-normal-G-6-PD serum as antibody. The normal and A+ enzymes also could not be differentiated by microcomplement-fixation techniques.[39]

Amino acid analysis showed no essential differences in amino acid composition between the mutant A+ and the normal (B+) enzyme. Chromatography and

TABLE 3

COMPARISON OF NORMAL (B+) AND COMMON NEGRO VARIANT (A+) OF G-6-PD

Physical Characteristics	Normal Enzyme (B+)	Negro Variant (A+)
Molecular weight	230,000–240,000	230,000–240,000
Sedimentation constant, $S_{20,w}$	10.0	9.0
Stokes radius, mμ	5.5	6.2
Subunit molecular size	ca. 40,000	ca. 40,000
Number of subunits per enzyme	6	6
Specific enzyme activity	700–800	700–800
Optimal pH	8.0	8.8
Michaelis constants		
for Glucose-6-phosphate	$3.9–5.2 \times 10^{-5}$	4.8×10^{-5}
for NADP	$4.4–5.7 \times 10^{-6}$	7.9×10^{-6}
for Galactose-6-phosphate	8.0×10^{-3}	6.2×10^{-3}
for 2-deoxy-D-glucose-6-phosphate	6.0×10^{-3}	4.4×10^{-3}
for NAD	4×10^{-3}	7.8×10^{-3}

electrophoresis of tryptic peptides of the A+ enzyme revealed 40 peptide spots (FIGURE 2), as did the normal enzyme. All but one peptide spot were identical in the two enzymes. Amino acid analysis of the shifted spot and its normal counterpart showed that an asparagine residue in the normal enzyme had been replaced by an aspartic acid residue in the A+ enzyme. The mutant enzyme, therefore, differs from the normal enzyme by a single amino acid substitution produced by a single-step transition for adenine/thymine → guanine/cytosine (A/T→G/C) in the gene. The DNA codons of asparagine are thymine-thymine-adenine (TTA) or thymine-thymine-guanine (TTG); those for aspartic acid are cytosine-thymine-adenine (CTA) or cytosine-thymine-guanine (CTG).

Negro Variant of G-6-PD Associated with Enzyme Deficiency (A–)[16]

Ten to 12 percent of American Negro males have a glucose-6-phosphate dehydrogenase deficiency. The variant is known as the A– enzyme and the enzyme activity in the red cells of these individuals ranges from 10–20 percent of normal. Sufficient material to characterize the A– enzyme in a manner similar to that described for the normal and A+ enzymes have not yet been obtained. A fast G-6-PD band (A–), identical in mobility to the band of the A+ enzyme, can be visualized in enzyme electrophoresis in individuals with the Negro type of G-6-PD deficiency. The mutant A– enzyme is not only identical in electrophoresis to the A+ enzyme, but also does not differ significantly from the A+ and normal enzymes in various enzymic characteristics such as Michaelis constants for glucose-6-phosphate, NADP and NAD, utilization of galactose-6-phosphate and 2-desoxy-glucose-6-phosphate, and optimal pH.[40] However, as frequently happens in studies dealing with protein mutations, use of a different biochemical method can result in separation of protein molecules which seemed identical by various electrophoretic techniques. By the use of CM-Sephadex chromatography, the A– enzyme can be clearly separated from the A+ enzyme: at pH 5.7, the A– enzyme is eluted at a slightly slower rate than the A+ enzyme, and at a slightly faster rate than the normal (B+) enzyme. The demonstration of these differences in chromatographic behavior strongly suggests that the A– enzyme represents yet another structural mutation at the G-6-PD locus. Further studies have given evidence that the A– enzyme is far more easily and irreversibly inactivated *in vitro* than the normal (B+) enzyme: about 80 percent of A− enzyme activity was lost by removal of NADP by dialysis for three days at 4° C.

Serologic studies using the anti-normal G-6-PD serum have shown that the A− enzyme was neutralized at the same rate as the normal and A+ enzymes. This finding indicates that, per molecule, A− enzyme must be as active as the normal (B+) and A+ enzymes. When red cells from Negro males with the A− mutation were fractionated using the two-phase centrifugation technique of Danon *et al.*,[41] the enzyme activity of the young cells was almost normal and contained more than ten times as much enzyme activity as the total unfractionated cell population. By contrast, the young fraction of normal (B+) red cells separated by this method had only three times as much enzyme activity as the total red cell population.

Considering all these findings, it appears that the A− G-6-PD variant represents a structural mutation different from the A+ variant. The mutation does not affect the rate of synthesis and the enzymatic activity of the A− enzyme. However, the mutant A− G-6-PD is characterized by more rapid loss of enzyme activity on red cell aging. The mechanism of accelerated degradation is yet unknown but may be related to more rapid dissociation of the A− enzyme to subunits. It is of interest that enzyme deficiency can be demonstrated only in cells without a nucleus, such as the red blood cell. White cells apparently synthesize new G-6-PD during their life cycle and the more rapid decay of the mutant G-6-PD (observed in red cells) presumably is compensated by new synthesis of G-6-PD in white cells of A− individuals.

Mediterranean Variant of G-6-PD Deficiency (B−)

Fairly severe enzyme deficiency with 0–7 percent of normal enzyme activity in red cells is found in a large number of Greeks, Sardinians, Sephardic Jews, and Asiatic Indians. This Mediterranean variant of G-6-PD deficiency known as the B− enzyme is electrophoretically indistinguishable from the normal enzyme. Enzymic data, such as the Michaelis constants for glucose-6-phosphate and NADP, and somewhat higher relative activity for galactose-6-phosphate and 2-desoxy-glucose-6-phosphate, indicated structural differences between the Mediterranean type of enzyme deficiency and the normal enzyme.[20]

Further studies in this laboratory substantiated that the Mediterranean enzyme is a mutant structurally different from the normal enzyme, as well as from the A+ and A− mutants. The enzyme from subjects with the Mediterranean type of deficiency could be separated chromatographically from the normal enzyme, as well as from the A+ and A− enzymes. Using calcium phosphate-gel chromatography, the Mediterranean enzyme is eluted at a slower rate than the normal enzyme (FIGURE 3). In serologic experiments using the anti-normal G-6-PD serum only 3 units of the mutant Mediterranean enzyme were neutralized by 1 ml of anti-normal G-6-PD serum, whereas 1 ml of anti-normal G-6-PD serum neutralized 9 units of the B+, A+, and A− enzymes. The findings indicate that the specific activity of the mutant Mediterranean enzyme is only one-third of the normal enzyme. Additional studies have shown that the enzyme activity in the fractionated young erythrocytes of subjects with the Mediterranean type of deficiency was only one-third of that of young erythrocytes of normal individuals. This indicates that the enzyme deficiency is already present in young red cells, and that the degradation of the Mediterranean enzyme is much faster than that of the normal enzyme.

The exact biochemical nature of the Mediterranean mutation has not yet been

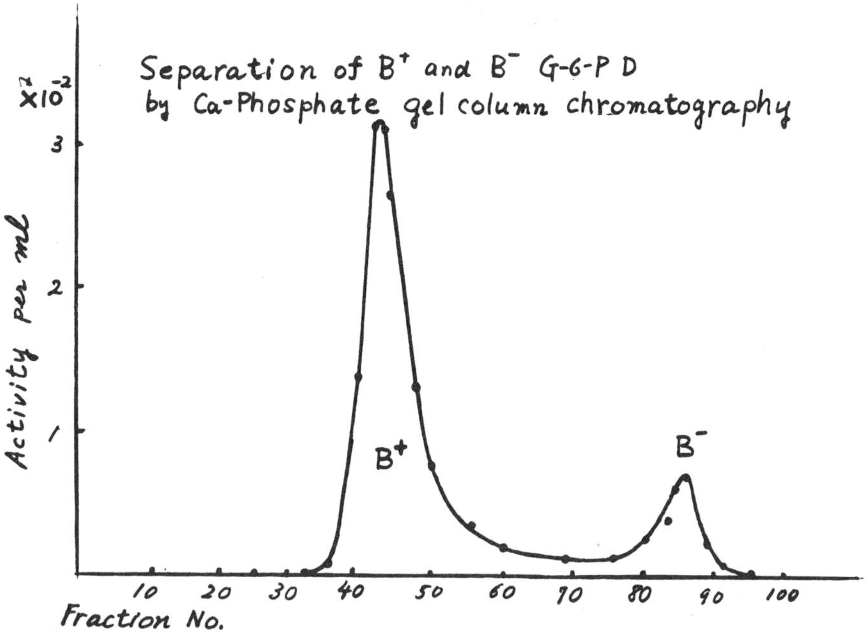

FIGURE 3. Elution pattern of normal (B+) and the common Mediterranean variant (B–) from a calcium phosphate gel column. Partially purified normal (B+, 1.1 units) and the variant (B–, 0.4 units) enzymes were placed on a column (1.5 × 30 cm), and eluted with increasing concentration of phosphate buffer. The exponential gradient was produced by adding 0.25 M phosphate buffer (pH 6.8) to a mixing chamber which contained 150 ml of 0.01 M phosphate buffer (pH 6.8). Flow rate 3.5 ml/tube/25 min.

identified due to lack of sufficient material for purification. Probably this mutation represents another structural mutation that interferes severely with the normal secondary and tertiary configuration of the G-6-PD molecule, which is necessary for normal enzyme activity.

SUMMARY

1. Genetic, serologic and enzymic evidence has demonstrated that red cell G-6-PD and white cell G-6-PD are structurally identical.

2. G-6-PD was purified from red blood cells and characterized. The enzyme is an hexamer of identical subunits, each having a molecular weight of 40,000.

3. The common Negro variant with normal enzyme activity (A+) was purified and found to differ from normal (B+) G-6-PD by a single amino acid substitution: asparagine to aspartic acid.

4. The common Negro variant associated with enzyme deficiency (A–) was found to be separable from the A+ enzyme by CM-Sephadex column chromatography. Its specific activity, serologic characteristics, and enzyme activity in young cells are similar to the normal enzyme, but there is a more rapid loss of enzyme activity on red cell aging, which causes the decreased activity.

5. The common Mediterranean mutation (B–) could be distinguished from the normal enzyme by chromatography (calcium phosphate gel), serologic, and enzymic techniques.

References

1. Koler, R. D., R. H. Bigley, R. T. Jones, D. A. Rigas, P. Vandellinghen & Thompson. 1964. Pyruvate kinase: molecular differences between human red cell and leucocyte enzyme. Cold Spring Harbor Symp. Quant. Biol. **29:** 213–221.
2. Appella, E. & C. L. Markert. 1961. Dissociation of lactate dehydrogenase into subunits with guanidine hydrochloride. Biochem. Biophys. Res. Commun. **6:** 171–176.
3. Cahn, R. D., N. O. Kaplan, L. Levine & E. Zwilling. 1962. Nature and development of lactic dehydrogenases. Science **136:** 962–969.
4. Kirkman, H. N., P. R. McCurdy & J. L. Naiman. 1964. Functionally abnormal glucose-6-phosphate dehydrogenases. Cold Spring Harbor Symp. Quant. Biol. **29:** 391–397.
5. Beutler, E. 1966. Glucose-6-phosphate dehydrogenase deficiency. *In* The Metabolic Basis of Inherited Diseases. J. B. Stanbury, J. B. Wyngaarden & D. S. Fredrickson, Eds. : 1060–1089. McGraw-Hill Book Co. New York, N. Y.
6. Bonsignore, *A*., G. Fornaini, A. Fantoni & G. Leoncini. 1965. Purification and properties of the glucose-6-phosphate dehydrogenase from the human erythrocytes and leucocytes. Italian J. Biochem. **14:** 217–230.
7. Shaw, C. R. & E. Barto. 1965. Autosomally determined polymorphism of glucose-6-phosphate dehydrogenase in *Peromyscus*. Science **148:** 1099–1100.
8. Shaw, C. R. 1966. Glucose-6-phosphate dehydrogenase: homologous molecules in deer mouse and man. Science **153:** 1013–1015.
9. Ohno, S., H. W. Payne, M. Morrison & E. Beutler. 1966. Hexose-6-phosphate dehydrogenase found in human liver. Science **153:** 1015–1016.
10. Boyer, S. H., I. H. Porter & R. G. Weilbacher. 1962. Electrophoretic heterogeneity of glucose-6-phosphate dehydrogenase and its relationship to enzyme deficiency in man. Proc. Natl. Acad. Sci. USA **48:** 1868–1876.
11. Nitowsky, H. M., R. G. Davidson, D. D. Soderman & R. Childs. 1965. Glucose-6-phosphate dehydrogenase activity of skin fibroblast cultures from enzyme-deficient subjects. Bull. J. Hopkins Hosp. **117:** 363–373.
12. Linder, D. & S. M. Gartler. 1965. Distribution of glucose-6-phosphate dehydrogenase electrophoretic variants in different tissues of heterozygotes. Amer. J. Hum. Genet. **17:** 212–220.
13. Porter, I. H., S. H. Boyer, E. J. Watson-Williams, A. Adam, A. Szeinberg & M. Siniscalco. 1964. Variation of glucose-6-phosphate dehydrogenase in different populations. Lancet **i:** 895–899.
14. Pinto, P. C. V., W. A. Newton & K. E. Richardson. 1966. Evidence for four types of erythrocyte glucose-6-phosphate dehydrogenase from G-6-PD-deficient human subjects. J. Clin. Invest. **45:** 823–831.
15. Justice, P., L-Yu Shih & D. Yi-Yung Hsia. 1966. Characterization of leucocyte glucose-6-phosphate dehydrogenase in normal and mutant human subjects. Clin Res. **14:** 318.
16. Yoshida, A., G. Stamatoyannopoulos & A. G. Motulsky. 1967. Negro variant of glucose-6-phosphate dehydrogenase deficiency in man. Science **155:** 97–99.
17. Yoshida, A. 1966. Glucose-6-phosphate dehydrogenase of human erythrocytes. I. Purification and characterization of normal (B+) enzyme. J. Biol. Chem. **241:** 4966–4976.
18. Kirkman, H. N. & H. D. Riley. 1961. Congenital nonspherocytic hemolytic anemia. Amer. J. Dis. Child. **102:** 313–320.
19. Kirkman, H. N., I. M. Rosenthal, E. R. Simon, P. E. Carson & A. G. Brinson. 1964. Chicago I variant of glucose-6-phosphate dehydrogenase in congenital hemolytic disease. J. Lab. Clin. Med. **63:** 715–725.
20. Kirkman, H. N., F. Schettini & B. M. Pickard. 1964. Mediterranean variant of glucose-6-phosphate dehydrogenase. J. Lab. Clin. Med. **63:** 726–735.
21. Ramot, B., S. Bauminger, F. Brok, D. Gafni & J. Schwartz. 1964. Characterization of glucose-6-phosphate dehydrogenase in Jewish mutants. J. Lab. Clin. Med. **64:** 895–904.
22. Kirkman, H. N., S. A. Doxiadis, T. Valaes, N. Tassopoulos & A. G. Brinson. 1965. Diverse characteristics of glucose-6-phosphate dehydrogenase from Greek children. J. Lab. Clin. Med. **65:** 212–221.
23. Luzzatto, L. & N. C. Allan. 1965. Different properties of glucose-6-phosphate dehydrogenase from human erythrocytes with normal and abnormal enzyme levels. Biochem. Biophys. Res. Commun. **21:** 547–554.

24. KIRKMAN, H. N., E. R. SIMON & B. M. PICKARD. 1965. Seattle variant of glucose-6-phosphate dehydrogenase. J. Lab. Clin. Med. **66:** 834–840.
25. YOSHIDA, A., G. STAMMATOYANNOPOULOS & A. G. MOTULSKY. Unpublished data.
26. SHOWS, T. B., R. E. TASHIAN & G. J. BREWER. 1964. Erythrocyte glucose-6-phosphate dehydrogenase in Caucasians: new inherited variant. Science **145:** 1056–1057.
27. MCCURDY, P. R., H. N. KIRKMAN, J. L. NAIMAN, R. T. S. JIM & B. M. PICKARD. 1966. A Chinese variant of glucose-6-phosphate dehydrogenase. J. Lab. Clin. Med. **67:** 374–385.
28. AZEVEDO, E., A. MORROW, H. N. KIRKMAN & A. G. MOTULSKY. To be published.
29. RAMOT, B. & F. BROK. 1964. A new glucose-6-phosphate dehydrogenase mutant (Tel-Hashomer mutant). Ann. Hum. Genet. Lon. **28:** 167–172.
30. MARKS, P. A., J. BANKS & T. R. GROSS. 1962. Genetic heterogeneity of glucose-6-phosphate dehydrogenase deficiency. Nature **194:** 454–456.
31. STAMATOYANNAPOULOS, G., A. PANAYOTOPOULOS, &TH. PAPAYANNOPOULOU. 1964. Mild glucose-6-phosphate dehydrogenase deficiency in Greek males. Lancet **ii:** 932–935.
32. STAMATOYANNOPOULOS, G., TH. PAPAYANNOPOULOU, CHR. BACOPOULOS & A. G. MOTULSKY, 1967. Detection of glucose-6-phosphate dehydrogenase deficient heterozygotes. Blood **29:** 87–101.
33. YOSHIDA, A. 1967. Human glucose-6-phosphate dehydrogenase II. Purification and characterization of Negro type variant (A+) and comparison with normal enzyme B+). Biochem. Genet. **1:** 81–99.
34. YOSHIDA, A. 1967. A single amino acid substitution—asparagine to asparatic acid—between normal (B+) and the common Negro variant (A+) of human glucose-6-phosphate dehydrogenase. Proc. Nat. Acad. Sci. **57:** 835–840.
35. LONG, W. K., H. N. KIRKMAN & H. E. SUTTON. 1965. Electrophoretically slow variants of glucose-6-phosphate dehydrogenase from red cells of Negroes. J. Lab. Clin. Med. **65:** 81–87.
36. NANCE, W. E. & I. UCHIDA. 1964. Turner's syndrome, twinning, and an unusual variant of glucose-6-phosphate dehydrogenase. Amer. J. Hum. Genet. **16:** 380–392.
37. RATTAZZI, M. C. 1966. Screening for electrophoretic variants of glucose-6-phosphate dehydrogenase in different populations. Absts. IIIrd Int Congr. Hum. Genet. : 82.
38. KIRKMAN, H. N. & E. M. HENDRICKSON. 1963. Sex-linked electrophoretic difference in glucose-6-phosphate dehydrogenase. Amer. J. Hum. Genet. **15:** 241–258.
39. SARICH, C. & A. C. WILSON. Unpublished observations.
40. KIRKMAN, H. N. & B. B. CROWELL. 1963. Molecular deficiency of glucose-6-phosphate dehydrogenase in primaquine sensitivity. Nature **197:** 286–287.
41. DANON, D. & Y. MARIKOVSKY. 1964. Determination of density distribution of red cell population. J. Lab. Clin. Med. **64:** 668–674.

CHROMOSOMAL ABERRATIONS AND SUPPRESSION OF LEUKOCYTE MITOSIS INDUCED *IN VITRO* BY A CIRCULATING FACTOR ASSOCIATED WITH ACUTE INFECTIOUS HEPATITIS*

Barbara Mella† and David J. Lang‡

Departments of Neurology and Pediatrics, Harvard Medical School and Department of Neurology and the Children's Service, Massachusetts General Hospital, Boston, Mass.

The chromosomes of human peripheral leukocytes were studied during a recent epidemic of acute infectious hepatitis at the Fernald State School for retarded children in Waverley, Mass. Blood and serum specimens were taken from patients during both the acute and convalescent stages of the disease. Clinical symptoms and liver function tests (primarily serum glutamic oxalacetic transaminase) were used to evaluate the progress of patients during the infection. Additional sera from patients with infectious hepatitis as well as sera from individuals with noninfectious hepatic disease, who demonstrated comparably disturbed liver function studies, were obtained from the Massachusetts General, Boston City, and Saint Elizabeth's Hospitals.

Methods

The method of Moorhead *et al.*[1] of culturing leukocytes and harvesting chromosomes was used, with two minor modifications. Eight drops of whole blood were added to the culture media in place of 1.0 ml of plasma and the cells were exposed to Colcemid® for only two hours.

All cells were scanned. The percentage of leukocytes in metaphase was estimated from a count of at least 200 cells. Chromosomal analysis was based on a count and study of 100 mitotic figures, or all the cells in mitosis if less than 100 were present.

The initial examination employed preparations of peripheral leukocytes taken from patients with acute infectious hepatitis. These studies were repeated on each patient during convalescence.

An indirect method was also utilized in which 0.1 ml of serum under study was added to cultures of leukocytes obtained from healthy individuals. Control preparations of normal blood and sera were simultaneously evaluated.

Results

No metaphase figures were seen in homologous leukocyte cultures obtained from 12 patients during the acute stages of infectious hepatitis. The cells present were pyknotic and deeply stained. Specimens of leukocytes obtained from healthy people demonstrated 8–20 percent metaphase figures. These data are summarized in TABLE 1.

TABLE 2 records the results obtained by the use of the indirect method. When the indirect technique was employed using sera taken from seven patients with acute infectious hepatitis, 0–0.5 percent of the cells were in metaphase. In every case, concurrent control cultures of leukocytes from the same donors were cultivated either without added serum, or with small aliquots obtained from normal

* Supported in part by NBEP 15f1–NB153201 NSRB, Children's Bureau Grant Project no. 238, and USPHS General Research Support grant no. FR 05486.

† Present address: 6120 Brandon Ave., Suite 302, Springfield, Va.

‡ Present address: Department of Pediatrics, Duke University Medical Center, Durham, N. C.

TABLE 1

EFFECT OF INFECTIOUS HEPATITIS ON AUTOLOGOUS LEUKOCYTE CULTURES IN 12 PATIENTS

Patients	Mean Percent Leukocytes in Metaphase
Acute hepatitis	0
Controls	18
Convalescent	9
Controls	15

TABLE 2

EFFECT OF HEPATITIS AND CONTROL SERA ON NORMAL HETEROLOGOUS LEUKOCYTE CULTURES

Serum Source	Number of Patients	Mean Percent Leukocytes in Metaphase
Acute hepatitis	7	<1
Convalescent hepatitis (three months)	4	12
Noninfectious liver disease	8	15
Normal controls	6	17

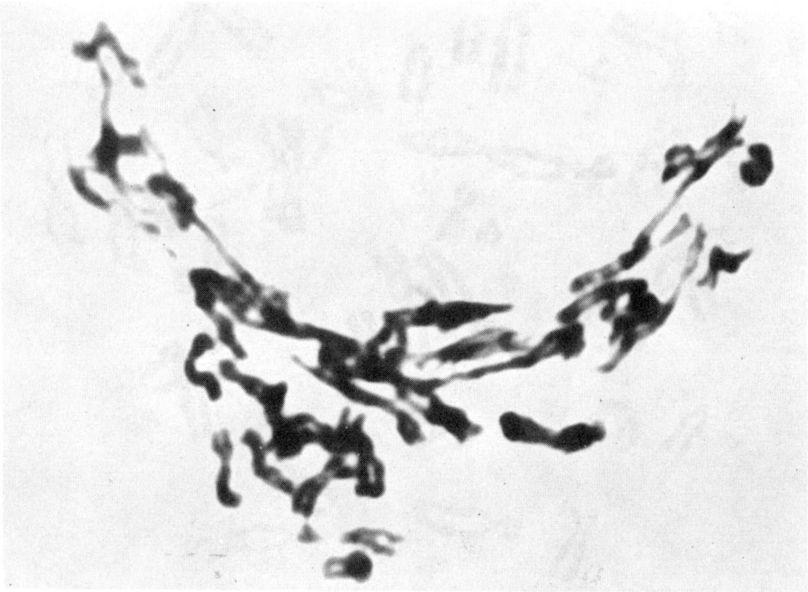

FIGURE 1. Increased chromosomal stickiness. × 780; orig. mag. × 1,200.

individuals, or from patients with noninfectious hepatic disease. These control cultures revealed 13–20 percent metaphase figures.

Suppression of mitotic activity in normal leukocyte cultures was achieved with dilutions up to 10^{-3} of several specimens of serum taken during the acute stages of hepatitis. When these sera were further diluted to 10^{-5}, 5–20 percent of the leukocytes were in metaphase; however, 40–90 percent of the cells in metaphase demonstrated multiple chromosomal breaks, increased stickiness, aneuploidy, or polyploidy. Similar chromosomal aberrations were seen in the peripheral leukocytes cultured during the early convalescent phase of infectious hepatitis. FIGURES 1–5 illustrate examples of the chromosomal abnormalities found.

Chromosomal analyses, which were normal, had been performed on three of these patients prior to the onset of hepatitis. In the cultures obtained before the illness, 23 percent of the leukocytes were in metaphase. During the acute phase of the disease no mitotic activity was seen. In early convalescence (one to two months) 13 percent of the cells present were in metaphase, but 40–90 percent of the chromosomes were abnormal. In late convalescence (five to six months) mitotic activity and chromosomal morphology had returned to normal. TABLE 3 summarizes the changes found. The numerical values reflect the results obtained after counting all stained cells. FIGURES 6 and 7 are representative of the appear-

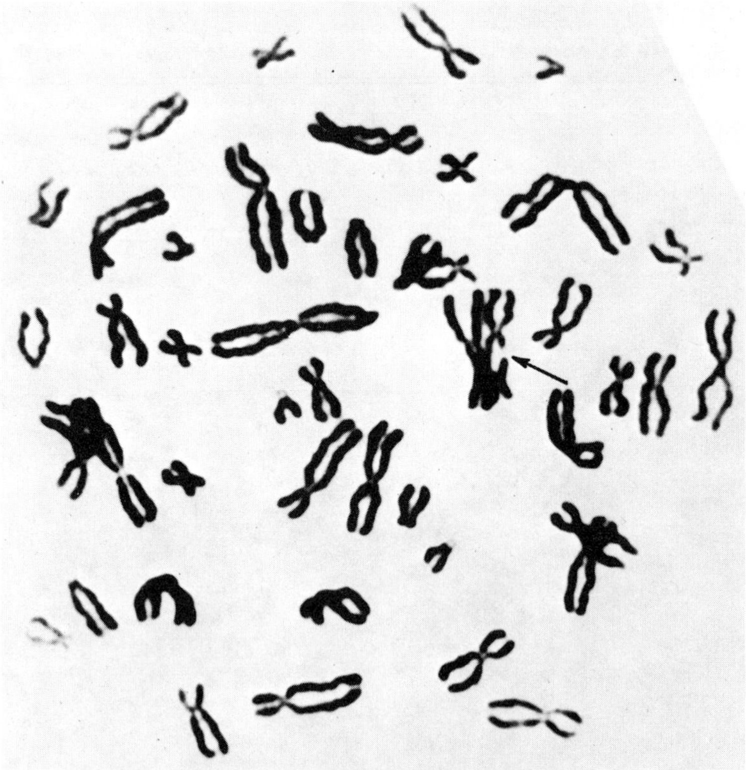

FIGURE 2. An example of chromosomal break. × 1,200.

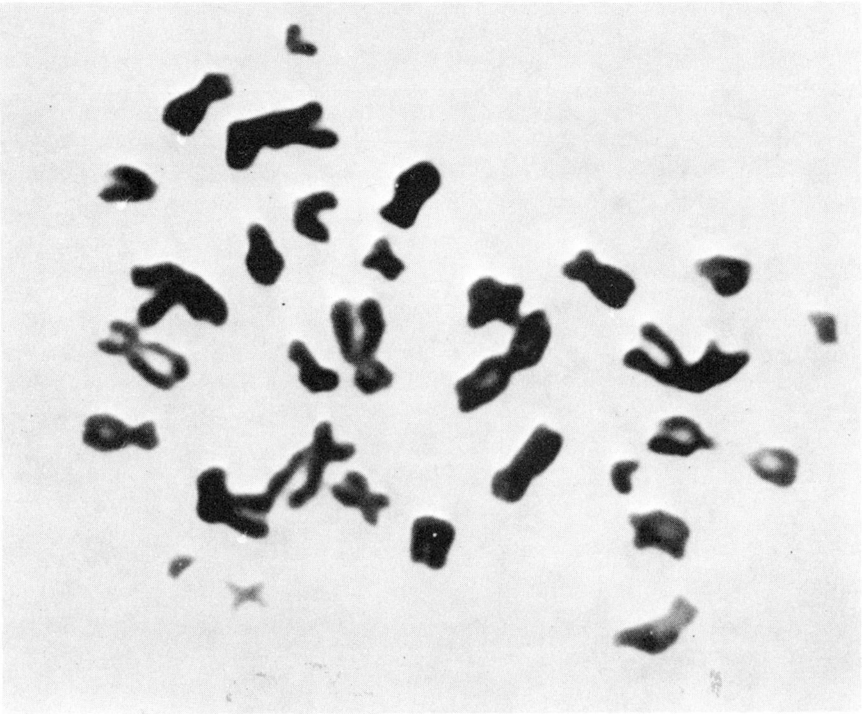

FIGURE 3. Aneuploidy. × 1,020; orig. mag. × 1,200.

ance of the leukocyte cultures in these three cases prior to, during, and after acute infectious hepatitis.

Discussion

The observed suppression of leukocyte mitosis by a factor in acute phase blood and serum of patients with infectious hepatitis has been discussed by the authors in a paper submitted for publication.[2] The fact that leukocyte cultures incubated with sera obtained from patients with noninfectious hepatic disease did not suppress mitosis suggests that elevated serum glutamic oxalacetic transaminase and bilirubin levels were not responsible for the observed effect.

Volunteer experiments have demonstrated a viremia during the acute phase of infectious hepatitis.[3] It seems possible that the virus of hepatitis multiplies in and damages leukocytes. The leukopenia often present during acute infectious hepatitis[4] may be a manifestation of cell injury or interference with leukocyte replication. Preliminary results of attempts to neutralize these effects with convalescent serum and to pass this factor in serial cultures of normal leukocytes have been encouraging.

Chromosomal abnormalities have been noted by other investigators in association with or following infection by hepatitis or other viruses.[5,6] The suppression of mitotis in leukocyte cultures obtained during the acute phase and the presence of chromosomal abnormalities in the convalescent phase of infectious hepatitis have not previously been reported. The addition of several sera diluted to 10^{-5}

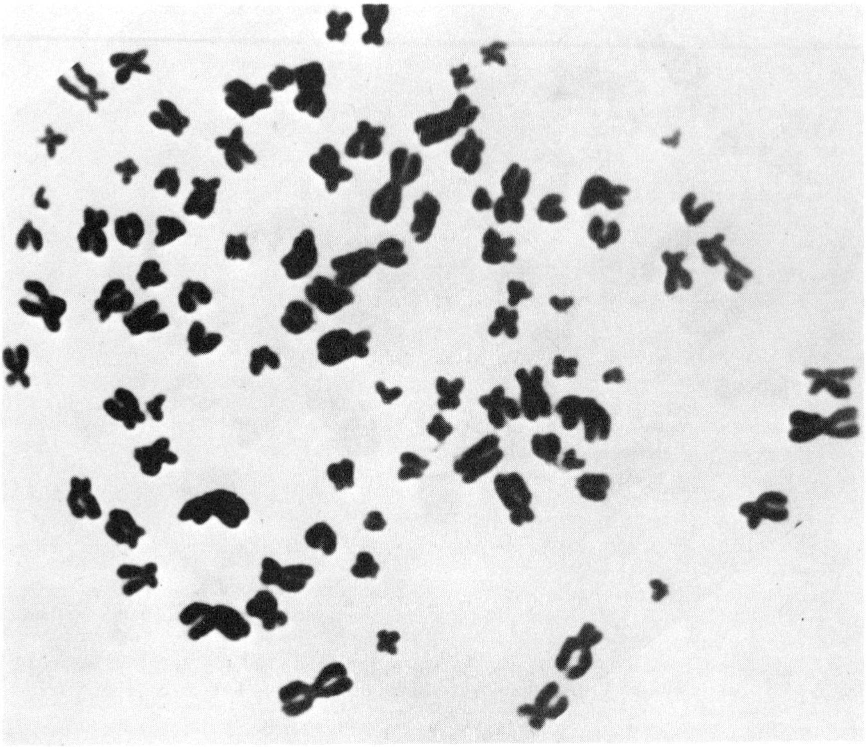

FIGURE 4. Polyploidy. × 1,200.

TABLE 3

THE EFFECT OF INFECTIOUS HEPATITIS UPON AUTOLOGOUS LEUKOCYTE CULTURES IN THREE PATIENTS

Patients	Mean Percent Leukocytes in Metaphase	Percent Chromosomes with Aberrations
Prehepatitis	23	8–11
Acute hepatitis	0	—
Controls	9	3–4
Convalescent (one to two months)	4	40–90
Controls	13	2–6
Convalescent (five to six months)	20	3–10
Controls	17	3–4

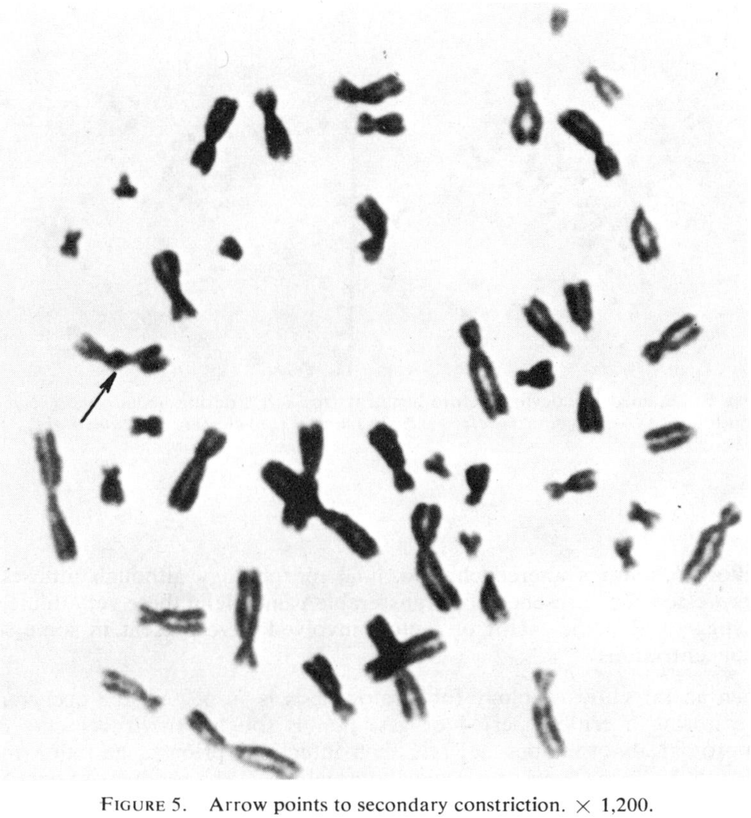

FIGURE 5. Arrow points to secondary constriction. × 1,200.

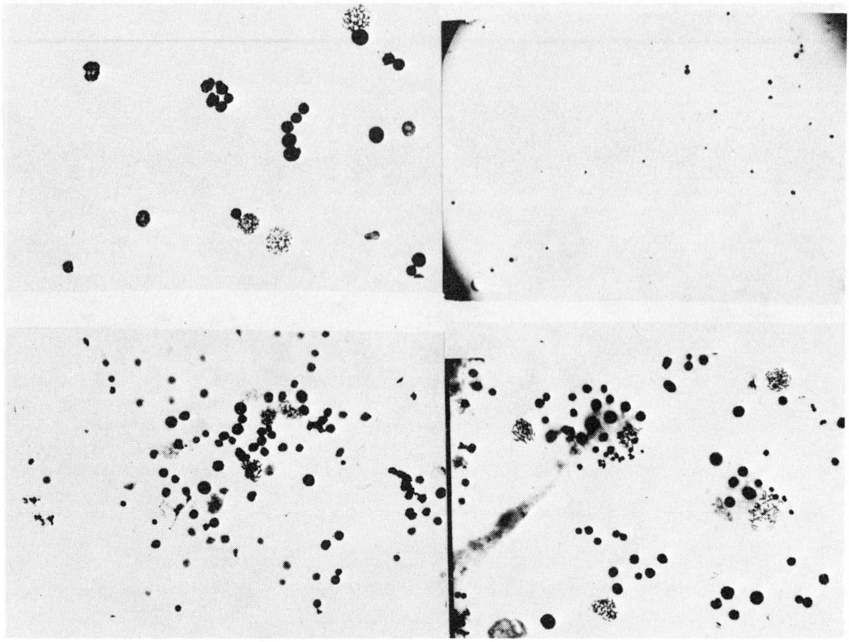

FIGURE 6. Stained leukocytes: before hepatitis (*top left*), during acute illness (*top right*), one month convalescent (*bottom left*), and six months convalescent (*bottom right*). × 109; orig. mag. × 128.

to leukocyte cultures altered chromosomal morphology although mitoses were not suppressed. The presence of a transferable principle in these very dilute specimens suggests that the factor or factors involved were present in some sera in high concentrations.

When an infectious etiology for teratogenesis is suspected, the occurrence of disease during a critical period of gestation is sought. If viruses may induce chromosomal abnormalities *in vivo,* then infections prior to gestation may be relevant to the appearance of genetic abnormalities in the products of conception. The observation of chromosomal abnormalities shortly after acute infectious hepatitis is of interest in view of a recent report suggesting a correlation between the occurrence of acute infectious hepatitis and Down's syndrome nine months later.[6]

Summary

A transferable factor has been demonstrated in the serum of infectious hepatitis patients which suppresses mitotic activity and alters chromosome morphology of cultured peripheral leukocytes. The possible virologic and genetic importance of these findings has been discussed.

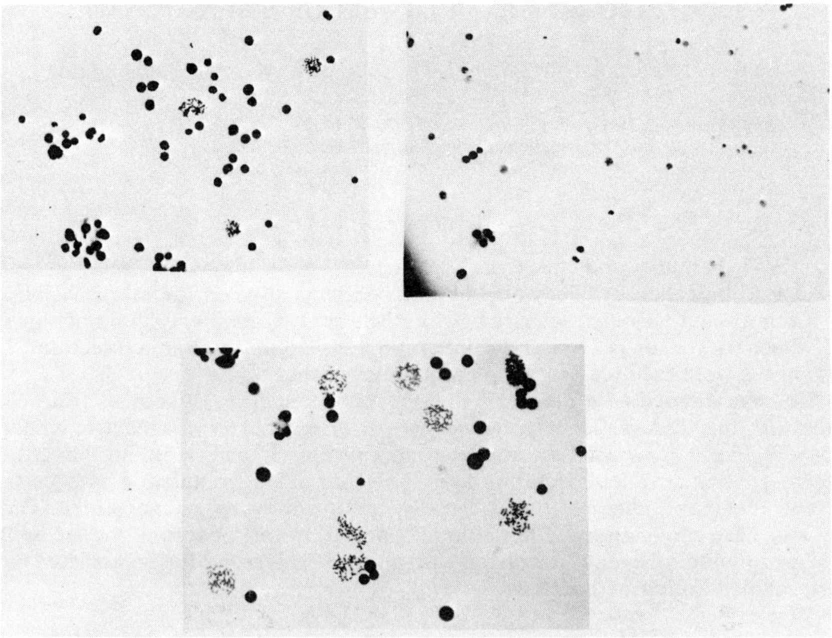

FIGURE 7. Stained leukocytes: before hepatitis (*top left*), during acute illness (*top right*), and six months convalescent (*bottom*). × 109; orig. mag. × 128.

References

1. MOORHEAD, P. S., P. C. NOWELL, W. J. MELLMAN, D. M. BALLIPS & D. A. HUNGERFORD. 1960. Chromosomes preparations of leukocyte cultures from human peripheral blood. J. Exp. Cell Res. **20:** 613–616.
2. MELLA, B. & D. J. LANG. 1967. *In vitro* suppression of leukocyte mitosis in association with acute infectious hepatitis. Science **155:** 80.
3. KRUGMAN, S. & R. WARD. 1964. Infectious Diseases of Children. 3rd edit. Chap. **8:** 104. C. V. Mosby. St. Louis, Mo.
4. GRESSER, I. & D. J. LANG. 1966. Relationship between viruses and leukocytes. Progr. in Med. Virology **8:** 62–130.
5. EL-ALFI, O. S., P. M. SMITH & J. S. BIESELE. 1965. Chromosomal breaks in human leukocyte cultures induced by an agent in the plasma of infectious hepatitis patients. Hereditas **52–3:** 285–294.
6. NICHOLS, W. W. 1966. The role of viruses in the etiology of chromosomal abnormalities. Am. J. of Human Genetics **18:** 80–92.
7. STOLLER, A. 1965. Incidence of infective hepatitis followed by Down's syndrome nine months later. Lancet **ii:** 1221–3.

THE METABOLIC PATTERN AND PHAGOCYTIC FUNCTION OF LEUKOCYTES FROM CHILDREN WITH CHRONIC GRANULOMATOUS DISEASE*

Beulah Holmes, Arthur R. Page, Dorothy B. Windhorst, Paul G. Quie
James G. White, and Robert A. Good

Pediatric Research Laboratories of the Variety Club Heart Hospital and the Departments of Pediatrics and Microbiology, University of Minnesota, Minneapolis, Minn.

INTRODUCTION

In 1957, Berendes and colleagues[1] defined fatal granulomatous disease of childhood as a clinical entity. They noted that this disease affected several male siblings in a family and was characterized by cervicle lymphadenitis, granulomatous involvement of the lungs, liver and spleen, and a susceptibility to skin infections. No organisms were cultured from the granulomas at that time.

We have discovered a defect of the polymorphonuclear leukocytes from children with this disease. Their polymorphonuclear leukocytes phagocytize bacteria normally, but have a decreased capacity to kill certain bacteria. In addition, their polymorphonuclear leukocytes fail to show normal degranulation and certain of the metabolic changes that normally occur following phagocytosis. These patients have provided us with a unique opportunity for separating the metabolic and morphological events associated with phagocytosis from those associated with intracellular killing of bacteria.

MATERIALS AND METHODS

Phagocytosis and Intracellular Killing of Bacteria

Preparation of leukocytes and bacteria for the bactericidal tests were identical to those previously described.[2] In the family studies, penicillin and streptomycin were added after 30 minutes incubation of the leukocyte-bacteria mixtures. Samples were removed at intervals and washed, lysed, and diluted for determination of the total number of viable bacteria.

Leukocyte Metabolism During Phagocytosis

A detailed description of the methods used for the evaluation of metabolism of leukocytes during phagocytosis has been presented elsewhere.[3]

RESULTS

Phagocytosis Studies

In the test system used for the evaluation of leukocyte killing of *Staphylococcus aureus,* the leukocyte-bacteria mixtures were incubated for 30 minutes prior to the addition of antibiotics. This time interval allows phagocytosis to occur in the absence of interference by antibiotics.

A comparison of the capacity to kill *S. aureus* of leukocytes from a patient with chronic granulomatous disease controls is demonstrated graphically in FIGURE 1. Two representative experiments are shown. The difference in rate of

* Supported by USPHS grants nos. AM–05830, HE–06314, AI–00798, HE–02085, and the National Foundation and the American Heart Association.

inactivation of *S. aureus* is due to intraleukocyte survival of the organism. After 24 hours incubation, less than a one log decrease in the total number of bacteria had occurred in the leukocyte cultures from the patient, whereas a decrease of two to three logs had occurred in the control cultures. By this time all extracellular bacteria had been inactivated by the antibiotics in the medium. Differences in the number of bacteria at the initial sampling period are due to differences in killing of bacteria during the 30 minutes of incubation prior to the addition of antibiotics. The total number of bacteria at the first sampling interval, in cultures from patients with granulomatous disease, was always similar to the total number of bacteria added. However, in controls, a variable decrease in total number of bacteria occurred from the time of addition of bacteria to the first sampling interval.

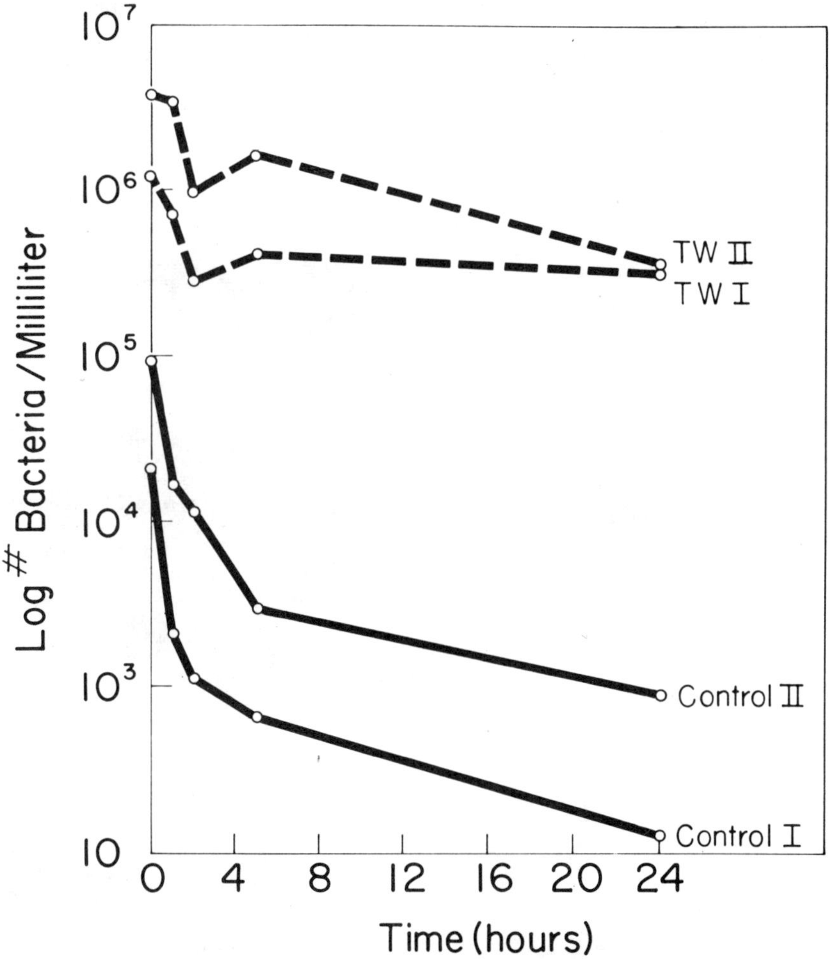

FIGURE 1. Viable bacterial counts from two separate experiments (I & II) showing the fate of *Staphylococcus aureus* during incubation in the presence of leukocytes from a patient (T.W.) with chronic granulomatous disease and controls.

An identical defect in capacity of leukocytes to kill *S. aureus* was found for the other five patients with granulomatous disease. Similar results were obtained when *Aerobacter aerogenes* was used as the test organism. Quie *et al.*[4] have also found the leukocytes of patients with chronic granulomatous disease to be defective in killing *Paracolon hafnia*.

Examination of stained smears revealed a conspicuous difference between leukocytes from patients and controls in the cellular reaction to phagocytosis. There was a lack of vacuolation and degranulation of leukocytes from patients after 30 minutes incubation with *S. aureus*. By contrast, leukocytes from controls were heavily vacuolated after the same period of incubation, and there was evidence of degranulation. In an electron microscopic study, Quie and co-workers[4] have clearly shown that degranulation does not normally occur following phagocytosis by leukocytes from patients (FIGURE 2a & b).

Bactericidal capacity of leukocytes from siblings and parents of patients has also been investigated. As shown in FIGURE 3, in all five families, the mother of the affected child has an intermediate abnormality in killing *S. aureus*. The same

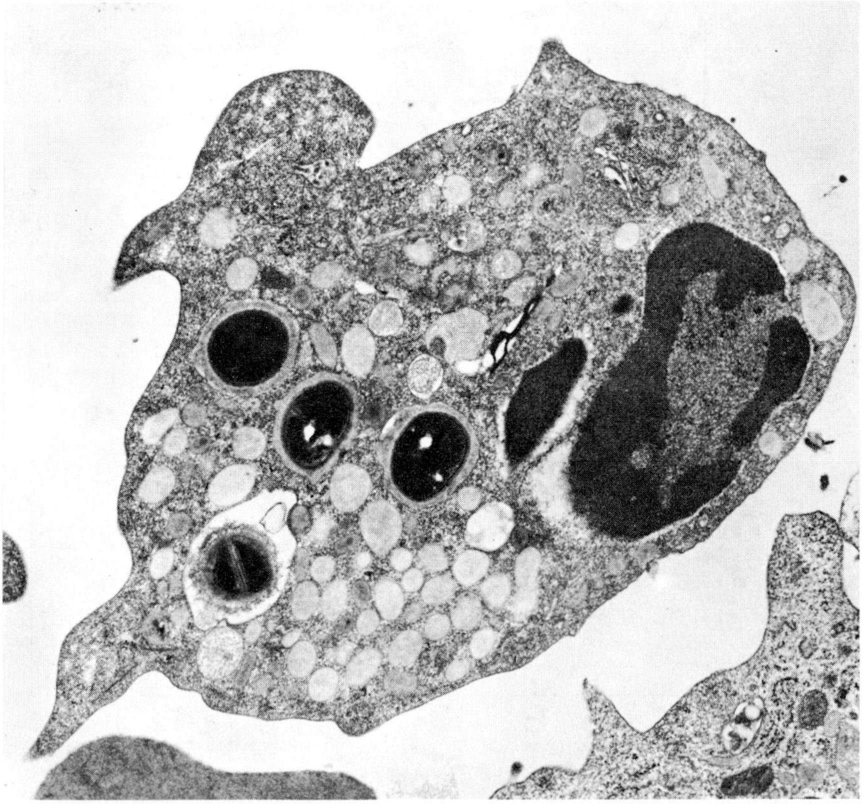

FIGURE 2a. Polymorphonuclear leukocyte from a child with chronic granulomatous disease incubated with staphylococci for one hour. Several bacteria are visible in the cytoplasm. Little degranulation is evident. × 20,250; Orig. mag. × 22,500.

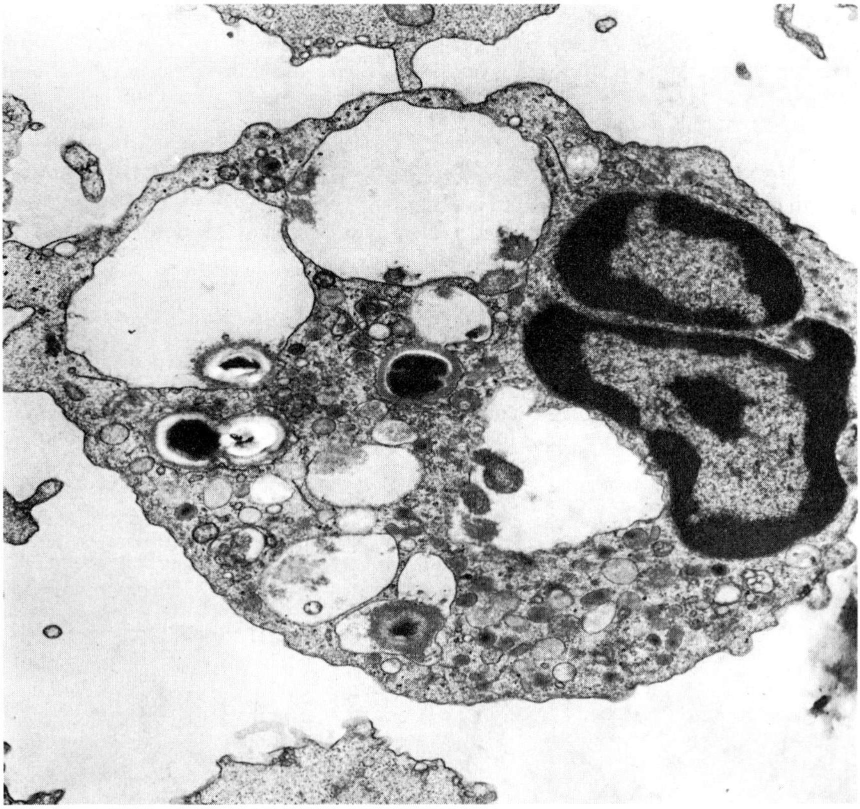

FIGURE 2b. Polymorphonuclear leukocyte from at normal control incubated with staphylococci for 30 minutes. Many bacteria in various stages of destruction are evident within the cell. Note the cytoplasmic vacuoles around or adjacent to the degenerating bacteria. × 16,200; Orig. mag. × 18,000.

was true of the one maternal grandmother available for study. The first sampling interval shown in this Figure was at the time of addition of bacteria to the leukocyte culture and 30 minutes before addition of antibiotics. The pedigrees and results of the phagocytosis test for all immediate family members of the affected children are shown in FIGURE 4. In the five families studied, 11 adults were tested (five males and six females). Of these, the leukocytes of all five males were normal and the leukocytes of all six females were intermediate in capacity to kill *S. aureus*. Nineteen children (patients and their siblings) were studied; nine were male and ten were female. Six of the males were clinically affected; the leukocytes of the remaining three were normal in bactericidal capacity. The leukocytes of six females were normal and four were intermediate in killing bacteria. These family studies provide evidence of the heterozygous expression of the trait in mothers and sisters of affected children and a clear demonstration of the trait's sex-linked recessive character.

Metabolic Studies

The metabolic concomitants of phagocytosis by polymorphonuclear leukocytes have been studied extensively during the past several years. The most striking changes in metabolism during particle uptake are the considerable increases in oxygen consumption[5,6,7] and the amount of glucose metabolized via the hexose monophosphate pathway.[7,8] There are less conspicuous increases in lactic acid production, glucose consumption,[6,7] and glycogen breakdown[6] during phagocytosis. The incorporation of radioactive precursors into lipid is increased, although no net increase in total lipid is observed.[9,10] There is also a marked increase in formate oxidation following particle uptake, which is thought to reflect an increase in hydrogen peroxide formation.[11]

The Effect of Particle Ingestion on Glycolysis and Lipid Turnover

Glucose consumption and lactate production were measured following 20 minutes of incubation with or without latex particles of leukocytes in 1 mM glucose. The resting and stimulated rates for both glucose consumption and

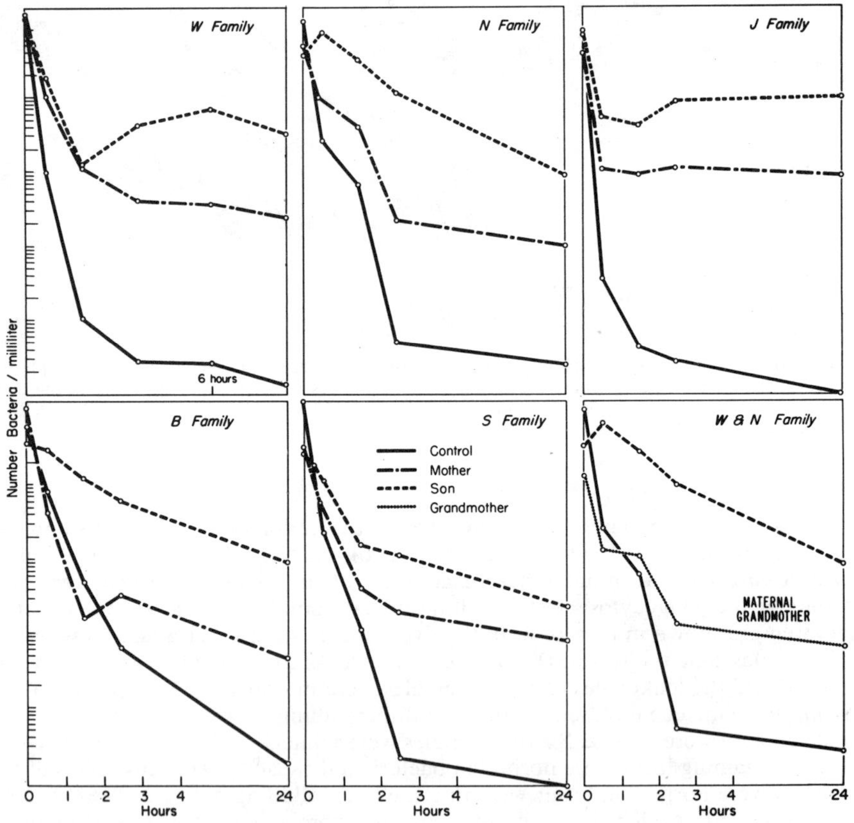

FIGURE 3. The killing of *S. aureus* by leukocytes from immediate family members of patients with chronic granulomatous disease.

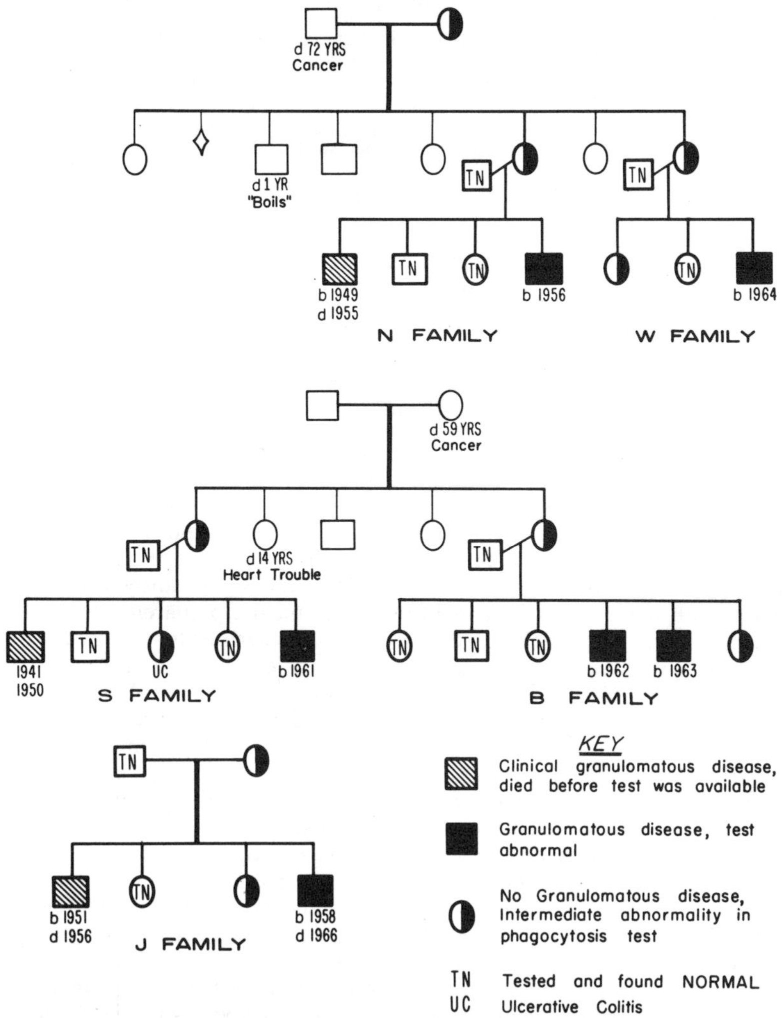

FIGURE 4. Pedigrees of families of children affected with chronic granulomatous disease, showing the capacity of leukocytes from family members to kill *S. aureus*.

lactate production did not differ significantly between patients and controls. Results are summarized in TABLE 1. Little or no breakdown of glycogen due to particle ingestion was detected in either the patient or control group.

The extent of incorporation of phosphate-^{32}P and uniformly labeled glucose-^{14}C into lipid of resting and phagocytizing leukocytes is also shown in TABLE 1. A marked increase in incorporation of both phosphate-^{32}P and uniformly labeled glucose-^{14}C was observed in phagocytizing cells compared with resting cells. This was true with leukocytes from both controls and patients with chronic granulomatous disease. No increase in incorporation of acetate-1-^{14}C into lipid of normal leukocytes during phagocytosis was detected in our experiments.

TABLE 1

METABOLIC CHANGES DURING PHAGOCYTOSIS BY LEUKOCYTES FROM PATIENTS AND CONTROLS

	Percent Change in Metabolism during Uptake of Latex Particles				
	Lactic Acid Produced	Glucose Consumed	Glycogen Degraded	Increased ^{32}P Incorporation into Lipid	Increased Glucose-U-^{14}C Incorporation into Lipid
Controls	17.40 (10)*	11.11 (5)	2.45 (4)	42.5 (2)	60.2 (2)
Patients	19.30 (15)	12.79 (8)	3.92 (4)	52.0 (2)	51.4 (3)
p	0.80	0.80	—	—	—

* Number of experiments performed is given in parentheses.

The Effect of Particle Ingestion on Respiration, Oxidation of Specifically Labeled Glucose, and Formate Oxidation

The amount of increase in oxygen consumption by leukocyte suspensions from patients with chronic granulomatous disease compared with normal controls incubated in the presence of latex particles is shown in TABLE 2. Patients with granulomatous disease have consistently failed to show the normal respiratory increment during particle uptake. The increase in the amount of oxygen consumed during phagocytosis by leukocytes from patients was significantly lower than that observed with controls ($p < 0.001$). Stained smears, prepared after cells were incubated with latex particles in the respiration experiments, revealed no difference in particle uptake between leukocytes of patients and controls.

A comparison of the pattern of $^{14}CO_2$ production from glucose-1-^{14}C and glucose-6-^{14}C by leukocytes incubated with and without latex particles is also shown in TABLE 2. In the presence of 1 mM glucose (1 μc/ml), 5–10 $\times$ 10^6 leukocytes were incubated for 20 minutes. The resting level of $^{14}CO_2$ production from glucose-1-^{14}C was normal in the leukocytes of patients, but very little increase in oxidation occurred during phagocytosis. The average percent increase during phagocytosis was 127 in the patient cells compared to 966 in the control cells. This is a statistically significant difference ($p < 0.001$). The resting values for $^{14}CO_2$ production from glucose-6-^{14}C were also normal in the leukocytes from patients. There was no significant difference between patient and control cells in stimulation of C-6 oxidation during phagocytosis.

In addition, leukocytes from patients did not show the normal increment in $^{14}CO_2$ formation from glucose-3, 4-^{14}C during phagocytosis. Leukocytes were incubated in the presence of 1 mM glucose (0.8 μc/ml) for 15 minutes in these experiments. The increase in $^{14}CO_2$ formation from glucose-3, 4-^{14}C was at least two times greater in leukocytes from controls than from patients. However, the resting rate in the leukocytes of patients was higher than normal.

Iyer *et al.*[11] have used formate oxidation as a measure of increased hydrogen peroxide formation during phagocytosis. In our experiments 2 $\times$ 10^7 leukocytes were incubated in the presence of 5 mM glucose and 3 μc/ml of sodium-formate-^{14}C. Results of the comparison of $^{14}CO_2$ production of resting leukocytes with phagocytizing leukocytes is shown in TABLE 2. Normal leukocytes incubated with latex particles oxidized from two to four times more formate than normal resting cells. Leukocytes from patients with granulomatous disease did not demonstrate any increase in formate oxidation during phagocytosis in the majority of the experiments.

Killing of S. aureus by Normal Leukocytes under Anaerobic and Aerobic Conditions

Under anaerobic conditions phagocytosis takes place normally.[12] There is a normal increase in glucose consumption, lactate production, and lipid turnover.[7,13] However, oxygen consumption, hexose monophosphate shunt activity, and formate oxidation do not increase.[7,11,13] Because this situation appeared to be identical to that of leukocytes from patients with chronic granulomatous disease, this culture system seemed suitable for evaluating bactericidal activity of normal leukocytes.

The results of a typical experiment are shown in FIGURE 5. Leukocytes incubated under anaerobic conditions consistently demonstrated a defect in killing of bacteria compared with leukocytes incubated aerobically. In stained smears, incubated in air and under nitrogen, intact bacteria were seen within the polymorphonuclear leukocytes in approximately equal numbers. However, cells that were incubated anaerobically did not show the vacuolization characteristic of

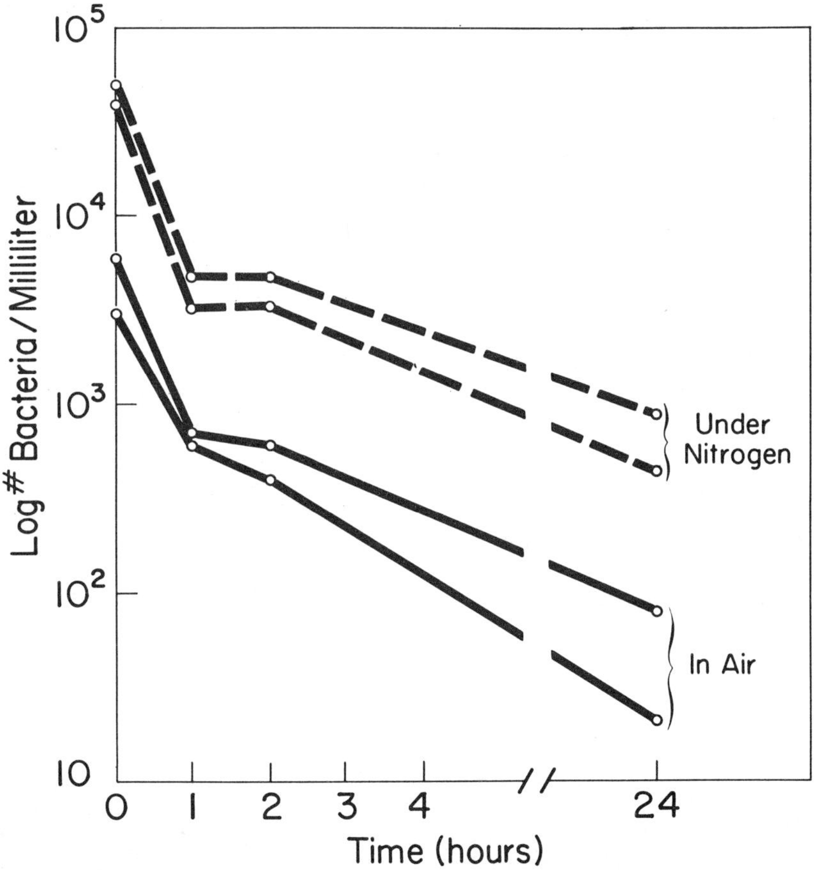

FIGURE 5. The killing of *S. aureus* by leukocytes incubated under anaerobic and aerobic conditions.

TABLE 2

METABOLIC CHANGES ASSOCIATED WITH PARTICLE UPTAKE BY LEUKOCYTES FROM GRANULOMATOSIS PATIENTS

	O_2 Consumed		$^{14}CO_2$ Production from Glucose-1-^{14}C		$^{14}CO_2$ Production from Glucose-6-^{14}C		$^{14}CO_2$ Production from Glucose-3,4-^{14}C		$^{14}CO_2$ Production from ^{14}C Formate	
	No. of Exp.	Percent of Change	No. of Exp.	Percent of Change	No. of Exp.	Percent of Change	No. of Exp.	Percent of Change	No. of Exp.	Percent of Change
Patient cells	29	26	7	127	6	125	7	52	10	24.6
Range		(0–186)		(0–208)		(11–333)		(3–115)		(−42)–(+156)
Control cells	18	411	7	966	6	300	7	272	10	211
Range		(108–2065)		(726–1749)		(86–462)		(156–509)		(90–319)

TABLE 3

CELLULAR RESPONSE TO PHAGOCYTOSIS OF *Staphylococcus aureous* BY LEUKOCYTES INCUBATED UNDER ANAEROBIC AND AEROBIC CONDITIONS

	Time of Incubation			
	30 Minutes		One Hour	
	Aerobic	Anaerobic	Aerobic	Anaerobic
Number of polymorphonuclear leukocytes containing bacteria*	22	11	33	20
Number of polymorphonuclear leukocytes with vacuoles	21	1	27	1

* 100 polymorphonuclear leukocytes were counted.

normal cells during phagocytosis. A tabulation of the marked difference in morphology of cells incubated with bacteria aerobically and anaerobically is shown in TABLE 3. The normal cells incubated anaerobically were similar in their appearance to the cells from the granulomatous patients mentioned earlier.

Possible Enzymatic Abnormality of Leukocytes from Patients with Chronic Granulomatous Disease

It has been demonstrated by Beck[14] that the availability of oxidized NADP is a factor that controls the relative activity of the hexose monophosphate pathway of glucose metabolism. We have investigated several enzymes that might contribute to the turnover of this coenzyme in the leukocyte. The details of these studies have been published elsewhere;[3] however, it would be of value to summarize our results at this time.

The two most obvious possibilities are an abnormality of NADH or NADPH oxidase activity[11,15] or a failure of the stimulation of fatty acid synthesis during phagocytosis. In our investigation, the NADPH and NADH oxidase activities of leukocyte homogenates from patients were found to be similar to those of normal controls. The abnormality in CO_2 formation from carbons 3 and 4 of glucose in leukocytes from our patients may be of importance. A defect in production of acetate for fatty acid synthesis would explain the failure to regenerate NADP since NADPH is utilized in fatty acid synthesis. However, we were unable to demonstrate an increase in incorporation of acetate-^{14}C into lipid of normal cells during phagocytosis, and only a small increase has been observed by other investigators.[9]

Evans and Karnovsky[15] and Cagan[16] have proposed that NADP is regenerated via a NADPH-specific lactic dehydrogenase. It was considered that if NADH was reoxidized by the NADH oxidase during phagocytosis, pyruvate might be available to reoxidize NADPH. It has been demonstrated that pyruvate stimulates the conversion of the C-1 carbon of glucose to CO_2 in resting leukocytes.[13,17] Considerable NADPH-linked lactic dehydrogenase activity was found to be present in the supernatant fraction of leukocyte homogenates and was shown to be most active at an acid pH.[15] We demonstrated that pyruvate stimulates the direct oxidation of glucose by leukocytes from patients to levels comparable to those of normal cells. If the mechanism whereby pyruvate-stimulated oxidation of the C-1 carbon of glucose to CO_2 is indeed via a NADPH-linked lactic dehydrogenase, the enzyme would appear to be normal in leukocytes from children with chronic granulomatous disease.

Four other possible pathways for regeneration of NADP are malic enzyme, glutamic dehydrogenase, transhydrogenase, and glutathione reductase. We studied the incorporation of sodium bicarbonate-^{14}C and pyruvate-2-^{14}C into Krebs cycle intermediates and amino acids of leukocytes. We found that the CO_2 fixation into organic acids and amino acids by leukocytes from patients was identical in extent and pattern to that of normal cells. There is evidence that CO_2 fixation by cells is not due to malic enzyme, but rather to the activity of pyruvate carboxylase,[18] a carboxylation reaction that is not reductive. Since CO_2 fixation is normal in the cells of patients, this is probably not an important source of NADP. Glutamic dehydrogenase has not been shown to be NADPH-specific in mammalian cells,[19] although there is evidence that NADPH can take part in the reaction as well as NADH. In our column chromatography studies, a normal level of incorporation of CO_2 and pyruvate-2-^{14}C into glutamic acid by leukocytes from patients was observed. The possibility that transhydrogenase activity supplies NADP for the hexose monophosphate shunt has been suggested.[17,20] However, transhydrogenase activity has been found to be extremely low in human leukocytes and completely lacking in guinea pig leukocytes.[17,21] Cagan[22] has measured the activity of glutathione reductase in guinea pig leukocytes, and both the oxidized and reduced forms of glutathione have been found to be present in human leukocytes.[23] It is possible that NADP is made available by the reduction of oxidized glutathione by NADPH.

Discussion

Results of the present study clearly show that the previously described clinical entity, chronic granulomatous disease of childhood, can now be defined in terms of an abnormality in leukocyte function. The fact that the leukocytes from these children phagocytize certain bacteria without killing them is probably the pathogenesis of their clinical problems. It seems possible that these patients react to organisms of low virulance in a manner similar to the normal person infected with tubercle bacilli or *Brucella,* organisms that can survive intracellularly.[24,25]

The familial incidence of this disease suggested a sex-linked recessive mode of inheritance.[26,27,28] The finding of a less severe bactericidal defect of the leukocytes from the mothers and some of the female siblings of the patients definitely establishes this syndrome as a sex-linked recessive trait.

Much is known about the morphological and metabolic changes associated with the phagocytosis of bacteria by normal polymorphonuclear leukocytes.[29,30] It has been shown that following phagocytosis, leukocyte granules rupture and empty their contents into the phagocytic vacuole immediately surrounding the ingested bacterium. It has been assumed that degranulation is responsible for the intracellular killing and digestion of bacteria.

Results of the many investigations of the metabolic properties and bactericidal capacity of leukocytes have indicated that it is impossible to alter the fate of intracellular bacteria by any reasonable manipulation. In every case, the rate of uptake of bacteria has controlled the rate of intracellular killing of bacteria by leukocytes.[6] As a result, there is essentially no information about the nature of the metabolic changes associated with only the intracellular phases of phagocytosis in normal leukocytes, whereas a large volume of information is available on the overall metabolic changes during phagocytosis. Studies of the metabolic changes associated with phagocytosis have established that particle ingestion is dependent on glycolysis; however, the importance to the cell of other changes in metabolism during phagocytosis has not been defined.

We have demonstrated that the leukocytes from patients with chronic granulomatous disease show normal increases in lactic acid production, glucose consumption, glycogen breakdown, Krebs cycle activity, and lipid synthesis during phagocytosis. However, the leukocytes from our patients fail to show the normal stimulation of the hexose monophosphate pathway, oxygen consumption, and formate oxidation during phagocytosis. Thus, it appears that the known metabolic events associated with phagocytosis are related to two separate cellular functions: (1) glycolysis, lipid turnover and Krebs cycle stimulation are related to the uptake of particles; whereas (2) the stimulation of the hexose monophosphate pathway, respiration, and hydrogen peroxide formation are associated with the intracellular killing of bacteria and the degranulation of leukocytes following phagocytosis. The results of our anaerobic experiments support the latter suggestion. Under anaerobic conditions, leukocytes have been shown to phagocytize bacteria normally[12] and to show a normal increase in lactic acid production, glucose consumption, and lipid turnover.[7,13] However, under these conditions, the stimulation of the hexose monophosphate pathway, oxygen consumption, and formate oxidation does not take place.[7,11,13]

We have shown that normal human leukocytes do not kill *S. aureus* normally under anaerobic conditions. We have also come to the conclusion, based on morphological investigations, that leukocytes incubated under anaerobic conditions are not stimulated to degranulate during phagocytosis. We have, therefore, effectively reproduced the metabolic and functional parameters of the leukocyte abnormality observed in patients with chronic granulomatous disease *in vitro*. It has been demonstrated recently that guinea pig polymorphonuclear leukocytes incubated under anaerobic conditions do not kill *E. coli* at a normal rate.[31] However, these investigators claimed that degranulation of leukocytes occurs normally in anaerobic cultures during phagocytosis, a finding at variance with our observations.

Our efforts to define the precise enzymatic defect of leukocytes from patients with chronic granulomatous disease have not yet been successful. However, we take our observations as sound evidence for predicting a defect in a single enzyme. An obvious possibility is a defect in an enzyme that utilizes NADPH. It has been demonstrated that the availability of the oxidized form of this coenzyme is involved in the regulation of the hexose monophosphate pathway.[14] We have investigated several of the possible enzymes involved and found them to be normal. There are undoubtedly many other enzymes, not yet defined, that utilize NADPH. There are several known oxidases[32] in leukocytes, and it is tempting to assume that an oxidase is missing which utilizes NADPH. This enzymatic defect would account for the failure of stimulation of the hexose monophosphate pathway and respiration, as well as for the failure of increased hydrogen peroxide formation. We have measured NADPH oxidase activity by the method of Evans and Karnovsky[17] and found normal levels of activity in the leukocytes of our patients.

We think that the failure of the leukocytes of patients with chronic granulomatous disease to show an increase in hydrogen peroxide formation is of central importance. Hydrogen peroxide may be bactericidal for certain bacterial species.[31] In addition, the formation of hydrogen peroxide and subsequent peroxidation of the lipid of red blood cells has been shown to lead to red cell lysis.[33,34] This suggests a possible relationship of lipid peroxidation to lysosomal lysis.

Although we have not yet defined the enzymatic abnormality of leukocytes from patients with chronic granulomatous disease, we have demonstrated a functional abnormality of the leukocytes from these patients and an associated metabolic defect. Further investigation of the metabolism of leukocytes from patients with chronic granulomatous disease may lead to a clear understanding of leukocyte function in relation to the intracellular killing of bacteria.

Summary

1. Fatal granulomatous disease is a definable clinical entity.

2. The syndrome has been shown to be inherited as a sex-linked recessive trait.

3. The leukocytes of these children have a normal capacity of phagocytosis but are defective in killing of certain bacterial strains.

4. The leukocytes of these children are defective in the degranulation process that normally follows phagocytosis.

5. The defect in killing is associated with a metabolic defect.

6. We have reproduced the functional defect with normal leukocytes incubated under anaerobic conditions.

References

1. Berendes, H., R. A. Bridges & R. A. Good. 1957. A fatal granulomatosis of childhood: The clinical study of a new syndrome. Minnesota Med. **40:** 309.
2. Holmes, B., P. G. Quie, D. B. Windhorst & R. A. Good. 1966. Fatal granulomatous disease of childhood: An inborn abnormality of phagocytic function. Lancet **i:** 1225.
3. Holmes, B., A. R. Page & R. A. Good. 1967. Studies of the metabolic activity of leucocytes from patients with a genetic abnormality of phagocytic function. J. Clin. Invest. **46:** 1422.
4. Quie, P. G., J. G. White, B. Holmes & R. A. Good. 1967. *In vitro* bactericidal capacity of human polymorphonuclear leukocytes: Diminished activity in chronic granulomatous disease of childhood. J. Clin. Invest. **46:** 668.
5. Baldridge, C. W. & R. W. Gerard. 1933. The extra respiration of phagocytosis. Amer. J. Physiol. **103:** 235.
6. Cohn, Z. A. & S. I. Morse. 1960. Functional and metabolic properties of polymorphonuclear leucocytes. J. Exp. Med. **111:** 667.
7. Sbarra, A. J. & M. L. Karnovsky. 1959. The biochemical basis of phagocytosis. I. Metabolic changes during the ingestion of particles by polymorphonuclear leucocytes. J. Biol. Chem. **234:** 1355.
8. Stahelin, H., M. L. Karnovsky, A. E. Farnham & E. Suter. 1957. Studies on the interaction between phagocytes and tubercle bacilli. III. Some metabolic effects in guinea pigs associated with injection with tubercle bacilli. J. Exp. Med. **105:** 265.
9. Sbarra, A. J. & M. L. Karnovsky. 1960. The biochemical basis of phagocytosis. II. Incorporation of C^{14}-labeled building blocks into lipid, protein, and glycogen of leucocytes during phagocytosis. J. Biol. Chem. **235:** 2224.
10. Elsbach, P. 1959. Composition and synthesis of lipids in resting and phagocytizing leucocytes. J. Exp. Med. **110:** 969.
11. Iyer, G. Y. N., M. F. Islam & J. H. Quastel. 1961. Biochemical aspects of phagocytosis. Nature **192:** 535.
12. Nungester, W. J. 1951. Mechanisms of man's resistance to infectious diseases. Bacteriol. Rev. **15:** 105.
13. Rossi, F. & M. Zatti. 1964. Changes in the metabolic pattern of polymorphonuclear leucocytes during phagocytosis. Brit. J. Exp. Path. **45:** 548.
14. Beck, W. S. 1958. Occurrence and control of the phosphogluconate oxidation pathway in normal and leukemic leukocytes. J. Biol. Chem. **232:** 251.
15. Evans, W. H. & M. L. Karnovsky. 1961. A possible mechanism for the stimulation of some metabolic functions during phagocytosis. J. Biol. Chem. **236:** PC30.
16. Cagan, R. H. & M. L. Karnovsky. 1964. Enzymatic basis of respiratory stimulation during phagocytosis. Nature **204:** 255.
17. Evans, W. H. & M. L. Karnovsky. 1962. The biochemical basis of phagocytosis. IV. Some aspects of carbohydrate metabolism during phagocytosis. Biochem. **1:** 159.
18. Scrutton, M. C., D. B. Keech & M. F. Utter. 1965. Pyruvate carboxylase. IV. Partial reactions and the locus of activation of acetyl coenzyme A. J. Biol. Chem. **240:** 574.
19. Euler, H. Von, E. Adler, G. Gunther & N. B. Das. 1938. Uber den enzymatischen Abbau und Aufbau der Glutaminsaure. II. In tierischen Geweben. Z. Physiol. Chem. **254:** 61.

20. ROSSI, R. & M. ZATTI. 1961. Pathways of glucose oxidation in leucocytes. Exp. Cell Res. **25:** 182.
21. SILBER, R., F. M. HUENNEKENS & B. W. GABRIO. 1963. Studies on normal and leukemic leucocytes. V. Pyridine nucleotide transhydrogenases. J. Clin. Invest. **42:** 1908.
22. CAGAN, R. H. 1966. Personal communication.
23. HARDIN, B., W. N. VALENTINE, J. H. FOLLETTE & J. S. LAWRENCE. 1954. Studies on the sulfhydryl content of human leucocytes and erythrocytes. Amer. J. Med. Sci. **228:** 73.
24. SUTER, E. 1953. Multiplication of tubercle bacilli within mononuclear phagocytes in tissue culture derived from normal animals and animals vaccinated with BCG. J. Exp. Med. **97:** 235.
25. HOLLAND, J. J. & M. J. PICKETT. 1958. A cellular basis of immunity in experimental brucella infection. J. Exp. Med. **108:** 343.
26. BRIDGES, R. A., H. BERENDES & R. A. GOOD. 1959. A fatal granulomatous disease of childhood. J. Dis. Child. **97:** 387.
27. LANDING, B. H. & H. S. SHIRKEY. 1957. A syndrome of recurrent infection and infiltration of viscera by pigmented lipid histiocytes. Pediatrics **20:** 431.
28. CARSON, M. J., D. L. CHADWICK, C. A. BRUBAKER, R. S. CLELAND & B. H. LANDING. 1965. Thirteen boys with progressive septic granulomatosis. Pediatrics **35:** 405.
29. HIRSCH, J. G. & Z. A. COHN. 1960. Degranulation of polymorphonuclear leucocytes following phagocytosis of microorganismis. J. Exp. Med. **112:** 1005.
30. KARNOVSKY, M. L. 1962. Metabolic basis of phagocytic activity. Physiol. Rev. **42:** 143.
31. SELVARAJ, R. J. & A. J. SBARRA. 1966. Relationship of glycolytic and oxidative metabolism to particle entry and destruction in phagocytosing cells. Nature **211:** 1272.
32. DITTRICH, H. 1962. Physiology of neutrophils. *In* The Physiology and Pathology of Leukocytes. H. Braunsteiner, Ed. : 130–151. Grune & Stratton, Inc. New York, N. Y.
33. MENGEL, C. E. & H. KANN, JR. 1965. A role of peroxidation of erythrocyte lipid in PNH hemolysis. Abstr. J. Lab. Clin. Med. **66:** 1002.
34. DODGE, J. T., G. COHEN, H. J. KAYDEN & G. B. PHILLIPS. 1966. Peroxidation of membrane lipids: A mechanism for cell damage in acanthocytosis. Abstr. J. Clin. Invest. **48:** 1000.

PART III. LEUKOCYTE ALKALINE PHOSPHATASE

THE REGULATION OF LEUKOCYTE ALKALINE PHOSPHATASE*

F. Rosner,† S. L. Lee,† F. S. Schultz,† and P. C. Gorfien‡
Maimonides Hospital, Brooklyn, N. Y.

INTRODUCTION

We have noted sex differences in leukocyte alkaline phosphatase activity in healthy individuals that appear to be a function of androgenic, and possibly estrogenic stimulation.[1] The activity of this enzyme is significantly higher in women than in men but no differences between boys and girls occur until puberty. After menopause, values for women approach those of men. *In vivo* and *in vitro* studies, attempting to delineate some of the regulatory mechanisms of leukocyte alkaline phosphatase activity, are the subjects of this presentation.

MATERIALS AND METHODS

Sources

Blood was obtained from healthy children in a Well-Baby Clinic. Healthy adult subjects consisted of physicians, medical students, nurses, technicians, and other hospital personnel. Subjects with acute infections or fever were excluded. Peripheral blood smears were scanned to rule out hematological abnormalities. In addition, patients with a variety of hematological and nonhematological disorders were studied.

Leukocyte Alkaline Phosphatase

Leukocytes were separated from whole blood by differential sedimentation using 6 percent dextran. After several washings with normal saline, hypotonic saline was added to lyse the few remaining erythrocytes and, thus, pure leukocyte suspensions were obtained. The number of neutrophils in the white cell suspensions was determined by multiplying the percentage of neutrophils obtained by differential counts on peripheral blood smears by the total count of the leukocyte suspension. Alkaline phosphatase activity was measured biochemically according to the sigma method[2] using glycine-buffered *p*-nitrophenyl phosphate (pH 9.3) as substrate. Results are expressed as milligrams of phosphorus liberated per hour per 10^{10} polymorphonuclear leukocytes. All determinations were performed in duplicate.

Histochemical demonstration of leukocyte alkaline phosphatase was achieved by slight modification of the Gomori technique.[3]

Preparation of Glassware

All glassware, including pipettes, was first cleansed in the usual manner with commercial detergent (Haemo-Sol; Meinecke & Co., Baltimore, Md.) in a laboratory glassware washer (Heinicke Instruments; Hollywood, Fla.). This

* This work was supported by grant No. AM07439 from the National Institute of Arthritis and Metabolic Diseases, National Institutes of Health, United States Public Health Service, Department of Health, Education and Welfare, Washington, D. C.
† Division of Hematology, Department of Medicine.
‡ Pediatric Research Laboratories.

clean glassware was immersed for a minimum of 12 hours in 10 percent hydrochloric acid, rinsed thoroughly in twice deionized water (Crystalab Deeminizer; Hartford, Conn.) and oven dried.

Measurement of Zinc and Magnesium

Leukocyte zinc was measured histochemically, employing the dithizone reaction, as described by Szmigielski and Litwin.[4] In addition, both zinc and magnesium levels in leukocytes were determined by atomic absorption spectrophotometry as follows: 1 ml samples of leukocyte suspensions were added to 2 ml aliquots of 10 percent trichloracetic acid at 20° C. Complete deproteinization occurred. After centrifugation at 2,500 rpm for 20 minutes, zinc levels were measured on the supernatants. For magnesium determinations, supernatants were further diluted 15 times in order to be in the range of measurability of the instrument, since magnesium concentration in human blood is much higher than that of zinc.

Further washings of the precipitate with trichloracetic acid failed to release additional zinc or magnesium. Various other concentrations of trichloracetic acid were tested at different temperatures without improving the yield of zinc or magnesium.

Operation of the Atomic-Absorption Spectrophotometer

The atomic-absorption spectrophotometer (Model No. 303, Perkin-Elmer Co., Norwich, Conn.) was operated exactly according to the instruction manual (Revised May, 1966) for magnesium determinations. For zinc measurements, the following operating conditions were applied: wavelength 214 mμ in the ultraviolet range with a slit opening of 5 (3 mm, 20 Å). The hollow-cathode source was 20 ma, the airflow rate was 5.5 and the acetylene flow rate was 7.0 on the flowmeter. For leukocyte magnesium determinations, noise suppression was set at 3 and scale expansion at 1. For leukocyte zinc measurement, noise suppression was set at 4 and scale expansion at 3.

Magnesium standards in varying concentrations were prepared by dissolving powdered magnesium oxide (Mallinckrodt) in a few drops of concentrated hydrochloric acid and diluted to volume with deionized water. Zinc standards were prepared in a similar manner using pure zinc metal (Fisher). Standard calibration curves were obtained and plotted daily for each analysis and separately for each setting on the instrument. Zinc and magnesium content of unknown samples were interpolated from these standard curves. Random samples were done in duplicate and triplicate and on separate days, with excellent reproducibility.

Recovery of Zinc and Magnesium from Leukocytes

In order to ascertain whether trichloracetic acid releases all the zinc and magnesium from leukocytes, numerous recovery experiments were carried out. Leukocyte suspensions from normal persons were separated into three aliquots. One aliquot was processed with trichloracetic acid as described above. A second aliquot was dry-ashed in a muffle oven, redissolved with 1 drop of concentrated hydrochloric acid and made up to 3 ml with 10 percent TCA. The third aliquot was "prespiked" with a known amount of zinc or magnesium standard and then ashed. Recovery was nearly identical in all three aliquots and ranged between 98 percent and 103 percent.

Results

Endocrine Studies

Leukocyte alkaline phosphatase levels were higher in children than in adults (TABLE 1). However, no significant difference between boys and girls was found. Statistically significant regression with age was found for both sexes.

Adult subjects were postpubertal men and women. The women were all premenopausal, and men up to the age of 60 years were included. There was a very significant difference ($p < .001$) in leukocyte alkaline phosphatase activity between the sexes (TABLE 1).

Elderly subjects were defined as women at least two years postmenopausal and men aged 65 years or above. Leukocyte alkaline phosphatase values for elderly women were nearly identical with those of elderly men (TABLE 1).

To test the hypothesis that androgens and possibly estrogens inhibit leukocyte alkaline phosphatase activity we studied the effect of various androgenic and estrogenic hormones on this enzyme.

In Vitro Studies

Ten different androgens and eight different estrogens obtained in pure crystalline form were dissolved in 95 percent ethyl-alcohol and added in varying concentrations to leucocyte suspensions. Alkaline phosphatase activity was measured in these white cells before and after the addition of the various hormones. Inhibition of enzyme activity by androgens was found in two out of five patients with polycythemia vera whom we tested (FIGURE 1). Such inhibition could not be demonstrated with estrogenic hormones (FIGURE 2).

In Vivo Studies

Female patients with carcinoma of the breast, all of whom were either postmenopausal or surgically castrated, were studied. Patients receiving androgenic hormones had lower leukocyte alkaline phosphatase levels than did those receiving no therapy (TABLE 2).

Elevated leukocyte alkaline phosphatase levels have been reported in pregnancy.[5-7] We have confirmed these findings (TABLE 3). Several normal women, tested during various phases of their menstrual cycle, showed no essential change in their leukocyte alkaline phosphatase levels.

TABLE 1

LEUKOCYTE ALKALINE PHOSPHATASE ACTIVITY IN NORMAL HEALTHY SUBJECTS IN VARIOUS AGE GROUPS

	Sex	Number of Subjects	Mean LAPA*	Significance of Differences Between Means
Children	male	26	66	$p > 0.5$
	female	20	70	
Adults	male	74	23	$p < .001$
	female	75	35	
Elderly subjects	male	43	21	$p > 0.5$
	female	65	22	

* Leukocyte alkaline phosphatase activity expressed as milligrams of phosphorus liberated per hour per 10^{10} polymorphonuclear leukocytes.

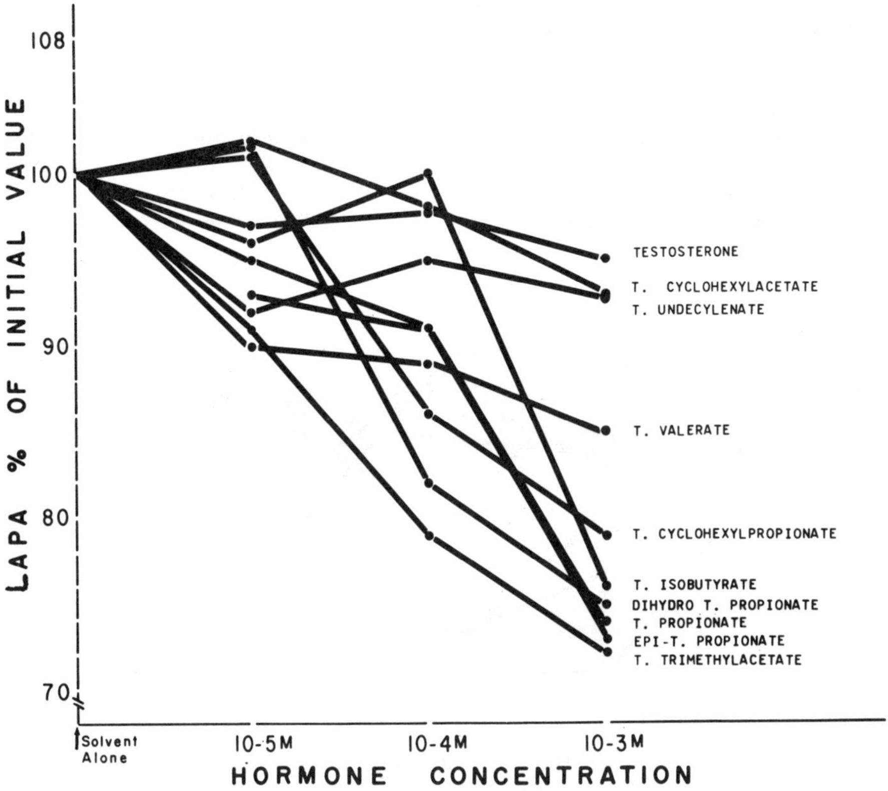

FIGURE 1. Inhibition of leukocyte alkaline phosphatase activity by androgens in a patient with polycythemia vera. (Reproduced by permission of Blood.)

Anatomic Localization of Leukocyte Alkaline Phosphatase Activity

Leukocyte alkaline phosphatase activity resides in the specific granules of polymorphonuclear leukocytes.[8] Its measure depends partly on the rate and extent of lysis of these granules.[9]

To help elucidate whether the observed sex differences are differences in release rather than content of leukocyte alkaline phosphatase, studies using 1 percent saponin to effect enzyme release from leukocyte granules were performed. A three- to fourfold increase in phosphatase activity was noted following saponin treatment of leukocytes (TABLE 4). The ratio of alkaline phosphatase activity between whole leukocytes and saponin lysate was similar in all groups tested. Preliminary studies indicate that resaponization of the saponin lysate sediment releases significant amounts of additional enzyme activity.

Further attempts at anatomic localization of leukocyte alkaline phosphatase activity were made. Toxic granulations of polymorphonuclear leukocytes occur in a variety of conditions in which leukocyte alkaline phosphatase activity is increased including infections, following surgery, and during pregnancy. Quantitative estimation of toxic granulations on Wright's-Giemsa-stained smears and calculation of alkaline phosphatase scores on duplicate smears, stained specifically for this enzyme, revealed no correlation between toxic granules and leukocyte alkaline phosphatase activity in a variety of disorders studied.

Leukocyte Zinc and Magnesium

Zinc and possibly magnesium are known to maintain or possibly enhance the activity of leukocyte alkaline phosphatase. Consequently, leukocyte zinc and magnesium levels were measured in patients with low, normal, and high levels of leukocyte alkaline phosphatase. No sex differences were found in leukocyte zinc

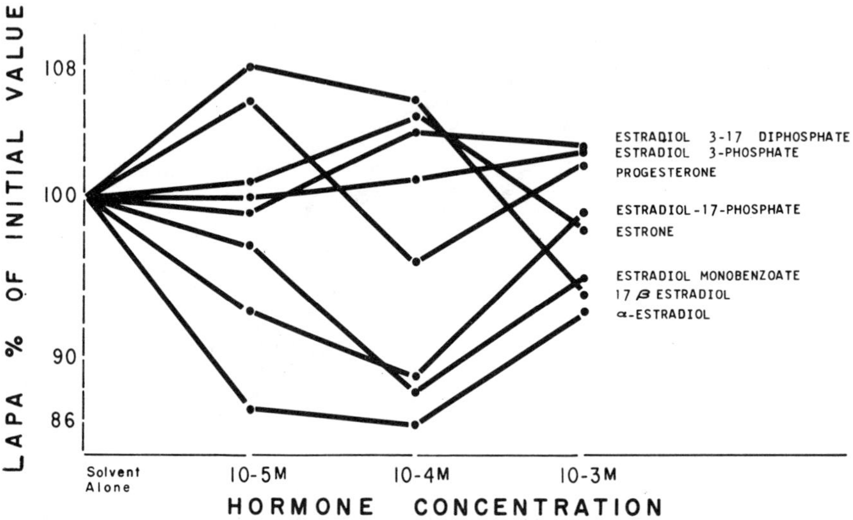

FIGURE 2. Lack of inhibition of leukocyte alkaline phosphatase activity by estrogens in a patient with polycythemia vera. (Reproduced by permission of Blood.)

TABLE 2

LEUKOCYTE ALKALINE PHOSPHATASE ACTIVITY IN PATIENTS WITH CARCINOMA OF THE BREAST

Treatment	Number of Patients	Mean Age (years)	Mean APA*
None	10	62	48
Androgen	6	62	31

* Leukocyte alkaline phosphatase activity expressed as milligrams of phosphorus liberated per hour per 10^{10} polymorphonuclear leukocytes.

TABLE 3

LEUKOCYTE ALKALINE PHOSPHATASE ACTIVITY IN PREGNANCY

	Number of Subjects	Mean Age (years)	Mean APA*	Significance
Nonpregnant	97	32	34	$p < .001$
Pregnant	34	26	47	

* Leukocyte alkaline phosphatase activity expressed as milligrams of phosphorus liberated per hour per 10^{10} polymorphonuclear leukocytes.

TABLE 4

INCREASE IN LEUKOCYTE ALKALINE PHOSPHATASE ACTIVITY FOLLOWING SAPONIFICATION OF LEUKOCYTES

		Number of Cases	Mean LAPA* Before Saponin	After Saponin
Young adult subjects	male	22	17	58
	female	22	29	79
Elderly subjects	male	8	18	60
	female	14	15	64
Pregnant women		34	47	126

* Leukocyte alkaline phosphatase activity expressed as milligrams of phosphorus liberated per hour per 10^{10} polymorphonuclear leukocytes.

TABLE 5

LEUKOCYTE ALKALINE PHOSPHATASE ACTIVITY, LEUKOCYTE ZINC AND LEUKOCYTE MAGNESIUM LEVELS IN NORMAL INDIVIDUALS AND IN PATIENTS

	Number of Cases	Mean LAPA*	Mean Leukocyte Zinc μg/100 ml	Mean Leukocyte Magnesium μg/100 ml
Young normal males	15	16	262	1788
Young normal females	14	26	243	1731
Pregnancy	25	89	187↓	2074
Myeloma	13	50	324	1987
Polycythemia vera	6	89	423↑	2682↑

* Leukocyte alkaline phosphatase activity expressed as milligrams of phosphorus liberated per hour per 10^{10} polymorphonuclear leukocytes.

and magnesium levels (TABLE 5). Furthermore, no correlation could be demonstrated between leukocyte zinc or magnesium levels and leukocyte alkaline phosphatase activity either biochemically or histochemically. In pregnancy, leukocyte alkaline phosphatase activity is high, whereas leukocyte zinc levels are low and leukocyte magnesium levels are normal. In polycythemia vera, leukocyte alkaline phosphatase activity is increased and leukocyte zinc and magnesium levels are also elevated. However, in multiple myeloma where leukocyte alkaline phosphatase activity is also increased, both leukocyte zinc and magnesium levels are normal. Lowered leukocyte zinc levels were found in patients with acute myeloblastic leukemia. Normal white blood cell zinc and magnesium levels were found in patients with pernicious anemia, secondary polycythemia, hepatic cirrhosis, lymphomas, chronic lymphocytic leukemia, infectious mononucleosis, disseminated carcinoma, diabetes, and a variety of other hematological and nonhematological disorders.

DISCUSSION

Leukocyte alkaline phosphatase activity is known to deviate from normal in certain disease states. It is increased in polycythemia vera, some cases of myeloid metaplasia, infections, leukocytosis, leukemoid reactions, trauma, surgery, and various "stressful" situations, such as myocardial infarction, diabetic acidosis, and gout.[5,10–14] It is also increased in response to adrenocorticotrophic hormone (ACTH) and adrenal steroids,[5,15] in pregnancy,[5–7] and in mongolism.[16–20] It is decreased in chronic myelogenous leukemia,[10–14] paroxysmal nocturnal hemoglobinuria,[21] and hypophosphatasia.[22]

No previous study mentions differences in leukocyte alkaline phosphatase activity between men and women. The fact that such differences exist, as we have just described, requires explanation. We wish to propose the thesis that androgens and possibly estrogens inhibit this enzyme. In animals, we know that androgens inhibit renal alkaline phosphatase activity in mice,[23-25] and certain estrogens inhibit renal alkaline phosphatase activity in rabbits.[26] Our studies indicate that human leukocyte alkaline phosphatase activity is inhibited by androgens. Low values in men, as compared with those in women, support this thesis, as do the fragmentary results from studies on hormone-treated breast-cancer patients and from test tube experiments with hormones.

Other influences on leukocyte alkaline phosphatase activity, probably also hormonal, are clearly present. Girls as well as boys show gradually decreasing activity with advancing age towards puberty, and women have levels which are distinctly lower than those of children. In women, levels of this enzyme rise in pregnancy and fall during menopause but have not been shown to vary during the menstrual cycle. In the test tube, none of the estrogens tested had any consistent effect on leukocyte alkaline phosphatase activity. How the female sex hormones influence leukocyte alkaline phosphatase activity is not clear. Perhaps estrogens and progestins have mutually antagonistic effects.

ACTH and adrenal steroids are known to stimulate leukocyte alkaline phosphatase activity.[5,15] Very high values of this enzyme in newborns,[27] high values in young children, and gradually decreasing levels toward puberty[7] suggest a possible stimulating role for growth hormone.

The absence of differences between prepubertal boys and girls and between old men and women suggests that leukocyte alkaline phosphatase activity is a secondary sex characteristic.

Might the sex differences be explained by differences in release of enzyme? Total enzyme content of leukocytes may be genetically determined. Saponin treatment of white blood cells to increase the rate of rupture of granules was found to increase the yield of leukocyte alkaline phosphatase three- to fourfold. However, proportionate enhancement of the enzyme activity occurred in all subjects studied. Furthermore, retreatment of the lysed "pellet" with saponin released significant additional activity. Release of more enzyme activity by saponin might simply mean more easily ruptured granules. Thus, until it is possible to release all the activity from all the granules of human leukocytes, the question of enzyme content versus enzyme release will remain unresolved.

Recent electron microscopic work by Breton-Gorius[28] indicates that neutrophils have at least two types of granules: large elongated, relatively lucent granules with an internal bar that appears to distend the envelope of the granulation, and small, very dense granules with amorphous structure. These latter do not seem to correspond to the classical neutrophilic granulations. Support for two or more types of neutrophilic granules also comes from preliminary work in our laboratory in which saponin was shown to effect increases in both leukocyte alkaline and acid phosphatase activities, whereas vitamin A only raised acid phosphatase levels. Anatomic localization of alkaline phosphatase in specific granules in leukocytes may thus be feasible.

Toxic granulations occur in numerous conditions in which leukocyte alkaline phosphatase activity is also increased. By histochemical techniques, we could not demonstrate any correlation between the level of this enzyme and toxic granules in a variety of disorders.

It has been suggested that zinc may play a significant role in human leukocyte alkaline phosphatase activity.[29] Some authors[30] postulate two leukocyte alkaline phosphatases in man, one requiring zinc and the other magnesium for their activation. In addition, zinc is known to be present in mature granulocytic leukocytes,[4] as is alkaline phosphatase. Eosinophils are rich in zinc,[4] yet deficient in alkaline phosphatase. We measured leukocyte zinc and magnesium levels in patients with a variety of illnesses in which leukocyte alkaline phosphatase activity was low, normal, or high. No sex differences were found, and no correlation between leukocyte zinc and magnesium levels and leukocyte alkaline phosphatase could be demonstrated either biochemically or histochemically.

Summary

Leukocyte alkaline phosphatase activity was found to vary between men and women. No significant differences between boys and girls occurred until puberty. After menopause, the values for women approached the values for men. Women treated with androgens had lower leukocyte alkaline phosphatase activity than did control women. These results suggested that androgens inhibit this enzyme. *In vitro* tests with various concentrations of androgens and estrogens suggested some direct inhibition by androgens, but not estrogens. Studies using saponin to effect enzyme release from leukocyte granules did not demonstrate whether the differences in leukocyte alkaline phosphatase activity between men and women are differences reflecting the rate of enzyme release or of enzyme content. Anatomic localization of this enzyme in toxic granulations of neutrophils could not be demonstrated. No sex differences in leukocyte zinc and magnesium values were found, nor could values for either of these trace metals be correlated with leukocyte alkaline phosphatase activity.

Acknowledgment

The authors are indebted to Mrs. Frances Rose for the typing of this manuscript.

References

1. Rosner, F. & S. L. Lee. 1965. Endocrine relationships of leukocyte alkaline phosphatase. Blood **25:** 356.
2. Sigma Technical Bulletin No. 104. 1962. Sigma Chemical Co., St. Louis, Mo.
3. Gomori, G. 1939. Microtechnical demonstration of phosphatase in tissue sections. Proc. Soc. Exp. Biol. Med. **42:** 23.
4. Szmigielski, S. & J. Litwin. 1965. The histochemical study of zinc content in granulocytes in normal adults and in hematological disorders. Blood **25:** 56.
5. Valentine, W. N., J. H. Folette, E. B. Hardin, W. S. Beck & J. S. Lawrence. 1954. Studies on leukocyte alkaline phosphatase activity: Relation to "stress" and pituitary adrenal activity. J. Lab. Clin. Med. **44:** 219.
6. Pritchard, J. A. 1957. Leukocyte phosphatase activity in pregnancy. J. Lab. Clin. Med. **50:** 432.
7. Quigley, H. J., E. A. Dawson, B. H. Hyun & R. P. Custer. 1960. The activity of alkaline phosphatase in granular leukocytes during pregnancy and the puerperium: A preliminary report. Amer. J. Clin. Path. **33:** 109.
8. Cohn, Z. A. & J. G. Hirsch. 1960. Isolation and properties of the specific cytoplasmic granules of rabbit polymorphonuclear leukocytes. J. Exp. Med. **112:** 983.
9. Hirsch, J. G. & Z. A. Cohn. 1960. Degranulation of polymorphonuclear leucocytes following phagocytosis of microorganisms. J. Exp. Med. **112:** 1005.
10. Valentine, W. N., W. S. Beck, J. H. Folette, H. Mills & J. S. Lawrence. 1952. Biochemical studies in chronic myelocytic leukemia, polycythemia vera and other myeloproliferative disorders. Blood **7:** 959.
11. Wiltshaw, E. & W. C. Moloney. 1955. Histochemical and biochemical studies on leukocyte alkaline phosphatase activity. Blood **10:** 1120.

12. MEISLIN, A. G., S. L. LEE & L. R. WASSERMAN. 1959. Leucocyte alkaline phosphatase in hematopoietic disorders. Cancer **12:** 760.
13. VALENTINE, W. N. & W. S. BECK. 1951. Biochemical studies on leucocytes. I. Phosphatase activity in health. Leucocytosis and myelocytic leucemia. J. Lab. Clin. Med. **38:** 39.
14. BECK, W. S. & W. N. VALENTINE. 1951. Biochemical studies on leucocytes. II. Phosphatase activity in chronic lymphatic leucemia, acute leucemia and miscellanous hematologic conditions. J. Lab. Clin. Med. **38:** 245.
15. VALENTINE, W. N., J. H. FOLETTE, D. H. SOLOMON & J. REYNOLDS. 1957. The relationship of leukocyte alkaline phosphatase to "stress," to ACTH, and to adrenal 17-OH-corticosteroids. J. Lab. Clin. Med. **49:** 723.
16. ALTER, A. A., S. L. LEE, M. POURFAR & G. DOBKIN. 1963. Studies of leukocyte alkaline phosphatase in mongolism: A possible chromosome marker. Blood **22:** 165.
17. TRUBOWITZ, S., D. KIRMAN & B. MASEK. 1962. The leucocyte alkaline phosphatase in mongolism. Lancet **ii:** 486.
18. LENNOX, B., H. ST. C. WHITE & J. CAMPBELL. 1962. The polymorph alkaline phosphatase in mongolism. Lancet **ii:** 991.
19. KING, M. J., E. M. GILLIS & A. G. BAIKIE. 1962. Alkaline phosphatase activity of polymorphs in mongolism. Lancet **ii:** 1302.
20. O'SULLIVAN, M. A. & C. V. PRYLES. 1963. A comparison of leukocyte alkaline phosphatase determinations in 200 patients with mongolism and in 200 "familial" controls. New Eng. J. Med. **268:** 1168.
21. TANAKA, K. R., W. N. VALENTINE & R. E. FREDRICKS. 1960. Studies on leukocytic and erythrocytic enzymes in paroxysmal nocturnal hemoglobinuria. Clin. Res. **8:** 132.
22. BEISEL, W. R., N. BENJAIN & K. F. AUSTIN. 1959. Absence of leukocyte alkaline phosphatase activity in hypophosphatasia. Blood **14:** 975.
23. KOCHAKIAN, C. D. 1945. Effect of various steroid hormones on "alkaline" and "acid" phosphatases of kidney of mouse. Amer. J. Physiol. **145:** 118.
24. KOCHAKIAN, C. D. 1947. Role of hydrolytic enzymes in some of the metabolic activities of steroid hormones. Recent Progr. Hormone Res. **1:** 177.
25. KOCHAKIAN, C. D. 1948. Histochemical study of "alkaline" phosphatase of the kidney of the castrated mouse after stimulation with various androgens. Amer. J. Physiol. **152:** 257.
26. ALDMAN, B., E. DICZFALUSY & T. ROSENBERG. 1948. In vitro inhibition of alkaline phosphatase by estrogenic hormones. Acta Chem. Scand. **2:** 529.
27. SCORZA, P., G. PACLUCCI & E. CACCIARI. 1961. Alcuni Enzima (Transaminasi glutammico-ossalecetics, transaminasi glutammico piruvica fosfatasi alcalina) Leuccocitari nel pato a termine e nell immaturo nei primi due mesi di vita. Boll. Soc. Ital. Biol. Sper. **37:** 323.
28. BRETON-GORIUS, J. 1966. Structures périodiques dans les granulations eosinophiles et neurophiles des leucocytes polynucléaires du sang de l'homme. Nouv. Rev. Franc. Hemat. **6:** 195.
29. VALENTINE, W. N., K. R. TANAKA & R. E. FREDRICKS. 1960. Studies on leukocyte alkaline phosphatase: Role of zinc and magnesium. J. Lab. Clin. Med. **55:** 303.
30. TRUBOWITZ, S., D. FELDMAN, C. BENANTE & D. KIRMAN. 1957. Metal requirements of alkaline phosphatases of human and rabbit leukocytes. Proc. Soc. Exper. Biol. Med. **95:** 35.

LEUKOCYTE ALKALINE PHOSPHATASE CYTOCHEMISTRY: APPLICATIONS AND METHODS*

Leonard S. Kaplow
Veterans Administration Hospital
West Haven, Conn.
and
Yale University, School of Medicine
New Haven, Conn.

Introduction

Almost 20 years ago O. P. Jones[1] in a special issue of *Blood* stated, "... the use of dry fixed smears is not necessarily limited to the field of descriptive or morphologic hematology but, with the proper selection of experimental material, may be utilized to good advantage in determining cell potentialities." In the same publication Dameshek wrote, "... morphology when appropriately interpreted, can be both physiology and chemistry ... far from being dead, morphologic hematology is undoubtedly in for a renaissance period, a period in which it is hoped that appropriate staining techniques will point directly to chemical and physiopathologic alterations."[2] That such an era has indeed emerged is evident from the titles of the papers presented in this monograph and is well exemplified by the cytochemical demonstration and assessment of leukocyte alkaline phosphatase activity (LAPA).

The demonstration of enzyme activity *in situ* is dependent upon fixation methods that will preserve cytological detail with minimal inhibition of enzyme activity and upon an enzyme-substrate reaction product which is either insoluble in its immediate environment or which can combine to form an insoluble product with other substances already present in, or to be added to, the incubation mixture. Preferably, this product should be colored so as to be visible under ordinary transmitted light, or a colorless product may be reacted on by other reagents so as to produce a final colored precipitate that is localized at the theoretical sites of enzyme activity.

There are important advantages to be gained in the study of blood, which are denied when working with solid tissues. Blood smears, monocellular in thickness, permit the briefest of fixation and staining times and require neither embedding nor mounting. Furthermore, cellular units are intact; the cell membrane is not cut as is unavoidable in tissue sections. The intracellular detail that can be discerned in properly prepared blood smears is generally superior to that seen on sectioned tissues. Above all, blood is a unique tissue. It is readily biopsied and a minute sample is not only representative of the circulating blood-cell population but may also reflect the physiological state of the whole organism.

Blood cells have been categorized according to their morphology and on the basis of their tinctorial staining characteristics (Giemsa-Wright's stain). Thus, mature neutrophilic granulocytes have been thought of as members of a homogeneous group of cells with similar function and similar capabilities. Cytochemical techniques readily destroy such concepts. This is well exemplified by staining for LAPA, which reveals that two adjacent neutrophils, lying within a single microscopic field, appearing almost identical by conventional staining techniques, may differ markedly in alkaline phosphatase activity (FIGURE 1). Whether these

* This study was supported in part by USPHS research grants nos. H–6240, HE–07456, and no. HE–09344 from the National Heart Institute.

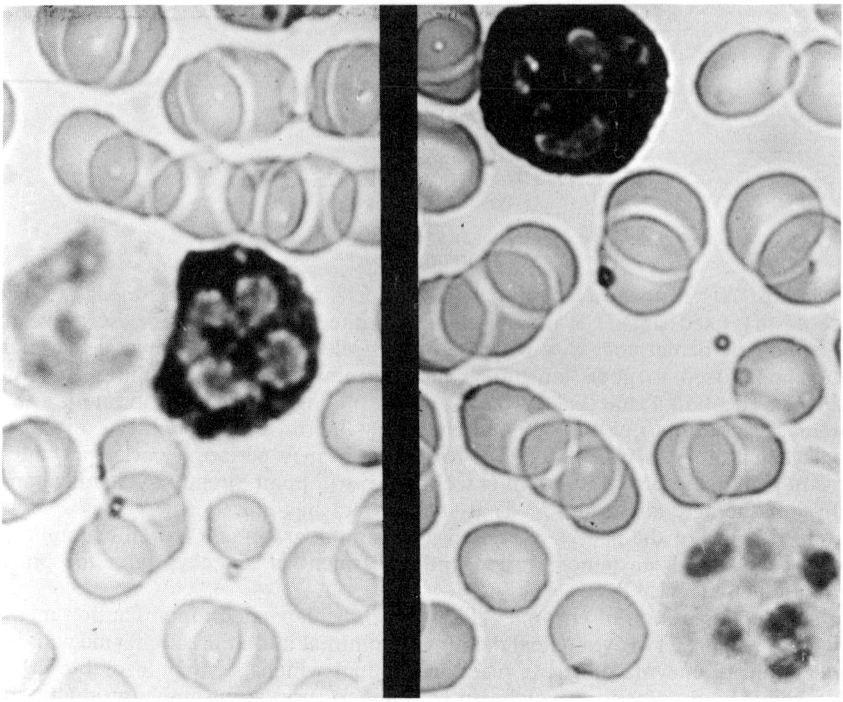

FIGURE 1. Peripheral blood neutrophilic granulocytes stained for alkaline phosphatase activity by azo dye technique.[68] Counterstained with Mayer's hematoxylin.

same cells differ in age, in function, or in other aspects of their physiological and chemical makeup remains uncertain.

Historical Background

Kay, in 1929, first suggested that alkaline phosphatase might be present in leukocytes.[3] A year later he reported that washed leukocytes suspended in plasma had activities three times greater than filtered plasma alone.[4] Kay's conclusions were soon confirmed by a number of investigators using quantitative biochemical techniques.[5-11]

It is ironic that Fiessinger and Boyer[12] came to an opposite opinion regarding the presence of alkaline phosphatase activity in leukocytes, because they were unable to detect an increase in serum alkaline phosphatase after adding to the serum a large number of leukocytes obtained from the buffy coat of a patient with chronic myelogenous leukemia. For a more complete review of the early biochemical studies on LAPA, reference should be made to the publication by Valentine and Beck[13] in 1951.

Takamatsu,[14,15] in 1938 and 1939, and Gomori,[16] in 1939, independently devised similar methods for demonstrating phosphatase activity histochemically. The technique they described is a three-step procedure now commonly referred to as the metal-salt method. Enzymatic hydrolysis of a suitable substrate, usually β-glycerophosphate, yields phosphate ions that combine with calcium ions already present in the incubation mixture to yield an insoluble, microscopically invisible form of calcium phosphate. Tissue sections are then exposed to solutions of silver, cobalt, or lead salts, resulting in the precipitation of the respective metal phosphates, which also are not detectable by ordinary light microscopy. In the final step, the cobalt or lead phosphate is reacted with ammonium sulfide to form black insoluble sulfide salts or, the silver phosphate is exposed to ultraviolet light resulting in the formation of metallic silver that can be readily seen microscopically (FIGURE 2). Gomori[17,18] proposed cobalt nitrate for alkaline phosphatase and a lead salt for acid phosphatase. The method was subject to much controversy because of spurious staining and nonoptimal staining conditions. Lison[19] has thoroughly reviewed this histochemical technique. Subsequent modifications, including shortened incubation times, use of activators, increased calcium concentration in the incubation mixture, better pH control, and the use of less inhibitory fixatives resulted in techniques that gave accurate and reproducible results and remain in use today.[20–22]

Takamatsu,[15] in his paper in 1939, concluded that peripheral blood leukocytes were devoid of phosphatase activity. However, in the same year in a joint paper with Takeuchi,[23] he observed activity in tuberculous guinea pig granulomata and suggested that activity originated in leukocytes. Gomori,[18] in 1941, described strong activity in guinea pig heterophils in blood smears and in tissue sections. He noted marked species differences in LAPA. In 1943, Fell and Danielli[24] also observed species differences using histochemical staining techniques. Of the various animals studied, they found the highest activity in leukocytes of guinea pigs. They also accurately noted that lymphocytes, monocytes, and eosinophils

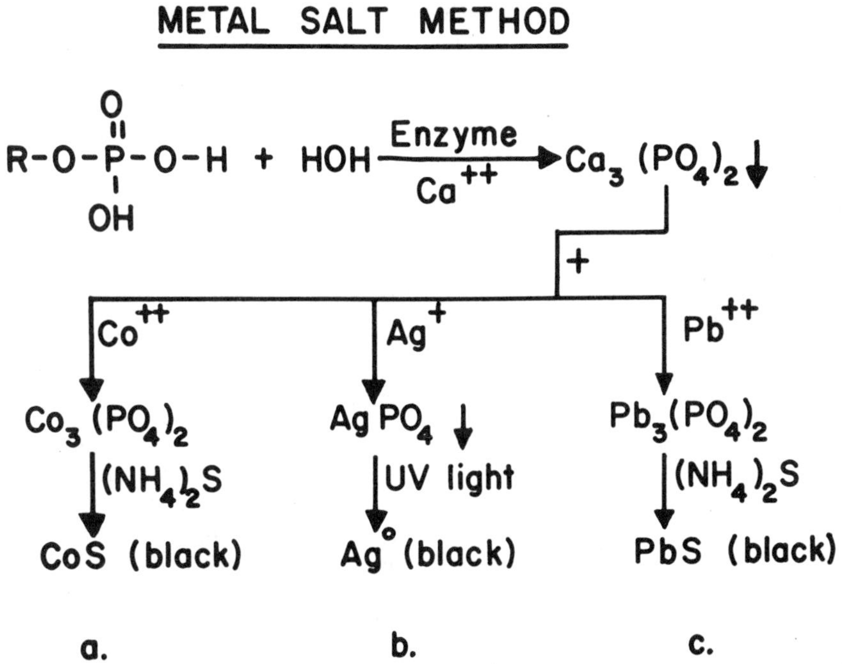

FIGURE 2. Schematic representation of chemical reactions involved in the Gomori-Takamatsu heavy-metal method[15,16] for demonstrating alkaline phosphatase activity.

did not stain for LAPA. Gomori,[25] in 1943, confirmed the findings of Takeuchi and Takamatsu with respect to the intense staining of tuberculous guinea pig lesions, particularly in regions of necrosis. He was also of the opinion that the enzyme originated from leukocytes. Takeuchi,[26,27] in 1943, published two additional papers in Japanese on LAPA. Wachstein,[28] in his classical paper of 1946, was the first to give a detailed report of human LAPA in normal and pathological states using the cobalt-salt method. Many of his findings remain valid and significant today; he noted increased activity in infectious diseases, purulent exudates, and in a single case of "leukemic myelosis." He also reported low levels in 13 cases of chronic myeloid leukemia. On the basis of these findings he speculated, ". . . only observation of other patients will show whether the phosphatase reaction can be of help in the differentiation of chronic myeloid leucemia from so-called nonleukemic myelosis." Wachstein also noted the absence of LAPA in the blood of the chicken, dog and mouse, and strong activity in the leukocytes of the rat, rabbit, guinea pig, and nucleated red cells of frogs. Wachstein did not fully appreciate the importance of his findings and stated, perhaps modestly, that "While no practical application of the phosphatase reaction for hematologic purposes can so far be recognized, the depression in activity in the granulocytes of chronic myeloid leucemia is of some interest." In the next seven years, a number of other publications appeared devoted to histochemical studies of LAPA.[29–35] For the most part optimal staining conditions were not used, so that results were conflicting and emphasis was placed on methods rather than on variations in health and in disease states. Plum,[33] however, did confirm some of Wachstein's findings, noting high values in myeloma, pernicious anemia, and polycythemia and low values in myelogenous leukemia. Takeuchi[36] and Kubo[37] also reported on human LAPA in various physiological and pathological states. Takeuchi and Utsunomiya[38] compared the various metal-salt methods using human and rabbit blood. Although they found the silver method to be more sensitive, most investigators have since used the cobalt technique. Friederici,[38a] in 1955, using a heavy-metal technique also studied human LAPA; he noted decreased activity in "anemia" and "leukemia," and also observed changes in activity in cultured bone marrow cells. Impetus to the cytochemical study of LAPA was given by the quantitative biochemical studies that were reported at this time, by Valentine and associates,[13,39–42] Moloney and associates,[43–45] and Williams and Mendel.[46,47]

A unique and totally different approach to the demonstration of alkaline phosphatase in tissue sections was introduced by Menten *et al.* in 1944.[48] They used the weakly soluble monoaryl salt, calcium β-naphthyl phosphate, as substrate and incorporated freshly diazotized α-naphthylamine in the incubation mixture. Upon enzyme hydrolysis, the liberated naphthol immediately coupled with the diazo compound to form a relatively insoluble red-colored azo dye deposit. The method is commonly referred to as the simultaneous azo dye coupling method. The technique as originally devised was relatively crude. The coupling salt was unstable, not available commercially, and had to be synthesized just prior to use. Numerous modifications soon followed, including the development and use of stable diazotates by Manheimer and Seligman in 1948.[49] Two years later, Friedman and Seligman[50] synthesized the readily soluble sodium salts of α- and β-naphthyl phosphate and recommended their use in histochemistry. In 1951, Gomori[21] demonstrated the superiority of the sodium salt of the α-ester of naphthyl phosphate over the calcium salt of the β-form. The compound used by Gomori was claimed to be more soluble, permitting higher substrate concentrations. The final reaction product (azo dye) was considered less soluble than previous coupling products and hence less diffusible and was said to yield sharper staining. Much attention was then devoted to the development and trial of other diazonium salts and other naphthoic compounds. In a sense, histochemists invaded the azo dye chemistry field borrowing and improvising terms, ideas, and compounds in efforts to devise methods for staining phosphatase and other hydrolytic enzymes. Comprehensive reviews of this period have been published by Pearse,[51] Deane *et al.*,[52] and Burstone.[53]

Vercauteren,[54] in a brief note in 1955, reported on the use of simultaneous azo dye coupling methods for demonstrating LAPA but did not indicate the technique used. In the same year Kaplow[55] described in detail a rapid (ten-minute incubation) method for demonstrating and assaying leukocyte alkaline phosphatase (LAP). Sodium α-naphthyl phosphate was recommended as the substrate and the diazonium salt of 4-benzoyl-2:5-methoxyaniline (Fast Blue RR) as the coupling salt (FIGURE 3). The incubation mixture was buffered to pH 9.6 with 0.05 M 2-amino-2-methyl-1,3-propanediol, and Mayer's aqueous hematoxylin was used as a nuclear counterstain. Excellent preservation of cellular morphology was obtained using cold 10 percent formalin in absolute methanol as a fixative. Enzyme activity was found limited to the cytoplasm only of some mature and rare band-form neutrophils (FIGURE 4). A "scoring" procedure was described in which 100 consecutive mature neutrophilic granulocytes were rated

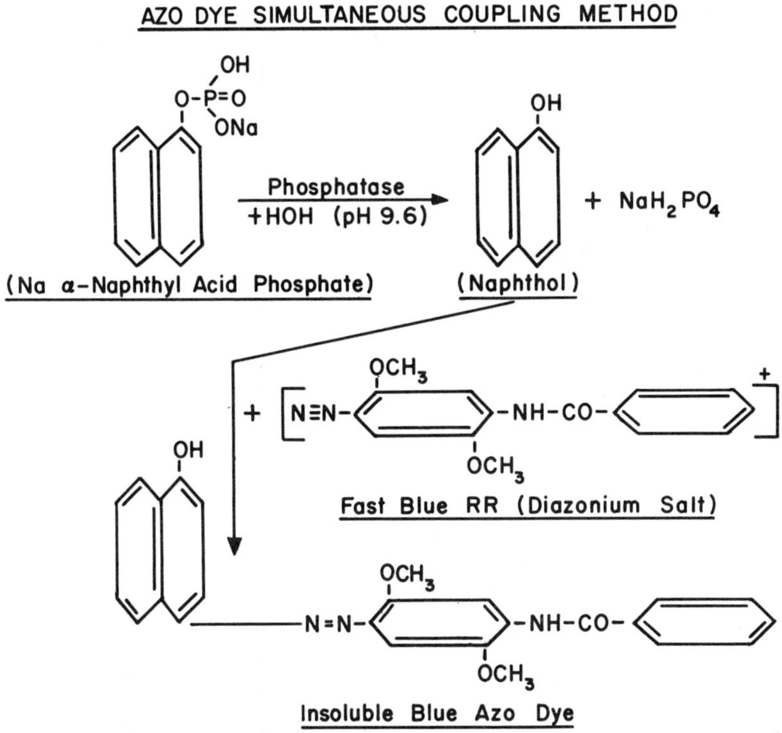

FIGURE 3. Schematic representation of chemical reactions involved in the azo dye technique for demonstrating alkaline phosphatase activity.

from 0–4 on the basis of intensity and appearance of the precipitated dye in the cytoplasm (FIGURE 5). The sum of the ratings was considered the "score" for a given blood smear and offered a convenient and practical means of assessing and comparing LAPA of blood from normal individuals and from patients with various diseases. A somewhat similar approach was taken in 1938 by Seabra[56] in assessing oxidase activity and was also recommended in 1955 for alkaline phosphatase activity by Brodel and Swisher,[57] who counted 100 leukocytes rather than 100 neutrophils. The scoring method has since been widely adopted. Unfortunately, there have been many modifications in the scoring technique. Ratings from 0–2 and from 0–6 have been reported.[58-63] Some investigators[63-65] have preferred to report their results as percent of neutrophils exhibiting positive staining rather than by scoring. As a result the literature now contains a variety of "scores," "indices," "rates," etc., with little meaning when compared with each other.

Effects of Anticoagulants

Although capillary blood is preferred for cytological study, it is often more practical to use anticoagulated venous blood. Trubowitz *et al.*[66] have shown that human LAP is predominantly zinc dependent, whereas rabbit LAP is magnesium dependent. They also clearly demonstrated that salts of ethylenediaminetetracetic acid (EDTA) inhibit LAPA by virtue of the zinc chelating effect of EDTA compounds. The suppression of LAPA by EDTA has been confirmed by a number

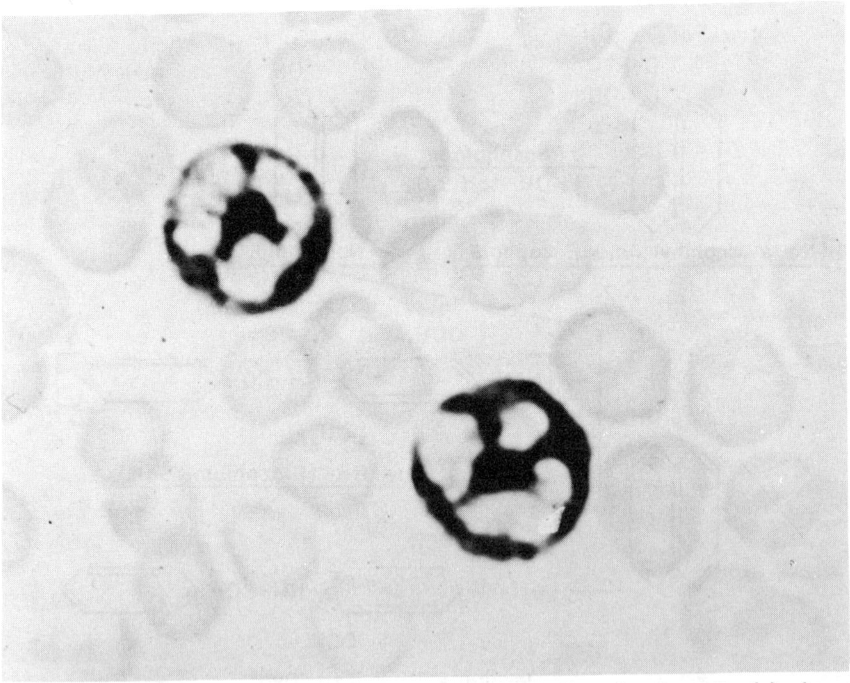

FIGURE 4. Peripheral blood granulocyte stained for alkaline phosphatase activity by azo dye technique. Not counterstained, demonstrating localization of final reaction product in the cytoplasm only.

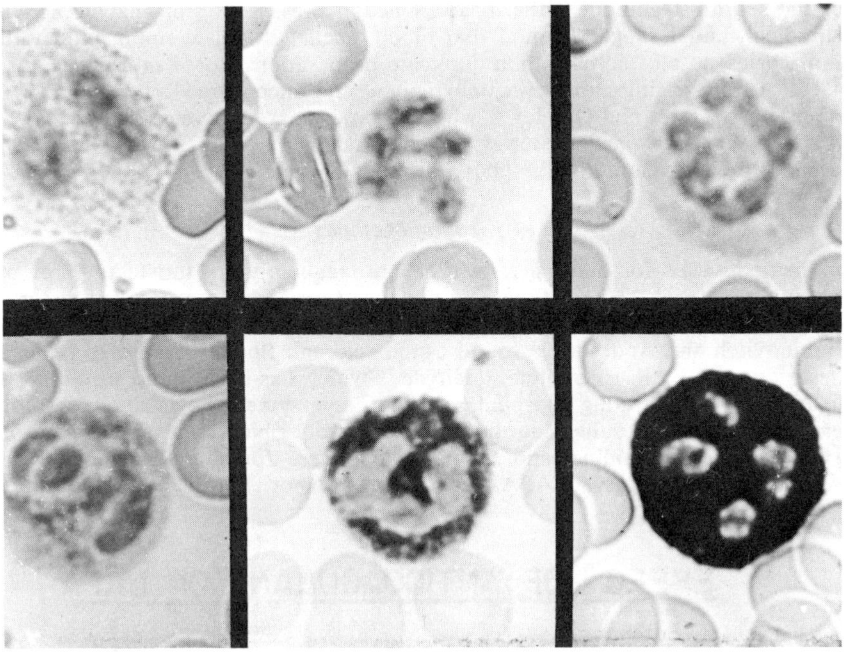

FIGURE 5. Composite photomicrograph showing unstained eosinophil in top upper left and 0, 1+, 2+, 3+, 4+ rated LAP positive neutrophils. Azo dye method.[91]

of other investigators.[67-69] Climie and associates,[70,71] however, claimed LAPA was not inhibited by EDTA. Knudtson and Evanger[60] found that agitation of citrate, oxalate, and heparinized blood at 37° C caused cytoplasmic swelling and cell membrane disruption, whereas neutrophils from similarly treated blood, anticoagulated with EDTA, remained well preserved. They also indicated that neutrophils with the lowest alkaline phosphatase activity were most susceptible to distortion by anticoagulants other than EDTA. Experiments in our laboratory have indicated that when blood smears are prepared shortly after venesection and properly fixed, cell morphology is good, regardless of the anticoagulant used. In our hands, heparin in a concentration of 25 units per ml blood has been found to be the most practical and least inhibitory anticoagulant for use in cytochemical studies of LAPA (FIGURE 6).

LAPA Stability on Stored Smears

Blood smears should preferably be stained for enzyme activity within eight hours after preparation. Instability of LAPA on stored smears has been noted by a number of investigators.[32,63,68,72] Our own studies have indicated a progressive decrease in activity with time, which may be delayed by prior fixation and storage below $^{-}10°$ C (FIGURE 7). Hoffman and Lucich,[72] and Whitt[73] also noted better preservation of activity following fixation. Rutenburg *et al.*,[74] using the granule count as a basis for scoring, reported no change in activity with storage of either unfixed smears at room temperature or fixed smears at 4° C for as long as four weeks. It is presumed that these findings are, at least partially, a reflection of the scoring technique rather than of actual preservation of enzyme activity. Knudtson and Evanger[60] found that blood smears stored at room temperature showed less loss of activity than duplicate preparations stored in a dessicator at 4° C. An interesting and as yet unexplained and unconfirmed phenomenon was reported by Harer and Quigley,[75] who observed marked increase in LAPA when fresh smears, still partially moist, were stored in the cold. Further studies are needed to clarify some of the above discrepancies.

Fixation Methods

Fixatives used for tissue preservation are frequently not satisfactory for preserving blood cells. Thus, 10 percent aqueous formalin causes marked distortion of erythrocytes. This occurs regardless of pH and of solute concentration.[55] Rabinovitch and Andreucci[32] found osmic acid and Bouin's fixative to be highly destructive of LAP. Even gluteraldehyde,[76] which has been found so useful as a fixative in demonstrating phosphatase and other enzymes by electron microscopy, has not given good results in our hands, when used for blood smears. Cold acetone, 10 percent formol-saline, and formol vapor were found by Rabinovitch and Andreucci[32] to preserve LAPA. Only formol vapor, however, was considered

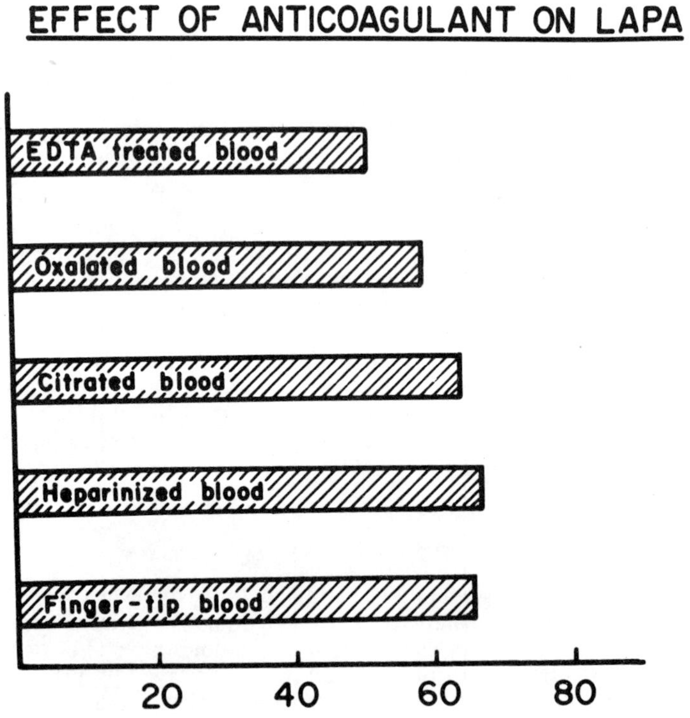

FIGURE 6. Comparison of inhibitory effects of commonly used anti-coagulants on leukocyte alkaline phosphatase activity. Azo dye technique.

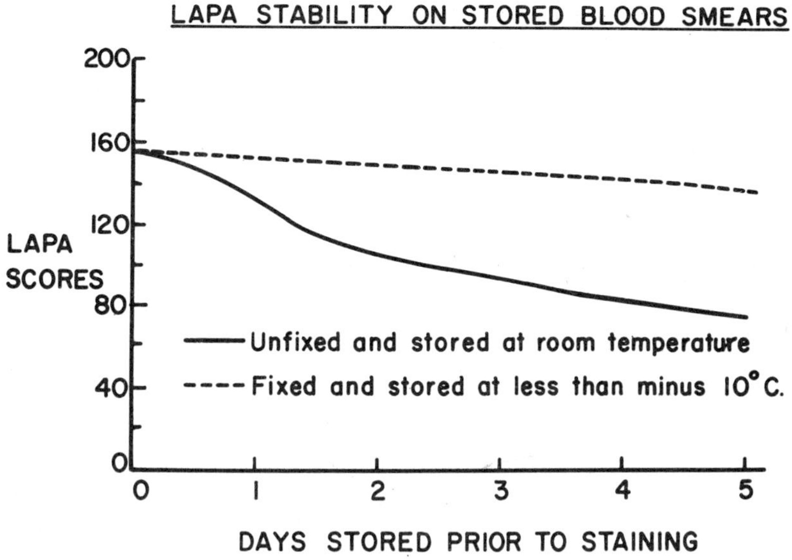

FIGURE 7. Effect of age of fixed and unfixed blood smears on LAPA. Azo dye methods.

satisfactory from the standpoint of preservation of cellular morphology. Some investigators have since used formol vapor as a fixative for LAPA staining.[61,61a,77–82] Boivin and Robineaux[83] critically studied a variety of fixatives for use with the Gomori-Takamatsu heavy-metal technique. They obtained best results when smears were fixed in either formol vapor or in a mixture of ethanol, formalin, and pyridine. In 1955, Kaplow[55] recommended fixation in cold 10 percent formalin in methanol for 30 seconds. This procedure causes minimal suppression of enzyme activity, and cell preservation is equivalent to that seen with Wright's-stained smears. It has been widely accepted and has become the most commonly used fixative in staining for LAPA. Plenert,[84] in 1959, in a comprehensive study of 23 fixative procedures also concluded that cold 10 percent formalin in methanol was the most satisfactory fixation procedure for demonstrating LAPA. Despite its usefulness, 10 percent formol-methanol has been criticized because of the tendency for blood films to wash off the slide during the staining procedure. It also has the disadvantage of having to be used at 0° to −10° C. Many investigators have modified the technique described by Kaplow, in efforts to overcome these objections. Hoffman and Lucich,[72] and Baxter[85] fixed for 90 rather than 30 seconds. Wulff and Riis[86] used 10 percent formalin in a mixture of equal parts of methanol and acetone and fixed for only seven to ten seconds in the cold. They obtained significantly higher scores compared to cold 10 percent formol-methanol fixation for 30 seconds. Climie *et al.*[70] suggested 50 percent formalin in methanol. Patterson and associates[87] also used this mixture but for only five seconds, followed by 25 seconds in 10 percent formol-methanol. Weissel[88,89] added small quantities of pyridine to the fixative mixture. Wyllie[90] recommended a three-step procedure using 10 percent formalin in equal parts of ethanol and methanol for 30 seconds, followed by 1:200 ammonia:acetone for 30 seconds, and finally, immersion in ether for 15 minutes. The present author has tried most of these modifications, and in general they all give excellent results.

It is evident that blood smears, monocellular in thickness, require only the briefest of fixation times to preserve morphology, and decreasing the fixation time results in increased enzyme activity. In 1960, Quaglino and Hayhoe[91] described the excellent results they obtained in staining for dehydrogenases on blood smears using 60 percent aqueous acetone. In 1963, Kaplow and Burstone[92] reported that 60 percent acetone buffered to pH 4.2 with citrate-citric acid was equally effective in preserving enzyme activity, and had the added advantage of more effectively maintaining adequate cellular morphology. This fixative has been found very suitable for a variety of hydrolases, as well as oxidases and dehydrogenases, and has been in use in our laboratory for a number of years as a fixative for LAPA. With this fixative, there is no tendency for smears to wash off the slides, and it has the added advantage of being stored and used at room temperature. The only disadvantage is the difficulty in recognizing eosinophils on acetone-fixed smears. Eosinophils do not stain for alkaline phosphatase activity and may be mistaken for unstained neutrophils. Except for bloods with eosinophilia, we now routinely fix for ten seconds at room temperature in 60 percent citrate-buffered acetone for LAPA staining. The fixative solution must be tightly stoppered and made up fresh monthly. Stock citrate and citric acid solutions are stable for long periods in the refrigerator. The fixative must not be used cold or marked erythrocyte lysis will result. The effects of formalin, methanol, and acetone on LAPA scoring are shown in FIGURE 8. It can be seen that methanol is more inhibitory than formaldehyde, and that this inhibition can be abolished by fixation in the cold. It is also

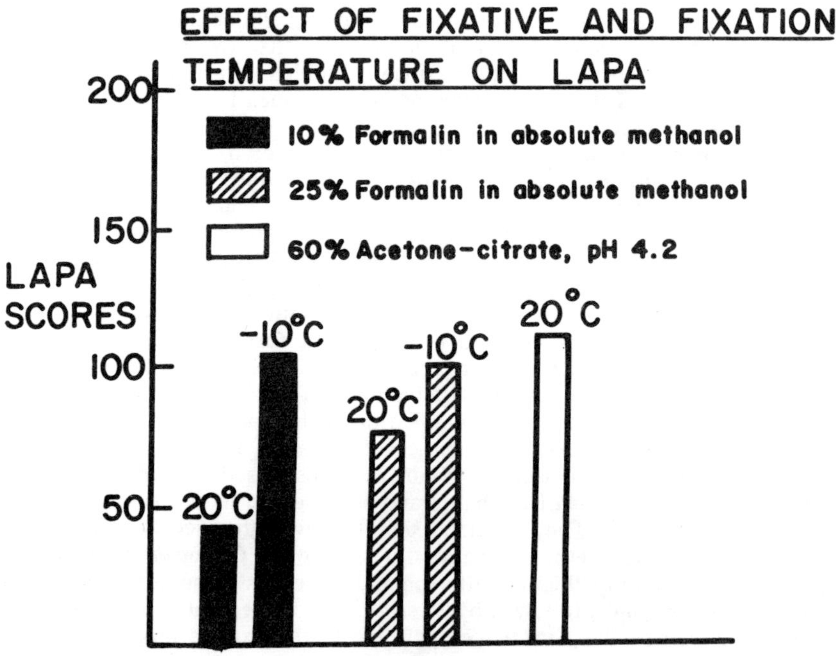

FIGURE 8. Comparison of inhibitory effects of 10 percent and 25 percent formol-methanol fixation at −10° C and at 20° C with fixation in 60 percent acetone, buffered to pH 4.2 with 0.03M citrate-citric acid.

apparent that acetone, even at room temperature, is less inhibitory than either methanol or formaldehyde. If cold 10 percent formol-methanol is used, it is advisable to use thin smears and to permit slides to stand at room temperature for two to six hours prior to fixation. This will greatly minimize loss of smears during the washing process.

Buffers and pH Optima

Gomori,[16] in his original paper, did not specify a particular pH or indicate the need for buffering the incubation mixture. Since then, however, there have been many studies on tissue alkaline phosphatase, both biochemical and histochemical, dealing with buffers and pH. It is generally agreed that for most tissues, the optimum pH is between 8.5 and 10.0, and is dependent to some extent on the substrate and substrate concentration, the buffer, and other aspects of methodology, as well as on the particular tissue source of the enzyme. The pH optima described for various solid tissues need not necessarily apply to leukocytes. Gomori[22] noted that aromatic phosphate esters tend to be hydrolyzed more readily at a higher pH than aliphatic esters. Kabat and Furth,[20] in 1941, used sodium veronal as a buffer. Gomori,[93] however, found veronal to be somewhat inhibitory. He proposed tris (hydroxymethyl) aminomethane as a buffer in the pH range 7.2–9.0 and 2-amino-2-methyl-1,3-propanediol (Ammediol) as a buffer in the pH range 8.0–9.7. Novikoff[94] confirmed Gomori's contention and also recommended the Ammediol buffer in the high alkaline range, pointing out that tris is relatively ineffective as a buffer at pH above 9.0. The optimum pH for LAP, as determined biochemically, lies between 9.0 and 9.9.[95,96] There have been relatively few cytochemical studies on pH optima and buffers for LAP. Kaplow,[55] in 1955, found 0.05 M Ammediol at pH 9.6 to be optimum, when Fast Blue RR salt was used as the diazotate and α-naphthyl phosphate as the substrate. In a later paper, Kaplow[68] reported that staining with Ammediol buffer gave consistently higher scores at various pH levels than staining with tris buffer, when Red Violet LB salt was used as the diazotate and naphthol-AS-BI phosphate as the substrate. Tomonaga *et al.*[63] found discrete staining with Ammediol buffer at pH 8.6 using naphthol-AS-MX phosphate and Fast Blue RR salt. Other investigators have obtained conflicting results. Ackerman,[97] working with the same reagents, preferred tris buffer and recommended pH 8.3. Rutenburg and associates,[74] using unsubstituted naphthol-AS phosphate and Fast Blue BBN, obtained most satisfactory staining with tris buffer at pH 9.1. My own more recent studies are in agreement with these findings, and very discrete staining is obtained with tris buffer and the appropriate reagents at these lower pH values. However, scoring may be more simple, using the more alkaline incubation mixtures buffered with Ammediol, provided the indicated substrates and diazotates are used. These differing results emphasize that optimal activity and the appearance of the final reaction product are dependent upon all of the ingredients of the incubation mixture and upon their effect upon each other. The only report on the effect of buffer concentration on LAPA was that of Kaplow,[68] who found no difference in enzyme activity using Ammediol buffers in concentrations between 0.017 M and 0.05 M. It is apparent that pH changes can be controlled by markedly dilute buffer systems.

Substrates

Both natural and synthetic substrates have been used in demonstrating LAPA cytochemically. Takamatsu[15] and Gomori[16] used the physiological substrate glycerophosphate for demonstrating tissue phosphatase, and this compound remains a popular substrate for staining for LAP by the heavy-metal technique. LAP is one of many phosphoesterases present in tissues and is nonspecific in its substrate requirements. To date, there are no critical studies indicating that LAP differs from other tissue nonspecific phosphatases in regard to substrate specificity. LAP does, however, differ from most tissue alkaline phosphatases in being predominantly zinc, rather than magnesium, dependent.[66] Kaplow,[98] using the azo dye coupling method in early studies, found magnesium ions to have no effect on LAPA. Plenert,[84] using a modified Gomori method, found higher activities when he added Mg^{++} in a concentration of 10^{-4}M than with higher or lower Mg^{++} concentrations. He did not, however, report on incubation mixtures in which Mg^{++} was omitted from the staining solution. In the same study, he found sodium α-naphthyl phosphate to be more rapidly hydrolyzed than the β-form. A review of the literature has failed to reveal the use of other substrates with the heavy-metal technique. Frankel and Peters[99] recently described the use of *p*-nitrophenyl phosphate for demonstrating tissue alkaline phosphatase. This phosphate ester is hydrolysed much faster than glycerophosphate,[100] nevertheless, there have been no previous reports on the use of this substrate for demonstrating LAPA. Preliminary studies in our laboratory suggest that this compound is not a suitable cytochemical substrate for LAPA.

Substrates used to demonstrate LAP by the azo dye coupling method fall into two groups, simple α-naphthyl phosphate and naphthol-AS phosphates. These latter substances are arylamides of 3-hydroxy-naphthoic acid (beta-oxynaphthoic acid or BONA). The AS is from the German *anilinsaure,* indicating the derivation of naphthol-AS compounds from aniline. Naphthol-AS phosphate is the simplest compound in this group. Substitutions anywhere on the aniline derived aryl ring yield more complex, so-called substituted naphthol-AS phosphates. Kaplow[55] originally advocated the use of the sodium salt of α-naphthyl phosphate at pH 9.6, and this has been the most widely used substrate on the basis of published reports. Rutenburg *et al.*[74] used unsubstituted naphthol-AS phosphate at pH 9.1 with good results. With the popularization of the substituted naphthol-AS phosphates for tissue phosphatase by Burstone[101,102] in 1958, a number of studies were published concerning the use of these compounds as substrates for LAP. Ackerman[97] recommended naphthol-AS-MX phosphate at pH 8.3 (tris). Kaplow[68] preferred naphthol-AS-BI phosphate at pH 9.6 (Ammediol). Tomonaga *et al.*[63] also used the phosphate ester of naphthol-AS-MX at pH 8.6 (Ammediol). All reported superior results using naphthol-AS derivatives as compared to α-naphthyl phosphate. The naphthol-AS phosphates are water insoluble and are generally dissolved in small portions of dimethylformamide, as suggested by Burstone.[101] Stock solutions of the naphthol-AS phosphates in appropriate buffers may be prepared and stored in the refrigerator,[63,68,74,97] making it unnecessary to weigh out minute quantities of substrate with each staining procedure. Kaplow[68] found that varying the substrate over a wide range of concentrations had no effect on enzyme activity. For consistent reproducible results, the buffers should be permitted to warm to room temperature before using.

The writer has had some experience with all the above mentioned substrates. In general, they all give excellent reproducible results, and the choice of substrate and coupling salt is often subjective and dependent upon personal aesthetic values.

Diazonium Salts

Diazonium salts are generally derived by treatment of aryl amines with nitrous acid. These compounds are widely used in the dye industry and are commercially designated by various code letters usually preceded in this country by "Fast" or "Diazo," in England by "Brentamine," and in Germany by "Echt." Stable diazotates of a wide variety and complexity are now available commercially. These compounds are stable as powders for long periods of time if stored in a dessicator in the cold and protected from light. They are water soluble but unstable in solution and decompose at varying rates depending upon temperature, pH, and chemical structure. The decomposition products may inhibit alkaline phosphatase activity and to a varying degree are capable of imparting a nonspecific stain to cells and tissues. Fortunately, this background color usually differs from the azo dye formed after coupling occurs.

Diazonium salts couple with aromatic amines, phenols, and some heterocyclic compounds forming insoluble colored azo dyes. This is the basis for the technique devised by Menten and co-workers[48] for demonstrating alkaline phosphatase in tissues. Rate of coupling varies with the particular diazonium salt as well as with the pH, substrate, and temperature of incubation. It also varies with the amount and type of diluent metal compounds (stabilizers) present in commercial preparations.

Although "diazonium" salts are used as a general term, many compounds are actually tetrazonium salts (dicouplers). They are capable of coupling in two positions and the color of the resulting azo dye may depend upon whether one or both diazo groups have coupled. In addition, polymerized azo dyes are also possible, or one diazo radical may bind to a tissue protein site. These reagents are high molecular weight compounds that theoretically may have difficulty in penetrating sites of enzyme activity.

Kaplow[55] used Fast Blue RR salt (4′-amino-2,5′ dimethoxybenzanilide) to demonstrate LAPA, with α-naphthyl phosphate as the substrate. This diazonium salt is a relatively rapid coupler, reasonably stable, and forms a brown-black insoluble azo dye. The diethoxy analog (Fast Blue BB or BBN) has very similar properties. Merker and Heilmeyer[103] proposed Variamine Blue B salt (4-amino-4′methoxy-diphenylamine) as a coupler for α-naphthyl phosphate. Hayhoe and Quaglino[104] preferred Fast Garnet GBC salt (*o*-aminoazotoluene), which is an extremely rapid coupler but very unstable in solution. It forms a yellow-brown, pink-tinged azo dye when coupled with α-naphthyl phosphate. Because Fast Garnet GBC salt breaks down so rapidly, requiring use immediately after preparation, and because the decomposition products impart a yellow background stain, I have not considered it the most suitable diazonium salt. In 1963, Fast Red Violet LB salt (5-chloro-*o*-toluidine-benzanilide) was recommended as a coupling reagent for use with the substituted naphthols.[68] This salt is particularly useful for coupling with naphthol-AS-BI, -MX, and -TR phosphates, with which it forms a bright-red azo dye. It is one of the more stable salts in solution and a rapid coupler. The formation of a red dye is an advantage in that it permits more contrast between cytoplasmic staining, due to enzyme activity, and blue counterstained nuclei. Whitt[73] suggested coupling Red Violet LB salt with α-naphthyl phosphate but this has not given satisfactory staining in our laboratory. The resultant azo dye is slow forming, dull in appearance, and lacks discreteness. Ackerman[97] and Tomonaga and associates[63] preferred Fast Blue RR or BB(N) as diazonium salts for use with the complex substituted AS-naphthol phosphates. Rutenburg *et al.*[74] also recommended Fast Blue BBN for use with the unsubstituted naphthol-AS phosphate. Thus, Fast Blue RR, BB(N), and probably Variamine Blue B salts are equally suitable for coupling with either α-naphthyl, unsubstituted naphthol-AS, or substituted naphthol-AS phosphates, if one desires a brown-black or blue azo dye. Red Violet LB salt may be used with substituted or unsubstituted AS phosphates for obtaining a red azo dye, but it is not very satisfactory for use with α-naphthyl phosphate. It should be emphasized that the azo dye formed is not only dependent upon the combination of diazonium salt and substrate selected but also on pH, buffer, buffer concentration, and time of incubation. For these reasons, one must closely follow recommended procedures in order to obtain satisfactory results.

Time and Temperature of Incubation

Incubation conditions considered optimal for biochemical enzymatic analyses are not necessarily the most satisfactory for cytochemical studies. In staining for LAPA, it can be advantageous to adjust conditions to suit the aims of a particular investigation. Thus, in attempting to determine the presence or absence of activity in a given cell type, maximum staining is desired, even at a sacrifice of discreteness of the final reaction product. Diffusion of the azo dye from one cell to another is less likely on blood smears, where cells are relatively widely dispersed, than in tissue sections where cells are contiguous. If one desires to demonstrate precise intracellular sites of activity, then conditions and reagents should be selected which yield insoluble discrete reaction products. For routine clinical studies, in which comparative scoring is to be used, optimal staining conditions are those capable of demonstrating the widest spectrum of scores as found in physiological and pathological states. In selected clinical conditions, in which LAPA scoring is used for diagnostic or prognostic purposes, it may be advantageous to incubate for longer or shorter than usual times, in order to increase the usefulness of LAPA scoring. For example, blood smears from untreated patients with chronic myelogenous leukemia incubated for one hour show little change in scores when compared with duplicate smears incubated for ten minutes (FIGURE 9), whereas normal and other pathological blood smears almost always show considerably higher scores after prolonged incubation. If, however, one desires to discriminate among disorders characterized by extremely high scores, very short incubation times may be necessary. As more experience is gained, it may prove advantageous to routinely incubate replicate blood smears for three different time periods. Bellotti and associates[105] have recently reported that very prolonged incubation times have permitted distinguishing normals with extremely low scores from patients with low scores due to chronic myelogenous leukemia.

Temperatures higher than ordinary room temperatures are not advisable with the azo dye method because of increased instability of the diazonium salt. Such temperatures are also unnecessary, since hydrolysis procedes at a rapid enough rate even at room temperature. Longer incubation times at lower temperatures have been recommended by Merker and Heilmeyer,[103] presumably to reduce decomposition of the diazonium salt. We have not found it necessary to incubate slides under controlled temperatures for routine studies. However, if wide fluctuations in ambient temperatures occur, then such precautions are necessary if consistent results are desired. Higher incubation temperatures (37° C) are commonly used with the metal-salt method, in part on theoretical grounds, since β-glycerophosphate is a physiological substrate, but mainly because of the relatively slow rate of hydrolysis.

Biochemical Assays and Cytochemical Scoring

Chemical analyses of leukocyte suspensions are the only means of obtaining quantitative data on LAPA, and a variety of methods have been described. For

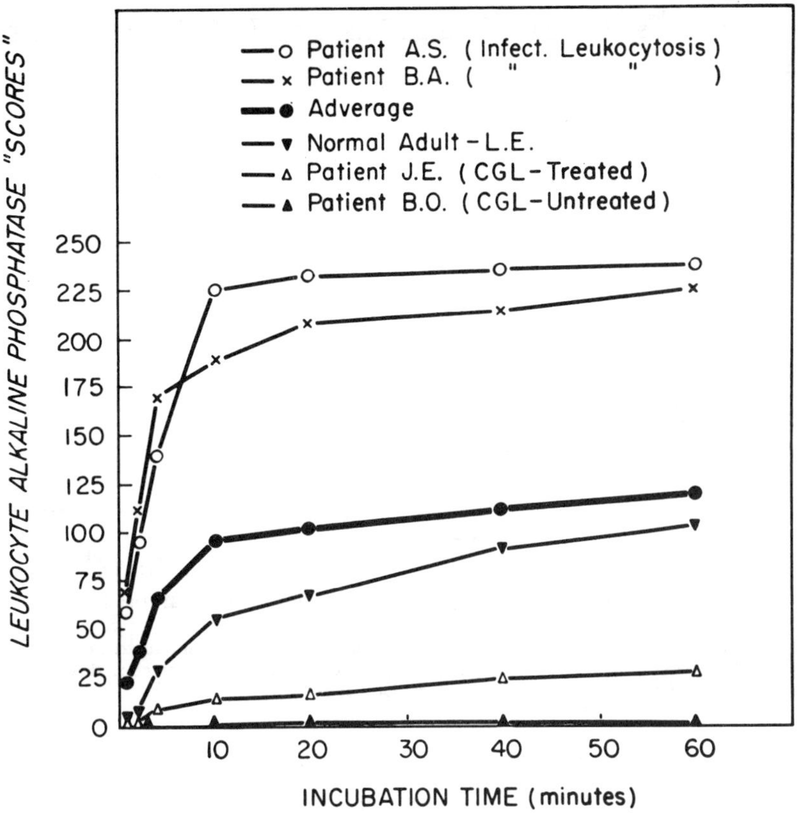

FIGURE 9. Effect of incubation time on LAPA. Azo dye method.[55] (Reproduced by permission of the Williams & Wilkins Co., Baltimore, Md.)

the most part these have been based on methods developed for assaying serum phosphatase levels. β-glycerophosphate was used as a substrate by Valentine and associates,[13] Williams and Mendel,[47] Moloney *et al.*,[44] and Trubowitz and colleagues.[66] In some of the early studies, results were expressed as milligrams of phosphorus liberated per hour per 10^{10} leukocytes. Cytochemical observations indicate that the enzyme is found exclusively in neutrophils, so that units of activity expressed as 10^{10} neutrophils are more meaningful. In 1958, Peacock *et al.*[106] described a biochemical method using *p*-nitrophenol phosphate as a substrate. Young and Prager[107] reported phosphatase activities as micromoles of phosphate liberated per hour per milligram of leukocyte protein. More recently, McCoy *et al.*[96] described a fluorometric method using disodium β-naphthol phosphate as a substrate and expressing results as micromoles of β-naphthol formed per milligram of leukocyte protein per hour. Alkaline phosphatase was solubilized by extracting leukocyte suspensions with 10 percent *n*-butanol. The authors suggest that by this technique, predominantly neutrophil protein is solubilized so that, despite the units used, the results are in reality more indicative of neutrophil rather than leukocyte activity. In general, studies comparing biochemical with cytochemical scoring methods of LAPA have indicated that both techniques yield

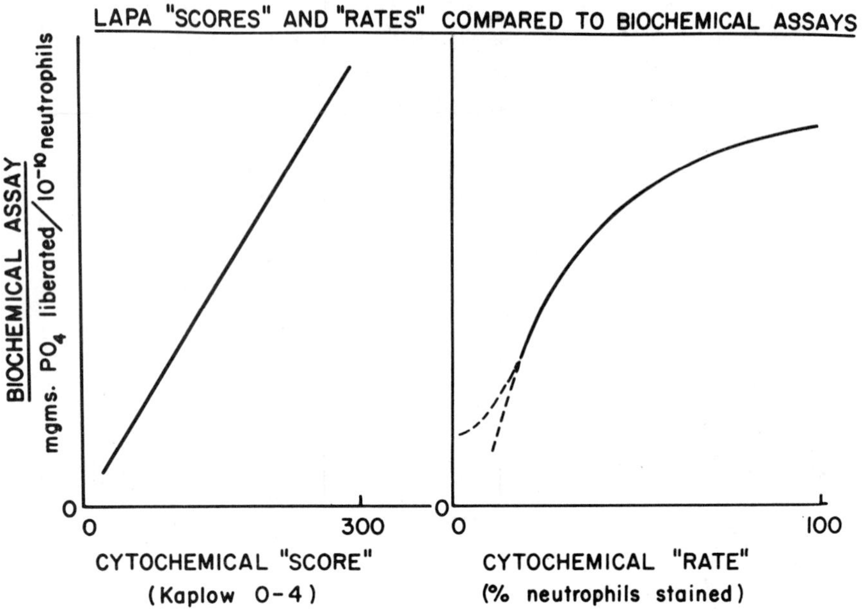

FIGURE 10. Relationship between biochemical assays of LAPA and cytochemical assays expressed as "score" (Kaplow 0–4) and "rate" (percent neutrophils stained). Based on data by Tomonaga *et al.*,[63] Wendt & Budde,[65] and McCoy et al.[96]

comparable results.[44,96,108–112] The close agreement between biochemical and cytochemical assays becomes evident when one plots LAPA scores (0–4 ratings) against biochemical results expressed as milligrams of phosphorus liberated per hour per 10^{10} neutrophils (FIGURE 10). The straight line that is obtained is in contrast to the curvilinear graph obtained by plotting similar biochemical results against LAPA "rates" (i.e., percent neutrophils stained). Such data tend to validate a scoring procedure in which different values are assigned to cells on the basis of intensity of staining. As previously indicated, many modifications of the scoring technique have been proposed. Because of the wide variation in normal adult LAP activities, some investigators[58–60,62] have preferred to use only 0–2 or 0–3 ratings in order to narrow the normal range. Such devices are, however, mathematical manipulations and the fewer the rating categories, the less linear is the relationship between cytochemical and biochemical results. Many European investigators have used a 0–5 scoring technique as described by Merker and Heilmeyer.[103] In practice, the results by this method are almost identical with 0–4 scoring, since cells rated 5 are so infrequently encountered. TABLE 1 indicates the similarity in range and means obtained by different investigators using both 0–4 and 0–5 ratings. Meislin *et al.*[108] did note a lack of agreement between the two methods in patients with chronic lymphatic and acute blastic leukemia. Their cytochemical studies indicated low normal LAPA, whereas chemical analyses revealed persistent elevated activities. They speculated that the higher values obtained by the chemical approach may have resulted from alkaline phosphatase present in nonneutrophil blood elements, in amounts too small to be detected by

TABLE 1

LAPA SCORES IN ADULT NORMALS

Authors	Year	Ref.	Subjects (No.)	Range	Mean ± S.E.	S.D.*	MPR†	Mean − MPR (Skewness)
Kaplow's Azo Dye Method[55]								
Patterson, R. B.	1963	87	36	20–149	70 ± 5.42	32.50	84.5	−14.5
Lacher, M. J.	1964	160	53	12–95	47 ± 2.51	18.28	53.5	− 6.5
Mitus, W. J.	1959	161	14	16–53	30 ± 2.90	10.85	34.5	− 4.5
Sherwood, L. M.	1959	67	26	4–96	36 ± 4.55	23.23	50.0	−14.0
Toderan, M. G.	1964	162	11	11–88	33 ± 7.32	24.29	49.5	−16.5
Harrop, J.	1961	163	14	7–120	52 ± 8.85	33.10	63.5	−11.5
Quigley, H. J.	1960	164	58	12–108	33 ± 2.73	20.80	60.0	−27.0
Kaplow, L. S.	1955	55	75	2–76	22 ± 1.78	15.40	39.0	−17.0
Tanzer, J.	1965	165	50	10–110	40 ± 3.14	22.22	60.0	−20.0
Berretta, L. R.	1962	166	5	24–42	34 ± 3.45	7.73	33.0	+ 1.0
Kotlarek, H. S.	1965	167	30	14–126	69 ± 5.00	27.40	70.0	− 1.0
Koler, R. D.	1958	113	35	5–175	73 ± 5.84	40.40	90.0	−17.0
Rieder, H.	1961	119	30	10–100	38 ± 4.01	22.00	55.0	−17.5
Mdzewski, B.	1964	168	10	11–27	21 ± 1.61	5.19	19.0	+ 2.0
Hausser, E.	1962	169	30	3–57	30 ± 2.89	15.84	30.0	0
Total:			477					
Averages:				10.7–94.8	41.9 ± 4.13	21.21	52.8	−10.9
Modified Kaplow Method – Merker and Heilmeyer[61]								
Bertolotti, E.	1965	61a	82	2–152	40 ± 3.35	30.36	77.0	−37.0
Alsleben, U.	1961	79	21	8–64.5	34 ± 3.21	14.70	36.3	− 2.3
Keiser, G.	1963	80	21	10–70	32 ± 4.09	18.73	40.0	− 8.0
Flury, R.	1964	81	25	20–76	45 ± 2.85	14.25	48.0	− 3.0
Immel, E.	1964	78	20	26–113	72 ± 5.12	23.20	69.5	+ 2.5
Merker, H.	1960	103	119	10–110	43 ± 1.78	19.44	60.0	−16.7
Total:			288					
Averages:				12.7–97.7	44.3 ± 3.40	20.11	55.2	−10.7
Overall Averages:				11.3–95.6	42.6 ± 3.92	20.90	53.5	−10.8

* Estimated values based on calculations using Tippett's numbers.

† Midpoint of range.

histochemical techniques. This is indeed a possibility despite almost unanimous agreement that in peripheral blood, alkaline phosphatase activity can be demonstrated cytochemically only in the neutrophil series.† Recently, in our own laboratory, very weak staining of platelets has been observed on rare occasions with smears fixed in 60 percent buffered acetone and with complex AS-naphthol phosphates used as substrates. McCoy and associates[96] noted that biochemical values were higher than cytochemical values in blood from pregnant women and from patients with polycythemia vera. Both conditions are frequently associated with thrombocythemia, and it is possible that platelet phosphatase activity may have been responsible for the discrepancies. It is also possible, as suggested by McCoy *et al.* that cytochemical methods may be incapable of distinguishing among bloods with very high LAPA. As can be seen in FIGURE 9, when LAPA scores are plotted against incubation times, a typical enzymatic curve is obtained. The reliability in the flat portion of the curve would be expected to be poor.

Tomonaga *et al.*[63] and Rutenburg *et al.*[74] devised scoring methods in which individual dye granules are counted in the cytoplasm of 100 neutrophils. Ratings are assigned on the basis of the number of granules per cell. This method, albeit less subjective, is technically more difficult and is open to serious criticism, since only number and not size of granules is taken into consideration. As one increases the incubation time, not only do new small dye granules appear, but granules previously present increase in size. It is thus evident that size of granules and number of granules are both indications of the degree of activity.

Despite the fact that scoring is a very subjective process, studies[70,98,113] have indicated that different observers can obtain very similar results when scoring duplicate blood smears for LAPA, provided certain precautions are observed. It is most important that cells be selected for rating in relatively thin areas of the blood smear only. In thick areas, leukocytes round up and present a greater volume per unit area and appear more intensely stained than in thin areas. For reproducible results, scoring should be done with oil immersion magnification ($\times$ 900). The substage condenser should be elevated to its maximum position, and the iris diaphragm opened enough to brightly light the whole field. Each scoring should be carried out under similar light conditions with respect to source and intensity. Although the newer azo dye substrates yield discrete granular deposits, scoring may be easier with the more diffuse staining obtained with α-naphthyl phosphate or with the heavy-metal method. Preference for a particular technique will vary with the individual.

Counterstains and Mounting Media

Counterstaining is essential in assaying LAPA cytochemically in order to visualize cells that have no activity. The ideal counterstain should stain nuclei only and give good contrast with but have no effect on the final reaction product. Since most azo dyes are soluble to some extent in organic solvents, only aqueous solutions are suitable for counterstaining. Kaplow[55] suggested Mayer's hematoxylin which stains nuclei blue-gray. Wasastjerna and co-workers[114] exposed smears for six minutes to a mixture of 0.5 percent celestine blue and 5 percent ammonium ferric sulphate prior to staining with hematoxylin. Hayhoe and Quaglino[104] preferred methyl green as a counterstain for the azo dye formed by

† [NOTE ADDED IN PROOF: Studies in this laboratory over the past year have consistently demonstrated that a small percentage (less than 0.8 percent) of the human peripheral blood buffy coat mononuclear cells that morphologically resemble lymphocytes contains weak to moderate cysoplasmic alkaline phosphatase activity (in press).]

Fast Garnet GBC and α-naphthyl acid phosphate. Another satisfactory stain is aqueous nuclear fast red (kernechtrot), which is particularly useful for blue, black, or brown azo dyes. Giemsa, safranin, and methylene blue have also been used as counterstains. However, since these agents are to some extent cytoplasmic as well as nuclear stains, they may mask cytoplasmic deposits.

A satisfactory mounting medium that will preserve activity for prolonged periods of time has not been described. The following materials have been tried and have affected either the azo dye or the counterstain: balsam, Permount®, damar, polyvinylpyrollidine, Diatex®, Valnor®, glycerol-gelatin, and Histoclad®. Unmounted stained slides remain unchanged for years. Brief exposure to oil and xylol has little effect on either the azo dye or the counterstain, although this varies somewhat with the substrate and diazonium used. It has been our practice to examine and score unmounted smears with the oil immersion lens and to then discard the slides. Recently, Peters[115] has described a technique for stabilizing intracellular azo dye deposits. The method involves coating blood smears with a thin covering of dilute glycerol-gelatin, which is then permitted to rapidly drain and dry. After application of additional mounting media, a cover slip is applied. The author indicates he has preserved alkaline phosphatase stained smears for four months by this method without any change in dye deposition.

Controls

Prefixed heat inactivated (one minute in boiling water) blood smears should be stained with each new batch of diazonium salt or substrate used, and each new shipment of diazonium should be tested for nonspecific staining by incubating in a mixture of buffer and diazonium salt without substrate. Positive controls should be run routinely along with unknowns. It is preferable to obtain positive controls from the same source. Guinea pig, rabbit, and rat neutrophils have very high activity and such blood is ideally suitable for positive controls. Blood from obstetrical cases in the third trimester or early postpartum period also can be used.

Intracellular Sites of Activity

There has been almost unanimous agreement that alkaline phosphatase activity in peripheral blood leukocytes is found exclusively in the cytoplasm of band- and segmented-neutrophilic granulocytes.‡ As previously mentioned, we have recent evidence of very faint staining in occasional platelets. Schubert and Martin[116] have reported strong activity in 19 percent of peripheral blood myeloblasts in a single case of chronic myelogenous leukemia in terminal blastic crisis. Quaglino,[117] using azo dye techniques, noted cytoplasmic staining in from 12 percent to over 50 percent of bone marrow erythroblasts and megaloblasts in two cases of hemolytic anemia and five cases of pernicious anemia. Most investigators[110,118–121] have found lower activity in bone marrow granulocytes than in circulating peripheral blood granulocytes, although Sirola and Sirola,[122] and Ciorapciu *et al.*,[123] using the heavy-metal technique, found greater numbers of cells showing LAPA in the bone marrow than in the peripheral blood. Rarely, metamyelocytes show weak activity in bone marrow.[97] Endothelial cells of the marrow vascular network stain intensely for LAPA.[97,121,124,125] Undritz[125] observed intense staining of osteoblasts. I have also seen intensely stained bone marrow cells, which have been interpreted as osteoblasts. Very strong staining

‡ See note added in proof on p. 928.

is frequently seen in bone marrow cells variously described as reticuloendothelial,[55,97,104,122] reticulum,[117,121] nonphagocytic-stellate,[126] and histiocytic-like.[44] These cells usually have a relatively small oval nucleus and a granular cytoplasm having poorly defined borders, which tends to stream out in long cytoplasmic projections. At times, these cells round up and may contain a few granules or vacuoles. Such cells are probably derived from the endothelial cells of the vascular network. In tissue culture, they go on to form alkaline phosphatase-positive, fibroblast-like cells, as has been so beautifully demonstrated by Farnes and Barker.[124] Ackerman[126] calls these cells "reticular" and subdivides them into nonphagocytic and phagocytic, which would appear to be a sound classification. However, most phagocytic reticulum cells do not stain for alkaline phosphatase but do stain intensely for acid phosphatase, whereas vascular-network reticuloendothelial cells stain only very weakly for acid phosphatase, although occasionally isolated stellate cells stain strongly for acid phosphatase.[127]

The precise ultrastructural localization of alkaline phosphatase in human neutrophils has not been definitely established. Wetzel and associates[128,129] have demonstrated three types of granules in rabbit heterophils, only one of which, intermediate in size, was shown to contain alkaline phosphatase activity and these were devoid of acid phosphatase activity, although larger granules corresponding to azurophilic granules as well as very small dense granules did contain acid phosphatase. Whether such findings hold true for human neutrophilic granules has not been ascertained. There have been very few biochemical enzyme studies on the isolated granules of human neutrophils. Kawabata[130] studied both human and horse leukocytes and obtained five cytoplasmic fractions by homogenization and differential centrifugation. Neutrophilic granules of varying electron density were found predominantly in fractions II and III. Alkaline phosphatase, however, was found almost equally distributed in all fractions. Young and Prager[107] found alkaline phosphatase in human neutrophils in a more slowly sedimenting fraction than acid phosphatase. Clarke[131] found highest alkaline phosphatase activity in a 27,000 $\times$ g fraction, which was said to contain mainly granules. These few studies suggest that alkaline phosphatase is localized in some type of neutrophilic granule. Whether this will prove to be a lysosomal-type particle remains to be seen.

LAPA in Various Animals

One of the unique facets in our knowledge of LAPA is the remarkable variation in activity found in leukocytes of different animals. Such variations were noted over 25 years ago by Gomori.[18] His findings have since been confirmed and expanded by numerous studies.[11,28,31,54,132–134] As can be seen in TABLE 2, different animals do not show a graded variation but seem to fall into three groups with either extremely high, very high, or extremely low or absent LAPA, as assayed by cytochemical methods. Lie-Injo Luan Eng[133] has shown that the leukocytes of at least one species of monkey (*Macaca mulatta*) has only faint traces of alkaline phosphatase activity, whereas leukocytes of all other monkeys studied have among the highest levels of activity known, in a range 30 times that seen in human leukocytes. Similarly, although the rat has very high LAPA, the mouse has none. This difference has been taken advantage of in marrow transplant studies,[135,136] in which mice subjected to lethal whole-body irradiation were infused with rat leukocytes, and the survival of the transfused cells was detected by LAPA staining. Studies of animal LAPA have indicated that alkaline phosphatase is not limited to neutrophils but is also present in the erythrocytes of the frog[28] and in the eosinophils of many animals.[132,134]

TABLE 2

LAPA IN VARIOUS ANIMALS*

Animal	Scores†		
	Very High	High‡	Low or Absent
Hamster	335		
Monkeys (most species)	320		
Guinea pig	320		
Rat		189	
Rabbit		171	
Steer		+	
Burro		+	
Ground hog		+	
Horse		+	
Cow		+	
Sheep		+	
Goat		+	
Man			11
Monkey *(Macaca mulatta)*			0.5
Mouse			0
Dog			0
Cat			0
Chicken			0
Pigeon			0

* Data from References 11, 18, 28, 31, 54, 132–134.

† 0–400 scoring.[11]

‡ LAPA also found in eosinophils of the rat, steer, burro, horse, cow, sheep, and goat,[132,134] and in erythrocytes of the frog.[28]

\+ = present.

Unfortunately, the extreme differences in animal LAPA make it doubtful whether the interpretation of the results of studies on animals may be applied to humans. As yet no convenient animal has been found with LAPA levels comparable to that seen in man, and in which LAPA changes under various physiological and pathological conditions as does human LAPA.

Normal Human LAPA "Scores"

There have been so many modifications in methods for cytochemically assessing LAPA, that in reviewing over 300 published papers devoted to studies on human LAPA, only 21 were found in which basically similar staining and scoring techniques were used and in which adult normal range and mean normal scores were reported. The findings in these studies are shown in TABLE 1, along with other statistically derived data. As can be seen, a very wide range of normal scores has been reported for apparently healthy human adults. The lowest reported score was two and the highest 175. The range of scores averaged from 11.3–96 for all 765 subjects included in the 21 studies. The average overall mean score was 42.6 and the average standard deviation (S.D.) for all the studies (estimated by use of Tippett's numbers) was 20.9. If the listed means are plotted against the S.D. of the same study, a linear relationship is evident (FIGURE 11). The regression line between S.D.'s and means passes approximately through the origin, indicating that the coefficient of variation (S.D. expressed as percent of mean) should be constant. The average S.D. is very close to 50 percent of the average mean. The variation in "normal" values reported by different investigators may be due either to a biased selection of population or from factors inherent in the staining or scoring procedures. It would seem more reliable for individual investigators to establish their standard deviation on the basis of 50 percent of their determined mean rather than by conventional mathematical treatment of their own data. In almost all 21 of the listed studies, the midpoint of the range is higher than the mean, indicating a skewed distribution of values, with a greater spread of scores in the high as opposed to the low range. Such relatively uniform skewness suggests that methods or factors other than biased population selection are responsible for the asymmetrical distribution.

Determination of an accurate normal range of LAPA scores which would define over 98 percent of the healthy adult population must await further studies and more sophisticated statistical analyses of the data. The problem is compounded by evidence of differences in LAPA between adult males and females,[137–141] as well as by variations of LAPA with age.[87,138,139,142–150] The high values found in infancy are the subject of a separate report which appears elsewhere in this monograph. Adolescents and the aged may have slightly lower mean LAPA scores than young adults.[61a,139,151] A graphic representation of probable normal LAPA ranges during life is shown in FIGURE 12. Most cytochemical studies have indicated that children have mean scores similar to adults.

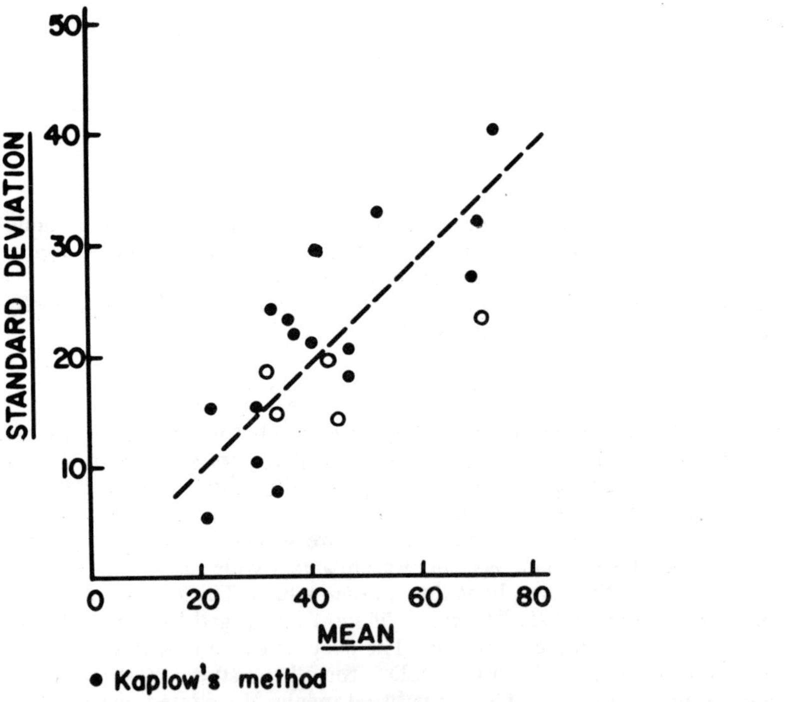

FIGURE 11. Relationship of mean adult scores and standard deviations (estimated by Tippett's numbers) of 21 investigations using similar staining and scoring techniques. (See TABLE 1).

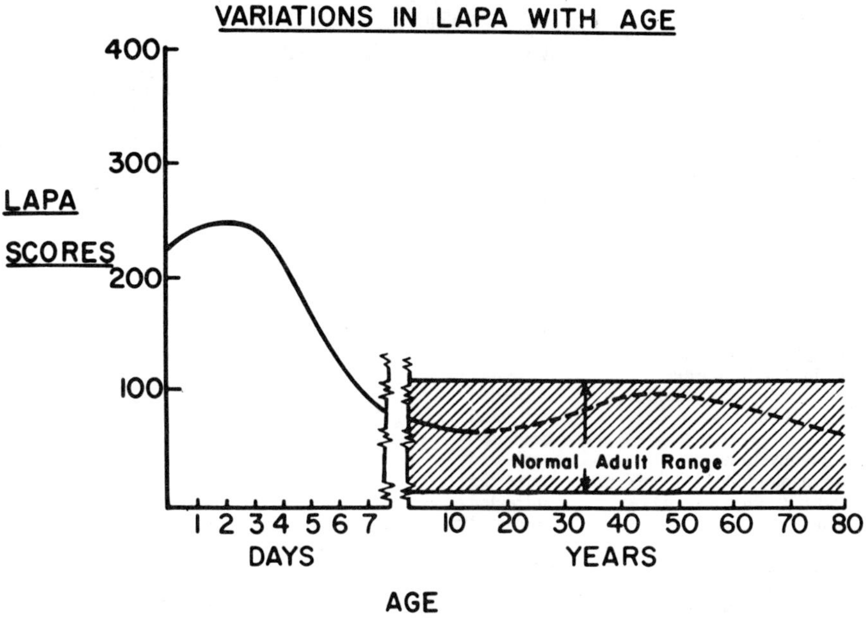

FIGURE 12. Approximate normal range and mean LAPA scores from infancy to old age (See text).

Alter[152] however, using biochemical methods, reported much higher scores in children under ten years of age than in older children or in adults. The possibility must be considered that biochemical analysis may be measuring alkaline phosphatase activity in cells other than neutrophils, or that cytochemical methods are incapable of demonstrating weak activity in sites other than the cytoplasm of the more mature neutrophilic granulocytes.

Evidence regarding a diurnal variation in LAPA has been conflicting. Wachstein[28] suggested such a possibility and Anstey *et al.*[153] reported marked daily fluctuations with a tendency for higher scores in the evening as compared with other times. Other studies,[90,104,108,140] however, have indicated only insignificant diurnal or day to day variations in the same individual, except for increased activity in the premenopausal female during the midmenstrual cycle, presumably associated with ovulation.[137,140]

Clinical Significance of LAPA Assays

Leukocyte alkaline phosphatase shows wide fluctuations in a variety of diseases. An attempt has been made to survey the literature on changes in LAPA in various diseases. Although hundreds of studies have been reviewed, many of the findings could not be included because of the mode of expression. Also, only those reports were tabulated in which the total number of cases studied was stated, and in which the number of cases with high, low, or normal LAP activities for each disease entity was specifically indicated or could be readily interpolated. In addition, patients receiving therapy or in remission from this disease at the time of the assay were either excluded or seperately summarized. Finally, studies were

TABLE 3

DISEASES ASSOCIATED WITH HIGH "LAPA"*

Disease	Stage or Rx Status	No. Studies	No. Cases	Findings (LAPA Scores, %)		
				Normal	High	Low
Cirrhosis (decompensated)	†	1	13	0	100	0
Lymphoma	untreated†	2	41	5	95	0
Bacterial infections	untreated†	18	703	2	95	3
Chronic lymphatic leukemia	treated	3	13	8	92	0
	untreated†	16	121	34	54	12
Leukemoid reaction	†	11	86	4	93	3
Polycythemia vera	untreated†	33	411	8	91	1
	treated	5	21	24	71	5
Acute lymphatic leukemia	untreated†	8	63	11	87	2
Reticulum cell sarcoma	untreated†	6	22	14	86	0
Acute monocytic leukemia	untreated†	4	7	14	86	0
Hodgkin's Disease	untreated†	20	227	18	81	1
	treated‡	6	103	63	34	3
Multiple myeloma	untreated†	13	68	18	79	3
Acute myelomonocytic leukemia	untreated†	2	32	19	75	6
Cirrhosis (compensated)	untreated†	5	49	27	71	2
Obstructive jaundice	untreated†	4	53	36	62	2
Myelosclerosis	†	20	154	23	62	15
Aplastic anemia	untreated†	9	57	17	62	21
Agranulocytosis	untreated†	4	20	50	50	0

* See Appendix 1.
† Or not indicated.
‡ Or in remission.

not included if varied scores were obtained when multiple determinations were carried out on the same patient.

TABLE 3 lists those diseases most frequently associated with high LAPA. Over 85 percent of patients with decompensated cirrhosis, bacterial infectious diseases, and untreated lymphoma had LAPA scores above the normal range. The data, however, is based on only one study (13 cases) of cirrhosis and two studies (41 cases) of lymphoma. Leukemoid reactions, untreated polycythemia vera, acute lymphatic and monocytic leukemias, reticulum cell sarcoma, Hodgkin's disease, and multiple myeloma were all associated with high levels of LAPA. It is of interest that in all the untreated disorders in the preceding list, only 3 percent or less of the patients studied had LAPA scores below the normal range. Thus, a low score in such instances would be stronger evidence for excluding a disease than an elevated score would be for incriminating a disease. Similarly, a low score was never found in the 20 cases of agranulocytosis included in the data, although only half of the patients studied had high scores.

TABLE 4 lists the eight disorders most commonly associated with low LAP activity. The data include a single report on eight patients with progressive muscular dystrophy and a single study on three patients with the nephrotic syndrome without complications. Further studies are needed to confirm these interesting findings. Only in hereditary hypophosphatasia has absent LAPA been an invariable finding. The well-documented frequent rise in LAPA seen in patients with chronic myelogenous leukemia in remission or in blastic crisis is evident from the tabulation.

TABLE 5 indicates diseases in which LAPA is usually normal. It is of particular interest that low values have not been reported in any of the tabulated cases of hemolytic anemia, nor have high values been reported in uncomplicated cases of infectious mononucleosis. Those diseases in which no significant relationship to LAPA levels is apparent are listed in TABLE 6. In addition to the more obvious specific conclusions that can be inferred from the accumulated data, certain generalizations are possible. Although LAPA changes are nonspecific in nature, activity tends to increase in bacterial infections and to remain within normal limits

TABLE 4

DISEASES ASSOCIATED WITH LOW "LAPA"*

Disease	Stage or Rx Status	No. Studies	No. Cases	Findings (LAPA Scores, %)		
				Normal	High	Low
Hereditary hypophosphatasia		4	4	0	0	100
Nephrotic syndrome	uncomplicated	1	3	0	0	100
Progressive muscular dystrophy	†	1	8	0	0	100
Chronic myelogenous leukemia	untreated†	34	516	6	2	92
	treated‡	21	166	32	7	61
	blastic crisis	7	52	15	56	29
Refractory anemia (siderotic)	untreated†	5	11	14	7	79
Paroxysmal nocturnal hemoglobinuria	untreated†	4	23	9	13	78

* See Appendix 2.
† Or not indicated.
‡ Or in remission.

TABLE 5

DISEASES ASSOCIATED WITH NORMAL "LAPA"*

Disease	Stage or Rx Status	No. Studies	No. Cases	Findings (LAPA Scores, %)		
				Normal	High	Low
Secondary polycythemia		14	117	84	4	12
Hemolytic anemia	untreated†	6	29	83	17	0
Infectious mononucleosis	untreated†	9	65	75	0	25
Viral hepatitis	untreated†	5	130	70	8	22
Lymphosarcoma	untreated†	8	45	69	11	20
	treated	2	11	73	27	0

* See Appendix 3.
† Or not indicated.

TABLE 6

DISEASES WITH VARIABLE "LAPA"*

Disease	Stage or Rx Status	No. Studies	No. Cases	Findings (LAPA Scores, %)		
				Normal	High	Low
Pernicious anemia	untreated†	9	32	53	31	16
	treated	3	17	82	12	6
Idiopathic thromobocytopenic purpura	untreated†	5	18	44	28	28
Iron deficiency anemia	untreated†	3	28	43	25	32
Acute myelogenous leukemia	untreated†	13	61	30	13	57
Acute undifferentiated leukemia	untreated†	9	111	26	40	34
Erythroleukemia	untreated†	6	12	25	33	42

* See Appendix 4.
† Or not indicated.

in viral afflictions. Activity increases with tissue necrosis regardless of etiology and in a variety of other stressful situations.

A number of studies[41,154–156] have demonstrated that a rise in LAPA occurs following surgery and peak activities are observed two to three days after the start of surgery. There is a gradual return to normal scores over the next four to six days. This response differs significantly from the changes in total leukocyte counts which occur following surgery, in which peak leukocytosis occurs less than 24 hours after the start of surgery. These findings are shown in FIGURE 13. This delayed response of LAPA to stress has also been shown in humans given intravenous endotoxin.[157–159] LAPA may be a more sensitive and reliable indicator of body stress than fever or leukocytosis. Some individuals, particularly the aged, are unable to respond to bacterial infections or other stressful situations by fever or leukocytosis. However, in such individuals, an elevated LAPA can be demonstrated.[41,154,155] Thus, LAPA assays can be useful in detecting postoperative complications, when the usual manifestations of infection are not present. The very delicate sensitivity of LAPA to stress also suggests another potential area of clinical usefulness. It is often difficult to interpret minimal elevations in total leukocyte counts, with or without changes in the differential count, and it is likewise difficult to interpret the significance of a modest shift to the left in the differential count in the face of a normal total leukocyte count. In such situations, an elevated LAPA would be strong evidence in favor of an active inflammatory process.

Changes in LAPA during pregnancy are shown in FIGURE 14. The role of LAPA in the diagnosis of pregnancy is discussed elsewhere in this monograph. LAPA assays have been suggested as being useful in the diagnosis of ectopic pregnancy[70,166,219,220] and in the detection of anovulatory menstrual cycles.[137,221] The report[222] that LAPA is normal in patients with choriocarcinoma and tends

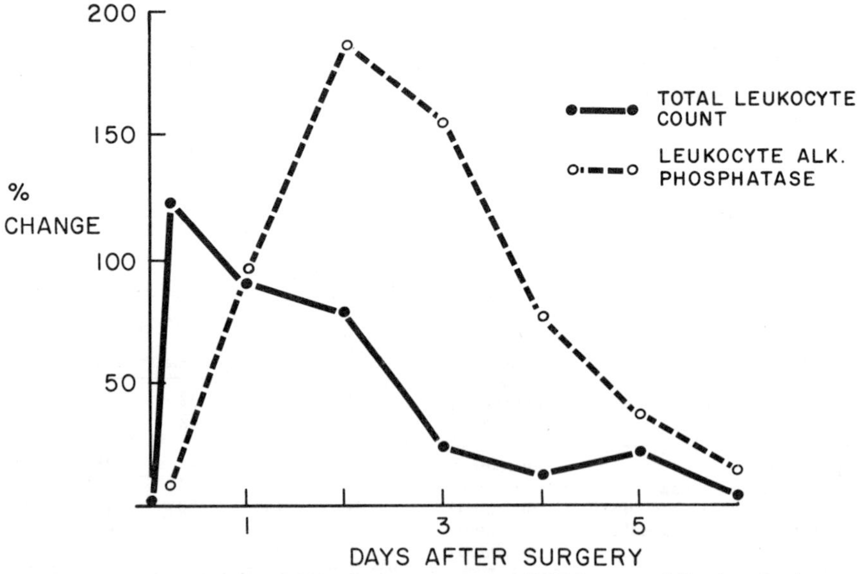

FIGURE 13. Variations in total leukocyte counts and LAPA scores following elective surgery.[154] (Reproduced by permission of Surgery, Gynecology & Obstetrics.)

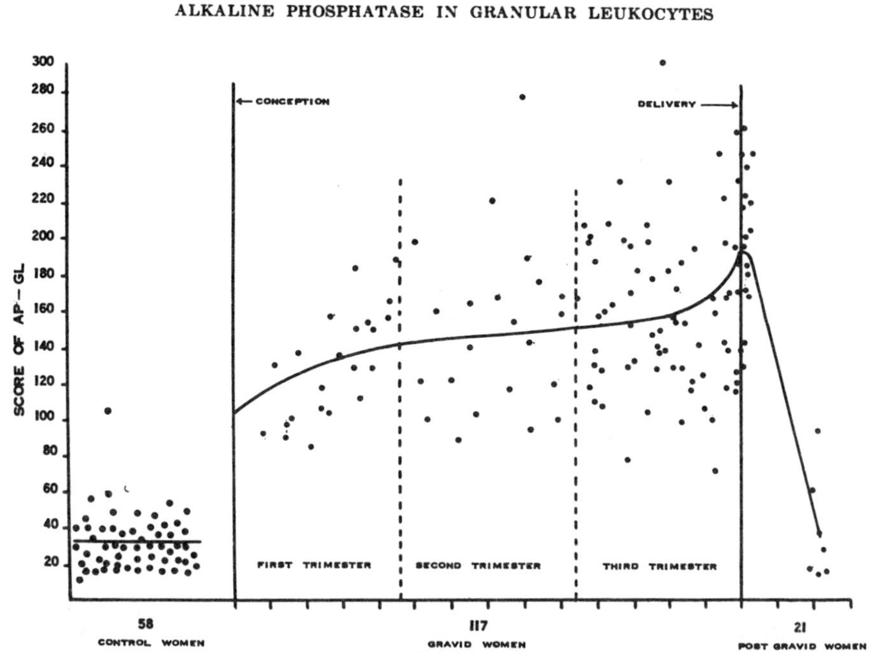

FIGURE 14. Variations in LAPA scores during pregnancy, delivery and the early puerperium. (Reproduced by permission of Quigley, *et al.*[164] and the Williams & Wilkins Co., Baltimore, Md.)

to be high in patients with hydatidiform mole may prove useful as an aid in distinguishing these two entities. Haering[223] has shown that LAPA tends to remain elevated in women who breast-feed, whereas LAPA returned to normal within a few weeks after delivery in women who did not breast-feed.

Other Applications of LAPA Staining

The cytochemical methods used to demonstrate LAP may be applied to material other than blood and to cells other than leukocytes. There have been a number of studies in which LAP staining techniques have been used to demonstrate alkaline phosphatase activity in cells in tissue culture. Such studies have been useful in determining cell lineage[124] and in detecting clonal derivatives.[224,225] Cytochemical methods have also been used to study organ and tumor imprints.[226] Such studies may reveal sites of myeloid extramedullary hematopoiesis. Perillie and Finch[227] studied LAP in inflammatory exudates evoked by the skin-window technique of Rebuck.[228] By this approach, they were able to obtain adequate numbers of mature leukocytes from patients with acute leukemia and to assay these cells for LAPA. Dannenberg and associates[229] investigated rabbit peritoneal-exudate cells for alkaline phosphatase activity using similar techniques.

Conclusions

It is fortuitous that of the many intracellular leukocyte enzyme systems, the only one known to fluctuate so widely in activity in health and in disease should also be one that may be so readily demonstrated and so easily assayed. Available cytochemical techniques for staining for leukocyte alkaline phosphatase activity are simple, inexpensive, and require only a drop of blood. The Gomori-Takamatsu heavy-metal technique is a three-step procedure and requires more reagents and significantly longer incubation times than the azo dye simultaneous coupling technique. The latter is a one-step procedure and requires only a short incubation time. The azo dye method, however, requires reagents that are potentially bladder carcinogens. They should be handled with appropriate respect. The final reaction product of the azo dye technique is more particulate than that obtained with the heavy-metal method. Both methods, when properly carried out, yield reproducible results, and the choice is often subjective and will vary with the investigator and the availability of reagents.

Our knowledge of LAPA is still very limited. The precise subcellular localization is uncertain. Some of the factors responsible for controlling LAPA are slowly coming to light, but nothing is as yet known about the function of this ubiquitous enzyme. Our knowledge of the significance of changes in LAPA in both physiological and pathological conditions is at a stage similar to the situation that existed many years ago with respect to leukocyte counts, when studies on that parameter of body stress were in their infancy.

Acknowledgments

The technical assistance of Mrs. Charlotte Ladd and Mrs. Janette Clinckenbeard is gratefully acknowledged. Dr. Arne Sollberger of the Veterans Administration Eastern Research Support Center, West Haven, Conn. aided in the statistical analysis and interpretation of the data. This manuscript could not have been completed without the assistance of Miss Mary Lucibello, Mrs. Greta Stanford, and my wife Dr. Sheila Briscoe Kaplow, all of whom aided in sorting and tabulating the data presented. The author is also indebted to Mrs. Osa Kelsey for her assistance in preparing the references and in typing the manuscript.

References

1. Jones, O. P. 1947. Morphologic hematology. Introduction. Blood (Special Issue No. 1) : 3–6.
2. Dameshek, W. 1947. Morphologic hematology. Preface. Blood (Special Issue No. 1) : 1-2.
3. Kay, H. D. 1929. Plasma phosphatase in osteitis deformans and in other diseases of the bone. Brit. J. Exp. Path. **10**: 253–256.
4. Kay, H. D. 1930. Plasma phosphatase. I. Method of determination. Some properties of the enzyme. J. Biol. Chem. **89**: 235.
5. Roche, J. 1931. Blood phosphatases. Biochem. J. **25**: 1724–1733.
6. Umeno, M. 1931. Studien über Phosphatase; über die Glycerophosphatase der Leucocyten im Blute. Biochem. Z. **231**: 339–345.
7. Iwatsuru, R. & Y. Minami. 1934. Studien über Phosphatase; die Phosphatase in Blut, Milz, Leber und Hieren bei akuter lymphatischer Leukamie. Biochem. Z. **268**: 394–398.
8. Iwatsuru, R. & K. Nanjo. 1939. Studien über die Phosphatasenaktivitat des Blutes, Serums und Harns bei chronischer myeloischer Leukamie. Biochem. Z. **300**: 422–428.
9. Rossiter, R. J. 1949. Effect of surface-active substances on the liberation of enzymes from rabbit polymorphonuclear leukocytes. J. Physiol. **108**: Proc. 14.
10. Cram, D. M. & R. J. Rossiter. 1949. Phosphatase of rabbit polymorphonuclear leukocytes. Canad. J. Res. Sect. E. **27**: 290–307.
11. Haight, W. F. & R. J. Rossiter. 1950. Acid and alkaline phosphatase in white cells: data for the lymphocyte and the polymorphonuclear leukocyte of man and the rabbit. Blood **5**: 267–277.

12. FIESSINGER, N. & F. BOYER. 1936. Les phosphatases des leucocytes. Enzymologia **1:** 172–176.
13. VALENTINE, W. N. & W. S. BECK. 1951. Biochemical studies on leukocytes. I. Phosphatase activity in health, leukocytosis and myelocytic leukemia. J. Lab. Clin. Med. **38:** 39–55.
14. TAKAMATSU, H. 1938. Manshu Igaku Zasshi **29:** 1351.
15. TAKAMATSU, H. 1939. Histologische und biochemische Studien uber die Phosphatase. I. Histochemische Untersuchungsmethodik der Phosphatase und deren Verteilung in verschiedenen Organen und Geweben. Trans. Soc. Path. Jap. **29:** 492–498.
16. GOMORI, G. 1939. Microtechnical demonstration of phosphatase in tissue sections. Proc. Soc. Exp. Biol. Med. **42:** 23–26.
17. GOMORI, G. 1941. Distribution of acid phosphatase in the tissues under normal and under pathologic conditions. Arch. Path. **32:** 189–199.
18. GOMORI, G. 1941. Distribution of phosphatase in normal organs and tissues. J. Cell. Comp. Physiol. **17:** 71–83.
19. LISON, L. 1960. Histochimie et Cytochimie Animales. 3rd edit. Vol. 2. Chap. 15. Gauthier Villars. Paris, France.
20. KABAT, E. A. & J. FURTH. 1941. A histochemical study of the distribution of alkaline phosphatase in various normal and neoplastic tissue. Amer. J. Path. **17:** 303–318.
21. GOMORI, G. 1951. Alkaline phosphatase of cell nuclei. J. Lab. Clin. Med. **37:** 526–531.
22. GOMORI, G. 1952. Microscopic Histochemistry. University of Chicago Press. Chicago, Ill.
23. TAKEUCHI, T. & H. TAKAMATSU. 1939. Histologische und biochemische Studien über die Phosphatase in tuberkulosen Herden. Trans. Soc. Path. Jap. **29:** 490–492.
24. FELL, H. B. & J. F. DANIELLI. 1943. The enzymes of healing wounds. I. The distribution of alkaline phosphomonoesterase in experimental wounds and burns of rats. Brit. J. Exp. Path. **24:** 196–203.
25. GOMORI, G. 1943. Calcification and phosphatase. Amer. J. Pathol. **19:** 197–209.
26. TAKEUCHI, T. 1943. Ketsueki tomatsu-hyohon ni okeru kekkyu-phosphatase no shomeihoho ni tsuite ni. Igaku to Seibutsugaku **3:** 279–283.
27. TAKEUCHI, T. 1944. Tomatsu-hyohon ni okeru kekkyu-phosphatase no kenbi kagakuteki shomeihoho no koan narabi ni honpo ni yoru phosphatase-hanno ni tsuite. Manshu Igaku Zasshi (J. Oriental Med.) **41:** 279–294.
28. WACHSTEIN, M. 1946. Alkaline phosphatase activity in normal and abnormal human blood and bone marrow cells. J. Lab. Clin. Med. **31:** 1–17.
29. WISLOCKI, G. B. & E. W. DEMPSEY. 1946. Observations on the chemical cytology of normal blood and hemopoietic tissue. Anat. Rec. **96:** 249–277.
30. WISLOCKI, G. B., H. BUNTING & E. W. DEMPSEY. 1947. Further observations on the chemical cytology of megakaryocytes and other cells of hemopoietic tissue. Anat. Rec. **98:** 527–537.
31. RHEINGOLD, J. J. & G. B. WISLOCKI. 1948. Histochemical methods applied to hematology. Blood **3:** 641–655.
32. RABINOVITCH, M. & D. ANDREUCCI. 1949. A histochemical study of acid and alkaline phosphatase distribution in normal human bone marrow smears. Blood **4:** 580–594.
33. PLUM, C. M. 1950. Alkaline phosphatase in cells of normal and pathological bone marrow compared with peripheral blood. Nord. Med. **43:** 69–70.
34. KERPPOLA, W. 1951. Observations on the phosphatase content of blood and bone marrow cells in normal and pathological hemopoiesis. Blood **6:** 454–465.
35. STORTI, E., S. PERUGINI & V. ROSSI. 1953. Quadro citotopochimico delle fosfatasi nelle cellule del sangue e degli organi emopoietici dell'uomo normale. Medicina (Parma) **3:** 333–356.
36. TAKEUCHI, T. 1951. Ketsueki koto ni kekkyu-phosphatase no saibokagakuteki kenkyu. Nihon Ketsueki-Gakkai Kyushu Chihokai Zasshi **2:** 36–42.
37. KUBO, H. 1951. Histochemical studies on phosphatase. Trans. Soc. Path. Jap. **40:** 1–12.
38. TAKEUCHI, T. & S. UTSUNOMIYA. 1952. Sensitivity of the cytochemical demonstration of alkaline and acid phosphatases in blood cells. Acta Path. Jap. **2:** 57–63.
38a. FRIEDERICI, L. 1955. Histochemische methoden in der Hämatologie. Klin. Wschr. **33:** 1020–1026.
39. BECK, W. S. & W. N. VALENTINE. 1951. Biochemical studies on leukocytes. II. Phosphatase activity in chronic lymphatic leucemia, acute leucemia, and miscellaneous hematologic conditions. J. Lab. Clin. Med. **38:** 245–253.
40. VALENTINE, W. N., W. S. BECK, J. H. FOLLETTE, H. MILLS & J. S. LAWRENCE. 1952. Biochemical studies in chronic myelocytic leukemia, polycythemia vera and other idiopathic myeloproliferative disorders. Blood **7:** 959-977.

41. Valentine, W. N., J. H. Follette, E. B. Hardin, W. S. Beck & J. S. Lawrence. 1954. Studies on leukocyte alkaline phosphatase activity: relation to "stress" and pituitary-adrenal activity. J. Lab. Clin. Med. **44**: 219–228.
42. Valentine, W. N., J. H. Follette, D. H. Solomon & J. Reynolds. 1957. The relationship of leukocyte alkaline phosphatase to "stress," to ACTH, and to adrenal 17-OH-corticosteroids. J. Lab. Clin. Med. **49**: 723–737.
43. Moloney, W. C. & R. D. Lange. 1954. Leukemia in atomic bomb survivors. II. Observations in early phases of leukemia. Blood **9**: 663–685.
44. Wiltshaw, E. & W. C. Moloney. 1955. Histochemical and biochemical studies on leukocyte alkaline phosphatase activity. Blood **10**: 1120-1131.
45. Wiltshaw, E. & W. C. Moloney. 1956. Studies on various factors influencing leukocyte alkaline phosphatase activity. J. Lab. Clin. Med. **47**: 691–699.
46. Williams, M. J. & J. L. Mendel. 1954. Studies on the alkaline and acid phosphatase content of leukocytes in various hematological disorders. Texas Rep. Biol. Med. **12**: 429–437.
47. Williams, M. J. & J. L. Mendel. 1954. Polycythemia vera terminating with myeloblastic leukemia. Correlation of morphologic findings with leukocytic phosphatase studies. Blood **9**: 189–195.
48. Menten, M. L., J. Junge & M. H. Green. 1944. A coupling histochemical azo dye test for alkaline phosphatase in the kidney. J. Biol. Chem. **153**: 471–477.
49. Manheimer, L. H. & A. M. Seligman. 1948. Improvement in the method for the histochemical demonstration of alkaline phosphatase and its use in a study of normal and neoplastic tissues. J. Nat. Cancer Inst. **9**: 181–199.
50. Friedman, O. M. & A. M. Seligman. 1950. Preparation of naphthyl acid phosphates. J. Amer. Chem. Soc. **72**: 624–625.
51. Pearse, A. G. E. 1960. Histochemistry, Theoretical and Applied. 2nd edit. Little, Brown & Co. Boston, Mass.
52. Deane, H. W., R. J. Barrnett & A. M. Seligman. 1960. Handbuch der Histochemie. Vol. VII, Enzymes, Part I, Chapter IV. Gustav Fischer Verlag, Stuttgart, Germany.
53. Burstone, M. S. 1962. Enzyme Histochemistry and its Application in the Study of Neoplasms. Academic Press, New York, N. Y.
54. Vercauteren, R. 1954. The intracellular distribution of alkaline and acid phosphatase in leukocytes. Naturwissenschaften **2**: 532.
55. Kaplow, L. S. 1955. A histochemical procedure for localizing and evaluating leukocyte alkaline phosphatase activity in smears of blood and marrow. Blood **10**: 1023–1029.
56. Seabra, P. 1939. Indice de oxidase. Bol. Acad. Nacl. Med. **3**: 9. Quoted by Seabra, P. 1955. Ann. N. Y. Acad. Sci. **59**: 1026.
57. Brodell, H. & S. N. Swisher. 1954. Studies of leukocyte alkaline phosphatase determined by a clinically applicable histochemical method. Clin. Res. Proc. **2**: 58–59.
58. Elves, M. W., S. Roath & M. C. G. Israels. 1963. A modified azo dye method for the localization and assessment of leucocyte alkaline phosphatase. Acta Haemat. **29**: 141–146.
59. Knoblauch, M. 1962. Über die alkalische Phosphatase der neutrophilen Leukocyten. Helv. Med. Acta **29**: 143–155.
60. Knudtson, K. P. & A. E. Evanger. 1962. Standardization of the leukocyte alkaline phosphatase test. I. In vitro studies on human leukocytes. Amer. J. Clin. Path. **38**: 264–269.
61. Merker, H. & L. Heilmeyer. 1959. Die Bedeutung der alkalischen leukocyten Phosphatase bei Reaktion und Erkrankungen des myeloischen Systems. Schweiz. Med. Wschr. **89**: 1051–1053.
61a. Bertolotti, E., G. F. Quazza, G. Lojodice & E. Brovarone. 1965. La fosfatasi alcalina nei granulociti neutrofili: valori normali nelle varie epoch della vita fino all'eta senile. Minerva Pediat. **17**: 915–924.
62. Nicolau, C. T. & S. T. Nicoara. 1962. The value of the leukocyte alkaline phosphatase index in normal and pathological states. Med. Int. **14**: 1173–1181.
63. Tomonaga, M., T. Sasaki & M. Okuzaki. 1963. Studies on leukocyte alkaline phosphatase. I. Use of the naphthol AS-MX phosphate-Fast Blue RR staining method. Acta Haemat. Jap. **26**: 179–192.
64. Lambers, K. 1958. Die alkalische Phosphataseaktivitat der Blutzellen bei Leukosen und anderen pathologischen Zustanden. Z. Klin. Med. **155**: 176–190.
65. Wendt, F. & C. Budde. 1964. Zur Bewertung der Aktivitat der unspezifischen alkalischen Phosphatase neutrophiler Granulozyten im zytochemischen Verfahren. Med. Welt. **10**: 473–478.

66. TRUBOWITZ, S., D. FELDMAN, C. BENANTE & D. KIRMAN. 1957. Metal requirements of alkaline phosphatases of human and rabbit leukocytes. Proc. Soc. Exp. Biol. Med. **95:** 35–38.
67. SHERWOOD, L. M. & R. E. KENDALL. 1959. A histochemical study of leukocyte alkaline phosphatase in health and disease. Hartford Hosp. Bull. **14:** 18–26.
68. KAPLOW, L. S. 1963. Cytochemistry of leukocyte alkaline phosphatase. Use of complex naphthol AS-phosphates in azo dye coupling technics. Amer. J. Clin. Path. **39:** 439–449.
69. VALENTINE, W. N., K. R. TANAKA & R. E. FREDRICKS. 1960. Studies on leukocyte alkaline phosphatase: Role of zinc and magnesium. J. Lab. Clin. Med. **55:** 303–310.
70. CLIMIE, A. R. W., W. L. HEINRICHS & I. J. FOSTER. 1962. Neutrophilic alkaline phosphatase test. A review with emphasis on findings in pregnancy. Tech. Bull. Regist. Med. Techn. **32:** 95–103.
71. HEINRICHS, W. L. 1962. The neutrophil alkaline phosphatase test in pregnancy. Harper Hosp. Bull. **20:** 107–116.
72. HOFFMAN, G. C. & V. J. LUCICH. 1960. The clinical application of a modified azo-dye technic for the determination of alkaline phosphatase activity in neutrophils. Cleveland Clin. Quart. **27:** 146–156.
73. WHITT, J. 1963. Evaluation of a histochemical method for determining leukocyte alkaline phosphatase activity and a discussion of normal values in adults and newborns. Amer. J. Med. Techn. **29:** 169–174.
74. RUTENBURG, A. M., C. L. ROSALES & J. M. BENNETT. 1965. An improved histochemical method for the demonstration of leukocyte alkaline phosphatase activity: Clinical application. J. Lab. Clin. Med. **65:** 698–705.
75. HARER, W. B., JR. & H. J. QUIGLEY. 1961. Alkaline phosphatase activity in granular leukocytes as a test for early pregnancy. Obstet. Gynec. **17:** 238–242.
76. SABATINI, D. D., K. BENSCH & R. J. BARRNETT. 1963. Preservation of cellular ultrastructure and enzymatic activity by aldehyde fixation. J. Cell Biol. **17:** 19–58.
77. DEVRIES, S. I. & E. P. ROMIJN. 1960. The value of quantitative cytochemical determinations, notably phosphatases, in hematological examinations. Nederl. T. Geneesk. **104:** 1929–1935.
78. IMMEL, V. E. & W. TILLING. 1964. Alkaline leukocyte phosphatase in the differential diagnosis of liver diseases. Med. Klin. **59:** 895–896.
79. ALSLEBEN, U. 1961. The behavior of alkaline leukocyte phosphatase (ALP) in various diseases and its differential diagnostic significance. Ther. Umsch. **18:** 52–64.
80. KEISER, V. G. & U. ALSLEBEN. 1963. Alkaline phosphatase of leukocytes and blood diseases (differential diagnostic and prognostic significance). Schweiz. Med. Wschr. **93:** 1–7.
81. FLURY, V. R. & T. WEGMANN. 1964. The behavior of leukocyte alkaline phosphatase in Hodgkin's disease. Schweiz. Med. Wschr. **94:** 958–961.
82. SCHUMACHER, K. 1964. The significance of leukocyte alkaline phosphatase activity for differential diagnosis and prognosis of malignant hemoblastosis. Med. Welt. **9:** 415–418.
83. BOIVIN, P. & R. ROBINEAUX. 1956. Histochemie des cellules sanguines. II. Phosphatase alcaline. Étude de la valeur localisatrice de la réaction de Gomori appliquée aux leucocytes. Sang **27:** 535–545.
84. PLENERT, W. 1959. Methodische Studien zur Zytochemie der Leukozytenphosphatasen. I. Einfluss von Fixierung und Metallionen auf die Aktivität der alkalischen Leukozytenphosphatasen in Blutausstrichen. Histochemie **1:** 171–177.
85. BAXTER, A. 1963. A critical study of a histochemical stain for evaluating leukocyte alkaline phosphatase activity in smears of human peripheral blood. Canad. J. Med. Techn. **25:** 54–63.
86. WULFF, H. R. & P. RIIS. 1961. Cytochemical demonstration of alkaline phosphatase in leukocytes: A diagnostic aid. Ugeskr. Laeger **123:** 1303–1307.
87. PATTERSON, R. B., D. M. HAYES & C. L. SPURR. 1963. Studies on alkaline phosphatase activity of leukocytes in various diseases. Southern Med. J. **56:** 1026–1029.
88. WEISSEL, M. 1963. Leukocyte alkaline phosphatase. I. Method of determination and behavior in normal persons. Z. Ges. Inn. Med. **18:** 547–555.
89. WEISSEL, M. 1963. Behavior of leukocyte alkaline phosphatase in various diseases. Z. Ges. Inn. Med. **18:** 577–585.
90. WYLLIE, R. G. 1964. A modified method for staining neutrophil alkaline phosphatase and normal levels. Med. J. Aust. **1:** 876–878.
91. QUAGLINO, D. & F. G. J. HAYHOE. 1960. Acetone fixation for the cytochemical demonstration of dehydrogenases in blood and bone marrow cells. Nature **187:** 85–86.

92. KAPLOW, L. S. & M. S. BURSTONE. 1963. Acid-buffered acetone as a fixative for enzyme cytochemistry. Nature **200:** 690–691.
93. GOMORI, G. 1946. Buffers in the range of pH 6.5 to 9.6. Proc. Soc. Exp. Biol. Med. **62:** 33–34.
94. NOVIKOFF, A. B. 1951. The validity of histochemical phosphatase methods on the intracellular level. Science **113:** 320–325.
95. TRUBOWITZ, S., D. FELDMAN, S. W. MORGENSTERN & V. M. HUNT. 1961. The isolation, purification and some properties of the alkaline phosphatase of human leukocytes. Biochem. J. **80:** 369–374.
96. MCCOY, E. E., J. PARK & J. ENGLAND. 1965. A fluorometric assay and properties of leukocyte alkaline phosphatase. Clin. Chim. Acta **12:** 453–461.
97. ACKERMAN, G. A. 1962. Substituted naphthol AS phosphate derivatives for the localization of leukocyte alkaline phosphatase activity. Lab. Invest. **11:** 563–567.
98. KAPLOW, L. S. 1955. A histochemical procedure for localizing and evaluating the alkaline phosphatase of hematopoietic cells in smears of blood and bone marrow. M.S. Thesis. Univ. of Vermont, and State Agricultural College, Burlington, Vt.
99. FRANKEL, H. H. & R. L. PETERS. 1964. A modified calcium-cobalt method for the demonstration of alkaline phosphatase. The use of paranitrophenyl phosphate as a substrate. Amer. J. Clin. Path. **42:** 324–327.
100. HUGGINS, C. & P. TALALAY. 1945. Sodium phenolphthalein phosphate as a substrate for phosphatase tests. J. Biol. Chem. **159:** 399–410.
101. BURSTONE, M. S. 1958. Histochemical comparison of naphthol AS-phosphates for the demonstration of phosphatases. J. Nat. Cancer Inst. **20:** 601–616.
102. BURSTONE, M. S. 1958. Histochemical comparison of naphthol AS-substrates. J. Histochem. Cytochem. **6:** 87–88.
103. MERKER, H. & L. HEILMEYER. 1960. Die alkalische Phosphatase neutrophiler Leukozyten. Zytoenzymatischer Nachweis und Aktivität bei Erkrankungen und Reaktionen des blutbildenen Systems. Deut. Med. Wschr. **85:** 253–258.
104. HAYHOE, F. G. J. & D. QUAGLINO. 1958. Cytochemical demonstration and measurement of leukocyte alkaline phosphatase activity in normal and pathological states by a modified azo dye coupling technique. Brit. J. Haemat. **4:** 375–389.
105. BELLOTTI, R., G. F. QUAZZA, B. VERRI, A. IESTER & A. LIOTTA. 1966. Study of the behavior of alkaline phosphatase of neutrophil granulocytes during a prolonged incubation of the smears in stain. Minerva Pediat. **18:** 851–854.
106. PEACOCK, A. C., G. BRECHER & E. M. HIGHSMITH. 1958. A simplified procedure for quantitative measurement of alkaline phosphatase in white blood cells. Amer. J. Clin. Path. **29:** 80–85.
107. YOUNG, J. E. & M. D. PRAGER. 1962. Some hydrolytic enzymes in normal and leukemic human leukocytes. J. Lab. Clin. Med. **60:** 385–395.
108. MEISLIN, A. G., S. L. LEE & L. R. WASSERMAN. 1959. Leukocyte alkaline phosphatase activity in hematopoietic disorders. A correlative study by biochemical and cytochemical techniques. Cancer **12:** 760–766.
109. TOMONAGA, M., M. ICHIMARU, S. TOYODA & B. WATANABE. 1960. Studies on catalase and alkaline phosphatase of leukemic cells. Proc. VIIIth Int. Con. Haemat. Tokyo, Japan.
110. TRUBOWITZ, S., D. FELDMAN, C. BENANTE & V. M. HUNT. 1959. The alkaline phosphatase content of the human polymorphonuclear leukocyte in blood and marrow. Amer. J. Clin. Path. **31:** 483–486.
111. KENNY, J. J. & W. C. MOLONEY. 1957. Leukocytic alkaline phosphatase. Behavior during prolonged incubation and infection in normal and leukemic leukocytes. Blood **12:** 295–302.
112. TRUBOWITZ, S., D. KIRMAN & B. MASEK. 1962. The leukocyte alkaline phosphatase in mongolism. Lancet **2:** 486–487.
113. KOLER, R. D., A. J. SEAMAN, E. E. OSGOOD & P. VANBELLINGHEN. 1958. Myeloproliferative diseases—diagnostic value of the leukocyte alkaline phosphatase test. Amer. J. Clin. Path. **30:** 295–301.
114. WASASTJERNA, C., B. JEGLINSKY & C. E. NYLUND. 1963. The effect of X-ray treatment on leukocyte alkaline phosphatase in cancer patients. Acta Med. Scand. **173:** 505–510.
115. PETERS, H. 1964. A method for impeding dye decomposition and gas bubble formation in histochemical preparations of enzymes. Histochemie **4:** 345–347.
116. SCHUBERT, J. C. F. & H. MARTIN. 1965. Zytochemischer Nachweis alkalischer Phosphataseaktivitat in Myeloblasten. Med. Welt. **13:** 531–533.
117. QUAGLINO, D. 1964. Alkaline phosphatase positivity in erythroblasts. Haemat. Latina (Milan) **7:** 263–271.

118. LAMBERS, K. 1962. Ubersichten. Zur Zytochemie der Blutzellen. Deut. Med. Wschr. **87:** 1913–1917.
119. RIEDER, H. & Z. A. ZAWADZKI. 1961. Uber alkalische Leukozytenphosphatase bei Blut- und Leberkrankheiten. Wein. Klin. Wschr. **73:** 476–481.
120. TSUKADA, T. 1962. Cytochemical studies on alkaline phosphatase activity of neutrophilic leukocytes. II. Mechanisms of the changes in the activity in various physiologic and pathologic conditions. J. Jap. Soc. Intern. Med. **51:** 900–909.
121. PLENERT, W. 1960. Cytochemische Phosphatasereaktionen und Knochenmarkspunktaten unter besonderer Berucksichtingung der Leukamie. Proc. 7th Congr. Europ. Soc. Haemat. (1959) Part II : 390–393. London, England.
122. SIROLA, I. & K. SIROLA. 1957. A histochemical study of alkaline phosphatase in the leukocytes of blood and bone marrow in various diseases. Acta Haemat. **18:** 313–324.
123. CIORAPCIU, S., M. COSTESCU & T. MOLDOVAN. 1965. Clinical and physiopathological considerations on the alterations of leucocyte alkaline phosphatase. Med. Intern. **17:** 807–815.
124. FARNES, P. & B. E. BARKER. 1963. Cytochemical studies of human bone marrow fibroblast-like cells. I. Alkaline phosphatase. Exp. Cell Res. **29:** 278–288.
125. UNDRITZ, V. E. 1965. Zur aktivität der alkalischen Phosphatase bei der chronischen myeloischen Leukämie. Schweiz. Med. Wschr. **95:** 1515–1519.
126. ACKERMAN, G. A. 1964. Histochemical differentiation during neutrophile development and maturation. Ann. N. Y. Acad. Sci. **113:** 537–565.
127. KAPLOW, L. S. & M. S. BURSTONE. 1964. Cytochemical demonstration of acid phosphatase in hematopoietic cells in health and in various hematological disorders using azo dye techniques. J. Histochem. Cytochem. **12:** 805–811.
128. WETZEL, B. K., R. G. HORN & S. S. SPICER. 1963. Cytochemical localization of nonspecific phosphatase activity in rabbit myeloid elements. J. Histochem. Cytochem. **11:** 812–814.
129. HORN, R. G., S. S. SPICER & B. K. WETZEL. 1964. Phagocytosis of bacteria by heterophil leukocytes. Acid and alkaline phosphatase cytochemistry. Amer. J. Path. **45:** 327–335.
130. KAWABATA, S. 1959–1960. A study of the isolated granules of leukocyte by cytochemical stainings. Nagoya J. Med. Sci. **22:** 396–411.
131. CLARKE, A. E. 1965. Hydrolytic enzymes of human polymorphonuclear leucocytes and rat monocytes. Aust. J. Exp. Biol. Med. Sci. **43:** 201–212.
132. MOLONEY, W. C. 1958. Leukocyte alkaline phosphatase activity in the rat. Ann. N. Y. Acad. Sci. **75:** 31–36.
133. LIE-INJO LUAN ENG. 1964. Alkaline phosphatase activity of the leucocytes in animals. Nature **204:** 191–192.
134. BELL, JR., J. T. 1962. Histochemistry of the circulating leukocytes of domestic animals. Anat. Record **142:** 214.
135. BURSTONE, M. S. 1958. The relationship between fixation and techniques for the histochemical localization of hydrolytic enzymes. J. Histochem. Cytochem. **6:** 322–339.
136. SANTOS, G. W. & L. J. COLE. 1958. Effects of donor and host lymphoid and myeloid tissue injections in lethally X-irradiated mice treated with rat bone marrow. J. Nat. Cancer Inst. **21:** 279–293.
137. BOREL, C., J. FREI & A. VANNOTTI. 1958. Étude enzymatique directe au niveau du leucocyte. Helv. Physiol. Pharmacol. Acta **16:** 53–55.
138. ROSNER, F. & S. L. LEE. 1965. Endocrine relationships of leukocyte alkaline phosphatase. Blood **25:** 356–369.
139. MAEDA, K. & J. OSHIMA. 1952. Histochemical demonstration of alkaline phosphatase in human blood smears. Kumamoto Med. J. **IV:** 127–128.
140. GORDON, S. & E. HUNTER. 1965. Re-evaluation of the leucocyte alkaline phosphatase test. Med. J. Aust. **2:** 13–16.
141. SRAMKOVA, L., K. KOUBA & N. BENDOVA. 1965. Alkaline phosphatase in neutrophil leukocytes of patients with infectious mononucleosis and the effect of corticosteroid therapy. Blood **26:** 479–488.
142. BRUNELLI, L. & G. CAMERINI. 1960. Contributo allo studio della fosfatasi alcalina dei granulocite nell'eta infantile. Minerva Pediat. **12:** 628–632.
143. BERTOLOTTI, E., G. F. QUAZZA & G. LOJODICE. 1964. La fosfatasi alcalina nei granulociti neutrofili. Suo comportamento nelle prime epoche della vita. (b) Studio negli immaturi di oltre un mese di vita. Minerva Pediat. **16:** 635–641.
144. BERTOLOTTI, E., G. LOJODICE & G. F. QUAZZA. 1964. La fosfatasi alcalina nei granulociti neutrofili. Suo comportamento nelle prime epoche della vita. Studio negli immaturi nel corso del primo mese di vita. Minerva Pediat. **16:** 72–77.

145. PLENERT, W. 1958. Cytochemische Studie über das Verhalten der alkalischen Phosphatase der Leukocyten beim Neugeborenen. Folia Haemat. **75**: 378–385.
146. BERTOLOTTI, E., G. LOJODICE & G. F. QUAZZA. 1964. La fosfatasi alcalina nei granulociti neutrofili. Suo comportamento nelle prime epoche della vita. (c) Studio nei lattanti nati a termine. Minerva Pediat. **16**: 1–20.
147. TEJADA, C., V. ARGUETA, M. SANCHEZ & C. ALBERTAZZI. 1964. Phagocytic and alkaline phosphatase activity of leukocytes in kwashiorkor. J. Pediat. **64**: 753–761.
148. O'KELL, R. T. & L. L. AXON. 1965. Leukocyte alkaline phosphatase in the newborn infant. Amer. J. Obstet. Gynec. **93**: 1181–1182.
149. LIE-INJO LUAN ENG & S. GOVINDASAMY. 1965. Leucocyte alkaline phosphatase, leucocyte count and haemoglobin level in Malayan new-borns and young infants. Med. J. Malaya **19**: 263–266.
150. RANDALL, D. L., C. W. REIQUAM, J. H. GITHENS & A. ROBINSON. 1965. Familial myeloproliferative disease. A new syndrome closely simulating myelogenous leukemia in childhood. Amer. J. Dis. Child. **110**: 479–500.
151. TOMONAGA, M., N. OZONO, K. ITO, N. TANAKA, K. OKADA, N. KAMADA, T. ITO, T. HATANO, & H. MATSUMOTO. 1963. Studies on blood picture in old age. J. Kyushu Hemat. Soc. **13**: 137–144.
152. ALTER, A. A., S. L. LEE, M. POURFAR & G. DOBKIN. 1963. Studies of leukocyte alkaline phosphatase in mongolism: a possible chromosome marker. Blood **22**: 165–177.
153. ANSTEY, L.. N. H. KEMP, J. L. STAFFORD & R. K. TANNER. 1963. Leukocyte alkaline phosphatase activity in polycythaemia rubra vera. Brit. J. Haemat. **9**: 91–100.
154. KAPLOW, L. S. & R. E. BECK. 1964. Leukocyte alkaline phosphatase response to surgical stress. Surg. Gynec. Obstet. **119**: 97–102.
155. WYLLIE, R. G. 1962. Neutrophil alkaline phosphatase: Response to acute inflammation. Aust. Ann. Med. **11**: 118–125.
156. VACCARI, F., B. SABOTTO & E. MANZINI. 1955. Alkaline phosphatase activity of leukocytes in shock. Blood **10**: 730–734.
157. PLENERT, W. 1962. Der Phasenwandel der Aktivität der alkalischen Granulocyten-Phosphatase im Kindesalter. A. Kinderheilk. **87**: 218–227.
158. NOWOTNY, P. 1965. Zytochemische Untersuchungen und Funktionsprüfungen des Knochenmarkes bei Hämoblastosen und Knochenmarksinsuffizienzen. Folia Haemat. **84**: 406–416.
159. MERKER, H. V. 1961. Der aktivitätswechsel der alkalischen Neutrophilen-phosphatase im Pyrexalreizversuch und die Bedeutung dieses Testes für die klinik einiger Blutkrankheiten. Folia Haemat. **6**: 153–163.
160. LACHER, M. J. & A. B. LEY. 1964. The value of leukocyte alkaline phosphatase determinations in the malignant lymphomas. Cancer **17**: 402–408.
161. MITUS, W. J., I. B. MEDNICOFF & W. DAMESHEK. 1959. Alkaline phosphatase of mature neutrophils in various "polycythemias." New Eng. J. Med. **260**: 1131–1133.
162 TODERAN, M. G. 1964. The alkaline phosphatase activity of white blood cells. A comparison of two histochemical methods. Canad. J. Med. Tech. **22**: 81–87.
163. HARROP, J. & A. A. COOPERBERG. 1961. The myeloproliferative disorders with special reference to histochemical features. Canad. Med. Ass. J. **85**: 824–826.
164. QUIGLEY, H. J., E. A. DAWSON, B. H. HYUN & R. P. CUSTER. 1960. The activity of alkaline phosphatase in granular leukocytes during pregnancy and the puerperium: A preliminary report. Amer. J. Clin. Path. **33**: 109–114.
165. TANZER, J., A. HAMPE, P. BENSIMON, M. BOIRON & J. BERNARD. 1965. L'evaluation cytochimique de la phosphatase alcaline leucocytaire dans la leucemie myeloïde chronique. Son interet pratique. Nouv. Rev. Franc. Hemat. **5**: 873–879.
166. BERRETTA, L. R. 1962. Sul valore semeiologico della fosfatasi alcalina leucocitaria nella diagnosi di gravidanza ectopica. Minerva Ginec. **14**: 1138–1140.
167. KOTLAREK-HAUS, S. 1965. The activity of leucocyte alkaline phosphatase in some internal disease. Pol. Tyg. Lek. **20**: 520–523.
168. MDZEWSKI, B. 1963. Alkaline phosphatase of mature granulocytes in some hematologic conditions. Pol. Arch. Med. Wewnet. **33**: 511–518.
169. HAUSSER, E. & J. STROUN. 1962. La phosphatase alcaline leucocytaire au cours des affections virales. J. Suisse Med. **42**: 1334–1338.
170. GULBRANDSEN, R. & H. PRYDZ. 1962. Determination of alkaline phosphatases in granulocytes as an aid to haematological diagnosis. Nord. Med. **67**: 633–637.
171. KOCH, E. & D. REMY. 1960. Die alkalische Leukocytenphosphatase in der Differentialdiagnose Hämatologischer Erkrankungen. Klin. Wschr. **38**: 26–27.
172. CATOVSKY, D., J. RYMAR & J. J. CRISCAUT. 1965. Determinacion citoquimica de fosfatasa alcalina, fosfatasa acida, arilsulfatasa y peroxidasas. Sangre **10**: 71–76.

173. Martinez-Maldonado, M., R. Menendez-Corrada & A. R. de Sala. 1964. Diagnostic value of alkaline phosphatase in leukocytes. Amer. J. Med. Sci. **248:** 73–81.
174. Kemp, J. A., J. W. Herndon & C. S. Wright. 1962. Vacillations in leukocytic alkaline phosphatase. Southern Med. J. **55:** 281–286.
175. Marmot, A. & L. Correale. 1961. La determinazione della fosfatasi alcalina leucocitaria nella diagnostica e nello studio delle leucopatie. Boll. Soc. Ital. Haemat. **9:** 83–90.
176. Schafer, K. H., H. Beckmann & R. Neth. 1965. Die anwendung cytochemischer Nachweisverfahren in der diagnostik hämatologischer Erkrankungen des Kindesalters. Monatsschr. Kinderheilk. **113:** 428–434.
177. Tsukada, T. 1962. Cytochemical studies on alkaline phosphatase activity of neutrophilic leukocytes. I. Variations of the activity in various pathologic conditions, with special reference to the hematologic disorders. J. Jap. Soc. Intern. Med. **51:** 890–899.
178. Krug, K. 1964. Die alkalische Leukozytenphosphatase und ihre Bedeutung für die moderne hämatologische Diagnostik. Fortschr. Med. **82:** 609–612.
179. Bressel, V. D., S. Witte & N. Henning. 1961. Die Bedeutung der alkalischen Leukozytenphosphatase bei retikulären und lymphatischen Systemkrankheiten und bei der Lymphogranulomatose. Blut. **7:** 14–26.
180. Sasso, G. F. & P. Mancini. 1964. Research on leukocytic alkaline phosphatase activity. II. Non-leukemic histiocytic sarcomatosis. Med. Clin. Sper. **14:** 63–70.
181. Pardo Menendez, V., J. M. Estevez & E. R. Unanue. 1959. Estudio citoquimico de los leucocitos: Fosfatasa alcalina en estado normal y patologico. Arch. Hosp. Univ. (Havana) **11:** 89–101.
182. Stahlberg, K. G., I. Olsson, G. Gahrton & A. Norden. 1963. Serum vitamin B_{12} determinations and cytochemical reactions in the differential diagnosis of acute leukaemia. Acta Med. Scand. **174:** 105–114.
183. Hayhoe, F. G. J., D. Quaglino & R. Doll. 1964. The cytology and cytochemistry of acute leukaemias. Her Majesty's Stationery Office. London, England.
184. Gahrton, G., A. Norden & K. G. Stahlberg. 1962. Cytochemical investigations and serum vitamin B_{12} determinations in a case of erythroleukaemia. Acta Med. Scand. **171:** 243–249.
185. Moloney, W. C., A. D. Dorr, G. Dowd & A. E. Boschetti. 1962. Myelogenous leukemia in the rat. Blood **19:** 45–59.
186. Kretchmer, N., M. Stone & C. Bauer. 1958. Hereditary enzymatic effects as illustrated by hypophosphatasia, Ann. N. Y. Acad. Sci. **75:** 279–285.
187. Kellsey, D. C. 1962. Hypophosphatasia and congenital bowing of the long bones. J. Amer. Med. Ass. **179:** 187–190.
188. Beisel, W. R., N. Benjamin & K. F. Austen. 1959. Absence of leukocyte alkaline phosphatase activity in hypophosphatasia. Blood **14:** 975–977.
189. Bertolotti, E. & G. F. Quazza. 1965. La fosfatasi alcalina nei granulociti neutrofili. Ricerche in corso di malattie renali. Minerva Pediat. **17:** 868–872.
190. Bertolotti, E., G. F. Quazza & L. Vignolo. 1962. La fosfatasi alcalina nei leucociti neutrofili. Attivita enzimatica bassa in bambini affetti da distrofia muscolare progressiva. Minerva Pediat. **14:** 1526–1530.
191. Ruvidic, R., M. Brozovic-Vasic & B. Brozovic. 1964. Cytochemical analysis of the alkaline phosphatase of leukocytes. Lijecn. Vjesn. **86:** 13–23.
192. Better, O., S. Brandstaetter, B. Padeh & G. Bianu. 1965. Myeloid metaplasia: Clinical, laboratory and cytogenic observations. Israel J. Med. Sci. **1:** 810–817.
193. Leonard, B. J., M. C. G. Israels & J. F. Wilkinson. 1958. Alkaline phosphatase in the white cells in leukaemia and leukaemoid reactions. Lancet **i:** 289–292.
194. Fiehrer, A. 1965. L'evaluation cytochimique des phosphatases alcalines des granulocytes neutrophiles sanguins par le score de Kaplow, en hematologie. Rev. Path. Comp. **65:** 353–360.
195. Kahn, P. 1965. Cytochemische untersuchungen bei akuten Leukosen. Klin. Wschr. **43:** 1038–1041.
196. Brozovic-Vasic, M. & R. Ruvidic. 1964. Leukocyte alkaline phosphatase in chronic granulocytic leukaemia. Acta Med. Iugosl. **18:** 157–167.
197. Krauss, S., J. E. Sokal & A. A. Sandberg. 1964. Comparison of Philadelphia chromosome-positive and -negative patients with chronic myelocytic leukemia. Ann. Intern. Med. **61:** 625–635.
198. Mitus, W. J., L. J. Bergna, I. B. Mednicoff & W. Dameshek. 1958. Alkaline phosphatase of mature neutrophils in chronic forms of the myeloproliferative syndrome.
199. Helbig, W. & M. Weissel. 1961. Die Behandlung der chronischen Myelose mit
Amer. J. Clin. Path. **30:** 285–294.
Myleran (Myeleukon). Muench. Med. Wschr. **103:** 2390–2395.

200. Xefteris, E., W. J. Mitus, I. B. Mednicoff & W. Dameshek. 1961. Leukocytic alkaline phosphatase in busulfan induced remissions of chronic granulocytic leukemia. Blood **18:** 202–206.
201. Dacie, J. V., M. D. Smith, J. C. White & D. L. Mollin. 1959. Refractory normoblastic anaemia: A clinical and haematological study of seven cases. Brit. J. Haemat. **5:** 56–82.
202. Heilmeyer, L., W. Keiderling, H. Merker, R. Clotten & H. Schubothe. 1960. Die Anaemia refractoria sideroblastica und ihre Beziehungen zur Lebersiderose und Hämochromatose. Acta Haemat. **23:** 1–21.
203. Heilmeyer, L., W. Keiderling, R. Bilger & E. Bernauer. 1958. Uber chronische refraktäre Anämien mit sideroblastischem Knochenmark (Anaemia refractoria sideroblastica). Folia Haemat. N.F. **2:** 49–60.
204. Lewis, S. M. & J. V. Dacie. 1965. Neutrophil (Leucocyte) alkaline phosphatase in paroxysmal nocturnal haemoglobinuria. Brit. J. Haemat. **11:** 549–556.
205. Hartmann, R. C. & J. V. Auditore. 1959. Paroxysmal nocturnal hemoglobinuria. I. Clinical studies. Amer. J. Med. **27:** 389–400.
206. Tanaka, K. R., W. N. Valentine & R. E. Fredricks. 1960. Diseases or clinical conditions associated with low leukocyte alkaline phosphatase. New Eng. J. Med. **262:** 912–918.
207. Hughes, J. T., R. M. Johnstone, A. C. Scott & P. D. Stewart. 1959. Leukaemoid reactions in disseminated tuberculosis. J. Clin. Path. **12:** 307–311.
208. Sauer, H. & J. G. Rausch-Stroomann. 1955. Uber die alkalische Leukocytenphosphatase bei der Polycythämie. Deut. Arch. Klin. Med. **202:** 282–290.
209. Nachlas, M. M., T. P. Goldstein, D. H. Rosenblatt, M. Kirsch & A. M. Seligman. 1959. Influence of chemical structure on the rate of azo coupling and its significance in histochemical methodology. J. Histochem. Cytochem. **7:** 50–65.
210. Anstey, L., N. H. Kemp, J. L. Stafford & R. K. Tanner. 1961. Histochemical changes in polycythemia vera. Proc. 8th Congr. Europ. Soc. Haemat no. 91 Vienna. 1961.
211. Stobbe, V. H. & Neumann. 1963. Die alkalische Granulozytenphosphatase bei Polycythaemia vera. Z. Ges. Inn. Med. **18:** 925–928.
212. Shubich, M. G. & A. D. Vakulenko. 1964. On the content of alkaline phosphatase in neutrophil leukocytes under normal conditions and in some diseases of the haematopoietic system. Tsitologiia **6:** 769–771.
213. Lille-Szyszkowicz, I., P. Gabay, R. T. Saracino & J. S. Bourdin. 1966. La phosphatase alcaline leucocytaire chez les malades atteints de tumeurs ou d'hemopathies malignes. Nouv. Rev. Franc. Haemat. **6:** 187–194.
214. Birk, W., L. Peschl & E. E. Reimer. 1960. Zur diagnostischen Bedeutung der Leukozytenphosphatase. Wien. Z. Inn. Med. **41:** 489–493.
215. Muller, V. D. 1964. Die aktivitat der alkalischen Leukozytenphosphatase unter zytostatischer Stosstherapie beim Malignomkranken. Med. Klin. **59:** 7–9.
216. Nakai, G. S., C. G. Craddock & W. G. Figueroa. 1962. Agnogenic myeloid metaplasia. A survey of twenty-nine cases and a review of the literature. Ann. Intern. Med. **57:** 419–440.
217. Leonard, B. J., M. C. G. Israels & J. F. Wilkinson. 1957. Myelosclerosis, A clinicopathological study. Quart. J. Med. **26:** 131–147.
218. Mohler, D. N. & B. S. Leavell. 1958. Aplastic anemia: An analysis of fifty cases. Ann. Intern. Med. **49:** 326–362.
219. Russo, A. & B. Macchioni. 1962. Value of alkaline phosphatase in diagnosis of ectopic pregnancy. Minerva Ginec. **14:** 1138.
220. Silva, Jr., A. R. & J. D. Corbit, Jr. 1961. Rapid laboratory test for differential diagnosis of ectopic pregnancy. Obstet. Gynec. **18:** 283–284.
221. Plum, C. M. 1950. Die alkalische Phosphatase in den Zellen des normalen und pathologischen Knockenmarkes und des peripheren Blutes. Acta Haemat. **4:** 73–80.
222. Goldstein, D. P. 1965. Studies on leukocyte phosphatase activity: Relation to female sex hormones and gonadotropins. Obstet. Gynec. **25:** 413.
223. Haering, M. 1964. Das Verhalten der alkalischen Leukozytenphosphatase (ALP) in der Schwangerschaft, unter der Geburt und im Wochenbett. Z. Geburtsh. Gynaek. **162:** 132–140.
224. Cox, R. P. & C. M. Macleod. 1964. Regulation of alkaline phosphatase in human cell cultures. Sympos. Quant. Biol. **29:** 233–251.
225. De Carli, L., J. J. Maio & F. Nuzzo. 1963. Alkaline phosphatase activity and chromosome variation in human cells in culture. J. Nat. Cancer Inst. **31:** 1501–1507.
226. Lennert, K., H. Loffler & L. D. Leder. 1961. Fermenthistochemische Untersuch-

ungen des Lymphknotens. I. Alkalische phosphatase in Schnitt und Ausstrich. Virchow. Arch. Path. Anat. **334:** 399–418.

227. PERILLIE, P. E. & S. C. FINCH. 1961. Alkaline phosphatase activity of exudative leukocytes in acute leukemia. Blood **18:** 572–580.
228. REBUCK, J. W. & J. H. CROWLEY. 1955. A method for studying leukocytic functions in vivo. Ann. N. Y. Acad. Sci. **59:** 757–794.
229. DANNENBERG, JR., A. M., M. S. BURSTONE, P. C. WALTER & J. W. KINSLEY. 1963. A histochemical study of phagocytic and enzymatic functions of rabbit mononuclear and polymorphonuclear exudate cells and alveolar macrophages. I. Survey of quantitation of enzymes, and states of cellular activation. J. Cell. Biol. **17:** 465–486.

Appendices: Lists of References Broken Down According to Specific Disease

Appendix 1 (See TABLE 3)

Cirrhosis (decompensated): 169.
Lymphoma: 72, 174.
Bacterial infections: 44, 55, 67, 68, 72, 74, 79, 85, 97, 104, 141, 155, 163, 169, 173, 175, 191, 194.
Chronic lymphatic leukemia (treated): 79, 80, 170. (untreated): 44, 59, 64, 77, 79, 80, 86, 89, 97, 160, 170, 172, 173, 177, 191, 194.
Leukemoid reactions: 72, 74, 87, 113, 170, 172, 173, 174, 191, 193, 207.
Polycythemia vera (untreated): 46, 55, 58, 59, 62, 72, 74, 79, 80, 85, 86, 89, 97, 113, 119, 153, 161, 162, 163, 170, 171, 172, 173, 174, 175, 177, 181, 191, 208, 209, 210, 211, 212. (treated): 58, 67, 173, 174, 191.
Acute lymphatic leukemia: 72, 74, 104, 170, 172, 181, 182, 183.
Reticulum cell sarcoma: 86, 89, 172, 177, 179, 180.
Acute monocytic leukemia: 72, 85, 170, 172.
Hodgkin's disease (untreated): 55, 59, 67, 72, 79, 80, 81, 86, 89, 104, 160, 162, 172, 173, 175, 177, 180, 191, 194, 213. (treated): 79, 80, 81, 89, 160, 175.
Multiple myeloma: 64, 77, 79, 86, 89, 97, 104, 172, 178, 179, 180, 214, 215.
Acute myelomonocytic leukemia: 170, 183.
Cirrhosis (compensated): 64, 78, 169, 178, 194.
Obstructive jaundice: 78, 118, 169, 178.
Myelosclerosis: 46, 58, 67, 72, 74, 80, 86, 89, 113, 163, 170, 171, 174, 175, 181, 192, 195, 198, 216, 217.
Aplastic anemia: 80, 86, 89, 172, 174, 176, 181, 191, 218.
Agranulocytosis: 89, 172, 177, 191.

Appendix 2 (See TABLE 4)

Hereditary hypophosphatasia: 174, 186, 187, 188.
Nephrotic syndrome: 189.
Progressive muscular dystrophy: 190.
Chronic myelogenous leukemia (untreated): 44, 59, 62, 64, 67, 68, 72, 74, 79, 80, 82, 85, 89, 97, 104, 109, 113, 119, 162, 163, 165, 169, 170, 171, 174, 175, 181, 191, 192, 193, 194, 195, 196, 197. (treated): 59, 64, 67, 72, 77, 82, 86, 97, 104, 109, 150, 165, 169, 170, 173, 174, 175, 181, 198, 199, 200. (blastic crisis): 80, 82, 165, 174, 183, 196, 198.
Refractory anemia (siderotic): 72, 159, 201, 202, 203.
Paroxysmal nocturnal hemoglobinuria: 170, 204, 205, 206.

Appendix 3 (See TABLE 5)

Secondary polycythemia: 59, 62, 67, 72, 74, 80, 119, 161, 170, 171, 172, 173, 174, 175.
Hemolytic anemia: 64, 72, 89, 104, 174, 176.
Infectious mononucleosis: 44, 72, 86, 97, 141, 169, 172, 174, 177.
Viral hepatitis: 64, 78, 118, 169, 178.
Lymphosarcoma (untreated): 86, 97, 104, 172, 173, 178, 179, 180. (treated): 86, 97.

Appendix 4 (See TABLE 6)

Pernicious anemia (untreated): 55, 64, 72, 89, 119, 170, 173, 174, 177. (treated): 64, 104, 170.
Idiopathic thrombocytopenic purpura: 72, 97, 104, 174, 177.
Iron deficiency anemia: 89, 119, 177.
Acute myelogenous leukemia: 46, 72, 74, 86, 97, 119, 170, 172, 173, 177, 181, 182, 183.
Acute undifferentiated leukemia: 59, 64, 80, 86, 176, 178, 181, 182, 183.
Erythroleukemia: 86, 174, 181, 183, 184, 185.

ISOZYMES OF HUMAN LEUKOCYTE ALKALINE PHOSPHATASE*

Richard B. Lyons†, David D. Weaver‡, and James H. Beck
Division of Experimental Medicine and Department of Anatomy
University of Oregon Medical School, Portland, Ore.

INTRODUCTION

Gomori (1941) was the first investigator to point out that leukocyte alkaline phosphatase (LAlP)§ is confined to neutrophils. Using the techniques described by Gomori, Wachstein (1946) pointed out that the degree of staining and presumably the amount of enzyme, was variable in individual neutrophils and that some, indeed, lacked the enzyme. This observation has been upheld and has served as a stimulus for publication of hundreds of papers on LAlP. Wachstein also observed that LAlP activity was increased in patients with infections and much decreased in persons with chronic granulocytic leukemia (CGL).

The clinical usefulness of LAlP determinations is much too extensive to be reviewed here. Relevant to the present paper, LAlP values were found to be increased in Down's syndrome or mongolism (Alter *et al.*, 1962; Trubowitz *et al.*, 1962), pregnancy (Pritchard, 1957), polycythemia rubra vera (Valentine *et al.*, 1952) and during treatment of various patients with several corticoid compounds (Valentine *et al.*, 1954). Decreased or "zero" values of LAlP were observed in patients with CGL (Wachstein, 1946) and in patients with hypophosphatasia (Beisel *et al.*, 1959). These findings have since been confirmed and extended by many investigators. Numerous other clinical conditions have been studied and LAlP determinations are now a useful diagnostic tool.

The relationship between trisomy G (mongolism) and CGL noted above has led several investigators to suspect that a control gene may be located on one of the G chromosomes. Numerous papers have appeared in support or in opposition to this hypothesis and will be discussed fully in this monograph. In hypophosphatasia, Beisel *et al.* (1959) found no native or inducible LAlP. Several investigators have observed, in other disorders, that patients with low or absent LAlP activity may show increased activity during corticoid therapy or infections. The LAlP score in normal persons is also variable. Therefore, when LAlP activity is low, control factors that regulate the quantity of enzyme in leukocytes seem to be responsive to altered physiological status and/or drug therapy.

The possible heterogeneity of human LAlP was documented by Trubowitz *et al.* (1957) from studies of magnesium and zinc requirements of the enzyme. They found evidence of two different enzymes, one requiring magnesium and the other requiring zinc for maximal activation. Preliminary observations noted by these workers indicated that the zinc-activated enzyme accounted for most of the increased LAlP activity found in leukemoid states and infection.

Robinson *et al.* (1965) were the first to demonstrate isozymes of LAlP using

* Supported by USPHS grants nos. CA07941–02 and 5T5GM59 and by the Oregon Heart Association and the American Cancer Society (Oregon Division).

† Present address: USPHS, Arctic Health Research Laboratory, College, Alaska.
‡ Present address: USPHS, Arctic Health Research Laboratory, College, Alaska.

§ The abbreviation, LAlP, is here substituted for the conventional "LAP" to avoid confusion with leucine aminopeptidate, which has also been given the designation "LAP," and to distinguish between LAlP and acid phosphatase (we propose LAcP for the latter) which is also contained in leukocytes.

starch-gel electrophoresis. They studied seven normal persons, five patients with CGL, and four patients with acute myelogenous leukemia. They reported no isozyme differences in their normal controls and found essentially normal patterns in the patients with acute leukemia. The major fast component in their normal and acute leukemic patients was seen to disappear in CGL and be replaced by a slower migrating component not observed in the control group. McCoy *et al.* (1965) reported several kinetic studies of pooled LAlP extracts as well as of gel eluates, but they noted no heterogeneity of the leukocyte enzyme. Berg *et al.* (1965), using agar-gel electrophoresis showed that LAlP, extracted by multiple freezing and thawing in saline, migrated with the α-2 globulins. Most of the LAlP activity, however, remained at the sample origin and was regarded as denatured or particle-bound enzyme.

Preliminary observations in our laboratory (Weaver, 1966) suggested that there were three major LAlP isozymes in normal persons. It was found that the gel patterns of a given individual were subject to temporal variation. Also, the isozymes found in patients with CGL did not differ from those observed in most of the normal controls. Stimulated by the observation of increased LAlP activity in mongoloid patients cited earlier, mongoloid LAlP patterns were then studied and no striking differences between them and normal controls were observed.

An additional number of normal and mongoloid patients was studied for this paper. An attempt has also been made to evaluate the effects of pregnancy and corticoid therapy on LAlP patterns and to obtain preliminary kinetic data on the three major isozymes.

Materials and Methods

Patients

Leukocyte extracts from 13 normal persons (five females and eight males) in good health were studied on at least one occasion. One female and two males were studied twice. One female was studied on two different days, and then four samples were drawn over a period of six hours on a single day.

Nineteen healthy patients at the Fairview Home in Salem, Oregon with clinical mongolism (five females and 14 males) were studied; of these, four females and five males were investigated on two different occasions. Leukocyte cultures were performed on all these patients, but adequate karyotypes were obtained in only 14; nine of these had typical trisomy G, three were mosaics (trisomy G/normal), and one had a normal karyotype. No translocation cases were encountered. One patient, with trisomy G in most cells, had tetrasomy G in two out of 20 cells examined.

Eight normal mothers in the immediate postpartum period (2–40 hours) were studied after delivery. The cases included both primiparous and multiparous mothers, and they all delivered a single normal infant (four females and four males) without obstetrical complications.

Three normal persons (one female and two males) received 40 mg oral prednisone per day for three days to observe possible qualitative as well as quantitative changes in LAlP. Four persons receiving long-term oral prednisone therapy were studied on a single occasion: two were females receiving less than 15 mg prednisone per day (one with Felty's syndrome and the other with chronic bronchial asthma), and two patients (one female and one male) with lupus erythematosis were receiving 30–40 mg of the drug daily.

Three adult patients with chronic granulocytic leukemia were studied once.

One patient was known to have had the disease for four years and the other two for one year. The latter two patients had received prednisolone therapy during the course of their disease but not for several months prior to our study. Two adult females with polycythemia rubra vera were also studied a single time. All five of the patients had received ^{32}P prior to our studies and several had received additional therapy.

Blood Collection

Sterile venous blood was collected in heparin (10 units heparin, Upjohn, per ml of blood) for leukocyte isolation, hematology, and karyotype (mongoloid patients only) or without anticoagulant to obtain serum. Slides were prepared immediately for differential white-blood cell counts and for estimation of LAlP using the naphthol-AS-BI plus fast red violet LB (Sigma Chemical Co.) method of Kaplow (1963). The remaining heparinized sample (30–120 ml) was then used for isolation of leukocytes.

Leukocyte Isolation and Enzyme Extraction

To each 30 ml of heparinized blood was added 6 ml of 5 percent dextran (Sigma, type 100C) in 0.7 percent NaCl, following the method of Peacock *et al.* (1958). The samples were mixed by inversion and allowed to settle for 45 minutes, followed by removal of the leukocyte-containing plasma. Cells were then sedimented by low speed (800 $\times$ *g*) centrifugation of the plasma for ten minutes. The pellicle of cells was resuspended in 0.9 percent NaCl and the above centrifugation repeated. After a third wash, the cells were either stored overnight at 4°C, or preferably, homogenized immediately. Leukocyte isolation, as described, provided an average yield of 64 percent in eight cases that were followed closely. These yields were considered sufficient, and larger quantities (120 ml) of blood were withdrawn from patients expected to have low Kaplow scores.

Homogenization in glass tubes (of the Potter-Elvehjem type), such as those employed for LAlP preparation by McCoy *et al.* (1965) and also by Robinson *et al.* (1965 & 1966), seldom produced sufficient cell disruption. However, a modification of the method described for other leukocyte enzymes by Bertino *et al.* (1963), employing a Virtis® "45" blade-type homogenizer, used previously in many studies of alkaline phosphatase by others, was found to produce satisfactory cell disruption. The cells were sheared in 4–5 ml of freshly mixed cold saline-butanol (29 percent *n*-butanol, v/v, in 0.9 percent NaCl). The homogenizer was operated at 70 volts and at a full rheostat setting for 15 seconds, followed by a setting of "25" for 45 seconds. More vigorous and more prolonged homogenization than that routinely employed (up to two minutes at a full rheostat setting with 70 volts line potential) did not significantly affect the gel patterns.

The extracts were centrifuged at 2–4° C in a Sorvall RC-2 centrifuge at 20,000 $\times$ *g* for 20 minutes. A clear aqueous layer, beneath the butanol phase and floating protein skin, was removed and found to possess virtually all the enzyme activity. The aqueous phase (usually about 3 ml) was then dialyzed 12–18 hours at 4° C in 4–6 changes of buffer (prepared by a 1:20 dilution of 0.1 M tris, pH 8.6) to remove the butanol. The dialyzed solutions were then concentrated to suitable activity (usually ¼–⅛ original volume) by vacuum dialysis at 4° C. As noted by McCoy *et al.* (1965), the extracted LAlP is more stable at 4° C than in the frozen state and, therefore, extracts were stored in glass ampules at 4° C. Bacterial contamination was not encountered in the extracts.

Starch-gel Electrophoresis

Horizontal starch-gels of uniform dimensions were prepared in 0.076 M tris-0.024 M citric acid, pH 8.6, and handled essentially following the technique of Poulik (1957). Sodium hydroxide was added to boric acid to provide an electrode buffer which was 0.3 M borate, pH 8.6. Samples were separated by a potential of 10 volts cm, as measured in the gel. Electrophoresis was continued until the borate buffer zone (borate line) had migrated 6 cm beyond the sample origin; albumin was located at the borate line.

Several modifications in conventional starch-gel electrophoresis were devised to provide more uniform results from day to day. Each modification was studied thoroughly by comparison with conventional techniques until found to produce identical and more consistent gel patterns before being used extensively. First, a Tygon®-coated aluminum plate was substituted for the conventional plastic cooling plate, because plastic did not provide adequate heat dissipation. An external refrigerated bath supplied 5° C water to the cooling plate. In addition, by adding two connecting tubes between the electrode chambers and by continuous external circulation of buffer from one chamber to the other, pH was kept constant during the electrophoresis. Finally, by using a specially constructed power supply (described in the following section), an exact voltage in the gel was maintained at all times during the separation. As an additional check on the comparative isozyme mobilities, known marker isozymes were routinely included as samples.

Horizontal gel slices were stained for protein with 1 percent amido black and for alkaline phosphatase. Enzyme was localized with the same stain employed for LAlP isozymes by Robinson *et al.*, 1965 (0.06 M borate buffer, pH 9.7; 50 mg percent β-naphthyl acid phosphate, Sigma; 50 mg percent fast blue RR, Sigma), except that magnesium was used at a final concentration of 2×10^{-3} M rather than 5×10^{-3} M for reasons appearing later.

Preparative gels to obtain quantities of enzyme for kinetic studies were run as above, except that a single sample was applied across the origin and only a small slice of gel stained for enzyme localization (Moss *et al.*, 1961). The portion of the gel containing the desired isozyme was isolated within 15–20 minutes after cessation of electrophoresis and minced in tris-HCl buffer, pH 7.4 (5×10^{-3} M tris). Strips of gel measuring approximatley $6 \times 10 \times 130$ mm were minced in 10 ml of buffer, stored overnight at 4° C, and centrifuged at $15{,}000 \times g$ for 20 minutes. A perfectly clear solution was obtained with sufficient activity for kinetic studies.

Power Supply

To achieve reproducible electrophoretic separation, voltage potentials should be measured in the gel where the electrophoresis is occurring rather than at the power supply because of inevitable losses encountered in the gel-wick-electrode chamber junctions, buffer-return bridges, and buffer-circulation systems. Therefore, a power supply was constructed, which will be described in more detail elsewhere (Johnston *et al.*).

The power supply (FIGURE 1) differs from conventional models in the possession of two small wire electrodes that are inserted several millimeters into the edge of the gel. When the power supply is activated, the voltage potential between the two gel wires is "sensed" and then "read" by a control amplifier unit. The desired gel potential is selected on a dial that regulates a low voltage power supply providing a reference for the control amplifier. A deviation from the desired gel voltage is detected by the control amplifier that in turn changes the conduction

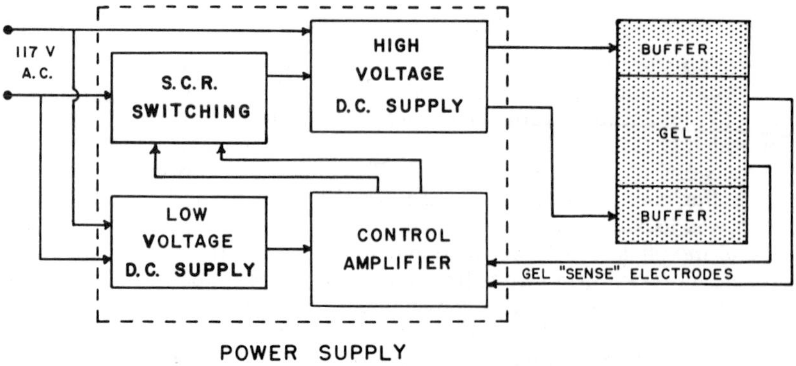

FIGURE 1. Simplified block diagram of silicon control rectifier (SCR) power supply. The four basic components of the power supply are separated to illustrate their relationship to one another and to the electrophoresis cell (dotted area).

angle of the silicon control rectifiers (SCR's) to compensate this deviation. The SCR's control the power to the high voltage supply and thence to the electrodes in the buffer chambers. The sensing circuit is of such high resistance that it has virtually no effect on the electric field of the gel, and enzyme bands that are more than a few millimeters away from the gel-sensing electrodes are not affected by the circuit.

Manual Enzyme Assay

Fluorometric procedures for assay of LAlP are known to have greater sensitivity than spectrophotometric methods. It also seemed desirable to use the same substrate in kinetic studies as that used to demonstrate the enzyme in starch gels. Methods used were essentially those used extensively, in the study of alkaline phosphatase from other human tissues by Moss and his associates (Moss, 1960; Moss *et al.*, 1961; Moss & King, 1962) and recently in human leukocytes by McCoy (1965).

A Model 111 Turner fluorometer with a cuvette kept at 37° C by a constant temperature device (door no. 110–655) was used in conjunction with a Corning 7–60 primary and a Wratten 2A secondary filter. Output from the fluorometer was directed to a Brush Mark 10 (or similar) strip chart recorder and the hydrolysis was monitored continuously. The above filters were selected to eliminate most of the activation and fluorescence of the substrate (β-naphthyl acid phosphate), while they transmit light of sufficient wave length to allow nearly maximum activation (ca. 350 mμ) and fluorescence (ca. 420 mμ) of the hydrolysis product (β-naphthol).

The reaction mixture consisted of 1.8 ml buffer, 0.1 ml substrate,¶ and 0.1 ml enzyme solution. Final concentration of tris was 0.1 M. The final pH was 10.0 (pH values are those measured at 25° C unless otherwise specified), and appro-

¶ Correspondence with the Sigma Co. revealed the substrate to be a monosodium salt (molecular weight = 246) with less than 0.1 percent free β-naphthol (dry weight) and no detectable free inorganic phosphate. Substrate concentration values given in this paper were corrected for apparent purity of the substrate by rapid complete hydrolysis of dilute (10^{-7} M) solutions with a concentrated enzyme preparation, followed by determination of the amount of observed and calculated β-naphthol released.

priate concentrations of substrate and enzyme were determined to achieve linear reaction velocities during the time of observation. The reaction was linear for surprisingly long periods (over 30 minutes).

The filter fluorometer was employed because consistent results could not be realized with a monochromator instrument due to fluctuation of the xenon arc, and low signal to noise ratio necessitated by the low concentrations of enzyme and substrate. The time required to complete studies of magnesium activation, phosphate inhibition, apparent Michaelis-Menten constants (K_m), and thermal stability made manual methods virtually impossible because of loss in enzyme activity, changes in actual substrate concentrations, fluctuation in instruments, etc. By the time studies were completed on one suspected isozyme, conditions were not exactly comparable for examination of another isozyme. Therefore, an automated fluorometric procedure was devised employing concentrations and volumes similar to those described earlier.

Automatic Assay Method ||

Several components of a Technicon Auto Analyzer were arranged as shown in FIGURE 2, utilizing the fluorometer and recorder described above. The thermoregulated cuvette door of the fluorometer was replaced by a 1 ml glass flow-cell door (no. 110–872).

The enzyme solution was sampled (Technicon Sampler II) at a rate of 40 samples per hour with a 2:1 wash ratio. Tris buffer (0.111 M, pH 10.0) was used in the regular wash reservoir, as well as between each enzyme sample cup, to obtain a better wash cycle between samples. Air was used to segment the enzyme sample stream, which was then mixed with buffer. For kinetic studies, the incubation buffer (same as wash buffer) was used either with or without added activator (magnesium) or inhibitor (inorganic phosphate). The substrate (same as that used for manual assay) was added by manually switching to increasing concentrations after termination of each enzyme sample series. The mixture next passed through a double (40 ft) coil in the 37.5° C bath. After incubation, the reaction was stopped with 0.2 M EDTA, pH 10.7, debubbled, and passed through the fluorometer flow cell. Total elapsed time between sampling of the enzyme and recording of the reaction was approximately 15 minutes. The above technique made it possible to study the reaction of several different isozymes at the same substrate concentration and in the same buffer within a few minutes of elapsed time. Appropriate dilutions of each isozyme were made to assure approximately equal activities at a given substrate concentration. The range of activity found useful in these studies was 1–3 micromoles of substrate hydrolyzed per minute per liter of enzyme.

Heat Inactivation

The three isozymes eluted from gels were diluted to nearly equal activities with 5×10^{-3} M tris, pH 7.4, and placed in a constant temperature bath at 56° C without added activators or inhibitors. Aliquots were withdrawn at appropriate time intervals and enzyme activity was then determined in triplicate using the automatic assay system.

|| Previously published automated assay procedures for enzyme kinetics (Pitot & Pries, 1964; Pitot *et al.*, 1965; Tappel & Beck 1965) were not suitable for various reasons. Therefore, existing procedures were modified and adapted for a fluorometric assay to add increased sensitivity.

Results

Gel Patterns

After starch-gel electrophoresis,** leukocyte extracts possessed one or more zones of alkaline phosphatase activity (FIGURE 3). For convenience of description, the common electrophoretic variants are referred to as fast (F), intermediate (I), and slow (S) with reference to their relative migration toward the anode. Occasionally, a band moving faster than the "fast" band was observed, which was referred to as an "ultra-fast" (UF) band, thus emphasizing the inadvisability of designations of this type. Comments on the justification for using the above reference system follow in the discussion. The leukocyte extracts were found to have one or more major bands of enzyme activity and frequently possessed one or more minor bands. TABLE 1 summarizes the data obtained from gel studies in terms of major and minor bands observed after repeated analysis of each extract. Patterns listed in the table are presented below for each category of patient. In several extracts, the I band was seen to have a slightly different mobility

** We have emphasized the importance of maintaining a constant gel and electrode buffer pH, gel temperature, and gel voltage to help minimize fluctuations in the electrophoretic separation, and Raymond (1964 and earlier) has also emphasized such control. Improved control during electrophoresis would also make comparisons among different investigators more meaningful.

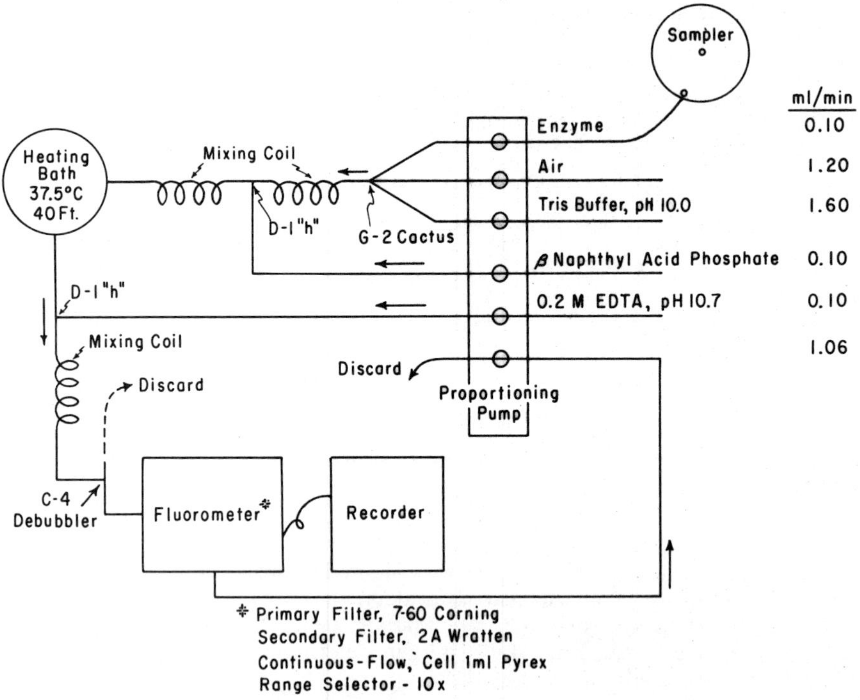

FIGURE 2. Manifold and flow diagram of automated assay procedure (see text for further description). Reagent concentrations and flow rates were those found most effective in present study; they are, of course, dependent upon many factors and must be adjusted for each assay system.

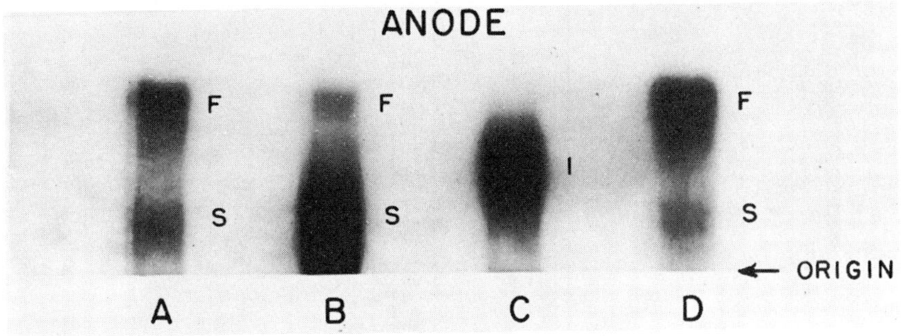

FIGURE 3. Starch-gel pattern of four leukocyte extracts stained for alkaline phosphatase. Designations of the gel patterns as summarized in TABLE 1 would be: A = major F, minor S; B = major S, minor F; C = major I; and D = major F, minor S. Conditions for electrophoresis similar to those of FIGURE 4.

than the typical I band seen in postpartum mothers. Such variations were uncommon and were thought to represent artifacts. However, heterogeneity of the I band remains a possibility in several extracts. Only the typical I isozyme was used in any of the kinetic studies.

The relative migration of major serum proteins, serum alkaline phosphatase, and placental phosphatase is shown in FIGURE 4, for comparison with the migration of LAlP. The placental tissue was homogenized exactly like the leukocyte preparations and handled in the same manner except that the placental extract was not concentrated. The placental pattern would correspond to the S, I, FI, or F pattern of Robson and Harris (1965).

No correlations were found between the total white-blood cell counts or differentials and the total leukocyte activity (Kaplow score) or gel pattern. Confirming the work of numerous investigators, Kaplow scores above those of normal controls were seen in most of the mongoloid patients, all of the postpartum mothers, in all persons receiving prednisone and in both patients with polycythemia rubra vera. Decreased Kaplow scores were observed in patients with chronic granulocytic leukemia. Extracts from several persons with Kaplow scores of zero revealed faint gel bands after suitable concentration, which was attributed to random sample error and/or inadequate staining or sensitivity encountered in the histochemical determination.

Normal and Mongoloid Patients

One of the most striking observations was the finding that the isozyme pattern of a given individual in the normal or mongoloid group often varied on subsequent extractions. Thus, a patient with a major F band on the first extraction might possess a major I band and a minor S band in the second extract. Other temporal changes in gel patterns were also observed. In order to test the consideration that the patterns were simple artifacts, leukocytes were withdrawn from a normal female every two hours to obtain four separate specimens on the same day. All of these specimens possessed identical gel patterns, although two other persons studied the same day possessed different isozyme patterns.

Isozyme variations followed no obvious pattern, and there was no apparent explanation for their occurrence. The variations were not confined to persons of either sex or of any particular age in the normal and mongoloid categories and were not related to the quantitative level of enzyme in the leukocytes (Kaplow score). Gel patterns of mosaic mongoloid patients resembled those of regular

TABLE 1
SUMMARY OF GEL PATTERNS

Category of Patients		Electrophoretic Pattern (No. of Cases in Each Group)												
		Major Bands						Minor Bands						
		F	I	S	F+I	F+S	I+S	F	I	S	F+I	F+S	I+S	UF
Normal female	*1st		4		1					2				2
	2nd					1								
	4 Consecutive						4	4						
Normal male	1st	3	5					1		4				1
	2nd	2								1				
Mongoloid female	1st	2	3							1		1		
	2nd	1	1				1			1			1	
Mongoloid male	1st	3	8		2	1			1	3				
	2nd	1	4		1					2		1		2
Postpartum			7				1			5				
† Prednisone therapy	a. Before	2			1					2				
	After		2				1			1		1		
	b. Low dose					1	1							
	c. High dose		1	1				1		1				
Chronic granulocytic leukemia			3							2				
Polycythemia rubra vera							2	2						

* Abbreviations: 1st = first extract examined, 2nd = second extract examined, 4 consecutive = four separate samples drawn from one patient on same day; for other abbreviations, see text.

† Prednisone therapy category separated into (a) = normal persons before and after treatment, (b) and (c) = patients receiving long-term low and high dose therapy, respectively. All patients possessed major bands but some did not possess minor bands.

trisomy-G mongoloid patients and there were no significant differences in Kaplow scores between the two groups. The patient with two tetrasomy-G cells had a Kaplow score much below that of normal controls, and the LAlP extract revealed major F and I bands and a minor S band. The most frequently observed major isozymes were the F and I types. In the normal and mongoloid patients, a major S band was always found in association with a major F or I band.

There was no appreciable difference between normal and mongoloid LAlP patterns. These findings suggested a physiological variation in both normal and mongoloid patients and stimulated the investigation of several other patient categories.

Pregnancy

All eight postpartum mothers were found to have a major I isozyme, and one also had a major S band. Most of the patients also possessed a minor S band. The F band was not observed in this group even as a minor component.

Prednisone Therapy

Prednisone administered to three normal persons for three days was associated with the appearance of a major I band in all three persons. There was a concomitant loss of the major F band in two cases and reduction to a minor F band in the third. One patient, possessing only a major F band before therapy, also had a major S band after treatment. Kaplow scores were elevated more than threefold in all three patients after drug treatment.

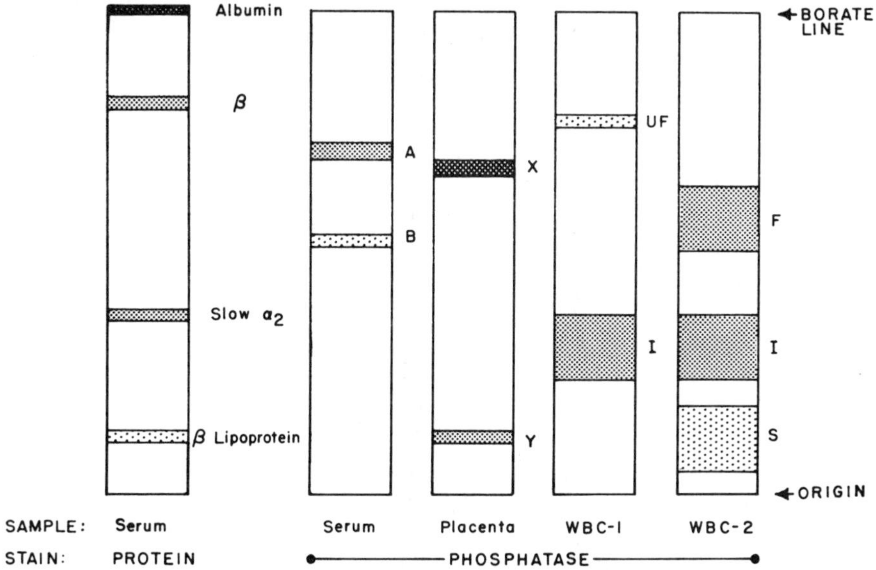

FIGURE 4. Diagram of gel patterns. Electrophoresis carried out at 10 v/cm, as described in text, until borate line migrated 5.9 cm beyond sample origin (anode at top of diagram). Protein stain of major serum bands, at left of diagram, included for comparison of same serum and several extracts stained for alkaline phosphatase. β = beta globulin; Slow α_2 = slow alpha-2 globulin. Serum contained phosphatase A and B bands; placenta contained a main fast component (X) and a less prominent band likely travelling with β-lipoprotein (Y); white blood cell-1 (WBC-1) extract had a major I and minor UF band; WBC-2 extract had major F and I bands and a minor S band. See TABLE 2 for further evaluation.

Out of four patients receiving long-term prednisone for treatment of an underlying disease, one possessed a major F band with an accompanying major S isozyme. No other major F bands were observed, but one other patient had a minor F band. A major F band was not found in patients receiving high doses of prednisone.

Leukemic and Polycythemic Patients

The patients with chronic granulocytic leukemia (CGL) had major I bands and completely lacked F bands; two of them had minor S bands. The two females with polycythemia rubra vera (PRV) both had major I and S and minor F isozyme patterns.

Kinetic Studies

Three main enzyme bands with different mobilities were encountered in gel studies, and several kinetic properties were studied to further elucidate the suspected heterogeneity. Data for the kinetic properties reported here were

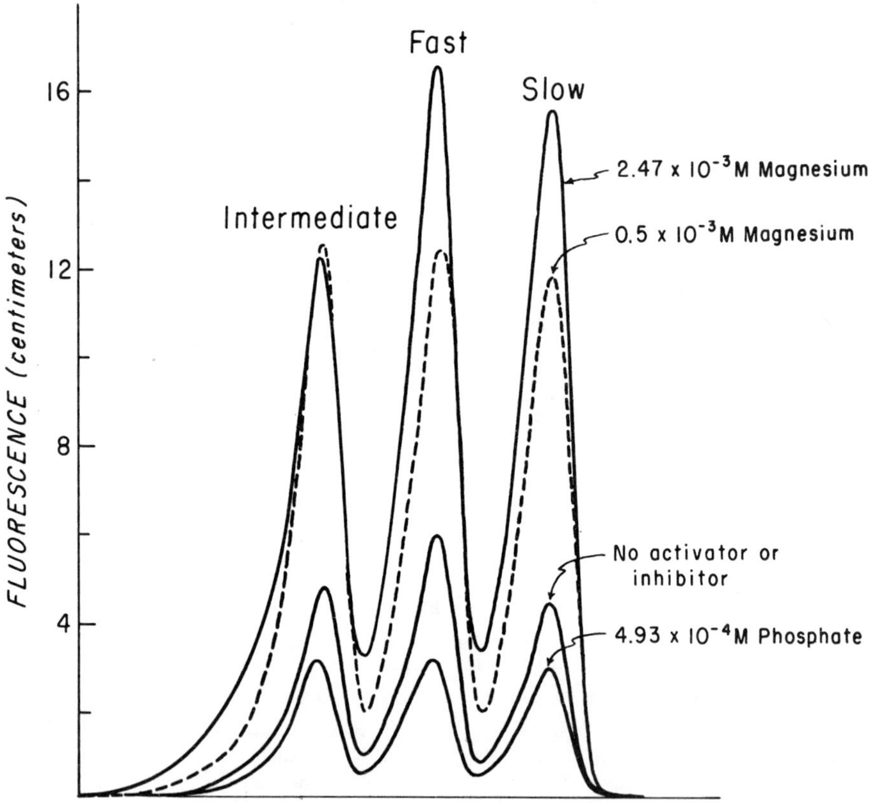

FIGURE 5. Tracing of chart record from automated assay of three isozymes at one substrate concentration (3.03×10^{-5} M in reaction coil). F isozyme original activity slightly greater than I or S. Final concentrations of phosphate inhibitor and magnesium activator as indicated. Recorder sensitivity was one mv per inch of chart and chart speed (abscissa) was 20 inches per hour.

obtained by automatic assays of preparative gel eluates of the three isozymes. Typical results from the automatic method are shown in FIGURE 5. Activity of each isozyme was studied in the presence of (1) no activator or inhibitor, (2) four concentrations of magnesium as activator, and (3) three concentrations of inorganic phosphate as inhibitor.

Apparent K_m values were obtained from double reciprocal plots (Lineweaver & Burk, 1934) of enzyme activity at five substrate concentrations without added activator or inhibitor from the relationship:

$$\text{slope} = \frac{K_m}{V_{max}}$$

where V_{max} is the reciprocal of the intercept on the *y* axis.

Upon addition of inorganic phosphate, the slopes were seen to increase, though V_{max} remained constant, thus suggesting competitive inhibition. For a competitively inhibited reaction:

$$\text{slope} = \frac{K_m}{V_{max}}\left(1 + \frac{[I]}{K_i}\right)$$

where K_m and V_{max} are determined from the uninhibited reaction, the given concentration of inhibitor [I] is known and K_i can be calculated. The value of K_i for the three concentrations of inhibitor was averaged for each isozyme.

Lineweaver-Burk plots of the F, I and S isozymes are shown in FIGURES 6, 7, and 8 respectively. The inhibition with three concentrations of phosphate is also shown. Calculations for the K_m and K_i values are presented in TABLE 2 based on the slope and intercept methods described above. The three K_m values are slightly different, and it is apparent from the K_i (TABLE 2) and from the data plotted in FIGURE 9 that the F isozyme is approximately twice as sensitive to inorganic phosphate as the S and I isozymes, which are not significantly different from one another.

Magnesium activation was evaluated by measuring activity of the three isozymes in the presence of four concentrations of activator. Activator studies were performed at four different concentrations of substrate. FIGURE 10 presents the data for magnesium activation at one substrate concentration. The ratio of activated enzyme to unactivated enzyme was plotted against concentration of activator. It can be seen that the I isozyme is very different from the F and S isozymes. The I type is maximally activated at 1×10^{-3} M Mg^{++} and higher concentrations are relatively inhibitory. In contrast, the F and S isozymes are maximally activated at approximately 3×10^{-3} M Mg^{++}. Not shown is the observation that in more dilute concentrations of substrate, the activity ratio reached a plateau at 3×10^{-3} M Mg^{++} for the F and S isozymes, and higher concentration of Mg^{++} did not decrease the activity. Higher concentrations of substrate than that shown in FIGURE 10 caused a sharper peak of activity at 3×10^{-3} M Mg^{++} for the F and S isozymes. The I isozyme activity ratio was not affected by changes in the concentration of substrate. Therefore, the I isozyme was affected very differently from the F and S isozymes by (1) the concentration of Mg^{++} for maximal activation and (2) the influence of substrate concentration on the Mg^{++} activation.

Thermal inactivation was evaluated for eluates of each isozyme containing approximately equal enzyme activities. The results (FIGURE 11) indicated that the F isozyme was reduced to half its original activity in about one-half the time required for similar inactivation of the S isozyme at the same temperature. The I isozyme had a heat lability intermediate between the F and S types (TABLE 2).

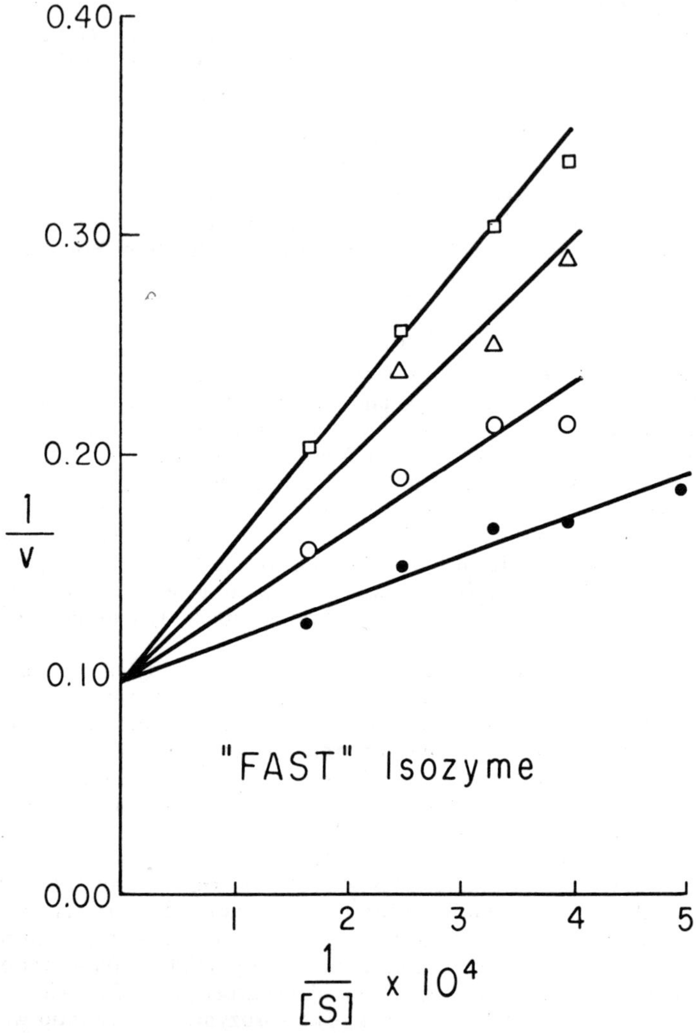

FIGURE 6. Lineweaver-Burk double reciprocal plot of Fast isozyme activity. Ordinate, 1/v = reciprocal of initial velocity and abscissa, 1/[S] = reciprocal of final substrate concentration. Symbols: ●——● = without activator or inhibitor; ○——○ = with added phosphate at 0.99 $\times$ 10^{-4} M final concentration; △——△ = with added phosphate at 2.47 $\times$ 10^{-4} M fiinal concentration; and □——□ = with added phosphate at 4.93 $\times$ 10^{-4} M final concentration. See text description of automatic assay procedure for details.

Discussion

Variable electrophoretic mobility does not establish the existence of multiple forms of an enzyme and, furthermore, does not indicate that such forms occur *in vivo*. Apparent isozymes may result from artifacts such as molecular aggregation or depolymerization. They may appear also when an enzyme binds to a carrier molecule (e.g., β-lipoprotein). It is also possible that isozymes with identical mobilities may be found to have different kinetic properties.

Confusion of alkaline phosphatase (AlP) isozyme nomenclature has developed in the literature primarily because different designations have been employed by

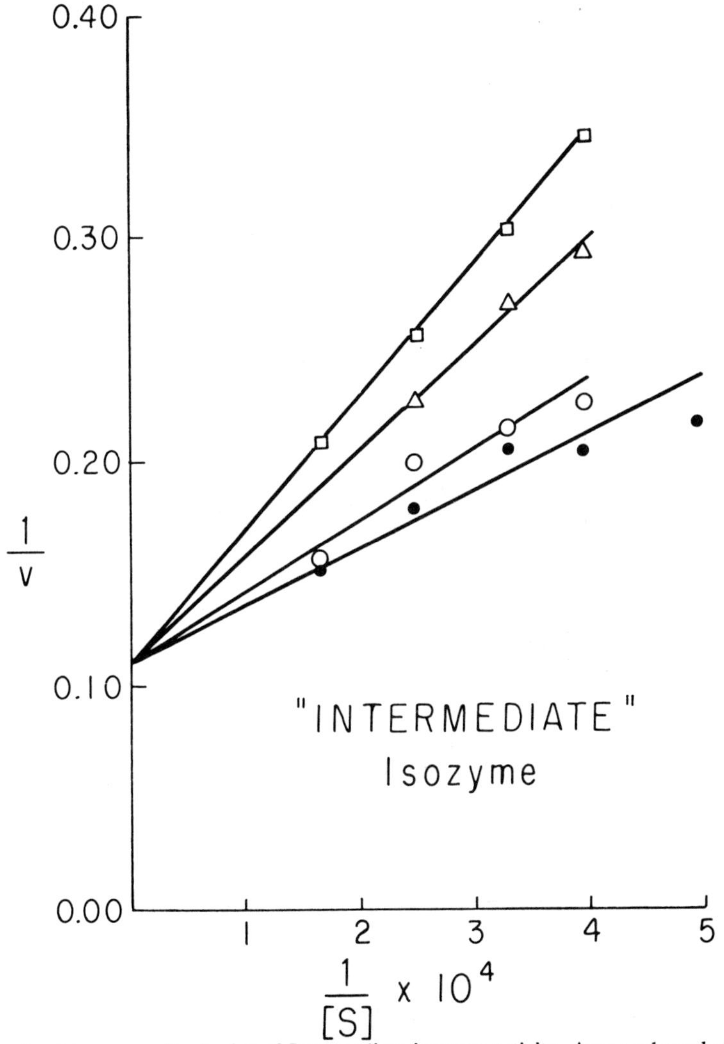

FIGURE 7. Lineweaver-Burk plot of Intermediate isozyme activity. Axes and symbols same as those in FIGURE 6.

different authors. It should be stressed that the F, I, S, and UF designations as used here are for simplicity of reference and no attempt has been made to give an unyielding identification to the bands. It is noted that Boyer (1961) gave A and B designations to fast and slow bands of placental extracts, and that Robson and Harris (1965), after examining 402 placentas, gave designations of fast (F), intermediate (I), and slow (S) to the placental patterns. In our FIGURE 4, the placental bands were labeled X and Y because the X band could have been the F, FI, I, or S of Robson and Harris, and the very slow (Y) band was not labeled by the latter authors. The X band in the placental extract of FIGURE 4 consistently

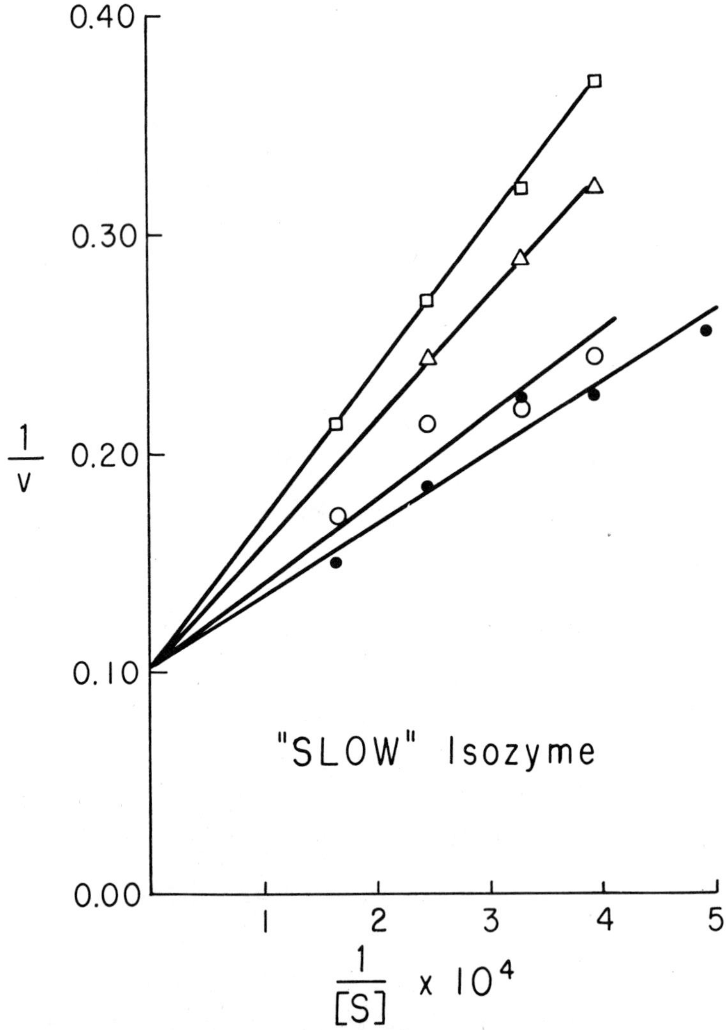

FIGURE 8. Lineweaver-Burke plot of Slow isozyme activity. Axes and symbols same as those in FIGURE 6.

TABLE 2

SUMMARY OF ISOZYME PROPERTIES

Isozyme*	R_f†	K_m (M)	K_i (M)	[Mg++] for Maximum Activation (M)‡	Thermal Denaturation Time (min)§
Fast	0.58	1.92×10^{-5}	1.58×10^{-4}	3×10^{-3}	11.5
Intermediate	0.31	2.56×10^{-5}	3.64×10^{-4}	1×10^{-3}	17.1
Slow	0.12	3.16×10^{-5}	3.77×10^{-4}	3×10^{-3}	22.8

* Isozyme = specific band eluted from preparative gel.

† R_f = ratio of isozyme mobility/distance traversed by borate buffer-zone in a separation where the latter was 59 mm. In the same gel separation, relevant R_f values of other alkaline phosphatase bands were: serum band A = 0.71, serum band B = 0.53, main fast placental band = 0.68, slow placental band = 0.12, ultra fast LAlP band = 0.78 (see also FIGURE 4).

‡ See FIGURE 10 for explanation.

§ Preincubation time at 56° C required for 50 percent inactivation of original activity. See FIGURE 11 for explanation.

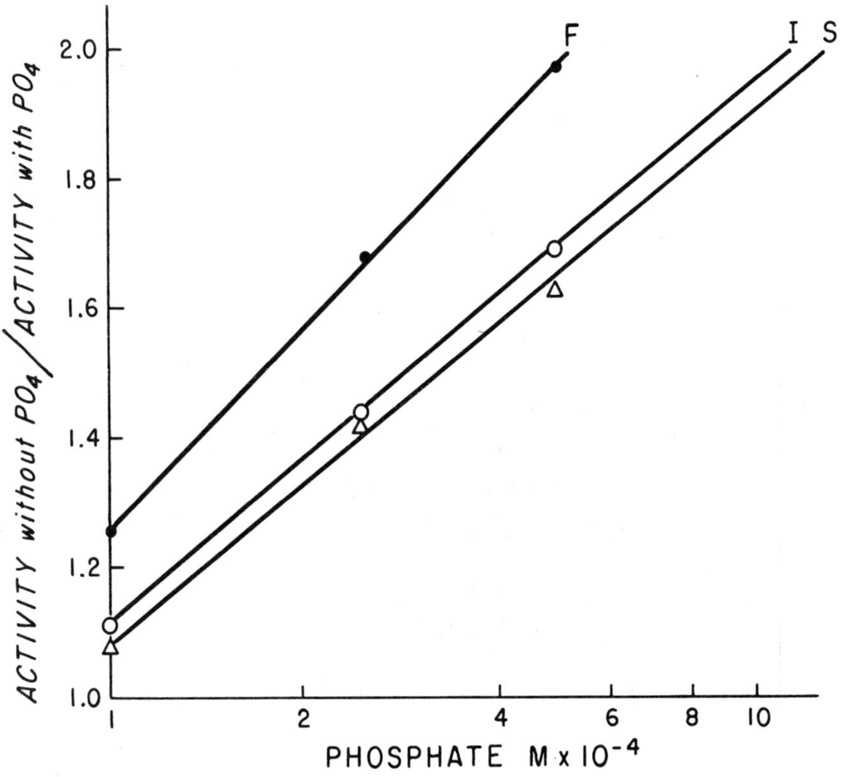

FIGURE 9. Effect of inorganic phosphate on isozyme activity. Final substrate concentration was 2.53×10^{-5} M. Similar data at other substrate concentrations can be obtained from FIGURES 6, 7, and 8. Activity of each isozyme without added phosphate is compared to the inhibited reaction at various phosphate concentrations. Symbols: ●——● = Fast isozyme; ○——○ = Intermediate isozyme; and △——△ = Slow isozyme.

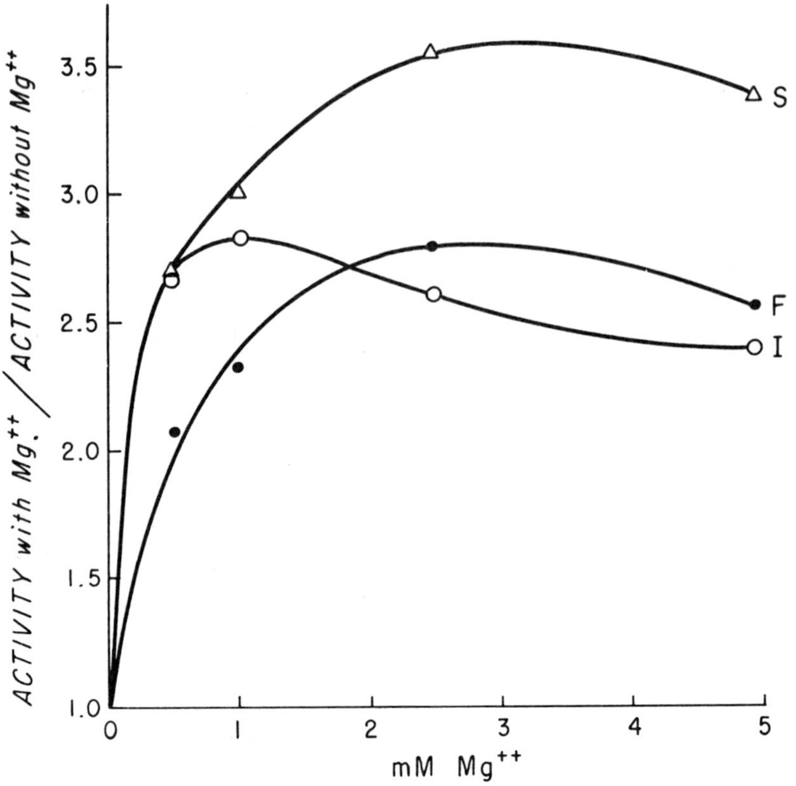

FIGURE 10. Effect of magnesium on isozyme activity at one substrate concentration (same as that of FIGURE 5). Activity of each isozyme with added Mg^{++} is compared to nonactivated reaction at various Mg^{++} concentrations. Two of the points for each isozyme were determined from data of FIGURE 5. Similar data obtained from three additional substrate concentrations is not shown (see text). Symbols same as those in FIGURE 9.

migrated faster than the F LAlP isozyme, and the Y band had the same mobility as the LAlP S isozyme (and β-lipoprotein). Unfortunately, designations of A, B, C, and D have also been used for the regular bands of serum AlP, and the A and B bands of serum do not correspond to Boyer's A and B bands of serum from pregnant mothers and placental extracts. Moss and King (1962) used designations of 1, 2, and 3 in their studies of liver, kidney, intestine, and bone AlP. However, the "1" band of liver did not have the same mobility or K_m as the "1" band of the other tissues, and the same was true for the other band designations. Other systems of nomenclature have been employed by other workers; none seem to be completely satisfactory. An attempt was made in this paper to refer to relative mobilities (R_f values shown in TABLE 2) and the designations seem adequate. In the discontinuous buffer system, the R_f values are dependent on the migration distance of the borate line. Thus, it is helpful to present the mobility of an isozyme band in relation to a serum protein or to an easily obtainable standard isozyme (e.g., serum bands A and B in FIGURE 4 and TABLE 2).

In our system, the LAlP F isozyme migrates slightly faster than the serum B

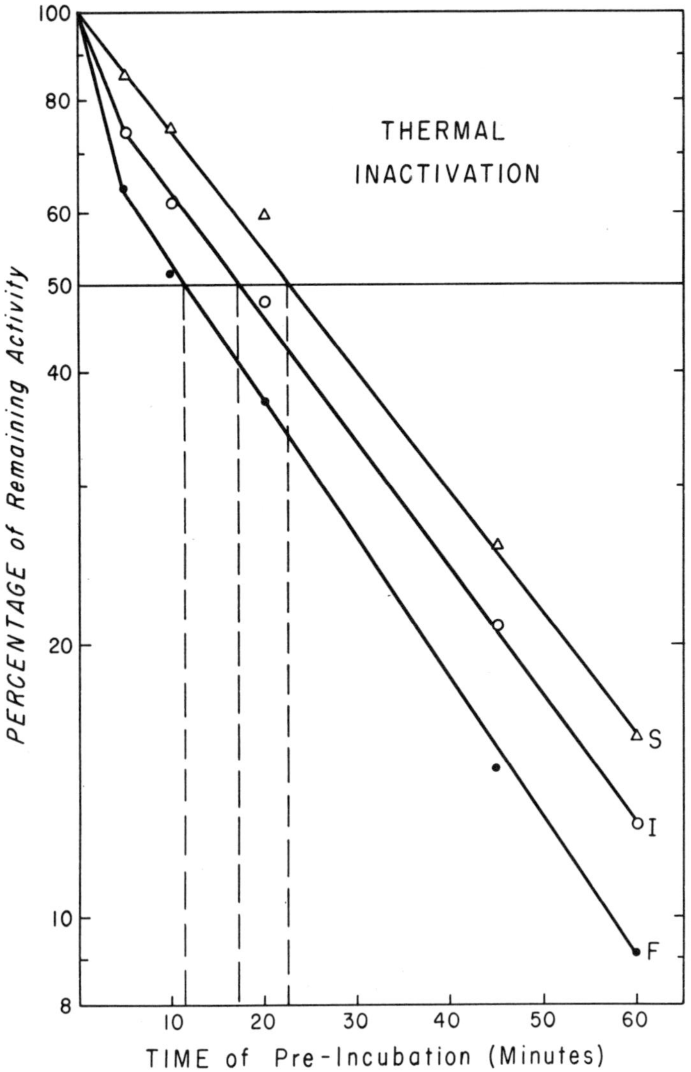

FIGURE 11. Thermal inactivation of the isozymes. Isozymes incubated as described in text without added substrate, activator, or inhibitor at 56° C. Aliquots removed at varying time intervals and subjected to automatic assay under the following conditions (final concentrations): 6.08×10^{-5} M substrate, 0.99×10^{-3} M Mg^{++}, and 9.87×10^{-2} M tris, pH 10.0. Symbols same as those in FIGURE 9.

band, the I isozyme migrates slightly behind the slow α-2 globulins of serum and the S isozyme has a mobility equal to that of serum β-lipoprotein (FIGURE 4). The F band of LAlP is clearly distinct from the fast (X) component of the placenta and the I isozyme, which is the major component of LAlP in postpartum mothers, does not have a mobility similar to any of the placental isozymes. This latter observation is interesting in view of the fact that serum AlP is elevated in pregnancy. Several investigators have shown that the elevated serum phosphatase in pregnancy is derived from the placenta. The present paper shows that the increased LAlP during pregnancy is due mainly to an isozyme not found in the placenta. The recent finding, of O'Kell and Axon (1965), that fetal LAlP is very high in cord blood, and their suggestion that the increased level is due to increased levels of maternal hormones would suggest that fetal LAlP is primarily the I isozyme. Unfortunatley, we were unable to obtain samples to evaluate this possibility.

As shown in TABLE 1, all three of the major LAlP isozymes were observed in the group of normal and mongoloid patients and in two patients with PRV. By contrast, the F isozyme was not observed in postpartum mothers or in the three patients with CGL. Prednisone administration was always associated with a diminution or disappearance of the F isozyme. Therefore, it is suggested that the F isozyme is most variable in occurrence and is decreased in the presence of high levels of glucocorticoids and, perhaps, in CGL.

There was no apparent correlation between the LAlP pattern and the total or differential white blood cell count, age or sex of patient, or the Kaplow score. McCoy *et al.* (1965) showed that the Kaplow score parallels the activity of LAlP extracts from a given patient. One would then expect that the gel pattern represents a majority of the activity observed histochemically. McCoy (1966) has also observed three major isozymes in LAlP extracts from normal and mongoloid subjects; he found no obvious differences between the normal patterns and those observed in approximately ten mongoloid patients. He studied several mothers in the early postpartum period and found results similar to those reported in the present paper. He also observed visible starch-gel patterns in concentrated samples of LAlP prepared from patients with Kaplow (histochemical) scores of zero.

Berg *et al.* (1965), using agar electrophoresis, reported only one isozyme in LAlP extracts. The latter workers did notice an additional precipitate of activity at the origin but regarded it as an artifact. They did not thoroughly examine the possibility that the additional activity was due to an isozyme. It is difficult to compare the work of Berg *et al.* with any starch-gel studies because of the different mobilities of proteins in the two media. Also, the latter authors extracted LAlP by alternate freezing and thawing which could well have eliminated some of the activity (McCoy *et al.*, 1965).

The absence of significant differences between LAlP patterns of mongoloid patients and those of normal patients suggests that the increased LAlP activity in mongolism is due to a regulator gene(s) or even to an entirely unrelated nonspecific effect. In the present study of LAlP in mongolism, there was no obvious correlation between the number of small acrocentric chromosomes and the Kaplow score or gel pattern of LAlP. It is quite likely that the correlation between small acrocentrics and AlP levels noted in EUE cells (human embryonic epithelium) by De Carli and associates (Maio & De Carli, 1962; De Carli *et al.*, 1963; De Carli *et al.*, 1964) is valid, and that individual variation in our mongolism category accounts for the discrepancy between the Kaplow score and the number of cells with extra G chromosomes. There is, however, an increased mean Kaplow score in the mongoloid patients studied in the present paper, which is in accord with the findings of De Carli's group.

The work of Robinson's group (Robinson *et al.*, 1965; Robinson *et al.*, 1966) is not easily compared with the present paper, since these authors did not include in their diagrams any reference points (e.g., serum protein bands and/or serum AlP bands) other than centimeters of migration. A photograph of their gel patterns would have been useful in assessing the intensity of their band at the origin, which we would regard as a possible artifact. Furthermore, the relative isozyme mobilities shown in their 1965 paper are not the same as those in the 1966 paper, although they indicate that the same methods were employed in each study. The 1966 paper does not indicate how many patients have been studied in the normal and CGL categories. It seems probable that Robinson *et al.*, have not yet examined enough normal persons to observe an isozyme with a mobility similar to that seen in their CGL, pregnant, and prednisone-treated patients. If we interpret their findings correctly, it seems that their results might be in essential agreement with our own in that the major isozyme in CGL is also seen in pregnancy, after corticoid administration, and in a number of normal persons. We are quite certain that the I band of our CGL patients is identical to the I band of normal persons. A change in CGL patterns is most likely a loss of the F isozyme.

Other studies of AlP in cultured human cells conducted by Cox and his colleagues have been summarized recently (Cox & MacLeod, 1964). Substrate induction and cysteine repression were employed by Cox (1965) to compare the response of cultured mongoloid fibroblasts to that of normal fibroblasts. He concluded that the extra G chromosomes did not affect either the absolute level or mode of regulation of AlP in the fibroblast cultures. The present paper substantiates Cox's observation that the enzyme in mongoloid patients is similar to that of normal persons, but there is a higher level of enzyme in leukocytes as noted previously.

The apparent loss of the LAlP F isozyme in pregnancy and its loss or diminution during prednisone therapy reported here also has a counterpart in studies of cultured human cells. Beckman and Regan (1964) studied RA cells (a continuous line from human amnion), WISH cells (also from human amnion), and HeLa cells. They found three major AlP isozymes in these cells after starch-gel electrophoresis. They also noted that the fastest migrating zone of AlP disappeared when cortisone was added to the culture and that the quantity of the intermediately migrating AlP was concomitantly increased. These observations correlate well with those of the present paper. Beckman and Regan also observed that the AlP pattern of their RA cell-line varied with time, just as we often observed in our normal and mongoloid patients upon subsequent extractions. They attributed the change in AlP patterns to "dynamic changes in a heterogenous cell population." It is possible that there are also clones of leukocytes in normal persons that are selectively produced in response to an altered environment and that the observed changes in LAlP gel patterns reflect such adaptations. Another interpretation for the variation is altered synthesis or masked activity of a particular isozyme in a homogenous cell population.

Cox and Griffin (1967) also studied HeLa cells and found that the fastest migrating isozyme was the most heat-labile isozyme and that it disappeared after addition of prednisolone to the culture medium.

Maio and De Carli (1962) found that EUE cell lines with undetectable AlP could be induced to synthesize considerable levels of enzyme by prednisolone and/or phenylphosphate.

In addition to electrophoretic mobility differences, there appear to be kinetic differences among the three major LAlP isozymes (TABLE 2). The K_m data are in fairly close agreement with the value of 1.38×10^{-4} M given for LAlP eluted from starch gel by McCoy *et al.* (1965), for the same substrate in a different buffer. Moss and King (1962) reported K_m values for human liver, intestine, kidney, and bone that were also slightly higher than those of the present paper for LAlP, but Moss and King used carbonate-bicarbonate and carbonate-veronal buffers with added magnesium (5 mM). Numerous manual and automated K_m determinations of eluted LAlP in our laboratory reveal that there is some variation ($1–8 \times 10^{-5}$ M), but the F isozyme has a K_m lower than that of the I isozyme which, in turn, is lower than that of the S isozyme. The K_m differences are small (TABLE 2) and may not be significant. Insufficient eluted enzyme was available to make a correction for the decrease in pH optimum subconsequent to lowered substrate concentrations. The K_m values reported by Moss and King were corrected for the pH optimum changes. The value given above for McCoy *et al.* was uncorrected, but they also reported a corrected value of 6.0×10^{-5} M.

Some of the differences encountered in kinetic properties reported in the literature may be due to the transferase action of the enzyme. This is especially true of techniques measuring inorganic phosphate production since the latter may be delayed by transfer reactions. Even the tris buffer used here and generally regarded as an "inert" buffer has recently been found to be phosphorylated by the transferase activity of alkaline phosphatase (Dayan & Wilson, 1964).

Activation of LAlP with magnesium definitely distinguished two different responses. The I isozyme was maximally activated at a lower concentration of magnesium than the F or S isozymes. The maximally effective concentration (3×10^{-3} M) for the F and S isozymes would actually result in less activity when added to the I isozyme than would the 1×10^{-3} M concentration. Furthermore, increasing substrate concentration had the effect of intensifying the peak of optimal magnesium concentration for the F and S isozymes but had no such effect on the I isozyme. Trubowitz *et al.* (1957) suspected the existence of a magnesium-activated LAlP isozyme as well as a zinc-activated isozyme. It is possible that their maximum concentration of magnesium (5×10^{-3} M) identifies the magnesium-activated isozyme as the F or S type. This thought is supported by their additional observation that the other isozyme was increased in leukemoid reactions and infections which would suggest similarities to the I isozyme. Unfortunately, later studies by Trubowitz *et al.* (1961), utilizing different techniques, failed to show substrate affinities (by mixing of substrates) indicative of two different isozymes. However, they did observe two active peaks upon ultracentrifugation and reserved the possibility of several different isozymes.

The F isozyme is about twice as sensitive to inorganic phosphate as either the I or S isozymes (FIGURE 9 and TABLE 2). The substrate had no detectable free inorganic phosphate and the concentration of phosphate required for significant inhibition would not have been produced by substrate hydrolysis during the period of observation. An explanation for the differences in phosphate sensitivity is not yet apparent, but environmental concentration of phosphate may have a role in regulating the synthesis and/or activity of the isozymes.

The studies of thermal inactivation also seemed to differentiate the isozymes (FIGURE 11 & TABLE 2). Herz and Nitowsky (1962) reported heat inactivation studies of cultured human cells. Posen *et al.* (1965) performed similar studies on various human sera as well as on bile and fetal bone extracts. Moss and King (1962) investigated the heat stability of human bone, kidney, intestine, and liver isozymes eluted from starch gels. Since the previously reported data are not exactly comparable, the only relevant comment is that the 50 percent inactivation time at 56° C for most of the specimens examined by the three groups are in the range of times reported in the present paper. Heat sensitivity would, of course, depend largely on such factors as enzyme concentration, total protein concentration, ionic strength, and composition of the incubation buffer. These factors were not similar in any of the above studies. Of the three investigations cited, our findings most closely resemble those of Moss and King.

As shown in TABLE 2, the F and I isozymes seem to be distinctive with respect to phosphate inhibition and magnesium activation, respectively. Further, the F and I isozymes have different heat stabilities and, perhaps, K_m values. The S isozyme, on the other hand, differs from the other two in respect to heat stability and K_m but resembles the F isozyme in its behavior with magnesium and the I isozyme in its behavior with phosphate. It seems conceivable that such relationships could implicate a binding of one or both of the faster migrating isozymes to a carrier molecule like β-lipoprotein, and that the S isozyme is really a complex with several indistinct properties. Other workers have noted instability of the β-lipoprotein fraction. Moss and King (1962) found that eluted, concentrated isozyme from the β-lipoprotein region would, upon reelectrophoresis, produce the original band plus bands with faster mobilities. Extending their work, we studied the placental extract shown in FIGURE 4. The Y band and the faster X band were separated by a prolonged electrophoresis, eluted from the gel, concentrated, and again separated on a starch gel. The results were most revealing: The X band eluate contained only an X band after the second electrophoresis, whereas the Y band eluate was clearly separated into a Y band and a less intense X band. Thus, a dissociation apparently took place which removed from the Y band eluate some molecules with a mobility identical to that of the X band. Similar studies with the LAlP isozymes were attempted but were not successful due to insufficient activity upon reelectrophoresis. It would be possible, though technically tedious, to perform such studies.

SUMMARY

Leukocyte alkaline phosphatase (LAlP) was examined in normal, mongoloid, postpartum, prednisone treated, chronic granulocytic leukemic (CGL) and polycythemic patients. The results suggested the existence of three major isozymes (fast, F; intermediate, I; and slow, S) in the normal, mongoloid and polycythemic patients. The F isozyme was not observed in postpartum mothers or patients with CGL and was reduced or absent in those receiving prednisone. Temporal variation in the LAlP patterns was observed. During pregnancy, the increased LAlP is due to an increase in a specific (I) LAlP not related to the increased serum enzyme (from placenta) present in these patients.

Kinetic studies revealed slightly differing K_m values for the F (1.92×10^{-5} M), I (2.56×10^{-5} M) and S (3.16×10^{-5} M) isozymes. Magnesium activation was maximal at higher concentrations (3×10^{-3} M) for the F and S isozymes than for the I isozyme (1×10^{-3} M). The K_i values were higher (about 3.7×10^{-4} M) for the I and S isozymes than for the F isozyme (1.58×10^{-4} M). The F isozyme was inactivated 50 percent in half the time required for similar inactivation of the S isozyme, and the I isozyme was intermediate between the two. The possibility that the S isozyme might represent a complex of the F and/or I isozyme with a carrier molecule was discussed. The apparent isozyme could also represent the combination of identical enzyme units into polymers and/or combination with other proteins, hormones, or even smaller molecules.

The authors are of the opinion that there are three major isozymes of LAlP and that their occurrence is probably subject to the physiological status, and/or environment of the individual. No obvious qualitative effect on the isozyme pattern produced by the extra chromosome in mongolism is apparent.

Specialized techniques for improved electrophoretic separations of LAlP and for the automated assay of gel eluates of phosphatase are presented. Possible artifacts encountered in the study are discussed and the results are compared to those in the literature.

Acknowledgments

The authors wish to express special gratitude to Dr. R. D. Koler, who made many valuable suggestions during the course of this work. We thank Dr. R. T. Jones and Mr. David Durfee for assistance in developing the automated assay procedure and Dr. R. H. Bigley for referring several of the patients. Many of the early modifications in the electrophoresis system were done in conjunction with Mr. John Brooke. Mr. Ernest Hage fabricated the special electrophoresis cells and helped design and construct numerous items of equipment. Mrs. Marleen Delay and Mr. Ronald Marcum made useful contributions to the study, including the karyotypes. Dr. Frank Jacobson kindly aided us in obtaining samples from patients at Fairview Hospital and Training Center in Salem, Ore.

[NOTE ADDED IN PROOF: Several papers on LAlP isozymes have been published since the preparation of this manuscript (Oct., 1966). These articles have been included in a recent review of the subject (Weaver, D. D. & R. B. Lyons. 1968. Leucocyte alkaline phosphatase isoenzymes. Lancet **i**: 1196–1197).]

References

ALTER, A., S. L. LEE, M. POURFAR & G. DOBKIN. 1962. Leucocyte alkaline phosphatase in mongolism, a possible chromosome marker. J. Clin. Invest. **41**: 1341.

BECKMAN, L. & J. D. REGAN. 1964. Isozyme studies of some human cell lines. Acta Path. Microbiol. Scand. **62**: 567–574.

BEISEL, W. R., N. BENJAMIN & K. F. AUSTEN. 1959. Absence of leukocyte alkaline phosphatase activity in hypophosphatasia. Blood **14**: 975–977.

BERG, G. Ü. ROORAND, S. WITTE, H. GÖTZ & D. BRESSEL. 1965. Über die Beziechungen zwischen neutrophilen Leukozyten und Serumglobulinfraktionen. Clin. Chim. Acta **12**: 282–291.

BERTINO, J. R., R. SILBER, M. FREEMAN, A. ALENTY, M. ALBRECHT, B. W. GABRIO & F. M. HUENNEKENS. 1963. Studies of normal and leukemic leukocytes. IV. Tetrahydrofolate-dependent enzyme systems and dihydrofolic reductase. J. Clin. Invest. **42**: 1899–1907.

BOYER, S. H. 1961. Alkaline phosphatase in human sera and placentae. Science **134**: 1002–1004.

COX, R. P. 1965. Regulation of alkaline phosphatase in skin fibroblast cultures from patients with mongolism. Exp. Cell Res. **37**: 690–692.

COX, R. P. & M. J. GRIFFIN. 1967. Alkaline phosphatase. **I**. Comparison of the physical and chemical properties of enzyme preparations from mammalian cell cultures, various animal tissues, and *Escherichia coli*. Arch. Biochem. Biophys. **122**: 552–562.

COX, R. P. & C. M. MACLEOD. 1964. Regulation of alkaline phosphatase in human cell cultures. Sympos. Quant. Biol. **29**: 233–251.

DAYAN, J. & I. B. WILSON. 1964. The phosphorylation of tris by alkaline phosphatase. Biochim. Biophys. Acta **81**: 620–623.

DE CARLI, L., J. J. MAIO & F. NUZZO. 1963. Alkaline phosphatase activity and chromosome variation in human cells in culture. J. Nat. Cancer Inst. **31**: 1501–1507.

DE CARLI, L., J. J. MAIO, F. NUZZO & A. S. BENERECETTI. 1964. Cytogenic studies with alkaline phosphatase in human heteroploid cells. Sympos. Quant. Biol. **29**: 223–231.

GOMORI, G. 1941. The distribution of phosphatase in normal organs and tissues. J. Cell. Comp. Physiol. **17**: 71–83.

HERZ, F. & H. M. NITOWSKY. 1962. Alkaline phosphatase activity of human cell cultures: kinetic and physical-chemical properties. Arch. Biochem. Biophys. **96**: 506–515.
JOHNSTON, G. I., R. B. LYONS & D. D. BAILEY. Manuscript in preparation.
KAPLOW, L. S. 1963. Cytochemistry of leukocyte alkaline phosphatase-use of complex naphthol AS phosphates in azo dye-coupling technics. Amer. J. Clin. Path. **39**: 439–449.
LINEWEAVER, H. & D. BURK. 1934. Determination of enzyme dissociation constants. J. Amer. Chem. Soc. **56**: 658–666.
MAIO, JOSEPH J. & L. L. DE CARLI. 1962. Distribution of alkaline phosphatase variants in a heteroploid strain of human cells on tissue culture. Nature (London) **196**: 600–601.
MCCOY, E. E. 1966. Personal communication.
MCCOY, E. E., J. PARK & J. ENGLAND. 1965. A fluorometric assay and properties of leukocyte alkaline phosphatase. Clin. Chim. Acta **12**: 453–461.
MOSS, D. W. 1960. Kinetics of phosphatase action on naphthyl phosphates, determined by a highly sensitive spectrofluorimetric technique. Biochem. J. **76**: 32.
MOSS, D. W., D. M. CAMPBELL, E. ANAGNOSTOU-KAKARAS & E. J. KING. 1961. Characterization of tissue alkaline phosphatases and their partial purification by starch gel electrophoresis. Biochem. J. **81**: 441–447.
MOSS, D. W. & E. J. KING. 1962. Properties of aklaline-phosphatase fractions separated by starch-gel electrophoresis. Biochem. J. **84**: 192–195.
O'KELL, R. T. & L. L. AXON. 1965. Leukocyte alkaline phosphatase in the newborn infant. Amer. J. Obstet. Gynec. **93**: 1181–1182.
PEACOCK, A. C., G. BRECHER & E. M. HIGHSMITH. 1958. A simplified procedure for quantitative measurement of alkaline phosphatase in white blood cells. Amer. J. Clin. Path. **29**: 80–85.
PITOT, H. C. & N. PRIES. 1964. The automated assay of complete enzyme reaction rates. I. Methods and results. Anal. Biochem. **9**: 454–466.
PITOT, H. C., N. PRIES, M. POIRIER & A. CUTLER. 1965. Rate analysis of enzyme reactions by continuous and interrupted flow procedures. *In* Technicon Symposium: Automation in Analytical Chemistry : 555–558. New York. Sept. 1965.
POSEN, S., F. C. NEALE & J. S. CLUBB. 1965. Heat inactivation in the study of human alkaline phosphatases. Ann. Intern. Med. **62**: 1234–1242.
POULIK, M. D. 1957. Starch gel electrophoresis in a discontinuous system of buffers. Nature (London) **180**: 1477–1479.
PRITCHARD, J. A. 1957. Leukocyte phosphatase activity in pregnancy. J. Lab. Clin. Med. **50**: 432–436.
RAYMOND, S. 1964. Acrylamide gel electrophoresis. Ann. N. Y. Acad. Sci. **121**: 350–365.
ROBINSON, J. C., J. E. PIERCE & D. P. GOLDSTEIN. 1965. Leukocyte alkaline phosphatase: electrophoretic variants associated with chronic myelogenous leukemia. Science **150**: 58–60.
ROBINSON, J. C., J. E. PIERCE, D. P. GOLDSTEIN & W. R. ROSSE. 1966. Leucocyte-alkaline-phosphatase isozymes. Lancet **ii**(7467): 805.
ROBSON, E. B. & H. HARRIS. 1965. Genetics of the alkaline phosphatase polymorphism of the human placenta. Nature (London) **207**: 1257–1259.
TAPPEL, A. L. & C. BECK. 1965. Automated enzyme reactions. *In* Technicon Symposium: Automation in Analytical Chemistry : 559–562. New York. Sept. 1965.
TRUBOWITZ, S., D. FELDMAN, C. BENANTE & D. KIRMAN. 1957. Metal requirements of alkaline phosphatases of human and rabbit leukocytes. Proc. Soc. Exp. Biol. Med. **95**: 35–38.
TRUBOWITZ, S., D. FELDMAN, S. W. MORGENSTERN & V. M. HUNT. 1961. The isolation, purification and some properties of the alkaline phosphatase of human leucocytes. Biochem. J. **80**: 369–374.
TRUBOWITZ, S., D. KIRMAN & B. MASEK. 1962. The leucocyte alkaline phosphatase in mongolism. Lancet **ii**: 486–487.
VALENTINE, W. N., W. S. BECK, J. H. FOLLETTE, H. MILLS & J. S. LAWRENCE. 1952. Biochemical studies in chronic myelocytic leukemia, polycythemia vera and other idiopathic myeloproliferative disorders. Blood **7**: 959–977.
VALENTINE, W. N., J. H. FOLLETTE, E. B. HARDIN, W. S. BECK & J. S. LAWRENCE. 1954. Studies on leucocyte alkaline phosphatase activity: relation to "stress" and pituitary-adrenal activity. J. Lab. Clin. Med. **44**: 219–228.
VALENTINE, W. N., K. R. TANAKA & R. E. FREDERICKS. 1960. Studies on leukocyte alkaline phosphatase: role of zinc and magnesium. J. Lab. Clin. Med. **55**: 303–310.
WACHSTEIN, M. 1946. Alkaline phosphatase activity in normal and abnormal human blood and bone marrow cells. J. Lab. Clin. Med. **31**: 1–17.
WEAVER, D. D. 1966. Histochemical, fluorometric and electrophoretic analysis of human leukocytic alkaline phosphatase. M.S. Thesis. University of Oregon Medical School, Portland, Ore.

LEUKOCYTE ALKALINE PHOSPHATASE ACTIVITY TEST FOR PREGNANCY

Charles T. Stubblefield*
Kansas City, Kan.

Activity of alkaline phosphatase in mature granular leukocytes in various hematological disorders has attracted considerable attention in recent years. Pritchard,[1] in 1957, using the quantitative chemical technique of Valentine and Beck,[2] first reported the increased alkaline phosphatase activity in pregnancy. Quigley *et al.*[3] used the semiquantitative cytochemical technique of Kaplow[4] on peripheral blood smears to study alkaline phosphatase activity in pregnancy. Later, Harer and Quigley[5] confirmed the increased leukocyte alkaline phosphatase activity (LAPA) in early pregnancy. The following study confirms the work of the above authors and further evaluates the LAPA, frog, and Ortho pregnancy tests.

Material and Methods

Subjects were obtained from the OB-GYN clinics at the Kansas City General Hospital during a three-month period. All new patients admitted to the OB clinics were given the frog (*Rana pipens*) test and the LAPA test; those in the first three months of pregnancy were given the Ortho human chorionic gonadotropin test.

The technique for the LAPA test is as follows: A routine peripheral smear is obtained, following a simple finger prick, similar to that used for differential blood count. The smear is dried at room temperature and prepared according to the modified technique of Kaplow.[4] This involves fixation of the smear in alcohol-formalin mixture for 30 seconds at 0–5° C. The next step is incubation for ten minutes in an alkaline-buffered substrate containing sodium α-napthyl-phosphoric acid and Fast Blue RR.

Hydrolysis of buffered napthylphosphate substrate yields napthyl, which forms a linkage with diamonium amino to give an insoluble, colored precipitate in the cytoplasm of the leukocyte. The nuclei are then counterstained with Mayer's hematoxylin.

After air drying, the slides were examined under oil immersion and 100 neutrophils evaluated. The cells were scored from 0–4, depending on the amount of alkaline phosphatase activity, as follows: 0, colorless cytoplasm; 1, diffuse pale brown with no granules; 2, brown with or without occasional clumps of brownish-black precipitate; 3, brownish-black, unevenly distributed granular precipitate; 4, uniform deep black granular precipitate. The 100 scores were totaled and the following criteria used in evaluating the results: 20–60, not pregnant; 60–80, equivocal, test should be repeated in one week; above 80, pregnant (positive).

The Ortho human chorionic gonadotropin (HCG) test is a two-stage test for detection of chorionic gonadotropin in the urine. The patient's urine is incubated for one hour with the Ortho test antiserum which contains antibodies against human chorionic gonadotropin. In the second stage, Ortho test antigen, a cloudy solution containing latex particles coated with HCG, is added to the incubation mixture. If the patient is pregnant, the Ortho antiserum will neutralize her chorionic gonadotropin. In the second stage, since there is nothing to cause precipitation of the antigen, the solution remains cloudy, giving a positive result. If the urine contains no chorionic gonadotropin, the Ortho antiserum from the

* Medical Building, Suite 104, 155 South 18th St., Kansas City, Kan.

first stage will cause precipitation of the Ortho antigen during the second stage, giving a clear solution for a negative result. For accurate results, the specific gravity of the urine must be above 1.015, and the sample tested within 12 hours of voiding; both of these are important for the accuracy of this test.

The third test is the standard frog *Rana pipens* test in which a mixture of 2 cc of the patient's serum and 2 cc of normal saline are injected into the dorsal lymph sac of a male frog. After two hours the frog is examined for sperm production.

Results

A total of 81 patients, who were definitely pregnant at the initial examination or on subsequent visits, were evaluated with the LAPA and frog tests; patients in the first trimester were also evaluated with the Ortho test. In the series of 81 patients, the LAPA test was accurate in 100 percent of the cases and frog test was accurate in only 65 percent of the cases. Those figures are broken down into the three trimesters in TABLE 1.

Out of the 81 patients, 11 were evaluated with the LAPA, frog, and Ortho tests. The LAPA and Ortho tests were positive in all cases, whereas there were two negative frog results. An additional ten Ortho evaluations could not be done because the specific gravity of the urine was below 1.015.

There were seven negative controls, members of the nursing staff of the hospital, who had an average LAPA score of 17 and negative frog and Ortho tests.

Of special interest was use of the LAPA and frog tests in 11 diagnostic problems. Five of these patients are discussed in the following section.

Case 1. A 33-year-old 300-pound woman, a type of patient frequently seen at General Hospital, who had spotting the past three months at menstrual period time. Her cervix was cyanotic and soft; the size of her uterus could not be determined because of her obesity. Her LAPA score was 44 and the frog test was negative. Six weeks later, she had a normal period.

Case 2. A 31-year-old woman (gravida 7, para 6, abortus 1) whose last menstrual period was three months ago. She had some spotting and cramping for the past two months. Earlier she had symptoms of pregnancy. Dilation and currettage revealed villi. Her LAPA score was 96 and the frog test was negative.

Case 3. A 19-year-old woman (gravida 2, para 2) with a history of irregular menses. She was admitted with a tender pelvis, 102° temperature, white blood cell count of 15,000 and an increased sedimentation rate. This woman had acute pelvic inflammatory disease. She had a false positive LAPA score of 96 with a negative frog test.

Case 4. An 18-year-old woman (gravida 1, para 1) whose last menstrual period was three weeks earlier. She had been on Enovid® pills for some time, but

TABLE 1

ACCURACY OF THE LAPA TEST COMPARED WITH THE FROG TEST IN DIAGNOSING PREGNANCY

No. of Pregnant Patients		LAPA Test Positive	Frog Test Positive	Frog Test Negative
1st trimester	14	14	11	3 (22 percent)
2nd trimester	26	26	20	6 (23 percent)
3rd trimester	41	41	22	19 (46 percent)
Total	81	81	53	28 (65 percent)

had forgotten to take them, and was afraid she was pregnant. The pelvic examination was negative as were her LAPA and frog tests. Later she had a normal period.

Case 5. A 22-year-old woman (gravida 3, para 2) whose last menstrual period was 6 weeks earlier. She was admitted with right lower quadrant pain and spotting for three days. The cervix was cyanotic and the lower uterine segment was soft. She had a right adenexal mass. The cul-de-sac tap was positive indicating blood in the abdomen. Her LAPA score was 96 and the frog test was negative. At surgery, she had an ectopic pregnancy.

Adding these 11 difficult cases to our statistics gives a total of 63 correct frog evaluations and 29 frog errors for an overall accuracy for the frog test of 68 percent. There were 89 correct LAPA determinations and three false positive results for an overall accuracy of 97 percent.

Discussion

Pritchard,[1] Quigley *et al.*,[3] and Harer and Quigley[5] have noted a steady rise in the LAPA scores during pregnancy with a sharp rise during labor. The scores tend to return to normal at six weeks postpartum. All of the reported series are small but tend to follow the same pattern. A slight rise was noted in the average of the trimester scores in our series; the average LAPA score for the first trimester was 135, the second 139, and the third 143. Samples taken during labor were the highest values we obtained; normal readings were obtained at the six-week check-up after delivery.

Because the LAPA score is positive soon after implantation and rises steadily throughout pregnancy, it is somewhat superior to tests depending on the chorionic gonadotropin level, which give reliable results only between the 40–100 day range. Our earliest positive score in this series was three weeks from conception, or a week after the first missed period. Unfortunately, we are handicapped in this clinic because our patients fail to come to the clinic early.

Another advantage of the LAPA test is that it is easy to perform. Smears can be properly stained and counted in less than one hour. The only requirements are a small amount of laboratory space, the stains, and a microscope, making it truly practical and economical for use in offices and small hospitals. The grading of the cells is based on the estimation of the density of the stain, and with practice every technician and office nurse can produce consistently reliable results.

The clinician using this test must realize that elevation of the LAPA scores may also be caused by myeloproliferative disorders, severe infections, extensive tissue damage, and infarction. As with any other laboratory procedure, one must correlate the patient's history and physical findings with the laboratory data to make the correct diagnosis.

The false positive LAPA values have been mentioned. In all the literature on the subject, few false negative LAPA scores are reported and, these occurred early in pregnancy. The frog and LAPA tests are of value in diagnostic problems when run together because the frog test seldom has a false positive and the LAPA test seldom has a false negative reading.

The cause of the increase in alkaline phosphatase activity in the granular leukocyte is unknown; it is independent of the serum alkaline phosphatase. As stated, there is a rise at the time of implantation and a gentle rise during pregnancy, which seems related to the trophoblastic tissue. It does not parallel chorionic gonadotropin activity which is most active between 40–100 days after implantation.

Several authors suggested increased corticosteroids as the cause of the higher

LAPA scores. Normal patients when given adrenal corticotrophic hormone, and high doses of corticosteroids will give a positive (above 80) LAPA score. Adrenal activity seems unlikely, however, because the increased corticosteroids of pregnancy are biologically inactive, and little increase is seen until the end of the first trimester. Others have suggested progesterone as the cause, since there is a steady rise in progesterone throughout pregnancy. Further evidence to support this is a series of 19 patients on Enovid®, 16 of whom had a positive (above 80) LAPA score. Further studies are necessary to determine the etiology of the increase in alkaline phosphatase activity in the granular leukocytes in pregnancy.

Summary

This paper is a study of alkaline phosphatase activity in granular leukocytes as a test for pregnancy in comparison with the frog and Ortho pregnancy tests. Analysis of the results show that the LAPA test is indeed accurate in the early detection of pregnancy. It stays positive during the entire pregnancy and compares favorably with accepted pregnancy tests.

I might add that we have now accumulated some 500 LAPA tests and are still enthusiastic, particularly in its diagnostic importance in ectopic pregnancy. However, the test is more cumbersome than most of the new pregnancy tests and may never assume more than a secondary role in the diagnosis of pregnancy.

References

1. Pritchard, J. A. 1957. Leukocyte alkaline phosphatase activity in pregnancy. J. Lab. Clin. Med. **50:** 432.
2. Valentine, W. N. & W. S. Beck. 1951. Biochemical studies on leukocytes. Phosphatase activity in health, leukocytes, and myelocytic leukemia. J. Lab. Clin. Med. **38:** 39.
3. Quigley, H. J., E. A. Dawson, E. H. Hyum & R. P. Custer. 1960. The activity of alkaline phosphatase in granular leukocytes during pregnancy and the puerperium. A preliminary report. Amer. J. Clin. Path. **33:** 109.
4. Kaplow, L. S. 1955. A histochemical procedure for localizing and evaluating leukocyte alkaline phosphatase activity in smears of blood and marrow. Blood **10:** 1023.
5. Harer, W. B. & H. J. Quigley. 1961. Alkaline phosphatase activity in granular leukocytes as a test for early pregnancy. Obstet. Gynec. **17:**

LEUKOCYTIC ALKALINE PHOSPHATASE IN MYELOPROLIFERATIVE SYNDROME*

W. J. Mitus and K. A. Kiossoglou

Blood Research Laboratory, New England Medical Center Hospitals and the Department of Medicine, Tufts University School of Medicine, Boston, Mass.

Myeloproliferative disorders are characterized by self-perpetuating nonreversible proliferation of bone marrow elements, including their supportive structures such as fibroblasts, reticulin fibers, and osteoblasts. This proliferation occurs not only in the marrow itself, but also in the extramedullary sites, most notably in the spleen and liver. Combinations of various factors, such as preponderance of particular cell type or types, the rate of progression, and the areas of involvement, result in a variety of clinical pictures, some clear cut, some overlapping, and some bizarre. According to Dameshek,[1] polycythemia vera, myelofibrosis with myeloid metaplasia, thrombocytosis, and chronic granulocytic leukemia are representatives of the chronic form of the syndrome, and Di Guglielmo's syndrome of acute erythremic myelosis, erythroleukemia, acute granulocytic leukemia, and acute myelofibrosis are examples of the acute form.

Studies of leukocytic alkaline phosphatase (LAP) in these various groups of disorders show that distinct patterns in the levels of this enzyme occur in many of them (Valentine *et al.*;[2] Mitus *et al.*[3]). This was utilized in differential diagnosis and found to be of value mainly in two areas: (1) in differentiating between chronic granulocytic leukemia and leukemoid reactions and (2) in differentiating between polycythemia vera and secondary erythrocytosis.[4] LAP levels are low in chronic granulocytic leukemia, high in leukemoid reactions, usually high in polycythemia vera, and normal in secondary erythrocytosis.

The purposes of this study were to investigate LAP levels in a large number of patients showing the myeloproliferative syndrome, in an effort to establish the diagnostic significance of this test and to correlate the LAP levels with the chromosomal patterns.

Material and Methods

Thirty-five patients with polycythemia vera, 40 patients with chronic granulocytic leukemia, 30 with myelofibrosis with myeloid metaplasia, 18 with erythremic myelosis or erythroleukemia, 28 with acute granulocytic leukemia, and three with acute myelofibrosis were studied for LAP levels. Diagnosis was established by the usual clinical and hematological criteria. Bone marrow aspiration or biopsy was done in all cases, and splenic puncture was performed in 20 patients with myeloid metaplasia with myelofibrosis. Blood volume studies using the ^{51}Cr method were performed in borderline cases of polycythemia vera. Only patients who could be positively diagnosed as having acute granulocytic leukemia were accepted for this study. Criteria for acceptance were presence of granules in the primitive cells, presence of Auer bodies, and/or positive peroxidase stain in the primitive forms. The LAP levels were estimated by the semiquantitative histochemical method of Kaplow;[5] the normal range of scores found was 15–60. Chromosome studies were performed according to the direct bone marrow method of Kiossoglou *et al.*[6] or, in cases in which no bone marrow could be aspirated, by the short term peripheral blood culture method of Moorhead *et al.*[7]

* Aided with funds from USHS grant no. RO 1 CA 04168–9.

RESULTS

Results for the conditions listed below are summarized in TABLES 1 and 2.

Polycythemia Vera

Thirty-four out of 35 patients had distinctly elevated values of LAP; the other had a level within the normal range. Chromosomal analyses were performed in ten patients (all had elevated LAP levels) and were found to be normal.

TABLE 1

LAP LEVELS IN MYELOPROLIFERATIVE DISORDERS

Diagnosis	No. of Patients	LAP Levels*
Polycythemia vera	34	high
	1	normal
Chronic granulocytic leukemia	38	low
	2	normal
Myelofibrosis with myeloid metaplasis	20	high
	4	normal
	6	low
Atypical myeloproliferative disorder	4	low
Acute granulocytic leukemia	9	high
	8	normal
	11	low
Di Guglielmo syndrome (erythremic myelosis, erythroid leukemia)	8	high
	3	normal
	7	low
Acute myelofibrosis	3	high

* Normal scores = 15–60. Scored according to Kaplow.[5]

TABLE 2

LAP LEVELS CORRELATED WITH CHROMOSOMAL FINDINGS IN MYELOPROLIFERATIVE DISORDERS

Diagnosis	No. of Patients	LAP Levels* High	LAP Levels* Normal	LAP Levels* Low	Chromosomes No Ph[1]	Chromosomes Ph[1]	Chromosomes C trisomy
Polycythemia vera	10	10			10		
Chronic granulocytic leukemia	1		1			1	
	1		1		1		
	1			1	1		
	23			23		23	
Myelofibrosis with myeloid metaplasia	4	4			1		3
Atypical myeloprolifera-ative disorder	4			4	1	1	2
Acute granulocytic leukemia	6	2	3	1		6	
	12	4	4	4	12		

* Normal scores = 15–60. Scored according to Kaplow.[5]

Chronic Granulocytic Leukemia

Out of the 40 patients with chronic granulocytic leukemia (all were adults), 38 had low LAP values and two had normal levels. Chromosomal studies were performed in 26 patients; 24 of whom had low LAP levels and the other two had levels within the normal range. The Philadelphia (Ph^1) chromosome was present in 24 patients. One patient with the Ph^1 chromosome had normal LAP levels. One patient with the classical symptoms of chromic granulocytic leukemia had no Ph^1 chromosome and his LAP level was within the normal range. Another patient with no Ph^1 chromosome showed low LAP scores.

Myelofibrosis with Myeloid Metaplasia

LAP levels were elevated in 20 out of 30 patients with myelofibrosis with myeloid metaplasia, low in six, and within normal range in four. Out of four patients studied for chromosomal patterns (all had high LAP levels), three had marked a neuploidy with C trisomy (previously reported by Kiossoglou *et al.*[8]). No Ph^1 chromosome was present in any of the four.

Atypical Myeloproliferative Disorder

Out of four patients classified as atypical myeloproliferative disorder (all with low LAP levels), hyperdiploidy with C trisomy was present in two, one had normal chromosomes, and one had the Ph^1 chromosome. This last patient was a 13-year-old boy with slight splenomegaly, generalized lymphadenopathy, and leukocytosis (31,000 white blood cells) with 15 percent myelocytes, promyelocytes, and blasts. Nucleated red cells were present in the peripheral blood. Bone marrow was hyperplastic, but all normal elements were present in usual proportions. Tumorous masses consisting of mixed marrow elements were present in the marrow and at autopsy were shown to have originated from the lymph nodes.[8]

Acute Granulocytic Leukemia

Out of the 28 patients studied, LAP levels were low in 11, normal in eight, and elevated in nine. Eighteen of these patients were studied for chromosomal patterns, and six had the Ph^1 chromosomes. Out of these six patients, two had low LAP levels, three were within normal range, and one showed elevated levels. Out of the 12 patients with no Ph^1 chromosome, LAP levels were low in four, normal in four, and elevated in four.

Di Guglielmo's Syndrome (Erythremic Myelosis, Erythroleukemia)

Out of the 18 patients studied, seven had low LAP levels, eight had high levels, and three had levels within the normal range. Chromosomal studies were done in 16 patients (previously reported by Kiossoglou *et al.*[9]). Hypodiploidy was present in six patients, hyperdiploidy in two and monosomy in the G series in three.

Acute Myelofibrosis

LAP levels were estimated in three patients and were found to be elevated in all three.

Discussion

Although LAP levels follow in broad outline the clinical patterns of chronic forms of myeloproliferative syndrome and suggest a diagnostic significance for this test, a small number of cases give results that are inconsistent with the general pattern. Such discrepant findings lower the value of the test. Nevertheless, in differential diagnosis of polycythemia, high LAP values strongly favor the diagnosis of polycythemia vera. In differentiating between leukemoid reactions and chronic granulocytic leukemia, low LAP values strongly support diagnosis of the latter, normal or high LAP levels, however, do not exclude it. The LAP test, like any other test, should be used with discrimination and interpreted with caution.

LAP levels do not correlate well with the chromosomal findings. The Philadelphia chromosome and low LAP values are frequently found together, but this association is not absolute. Low, normal, or even high LAP levels may be encountered in patients with the Ph^1 chromosome, and low LAP levels may be present in patients without the Ph^1 chromosome. Other chromosomal abnormalities encountered, including C trisomy, which is the most common, do not correlate at all with LAP levels. Since, however, LAP is measured in mature neutrophils, and chromosomes are obtained from immature forms, the cell "populations" may not be comparable. It is conceivable that two populations of cells, one leukemic and one normal, coexist in various proportions, and that this may be responsible for the discrepant findings. If caution should be used in interpreting LAP findings, even more caution must be used in interpreting the chromosomal changes and their biochemical effects.

References

1. Dameshek, W. & Gunz. 1967. Leukemia. 2nd edit. : 356. Grune & Stratton, Inc. New York, N. Y.
2. Valentine, W. N., W. S. Beck, J. H. Follette, H. Mills & J. S. Lawrence. 1952. Biochemical studies of chronic myelocytic leukemia, polycythemia vera and other idiopathic myeloproliferative disorders. Blood **7**: 959.
3. Mitus, W. J., L. J. Bergona, I. B. Mednicoff & W. Dameshek. 1958. Alkaline phosphatase of mature neutrophils in chronic forms of myeloproliferative syndrome. Amer. J. Clin. Path. **30**: 285.
4. Mitus, W. J., I. B. Mednicoff & W. Dameshek. 1959. Alkaline phosphatase of mature neutrophils in various "polycythemias." New Eng. J. Med. **260**: 1131.
5. Kaplow, L. S. 1925. A histochemical procedure for localizing and evaluating leukocyte alkaline phosphatase activity in smears of blood and marrow. Blood **10**: 1025.
6. Kiossoglou, K. A., W. J. Mitus & W. Dameshek. 1964. A direct method for chromosome studies of human bone marrow. Amer. J. Clin. Path. **41**: 183.
7. Moorhead, P. S., P. C. Nowell, W. J. Mellman, D. M. Battips & D. A. Hungerford. 1960. Chromosome preparations of leukocyte cultures from human peripheral blood. Exp. Cell. Res. **20**: 613.
8. Kiossoglou, K. A., W. J. Mitus & W. Dameshek. 1965. Cytogenetic studies in the chronic myeloproliferative syndrome. Blood **28**: 241.
9. Kiossoglou, K. A., W. J. Mitus & W. Dameshek. 1965. Chromosomal aberrations in acute leukemia. Blood **26**: 610.

LEUKOCYTE ALKALINE PHOSPHATASE IN THE INFANT

Richard T. O'Kell*
The Children's Mercy Hospital
Kansas City, Mo.

Introduction

Throughout pregnancy the maternal leukocyte alkaline phosphatase (LAP) level rises and at term it is quite high.[1] The LAP level is also elevated in the newborn infant[2] and has been reported to remain high during childhood.[3]

Material and Methods

The LAP levels were studied in 134 normal infants from birth to five months of age. These infants were from St. Luke's Hospital, The Children's Mercy Hospital, and Kansas City General Hospital and Medical Center, Kansas City, Missouri. At birth, blood was obtained from the fetal circulation of the placenta and anticoagulated with phenol-free heparin. Smears were prepared a short time later. All other smears were made from heel-stick capillary blood. The smears were air dried, fixed, and frozen.[2] After thawing, the smears were stained and scored according to Kaplow.[4]

Results

The infant's LAP level is elevated at birth (TABLE 1). During the first five days of life, there is a slow decline in the LAP level. Then, between the fifth and tenth days of life a rapid fall ensues, and by the fifteenth day normal scores (40 ± 20 in our laboratory) are reached. These levels persist at least to the fifth month of life. Of the several factors studied, only length of gestation and birth weight bear any relationship to LAP levels.

Gestation. According to the maternal histories, gestation varied from 30–44 weeks. Sixteen out of the 113 infants for which this information was available were born before the end of the 36th week of gestation. The mean LAP score for this group was 196. Twenty-four were born after the 41st week. The mean score for these infants was 260.

Birth Weight. Twenty-nine of the infants weighed less than 3,000 g and had a mean LAP score of 218, whereas 16 weighed more than 4,000 g and had a mean score of 251.

Labor and Delivery. Information concerning the course of labor and the type and complications of delivery was available for 113 infants. Oxytocins were used 37 times, all without discernible effect on the LAP level. Similarly, the type of delivery did not alter the LAP levels. One hundred and nine deliveries were vertex and four were by caesarean section.

Race. Out of the 134 infants, 120 were white and 14 were Negro. There were no perceptible differences in the LAP levels between the races.

Sex. Eighty infants were male and 54 were female. No differences in LAP levels were apparent between the sexes.

Rh_o (D) factor. The Rh_o (D) factor was available in 113 instances; 80 of the infants were D positive, 33 D negative. This factor appears unrelated to LAP levels.

* Present address: St. Luke's Hospital of Kansas City, Kansas City, Mo.

TABLE 1

LAP SCORES CORRELATED WITH AGE IN 134 INFANTS

No. Infants	Age in Days	Mean Scores*	Standard Deviation
40	0 (Birth)	253	34
15	3	220	28
15	4	219	38
10	5	202	47
10	10	75	26
12	15	32	8
8	30	52	12
8	60	40	9
8	90	48	10
8	150	40	7

* Scored according to Kaplow.[4]

DISCUSSION

The mechanism producing the rising LAP level during pregnancy is active in both the mother and her fetus. Estrogens and progesterone are the most likely mediators in this mechanism. Parallel to the rising LAP level is an increasing production of estrogens[5] and progesterone,[6] all of which freely pass the placenta.[7] The LAP level is likewise elevated in women with hydatidiform mole[8] and in women taking synthetic estrogens and progestational agents as contraceptives.[2] In this latter group the LAP level falls to normal shortly after withdrawal of the hormones. As the infant's urinary estrogens[9] and pregnanediol[10] progressively disappear during the first week of life, a slow decline is also occurring in the LAP level and soon after the complete disappearance of the hormones, a precipitous fall in the LAP level occurs. Certainly these are parallel, if not related, events. In a similar vein, the lesser amounts of estrogens and progesterone present in the earlier months of pregnancy can easily account for the lower LAP scores in premature infants. The levels of estrogens[5] and progesterone[6] also reach a plateau at about the same time the LAP level does.

SUMMARY

The infant's LAP level increases during gestation until about the 36th week and then remains stationary. A slow, progressive decline in the LAP level begins shortly after birth and continues for the first five days of life. Between days five and ten the fall is more rapid, and by day 15 normal levels are reached which persist for the next five months. The changes in LAP levels follow a course parallel to, and seemingly related to, those of estrogens and progesterone.

ACKNOWLEDGMENTS

The technical assistance of Mrs. Loretta Coleman and Mrs. Jean Nicolaisen is greatly appreciated.

REFERENCES

1. PRITCHARD, J. A. 1957. Leukocyte alkaline phosphatase activity in pregnancy. J. Lab. Clin. Med. **50:** 432.
2. O'KELL, R. T. & L. L. AXON. 1965. Leukocyte alkaline phosphatase in the newborn infant. Amer. J. Obstet. Gynec. **93:** 1181.
3. ALTER, A. A., S. L. LEE, M. POURFAR & G. DOBKIN. 1963. Studies of leukocyte alkaline phosphatase in mongolism: A possible chromosome marker. Blood **22:** 165.

4. Kaplow, L. S. 1955. A histochemical procedure for localizing and evaluating leukocyte alkaline phosphatase activity in smears of blood and marrow. Blood **10:** 1023.
5. Brown, J. B. 1956. Urinary excretion of estrogens during pregnancy, lactation and the re-establishment of menstruation. Lancet **i:** 704.
6. Coyle, M. G., F. L. Mitchell & C. S. Russell. 1956. A report on the chromatographic assay of urinary pregnanediol in pregnancy. J. Obstet. Gynec. Brit. Comm. **63:** 560.
7. Avery, G. B. 1964. A brief review of placental function. Clin. Proc. Child. Hosp. (Wash.) **20:** 111.
8. Goldstein, D. P. 1965. Neutrophil alkaline phosphatase activity in patients with choriocarcinoma and related trophoblastic tumors, undelivered hydatidiform mole, and in normal pregnancy. Amer. J. Obstet. Gynec. **92:** 1014.
9. Eastman, N. J. 1956. Williams Obstetrics. 11th edit. : 205. Appleton-Century-Crofts, Inc. New York, N. Y.
10. Roby, C. C., W. B. Ober & J. E. Drorbaugh. 1956. Pregnanediol excretion in the urine of newborn male infants. Pediatrics **17:** 877.

PART IV. NEUTROPHILS IN 21 TRISOMY AND THE LEUKEMIAS

THE PHILADELPHIA CHROMOSOME AND LEUKOCYTE ALKALINE PHOSPHATASE IN CHRONIC MYELOCYTIC LEUKEMIA AND RELATED DISORDERS*

Stephen Krauss

Department of Hematology
The Mount Sinai Hospital, New York, N. Y.

The term "myeloproliferative disease" embraces a number of distinct clinical entities characterized by increased proliferation of one or more hematic and, in some cases, fibroblastic cell lines, in the bone marrow and extramedullary sites. The unknown stimulus to proliferation is postulated to act at the level of a multipotential stem cell, which is capable of giving rise to the various cell types involved in these disorders. Evidence for a fundamental relationship among these diseases has rested chiefly on clinical and hematologic features common to them, the evolution of one clinical disorder into another in the same patient, and the presence of transitional cases combining at one time features of several disorders. The discovery of the minute acrocentric chromosome known as the Philadelphia or Ph^1 chromosome in patients with chronic myelocytic leukemia (CML),[1] together with the finding of low or absent leukocyte alkaline phosphatase (LAP) activity in these patients, has suggested that CML may differ fundamentally from other, apparently related myeloproliferative disorders. Moreover, on the basis of the association of these two findings, it has been postulated that the locus controlling the production of leukocyte alkaline phosphatase resides on the deleted portion of the affected G chromosome.[2] More recent data emphasize that neither observation is diagnostic of CML, and that overlap characterizes the biochemical and cytogenetic, as well as the clinical and hematologic aspects of myeloproliferative disorders. The author and his associates, using a direct technique for bone marrow and short-term culture for peripheral blood metaphase preparations,[3] have observed two groups of patients with CML which illustrate the difficulties in the use of biochemical and cytogenetic parameters for diagnosis. The first group consists of patients with the clinical and hematologic features of CML, but lacking the Ph^1 chromosome (Ph^{1-}); the second consists of patients demonstrating the Ph^1 chromosome (Ph^{1+}), but showing atypical clinical and pathological features.

Out of 33 patients with CML studied cytogenetically, 13 (38 percent) were Ph^{1-}.[4] These patients differed in several respects from the Ph^{1+} patients and from the classic picture of CML. The average age of the 12 males and one female in this group was 65 years (range, 52–76 years) compared with an average age of 52 years (range, 22–79 years) for the Ph^{1+} group of seven males and 13 females. The absence of younger females from the Ph^{1-} group was also noteworthy. Atypical clinical and hematologic findings characterized these Ph^{1-} patients. Thus, they were in general more ill when first seen. Findings in the peripheral blood (FIGURE 1) revealed leukocyte counts that, although, elevated, were usually below 100,000 and platelet counts that were generally below normal. Myeloblasts and promyelocytes (FIGURE 2) tended to persist and even to increase despite therapy. In the bone marrow, the myeloid:erythroid ratio, although elevated, was below the 20–30:1 range usually seen in CML. Blasts and promyelo-

* Supported by USPHS grant no. 2–T4–CA–5076.

cytes, similar in both Ph^{1+} and Ph^{1-} patients initially, tended to increase despite therapy in the Ph^{1-} patients.

Several subclassifications were recognized within this group, including radiation-induced leukemia, eosinophilic leukemia, and CML with myelofibrosis and myeloid metaplasia. The patient with radiation-induced leukemia was a 60-year-old white female, who had received 157 mc of radioactive gold intraperitoneally following a panhysterectomy for adenocarcinoma of the ovary. A leukocyte count at the time of therapy was 6,300. Three years later, splenomegaly and a leukocyte count of 45,000 were discovered in routine follow-up, and the bone marrow aspirate was typical of CML. Of the two patients with eosinophilic leukemia, the first was hematologically a case of typical CML associated with a striking proliferation of eosinophilic myelocytes and granulocytes in the marrow and a peripheral eosinophilia of 50 percent with a leukocyte count of 48,500. Unusual clinical aspects of his course included intractable pruritis, as well as angina pectoris and paroxysmal nocturnal dyspnea refractory to the usual forms of therapy. The prominence of cardiopulmonary signs and symptoms in eosinophilic leukemia has been noted previously. The second patient should perhaps best be

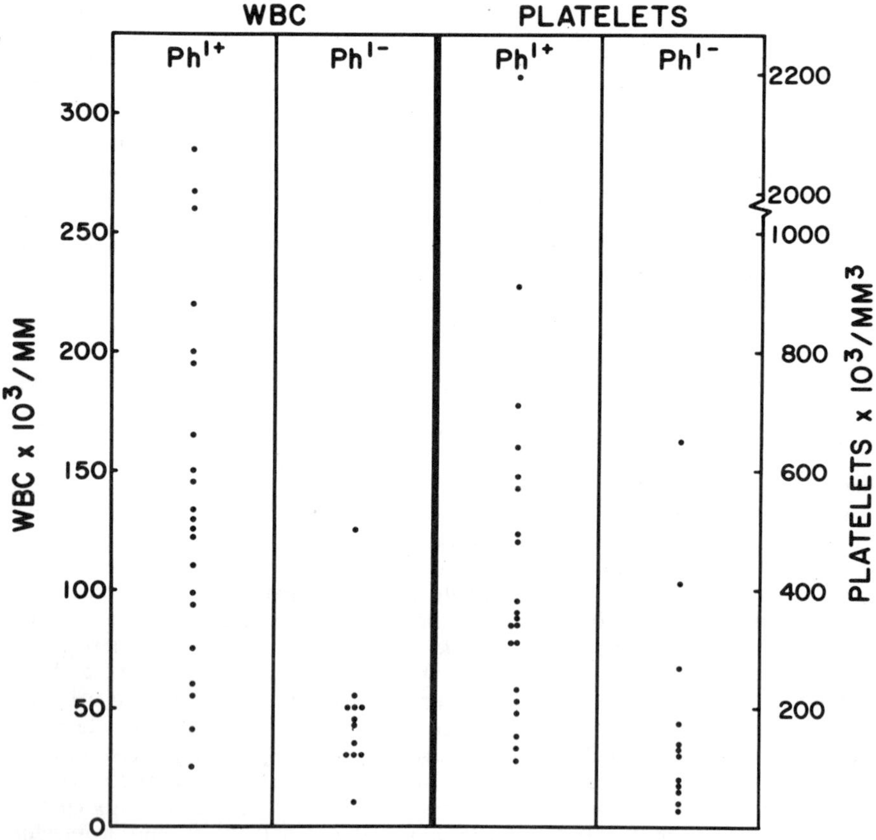

FIGURE 1. Initial leukocyte and platelet counts in peripheral blood of Ph^{1+} and Ph^{1-} patients.

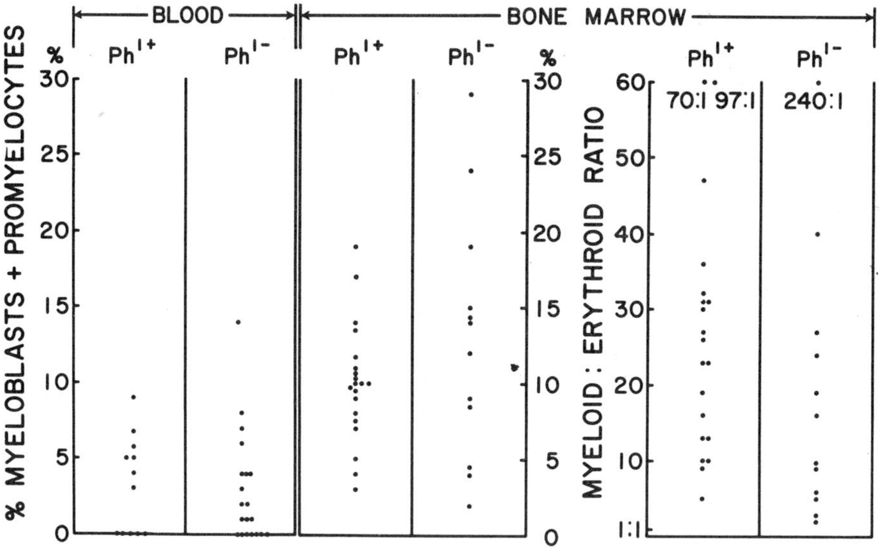

FIGURE 2. Initial hematologic findings: Immature granulocytes (peripheral blood and bone marrow) and myeloid:erythroid ratio (bone marrow) in Ph^{1+} and Ph^{1-} patients.

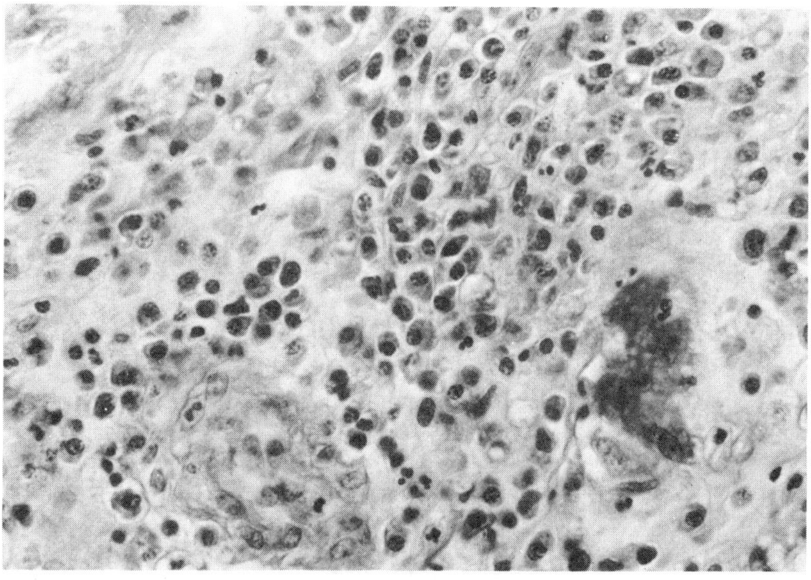

FIGURE 3. Extramedullary hematopoiesis in a testis of a Ph^{1-} patient (case 2, TABLE 1). Note normoblasts in center and left portion of field. H & E. × 400.

classified as "esosinophilic myeloma" by virtue of radiologic findings of widespread osteolytic lesions consisting of mature esosinophils.

The Ph^{1-} patient with CML and myelofibrosis had an initial leukocyte count of 163,000. In addition to the demonstration of fibrosis on bone marrow biopsy, surgical excision of a testicular mass revealed extramedullary hematopoiesis in that organ (FIGURE 3), as did splenic aspiration. In this patient, LAP activity was normal initially and then increased during chemotherapy. In all other Ph^{1-} patients, LAP activity was absent and remained so.

Prognostically, the absence of the Ph^1 chromosome in CML appeared to be of some importance. Using the life-table method (FIGURE 4), the cumulative probability of survival was plotted for both groups. This method takes into account only deaths due to leukemia. The high mortality among Ph^{1-} patients during the first year after diagnosis of leukemia is most striking. Blastic crises occurred in six out of 13 Ph^{1-} patients, whereas only two out of 20 Ph^{1+} cases have shown this evolution. Thus, when patients with CML are classified cytogenetically, it appears that the Ph^{1-} group shows more varied clinical and hematologic features, responds more poorly to therapy, and has a shorter survival time then the Ph^{1+} group.

Atypical features are not, however, confined to the Ph^{1-} group. Out of seven patients combining the clinical and hematologic features of CML with features of myelofibrosis with myeloid metaplasia (synonyms: agnogenic myeloid metaplasia, myelosclerosis with myeloid metaplasia), six were Ph^{1+}.[5] The salient hematologic and pathologic findings are tabulated in TABLE 1.

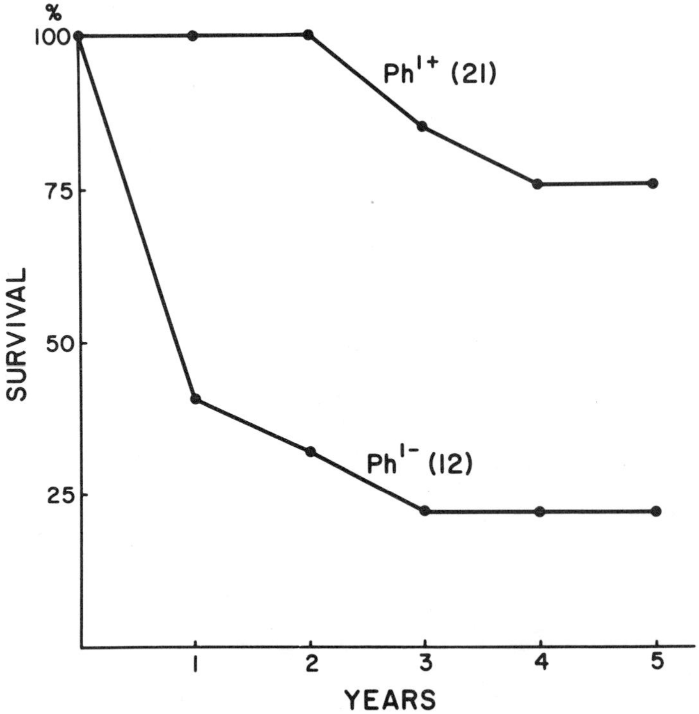

FIGURE 4. Survival time after diagnosis of CML in Ph^{1+} and Ph^{1-} patients, using the life-table method.

TABLE 1

CHRONIC MYELOCYTIC LEUKEMIA SIMULATING MYELOFIBROSIS WITH MYELOID METAPLASIA

			Hematologic Data (Initial Values at RPMI)											
Case	Age at D_x	Sex	WBC	Hb(g)	Platelet Count per mm^3	Percent Blasts	Nucleated RBC's per 100 WBC	Cellularity	M:E Ratio	Megakaryocytes	Bone Marrow Biopsy	Splenic Aspiration	Ph^1 Chromosome	Leukocyte Alkaline Phosphatase Activity
1	22	F	130,500	8.5	357,000	11	2	Normal	12:1	None seen	Osteosclerosis with tremendous increase in megakaryocytes	Cellular, megakaryocytes, many nucleated RBC's	Present	Less than normal (blood); absent (spleen); increased during therapy
2	72	M	163,050	11.9	615,000	1	1	Normal cellularity Several "dry taps"	24:1	Rare	Myelosclerosis and myelofibrosis	Extramedullary hematopoiesis in spleen and left testis	Absent (blood cultures only)	Normal (before therapy); increased (during therapy)
3	56	M	175,000	10.6	655,000	5	1	Normal	5.5:1	Normal	Myelofibrosis	Cellular, many megakaryocytes and normoblasts	Present	Absent
4	41	F	166,500	11.4	650,000	0	0	Increased	32:1	Increased	Myelofibrosis	Surgical specimen, megakaryocytes, foci of extramedullary erythropoiesis	Present	Absent
5	37	F	258,690	7.7	445,000	6	3	Repeated "dry taps"	—	—	Normal bone marrow, megakaryocytes normal	Not done. Extramedullary hematopoiesis in a subcutaneous mass	Present	Absent
6	68	M	220,000	9.0	220,000	2	0	Normal	36:1	Normal	No evidence of fibrosis	Very cellular, over 60 percent nucleated red cells, few megakaryocytes	Present	Absent
7	54	F	143,000	8.1	260,000	2	3	"dry taps"	—	—	Myelofibrosis	Not done	Present	Absent

The diagnosis of CML was based upon (1) marked leukocytosis exceeding 100,000 per mm^3 and greater than 200,000 per mm^3 in two patients, (2) preponderance of granulocytes and granulocyte precursors in the differential count with myeloblasts not exceeding 11 percent, and few nucleated red blood cells; (3) platelet count normal or slightly elevated, (4) mild to moderate anemia (7.7–11.9 g of hemoglobin per 100 ml) and (5) marked increase in the myeloid erythroid (M:E) ratio in the bone marrow in four patients in whom aspirates could be obtained.

In four of the seven patients, myelofibrosis and myeloid metaplasia were found prior to therapy. Among the features noted were: (1) Marked extramedullary hematopoiesis, including numerous erythroid precursors and megakaryocytes, seen upon splenic aspiration in four patients (FIGURE 5) and on pathologic sections following splenectomy in one. In two patients, extramedullary hematopoiesis was demonstrated in unusual sites (the left testis in case 2 and a subcutaneous mass in the buttock in case 5). (2) Fibrosis was found in iliac bone marrow biopsies in five patients (FIGURE 6). Case 5 showed a normal iliac bone marrow biopsy despite numerous "dry taps" on attempted marrow aspiration, and case 6 showed a normal biopsy despite marked extramedullary hematopoiesis in the spleen (FIGURE 7).

Other groups have reported findings similar to ours. Thus, 13 out of 73 patients with the clinical and laboratory features of CML studied at the National Cancer Institute were Ph^{1-}, showed lower leukocyte and platelet counts than the Ph^{1+} group, responded poorly to chemotherapy, and had a median survival time of 18 months compared to 45 months for the Ph^{1+} patients.[6] This series differs from ours in that proportionally fewer Ph^{1-} patients were seen (28 percent). In this group, which included a number of children under seven years of age, females rather than males predominated. These authors also noted that atypical features

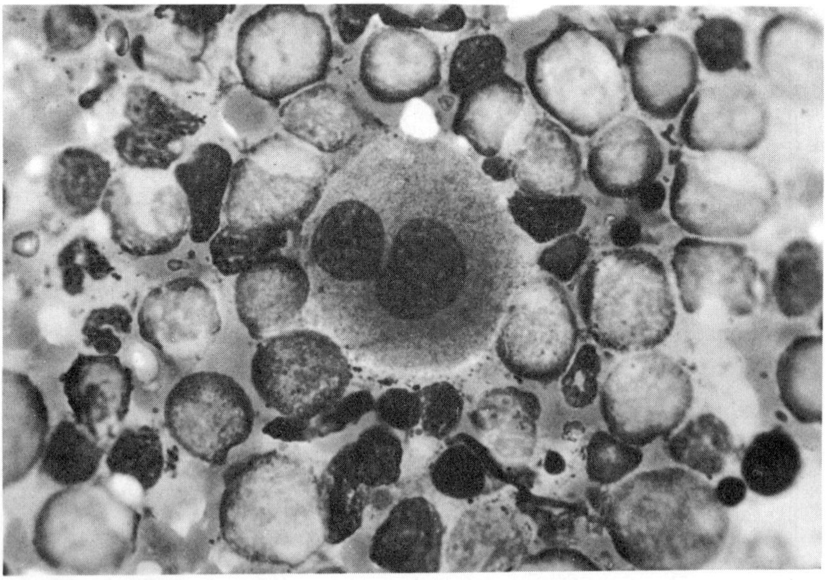

FIGURE 5. Splenic aspirate in a Ph^{1+} patient with fibrosis on marrow biopsy. Note megakaryocyte Wright-Giemsa. × 890.

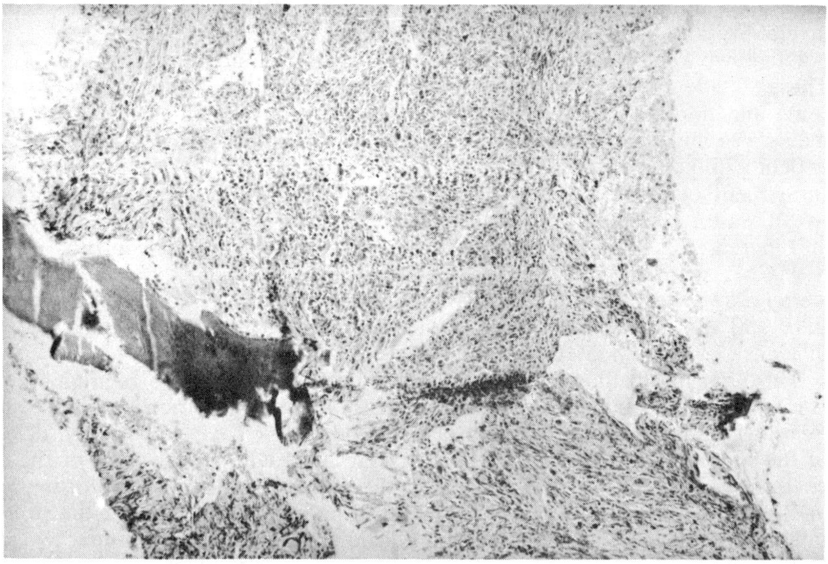

FIGURE 6. Vim-Silverman bone marrow biopsy of a Ph^{1+} patient (case 4, TABLE 1) showing areas of fibrosis, particularly at lower right and upper left H & E. × 90.

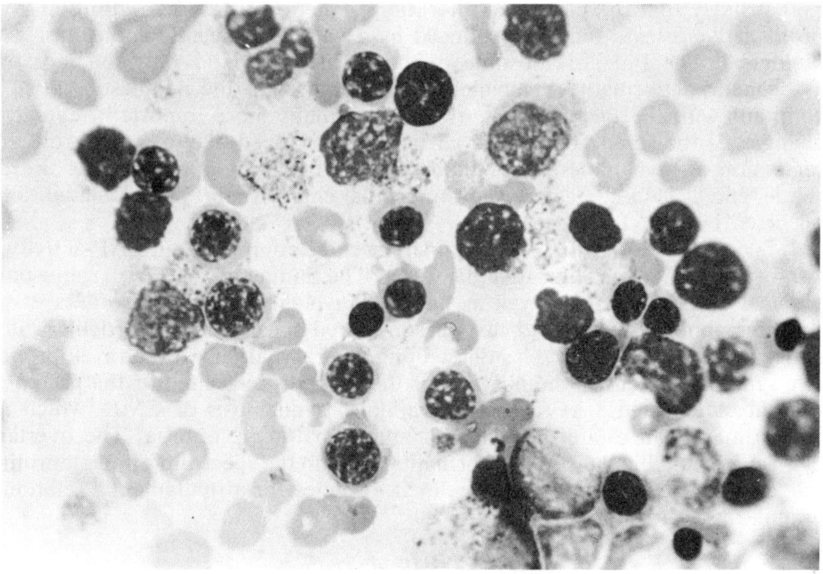

FIGURE 7. Splenic aspirate (case 6) on a Ph^{1+} patient without fibrosis on marrow biopsy. Note the many normoblasts Wright-Giemsa × 890.

were not confined to the Ph^{1-} group, since one of their Ph^{1+} patients showed myelofibrosis, relative leukopenia, and normal LAP activity.

Other workers have reported Ph^{1+} cases with features not typical of CML. These include a patient with eosinophilic leukemia with the Philadelphia chromosome and normal LAP activity;[7] two patients with myelofibrosis with myeloid metaplasia and the Ph^1 chromosome, both with diminished LAP activity;[8,9] one patient with polycythemia vera, the Ph^1 chromosome, and low LAP activity, who subsequently entered a phase of frank CML;[10] and a patient with myeloproliferative disease," resembling essential thrombocythemia, with the Ph^1 chromosome and increased LAP activity.[11] An additional report of interest concerns patients with CML with an onset over the age of 60 years. Although cytogenetic findings were not reported, these patients differed from classic CML in showing increased LAP activity, a lesser degree of splenic and hepatic enlargement, and a greater incidence of thrombocytosis than that seen in younger patients.[12]

This brief survey illustrates the difficulties in any attempted correlation between LAP activity, karotype and clinical diagnosis. A simple gene dose-enzyme content relationship based on the frequent association of low LAP activity and deletion of the long arm of chromosome 21[2] appears untenable in the light of the data cited above. In addition, the simple gene-dose theory cannot account for increases in LAP activity that may occur in CML during remission, or under the stress of intercurrent infections, inflammation, blastic crisis, or steroid therapy.

The relationship between the Ph^1 chromosome and the leukemic process itself also defies a simple explanation. Earlier speculation, based on a history of radiation therapy for ankylosing spondylitis in two Ph^{1-} patients with CML, suggested that this variant of CML was radiation-induced.[13] On the other hand, we have seen both Ph^{1+} and Ph^{1-} patients with CML which satisfy criteria for radiation-induced leukemia, and a Ph^{1+} patient with CML has been reported in a survivor of the atomic bombing of Hiroshima.[14]

It is likely that the presumed alteration of stem cell DNA resulting in myeloproliferative disease may be produced by a variety of agents, both physical and biological. The Ph^1 chromosome might be thought of as only the most gross cytogenetic abnormality associated with the onset of the neoplastic state, concomitant with the development of other, perhaps more important, cytogenetic changes. If the small acrocentric chromosomes indeed play a crucial role in the regulation of myelopoiesis and the development of myeloproliferative disorders, subtle, and as yet undetectable, chromosomal changes must be postulated to have occurred in Ph^{1-} patients.

It is concluded that there is no apparent correlation between LAP activity and karyotype in myeloproliferative disorders. The finding of the Ph^1 chromosome in atypical cases of CML as well as in other myeloproliferative disorders suggests that this abnormality should not be considered specific for a particular clinical entity, but rather may serve as one among several markers of the myeloproliferative syndrome. Neither the absence of the Ph^1 chromosome nor the presence of normal or elevated LAP activity invalidates a diagnosis of CML, which must rest primarily on established clinical and hematologic criteria. The overlap of cytogenetic and biochemical abnormalities within the spectrum of myeloproliferative diseases provides additional indirect evidence for a fundamental relationship among these disorders.

References

1. NOWELL, P. C. & D. A. HUNGERFORD. 1961. Chromosome studies in human leukemia. II. Chronic granulocytic leukemia. J. Nat. Cancer Inst. **27:** 1013.

2. ALTER, A. A., S. L. LEE, M. POURFAR & G. DOBKIN. 1963. Studies of leukocyte alkaline phosphatase in mongolism: A possible chromosome marker. Blood **22:** 165.
3. SANDBERG, A. A., T. ISHIHARA, L. H. CROSSWHITE & T. S. HAUSCHKA. 1962. Comparison of chromosome constitution in chronic myelocytic leukemia and other myeloproliferative disorders. Blood **20:** 393.
4. KRAUSS, S., J. E. SOKAL & A. A. SANDBERG. 1964. Comparison of Philadelphia chromosome-positive and -negative patients with chronic myelocytic leukemia. Ann. Intern. Med. **61:** 625.
5. KRAUSS, S. 1966. Chronic myelocytic leukemia with features simulating myelofibrosis with myeloid metaplasia. Cancer **19:** 1321.
6. TJIO, J. H., P. P. CARBONE, J. WHANG & E. FREI III. 1966. The Philadelphia chromosome and chronic myelogenous leukemia. J. Nat Cancer Inst. **36:** 567.
7. GRUENWALD, H., K. A. KIOSSOGLOU, W. J. MITUS & W. DAMESHEK. 1965. The Philadelphia chromosome in eosinophilic leukemia. Amer. J. Med. **39:** 1003.
8. BOWEN, P. & C. S. N. LEE. 1963. Ph[1] chromosome in the diagnosis of chronic myeloid leukemia: report of a case with features simulating myelofibrosis. Bull. Hopkins Hosp. **1:** 113.
9. FORRESTER, R. H. & J. M. LOURO. 1966. Philadelphia chromosome abnormality in agnogenic myeloid metaplasia. Ann. Intern. Med. **64:** 622.
10. KEMP, N. H., J. L. STAFFORD & R. TANNER. 1964. Chromosome studies during early and terminal chronic myeloid leukemia. Brit. Med. J. **1:** 1010.
11. HEATH, C. W. & W. C. MOLONEY. 1965. The Philadelphia chromosome in an unusual case of myeloproliferative disease. Blood **26:** 471.
12. CONRAD, M. E., H. RAPPAPORT & W. H. CROSBY. 1965. Chronic granulocytic leukemia in the aged. Arch. Intern. Med. **116:** 765.
13. TOUGH, I. M., A. G. BAIKIE, D. G. HARNDEN, W. M. COURT BROWN, K. E. BUCKTON, P. A. JACOBS & O. A. WILLIAMS. 1962. Chronic myeloid leukemia: cytogenetic studies before and after splenic irradiation. Lancet **ii:** 115.
14. TANAKA, N., K. ITO, N. KAMADA & K. OKADA. 1963. A case of an atomic bomb survivor with chronic granulocytic leukemia in the early stage. J. Kyushu Hemat. Soc. **13:** 124.

LEUKOCYTE ALKALINE PHOSPHATASE IN CHRONIC GRANULOCYTIC LEUKEMIA OF CHILDHOOD*

Robert B. Rosen and Hiroshi Nishiyama
City of Hope Medical Center
Duarte, Calif.

Although infrequent in childhood, chronic granulocytic leukemia (CGL) is by far the most common representative of the nonacute leukemias encountered at an early age. The majority of pediatric cases conform to the well-defined, classic disease as it is widely known in adults. However, an atypical variant usually found during the first few years of life has also been recognized. This so-called infantile or juvenile type differs from the usual disorder both clinically and hematologically. In addition, whereas no specific cytogenetic abnormality has been demonstrated in the atypical disease, the presence of the Philadelphia (Ph^1) chromosome appears to be a specific marker of classic CGL in childhood.[1,2]

One of the more familiar laboratory features of CGL is the reduction or absence of leukocyte alkaline phosphatase (LAP) activity in mature neutrophils.[3,4] This finding has been the subject of an extensive literature, but systematic studies on the enzyme specifically in affected infants and children have not been reported. The purpose of this presentation is to examine in detail the behavior of LAP during the course of CGL in childhood, based on experience with 19 patients. Certain theories concerning the production and regulation of LAP will also be considered in the light of observations on these patients.

Material and Methods

The patient groups were composed of 13 children with classic CGL ranging in age, at diagnosis, from 18 months to 16 years, and six children with atypical CGL, who were five to 16 months old. Clinical and hematological criteria for assignment of patients to the atypical category included a relatively acute course characterized by hemorrhage, infection, and unresponsiveness to busulfan; the presence of lymphadenopathy, hepatomegaly, and occasionally, facial rash; and findings of amegakaryocytic thrombocytopenia and a degree of anemia, granulocyte immaturity, normoblastosis, and monocytosis exceeding that of classic CGL.

Cytogenetic analyses were carried out on bone marrow metaphases by a modification of the direct method of Sandberg *et al.*[5] Every patient with classic CGL had the Philadelphia chromosome (Ph^{1+}); no such abnormality was found in any of the children with the atypical disease (Ph^{1-}).

Leukocyte alkaline phosphatase activity was determined by the semiquantitative histochemical technique and scoring method of Kaplow.[6] Capillary blood smears were fixed within one hour and stained no later than three hours after preparation. At least 300 neutrophils were counted from two or more thin blood films by the same observer (R.B.R.). Positive and negative controls were stained and scored simultaneously.

Results

LAP Activity in Untreated Classic and Atypical CGL

In eight children with classic (Ph^{1+}) CGL, the LAP scores prior to specific therapy were consistently lower (mean 3.5 ± 2.1) than in five infants with the

* This work was made possible, in part, by a supporting fund established in the name of Ernest W. Hahn.

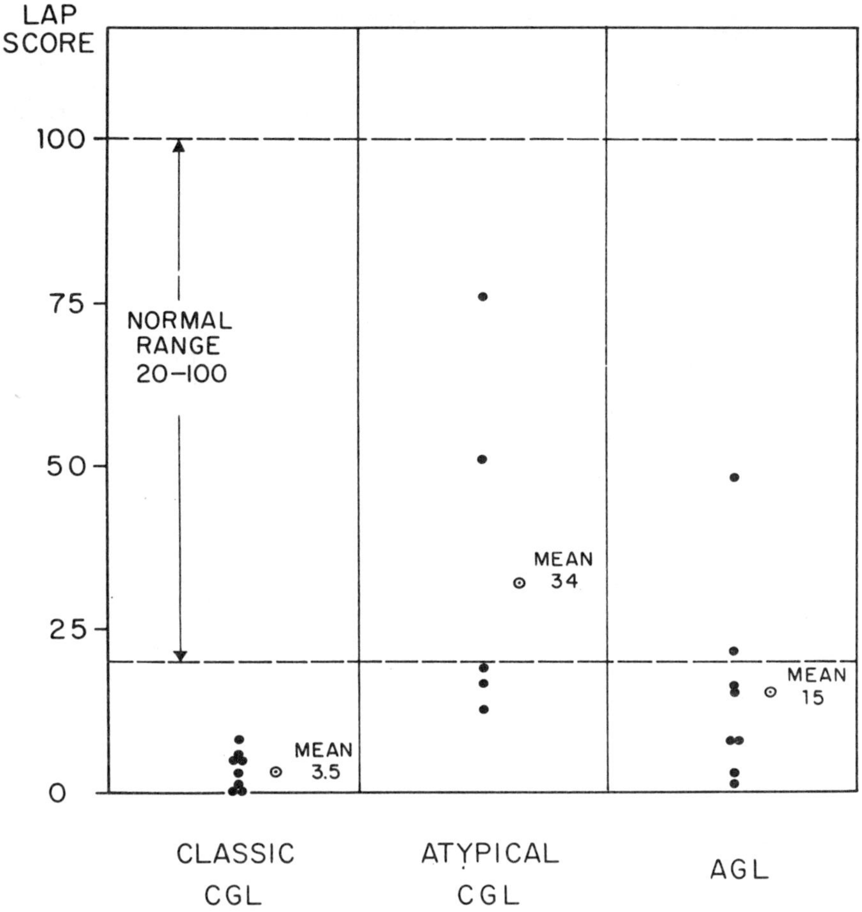

FIGURE 1. LAP scores in children with classic CGL, atypical CGL and *de novo* acute granulocytic leukemia (AGL), all prior to specific therapy.

atypical (Ph^{1-}) disorder (mean 34.2 ± 22.6) (FIGURE 1). The difference in means is significant by the "t" test at the 5 percent level. The activities in the classic cases were tightly clustered as opposed to greater scatter in the atypical variant. Two out of the five scores in the Ph^{1-} group were within the normal range (20–100) before antileukemic treatment and in the apparent absence of infection or other stressful situations. The higher values in these patients did not appear to be simply a function of age; one child in the Ph^{1+} group was barely 18 months old at the time of diagnosis and had very low scores (3–5). For comparison, LAP levels in eight children with acute granulocytic leukemia arising *de novo* are also plotted in FIGURE 1. The mean value in this situation (15.1 ± 14.1) was also lower than in the Ph^{1-} group of patients, although there was considerable overlap of individual scores. However, LAP activity in the Ph^{1-} group was not as high as in most Ph^{1+} cases after the latter had progressed to the acute phase, when values well above normal were usual.

LAP Activity During Course of Classic CGL

Enzyme activity in most patients with the more common type of childhood CGL was followed serially throughout various stages of the disease. FIGURE 2 depicts these findings. In only one out of eight children did the score rise to normal after induction of complete remission with busulfan. This particular patient remained in remission less than six months before pancytopenia ("marrow insufficiency") developed and the blast crisis supervened. The course in two other patients displayed a similar pattern of marrow insufficiency preceding acute transformation and in both, LAP activity increased during these periods.

Out of six patients studied during the acute phase of CGL, LAP scores were high in four and normal in two. One of the latter, however, was already in the terminal stages of the blast cell crisis when first evaluated. Two children remained in the myeloblast stage for more than 12 months and the earlier increased activity tended to abate as the disease neared termination. There was also a trend toward

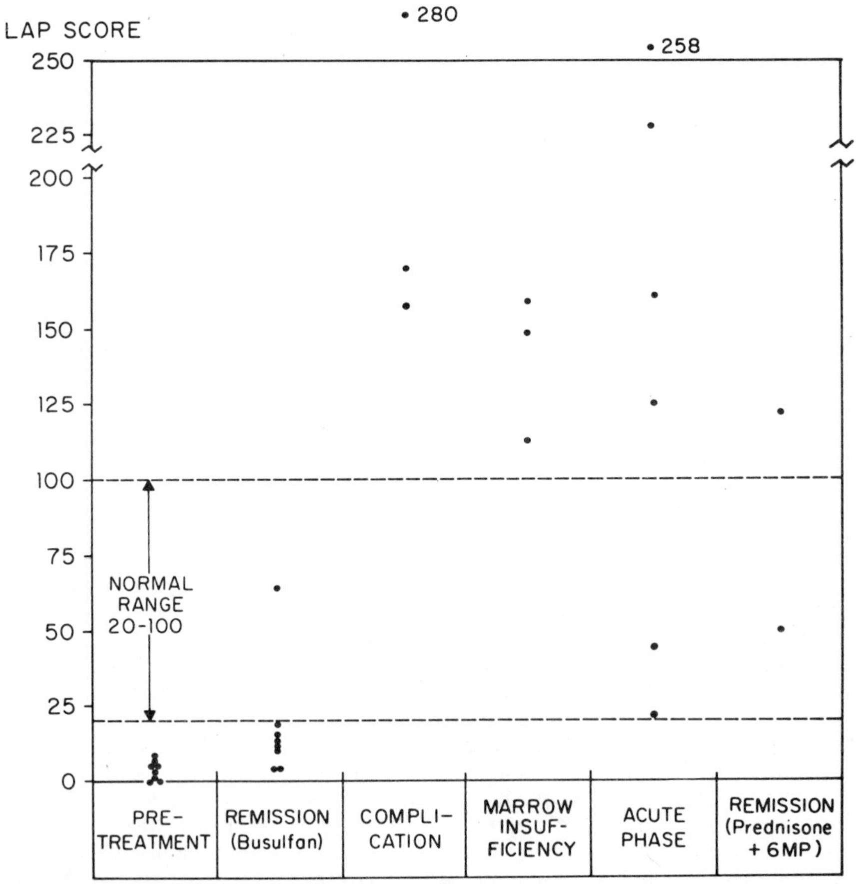

FIGURE 2. LAP activity during various landmarks of classic CGL in 13 children. Scores within each category represent the mean of several determinations in individual patients.

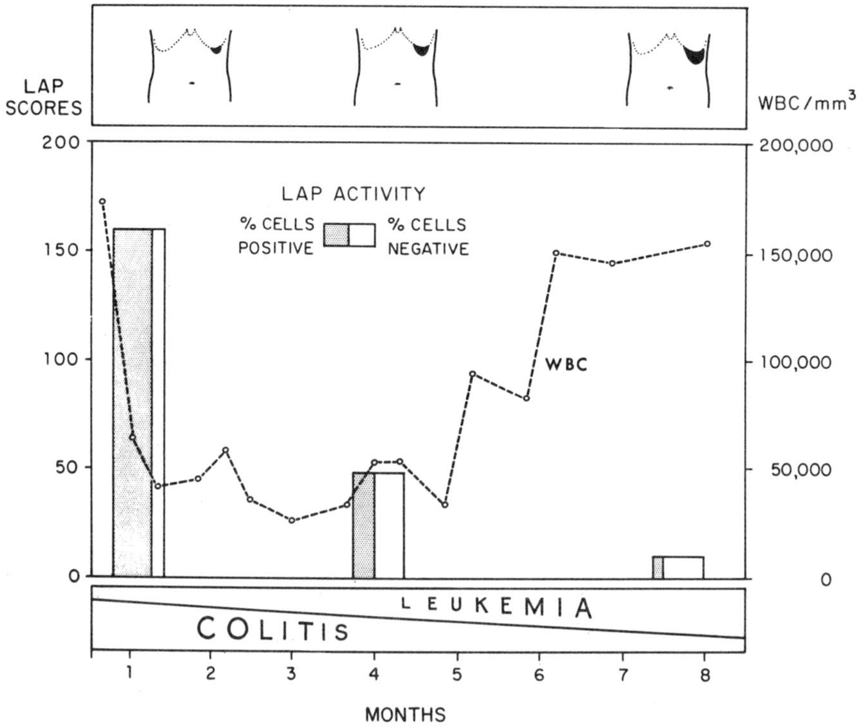

FIGURE 3. Concurrent CGL and ulcerative colitis in a 16-year-old male. Only anticolitis therapy was administered during the period shown. Busulfan therapy was started one month later and resulted in a complete remission of the leukemia. At the top, enlargement of the spleen below the costal margin is illustrated.

lower values during the few brief remissions which followed therapy with prednisone and 6-mercaptopurine.

Among the complications encountered in the course of the chronic stage, bronchopneumonia occurred in two children and was associated with transient but sharp rises in LAP activity. In one boy, early CGL coexisted with active ulcerative colitis;[7] the inflammatory stimulus evoked a brisk LAP response that subsided as the colitis was brought under control (FIGURE 3).

One child had at least eight separate bouts of leukemic meningitis over an 18 month period during the acute phase of CGL (FIGURE 4). Extremely high levels of LAP generally corresponded to episodes of central nervous system involvement and spinal fluid pleocytosis. After treatment with intrathecal methotrexate, LAP activity returned to normal on several occasions. In the final months of the disease, scoring became increasingly difficult because of progressive neutropenia, but as a rule the enzyme content of remaining polymorphs was reduced.

LAP Activity During Course of Atypical CGL

The Ph^{1-} variant of childhood CGL pursues a rather acute course dominated by hemorrhage and is, by and large, unresponsive to chemotherapy. Furthermore, in none of the five patients of our series, who have thus far died, has there been transition into the myeloblast phase that is commonly the terminal event in the usual form of CGL. For these reasons, it is not possible to make point-by-point comparisons between the Ph^{1+} and Ph^{1-} categories with respect to LAP activity at different landmarks of the disease. However, practically all the Ph^{1-} patients had recurrent infections, especially while being treated with busulfan, 6-mercaptopurine, and prednisone. They were particularly prone to bronchopneumonia, suppurative lymphadenitis and furunculosis. Paradoxically, these children did not react to infection with as high LAP activity as did some of the patients in the Ph^{1+} group. In the Ph^{1-} patients, LAP values usually rose to normal or to a moderately high level, but did not achieve the extremely high levels occasionally recorded in classic CGL during comparable bouts of infection.

Comparison of LAP Activity in Children and Adults with CGL

The above observations, at least as they pertain to the classic disease in children, generally accord with many of the results that have been reported in adults.[8-10] One difference, the failure of LAP to rise significantly during remission in most patients of this series, could possibly be related to the degree of response to busulfan therapy. In adults, LAP actively has been reported to increase more frequently with complete remissions than with only partial responses to chemotherapy.[8,9] Although the eight remissions in the children treated with busulfan were classified as "complete," they may not have been strictly comparable to those of the older individuals.

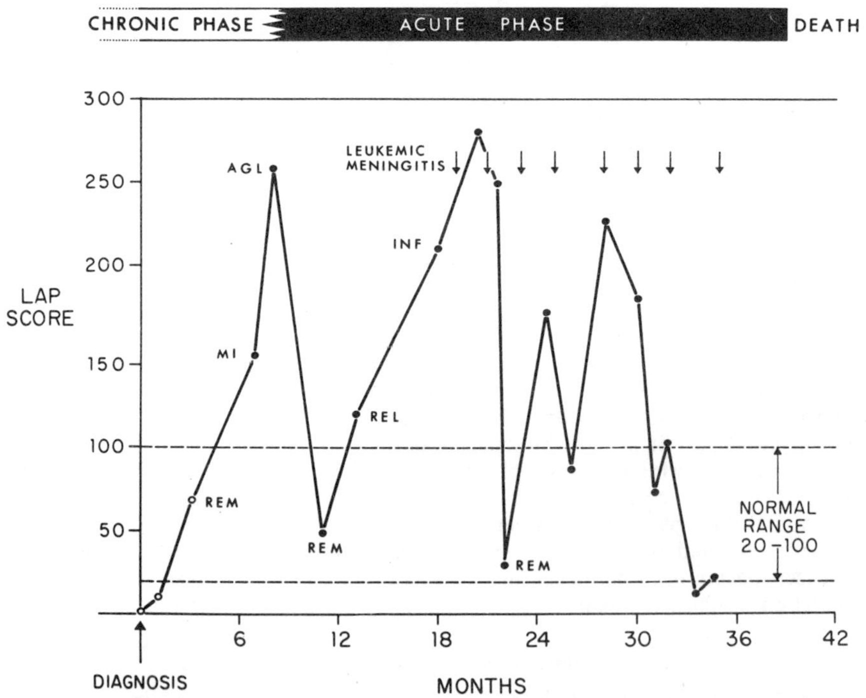

FIGURE 4. LAP activity during course of classic (Ph^{1+}) CGL in an 18-month-old male. Recurrent bouts of leukemic meningitis are indicated by arrows. REM = remission, MI = marrow insufficiency, AGL = acute phase, REL = relapse, INF = infection.

The other point of divergence is that higher LAP values were found in the Ph^{1-} children than in the Ph^{1+} children, as compared with the low activities reported in both Ph^{1-} and Ph^{1+} adults with CGL.[8–11] Theoretically, this discrepancy might be attributable to the presence of occult infection in the highly susceptible infants. Clinically, however, there was no evidence of intercurrent infection in any of these babies at the time of baseline LAP activity determinations. Age itself does not appear to be a factor, since in our experience LAP levels do not differ significantly in infants, children, or adults under similar circumstances. However, the higher LAP activity in the untreated atypical disease does suggest a fundamental difference between the so-called infantile or juvenile type of CGL and classic CGL. Considering also the clinical, hematological, and cytogenetic features of the atypical disease, its classification as a separate entity would seem appropriate.

Dynamics of LAP Activity

Attempts to explain the behavior of LAP and to interpret descriptive material such as that presented here have taken several directions. The theories that appear to be most widely held and to have stimulated the greatest interest involve the following concepts: (1) the existence of a mixed population of leukocytes, (2) the dependence of enzyme activity on cell age, and (3) the control of LAP synthesis by genes located on chromosome 21. These will be considered in order.

Multiple Population Theory

The increases in LAP activity during intercurrent infection[12] and remission[13,14] of CGL have been ascribed to the persistence or emergence of a functionally normal line of neutrophils. Indeed, multiple clones have been demonstrated cytogenetically in the blood or bone marrow of some patients with CGL.[15–17]

In the boy whose clinical course is shown in FIGURE 3, the possibility that the ulcerative colitis stimulated strong LAP activity in a residual population of "normal" polymorphs had to be considered, especially since the leukemia was in a relatively early stage at the time of diagnosis. Kemp *et al.*[16] have suggested that this might be the case in one of their patients with normal LAP activity and a Ph^{1-} (normal) cell line in the peripheral blood. However, in our patient no Ph^{1-} bone marrow metaphases were found; moreover, at the height of the inflammatory process (FIGURE 5), analysis of the distribution of LAP revealed activity in 73 percent of his circulating neutrophils. It is most unlikely that this number of cells could have descended from Ph^{1-} (normal) precursors when, in fact, all karyotyped bone marrow metaphases showed the Ph^1 abnormality.

Another indication that enzyme activity in CGL is not just confined to a minor population of strongly staining normal cells may be found in the relatively large number of LAP-positive neutrophils often present during infection and myeloblast crisis. Occasionally under these circumstances as many as 95 percent of the neutrophils stain for LAP (FIGURE 6). Inasmuch as during myeloblastic transformation the Ph^1 chromosome persists, or may even be augmented,[15] the overwhelming majority of LAP-positive cells must arise from genetically abnormal (Ph^{1+}) progenitors. Thus, although the concept of "end cell failure" in the CGL polymorph probably applies under certain conditions,[4] it is evident, as suggested by King *et al.*,[18] that cells derived from leukemic forerunners do retain the potential for LAP activity. Therefore, it is unnecessary to evoke a normal cell line to account for increases in LAP activity in the course of CGL. Interestingly, in one of our patients who did have a dual bone marrow population of Ph^{1-} and Ph^{1+}

cells, LAP activity was very low prior to therapy and remained so even during complete remission.

Cell Age Theory

Hook and Engle[19] have postulated that LAP activity is a function of cell age and have attributed the deficiency of enzyme in CGL to a prolonged neutrophil life-span.

To test this hypothesis, simultaneous neutrophil lobe counts and LAP cell ratings have been performed. In the patient with CGL complicated by active ulcerative colitis, "older" neutrophils with three or more nuclear segments actually displayed greater LAP activity than presumably younger cells with fewer lobes.[20] Under these conditions, the LAP content and morphological age of neutrophils did not appear to be inversely related.

This conclusion presupposes the validity of Arneth's time-honored concept that as neutrophils mature their nuclei undergo progressive segmentation. Recent studies utilizing tritiated thymidine have demonstrated no difference in the rela-

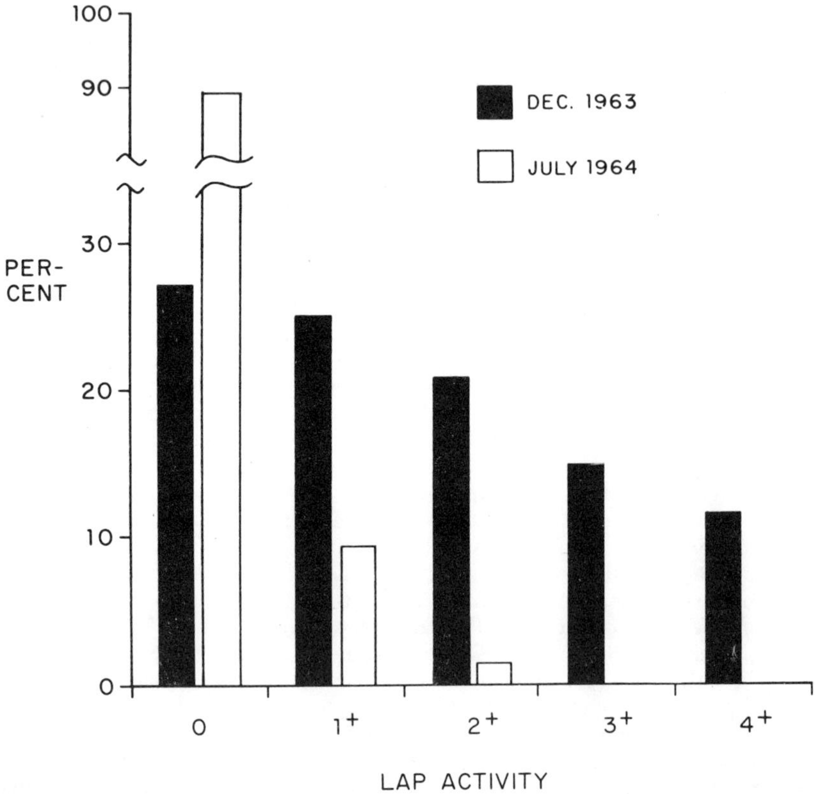

FIGURE 5. Distribution of alkaline phosphatase in neutrophils of same patient as in FIGURE 3 during active (Dec., 1963) and quiescent (July, 1964) stages of ulcerative colitis. Note the large percentage of LAP-positive cells associated with the acute inflammatory process despite the presence of the Ph[1] chromosome in 100 percent of this boy's bone marrow metaphases.

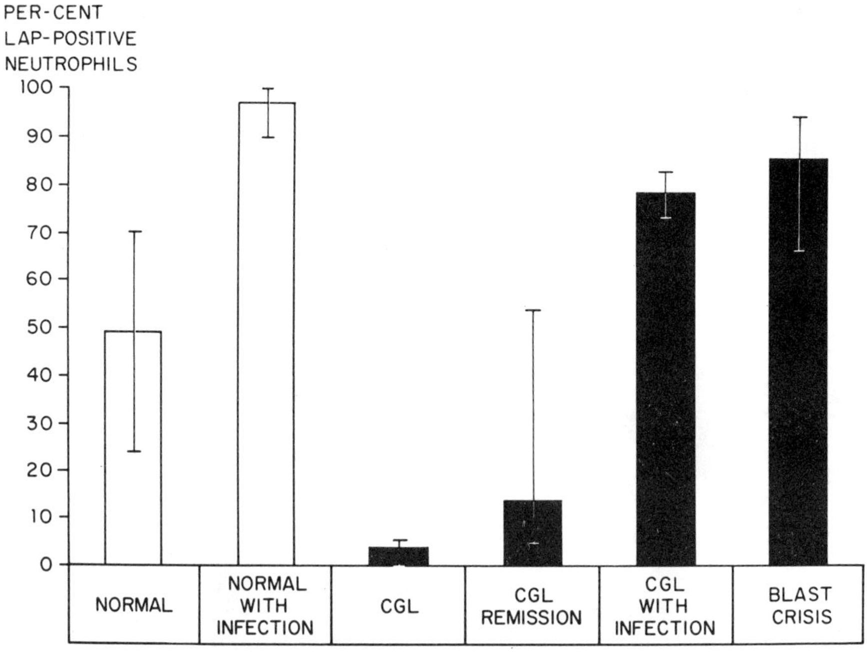

FIGURE 6. LAP responses in normal subjects and in children with classic (Ph^{1+}) CGL. The high LAP scores in CGL, complicated by infection and during the blast cell crisis, result from activity in many circulating neutrophils rather than intense staining of few cells.

tive age of neutrophils with two, three, four, five, or more nuclear lobes.[21] However, the earlier emergence time of labeled band-forms suggested that these unsegmented cells were indeed younger.

In subsequent studies, we therefore compared the LAP activity of segmented versus nonsegmented neutrophils in diverse conditions associated with enzyme elevations (FIGURE 7). Even under circumstances of a "shift to the left" in the differential formula, very few band-forms ("juvenile" neutrophils) earned a strong rating, whereas a disproportionate number of apparently older cells was consistently more heavily stained. Similarly, the total LAP score per 100 segmented neutrophils was higher than that of 100 nonsegmented neutrophils in each of the categories investigated.

These findings do not lend support to the contention that cell age per se, at least as reflected by nuclear segmentation, is an important determinant of LAP activity.

Gene Deletion Theories

The deletion of a segment of the long arm of chromosome 21 found with the low to absent LAP activity in CGL has been interpreted as a gene-dose effect.[22] If this were so, the irretrievable loss of a structural gene governing LAP synthesis should impose limitations on enzyme activity, so that fluctuations within a relatively narrow range about the 50 percent level should be expected. It is difficult to explain the observed values of LAP activity in untreated classic CGL if two genes confer 100 percent activity and the patient still possesses one gene. Furthermore, diminished enzyme levels have been reported in miscellaneous, nonleukemic conditions,[23] as well as in otherwise typical cases of CGL lacking the Ph[1] deletion.[24] Conversely, normal or greatly increased LAP activity may occur in CGL despite the persistence of the genetic defect throughout the course of the disease.

Such observations suggest that LAP production may be independent of genes on chromosome 21 or that regulation at the genetic level is sensitive, if not subordinate, to other factors of a physiological or endocrine nature that influence the cellular environment. As an alternative to the simple gene-dose theory, a

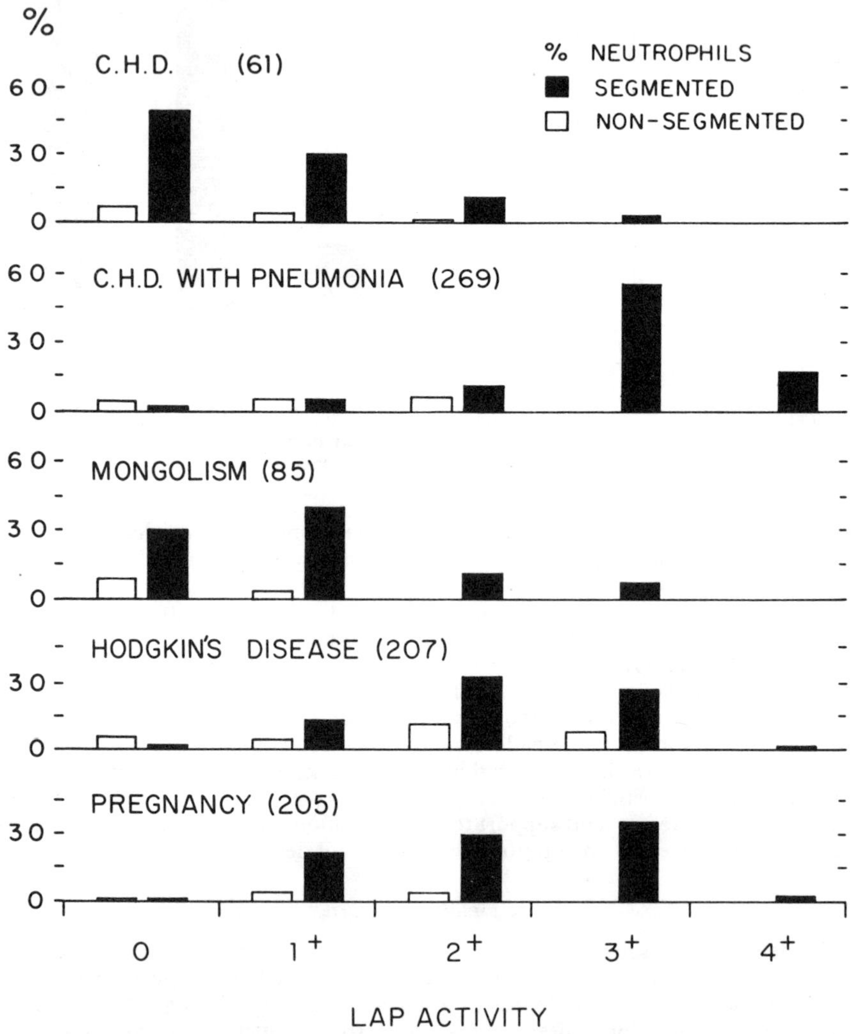

FIGURE 7. LAP in segmented and nonsegmented neutrophils of a hematologically normal child (C. H. D.), and in conditions with high levels of the enzyme. Figures in parentheses refer to total LAP scores. Segmented ("older") neutrophils contribute a major share of LAP activity even when there is a relative increase in nonsegmented ("juvenile") cells.

hypothesis based on the model of Jacob and Monod[25] has been proposed.[7] Sequential negative control of the structural gene for LAP by a pair of regulators is postulated. On this assumption, deletion of one of the regulators (modifier) from chromosome 21 in CGL, should result in inhibition of the corresponding structural gene and a decrease in enzyme production. Further, if the inhibitory substance were a diffusible protein it should also repress the modifier of the trans-chromosome, thereby additionally reducing total LAP activity to well below 50 percent of normal, as expected in uncomplicated CGL. Changes in the opposite direction associated with intercurrent infection and blast cell crisis, for example, require an increase in modifier substance on the intact chromosome which, in turn, would counteract the regulators and release from inhibition the structural genes for LAP on both chromosomes of the 21st pair.

This theory, although it can be made to account for a number of aspects of LAP behavior in CGL, remains speculative since the crucial modulators of gene action in man have not yet been identified.

Summary and Conclusions

Leukocyte alkaline phosphatase (LAP) activity has been assessed histochemically in a group of 19 pediatric patients with chronic granulocytic leukemia (CGL).

Prior to busulfan therapy, mean LAP scores were significantly higher in the atypical (Ph^{1-}) variant than in the classic (Ph^{1+}) disease. In the latter group enzyme activity usually remained low during remission, whereas moderate to marked increases accompanied intercurrent infection, marrow insufficiency, and myeloblast transformation. In the Ph^{1-} patients LAP activity also increased in infection, although to a lesser extent. On the basis of these and other differences, it is suggested that the atypical disease is a distinctive entity.

Of several theories advanced to explain the dynamic behavior of LAP, none appear to do so fully and all lack experimental confirmation. Multiple factors are probably operative in the control of LAP synthesis and, at most, genes on chromosome 21 constitute one facet of this complex system. In CGL, a direct relationship between the enzymatic (LAP) and cytogenetic (Ph^1 chromosome) abnormalities has not been established.

References

1. Reisman, L. E. & J. M. Trujillo. 1963. Chronic granulocytic leukemia of childhood. J. Pediat. **62:** 710–723.
2. Hardisty, R. M., D. E. Speed & M. Till. 1964. Granulocytic leukaemia in childhood. Brit. J. Haemat. **10:** 551–566.
3. Wachstein, M. 1946. Alkaline phosphatase activity in normal and abnormal human blood and bone marrow cells. J. Lab. Clin. Med. **31:** 1–17.
4. Valentine, W. N. & W. S. Beck. 1951. Biochemical studies on leucocytes. I. Phosphatase activity in health, leucocytosis, and myelocytic leucemia. J. Lab. Clin. Med. **38:** 39–55.
5. Sandberg, A. A., G. F. Koepf, L. H. Crosswhite & T. S. Hauschka. 1960. The chromosome constitution of human marrow in various developmental and blood disorders. Amer. J. Hum. Genet. **12:** 231–249.
6. Kaplow, L. S. 1963. Cytochemistry of leukocyte alkaline phosphatase. Amer. J. Clin. Path. **39:** 439–449.
7. Rosen, R. B. & R. L. Teplitz. 1965. Chronic granulocytic leukemia complicated by ulcerative colitis: Elevated leukocyte alkaline phosphatase and possible modifier gene deletion. Blood **26:** 148–156.
8. Block, J. B., P. P. Carbone, J. J. Oppenheim & E. Frei, III. 1963. The effect of treatment in patients with chronic myelogenous leukemia. Biochemical studies. Ann. Intern. Med. **59:** 629–636.

9. Frei, E., III, J. H. Tjio, J. Whang & P. P. Carbone. 1964. Studies of the Philadelphia chromosome in patients with chronic myelogenous leukemia. Ann. N. Y. Acad. Sci. **113**: 1073–1080.
10. Krauss, S., J. E. Sokal & A. A. Sandberg. 1964. Comparison of Philadelphia chromosome-positive and -negative patients with chronic myelocytic leukemia. Ann. Intern. Med. **61**: 625–635.
11. Tjio, J. H., P. P. Carbone, J. Whang & E. Frei, III. 1966. The Philadelphia chromosome and chronic myelogenous leukemia. J. Nat. Cancer Inst. **36**: 567–575.
12. Kenny, J. J. & W. C. Moloney. 1957. Leukocytic alkaline phosphatase. Blood **12**: 295–302.
13. Xefteris, E., W. J. Mitus, I. B. Mednicoff & W. Dameshek. 1961. Leukocytic alkaline phosphatase in busulfan induced remissions of chronic granulocytic leukemia. Blood **18**: 202–206.
14. Valentine, W. N., J. H. Follette, D. H. Solomon & J. Reynolds. 1957. The relationship of leukocyte alkaline phosphatase to "stress," to ACTH, and to adrenal 17-OH-corticosteroids. J. Lab. Clin. Med. **49**: 723–737.
15. Hammouda, F., D. Quaglino & F. G. J. Hayhoe. 1964. Blastic crisis in chronic granulocytic leukaemia. Cytochemical, cytogenetic, and autoradiographic studies in four cases. Brit. Med. J. **1**: 1275–1281.
16. Kemp, N. H., J. L. Stafford & R. Tanner. 1964. Chromosome studies during early and terminal chronic myeloid leukaemia. Brit. Med. J. **1**: 1010–1014.
17. Pedersen, B. & A. Videbaek. 1964. Several cell-lines with abnormal karyotypes in a patient with chronic myelogenous leukaemia. Scand. J. Haemat. **1**: 129–137.
18. King, M. J., E. M. Gillis & A. G. Baikie. 1962. Alkaline phosphatase activity of polymorphs in mongolism. Lancet **ii**: 1302–1305.
19. Hook, E. B. & R. R. Engel. 1964. Leucocyte life-span, leucocyte alkaline phosphatase, and the 21st chromosome. Lancet **i**: 112.
20. Rosen, R. B. & H. Nishiyama. 1965. Leucocyte life-span and leucocyte alkaline phosphatase. Lancet **i**: 554.
21. Fliedner, T. M., E. P. Cronkite, S. Å. Killmann & V. P. Bond. 1964. Granulocytopoiesis. II. Emergence and pattern of labeling of neutrophilic granulocytes in humans. Blood **24**: 683–700.
22. Alter, A. A., S. L. Lee, M. Pourfar & G. Dobkin. 1962. Leukocyte alkaline phosphatase in mongolism. J. Clin. Invest. **41**: 1341.
23. Tanaka, K. R., W. N. Valentine & R. E. Fredricks. 1960. Diseases or clinical conditions associated with low leukocyte alkaline phosphatase. New Eng. J. Med. **262**: 912–918.
24. Tough, I. M., P. A. Jacobs, W. M. Court Brown, A. G. Baikie & E. R. D. Williamson. 1963. Cytogenetic studies on bone marrow in chronic myeloid leukaemia. Lancet **i**: 844–846.
25. Jacob, F. & J. Monod. 1961. Genetic regulatory mechanism in the synthesis of proteins. J. Mol. Biol. **3**: 318–356.

KARYOTYPES OF HUMAN CULTURED CELL CLONES AND THEIR ALKALINE PHOSPHATASE ACTIVITY*

L. De Carli, Fiorella Nuzzo, A. Silvana Santachiara-Benerecetti, and J. Morrow†

Laboratorio Internazionale di Genetica e Biofisica
Pavia Section, Pavia, Italy

Introduction

Alkaline phosphatase (AP) has proved to be a suitable character for genetic studies in mammalian cell populations. It may be used for investigating the clonal distribution of cellular variants, the selection processes, and the correlation between chromosomal changes and variation of cell phenotype in heteroploid lines (Maio & De Carli, 1962; De Carli *et al.*, 1963). Finally, AP variations offer a system in which the regulatory processes of mammalian cells may be explored, since the enzyme is subjected to induction-repression mechanisms (Cox & MacLeod, 1962; Maio & De Carli, 1963). Our studies have concentrated so far on the relationship between karyotypes and enzyme levels with the aim of locating the character cytologically. The method is essentially based on a gene-dosage effect. The study of the karyotypes of a number of clonal cell lines derived from a human heteroploid line, the EUE, showed a positive correlation between the number of small acrocentric chromosomes‡ and the specific activities of AP (De Carli *et al.*, 1963). These findings supported the hypothesis that the chromosome which is triplicated in mongolism and deleted in chronic myeloid leukemia carries genes determining the synthesis of AP. Such a hypothesis was based on the observation of elevated levels of the enzyme in Down's syndrome and of reduced levels in peripheral leukocytes of leukemic individuals (Alter *et al.*, 1962; King *et al.*, 1962; Trubowitz *et al.*, 1962).

The significance of these findings to the existence of a gene-dosage effect has been questioned and attention has been drawn to some conflicting data. The most relevant objections are that: (1) a number of enzyme levels other than AP is elevated in leukocytes of mongoloids (Mellman *et al.*, 1964); (2) the AP levels of fibroblast cultures from individuals with trisomy G do not differ significantly from those of the normal controls (Cox, 1965); and (3) there are cases of myeloid leukemias in which the AP level is not reduced in leukocytes and in certain cases is even elevated above normal (Teplitz, *et al.* 1964). To overcome these discrepancies, Teplitz (1966) proposed that chromosome 21 carries a modifier gene instead of a structural one for the synthesis of AP.

It is difficult to determine (1) to what extent these conflicting data can invalidate the hypothesis of the location of the AP character on the chromosomes, and (2) how tenable are our formulations in reconciling the same data with the proposed model.

The study of gene dosage for a character such as AP, *in vivo* or in primary cultures, is hindered by many factors such as the polymorphic nature of the character (Boyer, 1961; Beckman *et al.*, 1966), tissue and developmental differences (Boyer, 1963), and physiological factors possibly operating at a regulatory level.

In view of all these variables, any scheme based on the relationship between

* This work was supported by a grant from EURATOM–CNR–CNEN, contract no. 012–61–12 BIAI.

† Present address: Department of Zoology, University of Kansas, Lawrence, Kan.

‡ In this paper, they will be referred to as G chromosomes.

the phenotypes and altered karyotypes *in vivo* cannot be a rigorous one. For some purposes, therefore, the *in vitro* systems represented by the heteroploid lines are more advantageous. In fact, the study can be restricted to cells belonging to the same individual and thus having the same genotype. In addition, any interference by physiological factors is eliminated and the environment is controllable. Finally, the correlation between the enzymic levels and the karyotypes can be studied over a wider range of chromosomal variants, than that which may be obtained *in vivo,* since most of the aneusomies for autosomes are not compatible with the life of the organism. The instability of the karyotypes *in vitro* may limit these possibilities; however, we have demonstrated that this instability does not affect all the groups of chromosomes of the human complement to the same extent (Nuzzo *et al.*, 1961). There are certain groups that are sufficiently stable to allow cytogenetic analysis. If a correlation can be established between the number of chromosomes belonging to a relatively stable group and the levels of a given cell character, we can measure the net effect of the addition or removal of a chromosome on the expression of the same character. This permits a more direct study of the gene-dosage effect. However, the data obtained from continuous cultures *in vitro* can in no way be extrapolated to the *in vivo* system. The adaptation *in vitro* of a cell is likely to change drastically the relative dosage of genes and their activity. Therefore, the study of the gene-dosage effect in cells continuously propagated *in vitro* necessarily develops on a different scale, but one that can be equally indicative for the cytological location of the characters.

The study of the correlation between the number of specific chromosomes and the enzyme levels requires information on the inheritability of the enzymic variants. In order to assess this condition, the clonal distribution of the AP character in the EUE population has been studied by repeating platings. The results of these studies have been reported previously (De Carli & Maio, 1963) and will be briefly summarized here. The purpose of this work is to compare the present situation of the EUE lines with the one described earlier. The following features are considered: the relative frequencies of AP variants, the karyotypes and their correlation with the enzyme activities, and the induction-repression phenomenon. New data will be presented on some physicochemical properties of the AP in the two lines, which will enable us to make some inferences about the number of enzyme variants contributing to the total activity. Finally, attention will be drawn to the possibility of producing or selecting AP negative variants using 8-azaguanine.

Materials and Methods

Cell Cultures

Abbreviations. EUE: the parental unselected line derived from human embryonic epithelium (Terni & Lo Monaco, 1958). E6D: collective name indicating the progeny of a clone with very low levels of AP derived from EUE and originally referred to as Sub 2 (De Carli *et al.*, 1963). The E6D has been recloned twice since its isolation. EUE AZA 10 and EUE AZA 100: EUE sublines selected for resistance to 8-azaguanine at 10 and 100 μg/ml, respectively.

Culture Conditions. Both the parental line and its clonal derivatives were grown under the standard conditions of our laboratory as described previously (Maio & De Carli, 1962). An exception has been made for the EUE AZA 10 and the EUE AZA 100, which were grown in Eagle's basal medium instead of lactalbumin medium, in order to prevent any competitive inhibition of 8-azaguanine. The substitution of this medium did not change the relative proportion of AP^+ and

AP⁻ cells nor did it affect the chromosomal distribution in the EUE parental strain.

Histochemical Methods. Alpha-naphthol phosphate coupled to Fast Blue RR has been used in histochemical staining, according to Gomori's method (1958). The test was usually made on colonies that were classified as positive, weakly positive, mixed, and negative. Cells or lines giving marked or weak histochemical reaction for AP are designated as AP^+; those in which the enzyme is histochemically undetectable are indicated as AP^-.

Biochemical Methods. The technique for quantitative assay of the enzyme is essentially based on the spectrophotometric determination of the product of hydrolysis of *p*-nitrophenyl phosphate. All the properties of the AP of EUE and E6D lines has been studied on crude cell extracts obtained by mechanical disruption. In most of the cases the enzyme was solubilized with butanol. Detailed methods are described elsewhere (Santachiara-Benerecetti *et al.*, 1967).

Cytological Analyses. Before 1966 all the cytological analyses were carried out on preparations on coverslips, according to the technique described in previous articles (Nuzzo *et al.*, 1961). Later analyses have been done on trypsinized cell suspensions, according to the method described by Hsu and Kellog (1960), with slight modifications.

RESULTS

Dynamics of the Alkaline Phosphatase Character in the EUE Population

When the EUE cell population was initially analyzed by scoring for AP activity of individual colonies derived from single cells, essentially two types of clones were recognized, namely: (1) AP-positive (AP^+) colonies showing a weak or marked reaction on histochemical staining. This was the prevalent type that constituted about 99 percent of the total colonies. (2) AP-negative (AP^-) colonies, in which the enzyme was histochemically undetectable (FIGURE 1). This latter type had a frequency of about 1 percent, which remained constant for months. However, the negative clones were not all equally stable; only a fraction (about 30 percent) of them yielded 100 percent negative cells on successive platings. The remainder continued to segregate both positive and negative cells in variable proportions. These clones were called "mixed." The AP^+ cells proved to possess a selective advantage over the negative ones; in fact when the mixed clones were grown in mass cultures, the composition of the cell population returned to that of the unselected line after a few passages. The advantage of the AP^+ cells is due to their higher growth rate. Results of the experiments of successive clonings are diagrammed in FIGURE 2. From the three examples of mixed clones reported in the scheme, it is evident that the tendency to segregate AP^+ and AP^- cells, but not the proportion of the two cell types, is inheritable.

After almost three years of culture under standard conditions, the composition of the EUE population, as described before, underwent small changes. A small reduction of the frequency of AP^- cells (from around 1 to 0.6 percent) has been observed. This reduction took place mainly at the expense of the unstable negative clones, defined as "mixed," which have almost completely disappeared from the population. The actual distribution of the AP variants in the EUE population is reported in TABLE 1, where a more detailed classification of the various types is used, inclusive of the positive, weakly positive, negative, and mixed types.

Two important features emerge from these population studies: the constant frequency of AP^- cells in the EUE line in spite of their selective disadvantage and the instability of the so called "mixed" clones. For the maintenance of an equilibrium under these conditions, a continuous production of negative cells is required. Such dynamics are adequately explained on the basis of the chromosomal mechanisms that are described in the following section.

Cytogenetical Studies on EUE Parental Line and Its Clonal Derivatives

Karyotype analyses, of the EUE parental line with high AP and a number of clonal sublines with low and intermediate activity, allowed us to construct a dose-response curve, in which the number of G chromosomes was plotted against the logs of AP specific activities (FIGURE 3). The EUE unselected line showed a modal number of four small acrocentric chromosomes, whereas the negative lines had two small acrocentrics. Lines with intermediate levels of AP showed three small acrocentrics. This latter class of variants was distributed over a wide range of AP specific activities (De Carli *et al.*, 1964). The function so obtained deviated significantly from linearity. This was attributed to the phenomenon of regulation that is suggested by the observations of induction in lines with low

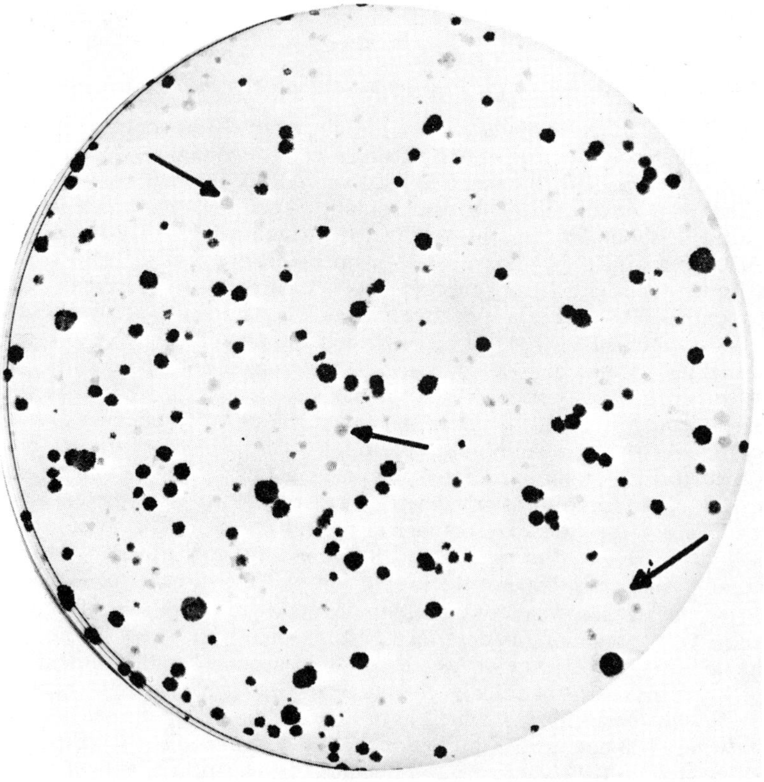

FIGURE 1. Plate of colonies from single cells of an artificial mixture of AP^+ and AP^- cells. AP is revealed by the histochemical staining reaction (see MATERIALS AND METHODS). The negative colonies, some of which are indicated by arrows, have been visualized with a contrast color which was obtained by staining with acridine orange when the histochemical reaction was completed.

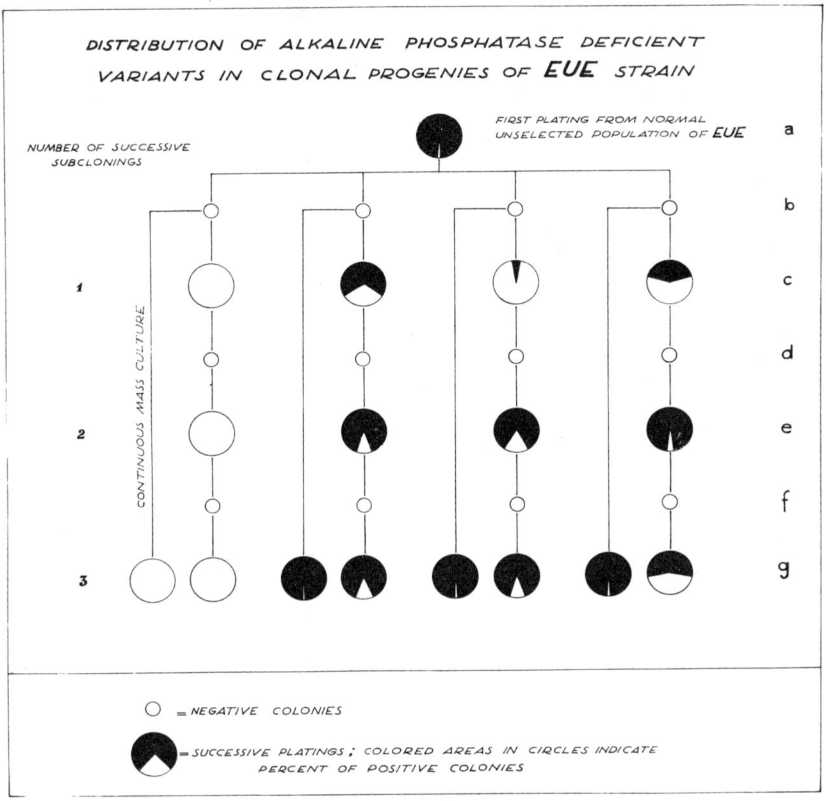

FIGURE 2. *Symbols*: Large circles = plates of colonies from single cells; small circles = individual colonies isolated from plates; dark areas = fraction of AP^+ colonies in a plate. *Explanation of the diagram*: From a plate of colonies of EUE parental line (a), four colonies are isolated (b), all recognized as AP^- by the vital-staining reaction for alkaline phosphatase (Maio & De Carli, 1962). These colonies are dissociated into single cells with trypsin, part of the cell suspension is plated (c), and part inoculated in tubes and subsequently in bottles to give mass cultures. The clonal isolation of AP^- variants is repeated twice (d–f). Finally, the proportion of $AP+$ and AP^- cells is determined by cloning both the last AP^- clonal derivative and a sample of the mass cultures derived from the original colonies (g).

TABLE 1

RELATIVE FREQUENCIES OF ALKALINE PHOSPHATASE VARIANT COLONIES IN SINGLE CELL CULTURES OF EUE LINE (1966 SCORING)

Types of Colonies Stained Histochemically	Frequencies	Confidence Limits at 0.05 p
AP positive	0.872	0.839 –0.902
AP weakly positive	0.120	0.101 –0.141
Mixed	0.0009	0.0004–0.0045
AP negative	0.006	0.003 –0.013

"constitutive" levels and of repression in lines with high levels by organic monophosphates and steroid hormones (Maio & De Carli, 1963).

Cultures of the EUE parental line and some lines with reduced activity levels have been maintained for more than two years. Our study has concentrated mainly upon the stable negative lines, one of which was maintained in parallel with the EUE line. During the three-year period, a complete reversion to the positive type was never observed in the negative subline, as should have occurred if some sporadic revertants had emerged and overgrown the rest of the culture, due to their higher growth rate. However, after several months of mass culture, a slow increase in enzyme activity, which was also detectable histochemically, was observed in the negative subline. The line was thereupon recloned and the level of activity was restored to the previous low value. This process has been repeated twice in two years. Analysis of the karyotypes was carried out in parallel with determination of the AP specific activity at intervals of one year on the EUE line and on the negative subline which had undergone successive recloning. The results are summarized in TABLE 2.

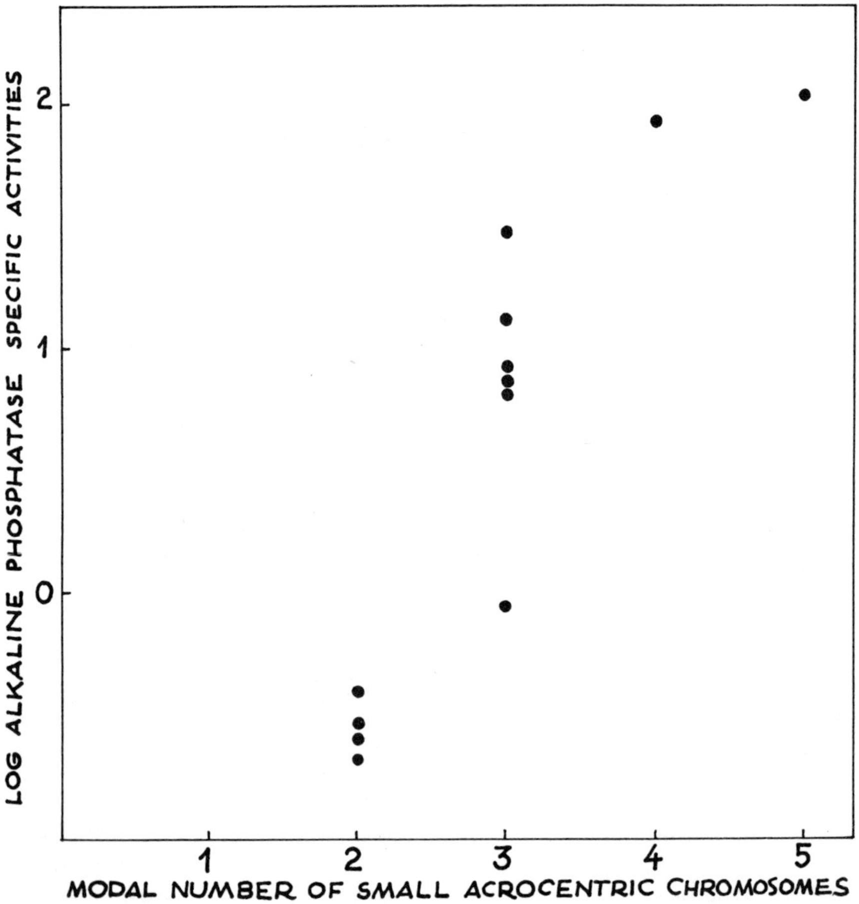

FIGURE 3. Variation of AP in EUE lines with different numbers of G chromosomes.

TABLE 2

CORRELATION BETWEEN KARYOTYPES AND ALKALINE PHOSPHATASE ACTIVITIES UNDER CONSTITUTIVE AND INDUCTION-REPRESSION CONDITIONS IN THE EUE LINE AND ITS CLONAL DERIVATIVE E6D (VALUES OBTAINED IN DIFFERENT YEARS)

		No. of Chromosomes				Alkaline Phosphatase Activities*	
		Total		G group			
	Years	Mode	Average	Mode	Average	Constitutive	Induced or Repressed†
EUE	1963–1964	67–68	67.27	4	4.17	86.0	30.8
	1965	64	63.76	3	3.20	51.0	—
	1966	64	63.40	3	3.33	40.5	28.5
E6D	1963–1964	59	58.66	2	2.07	0.2	1.1
	1966	53	53.01	2	2.05	0.14	0.70

* Representative values for each period are given.
† Prednisolone at 10 μg/ml has been used as an inducing or repression agent.

Representative metaphases and karyotypes of the EUE line and E6D subline, for the years 1963 and 1966 are shown in FIGURE 4. As can be seen in TABLE 2, the number of G chromosomes in the EUE line shifted from a mode of four to a value of three during the three-year period. The average number is 4.17 and 3.33, respectively. A consistent reduction in AP activity was also observed, from specific activity values in the range of 86–168, as reported previously for the AP positive line (Maio & De Carli, 1963; De Carli *et al.*, 1963), to the present values in the range of 40–77. The negative subline, after two clonal

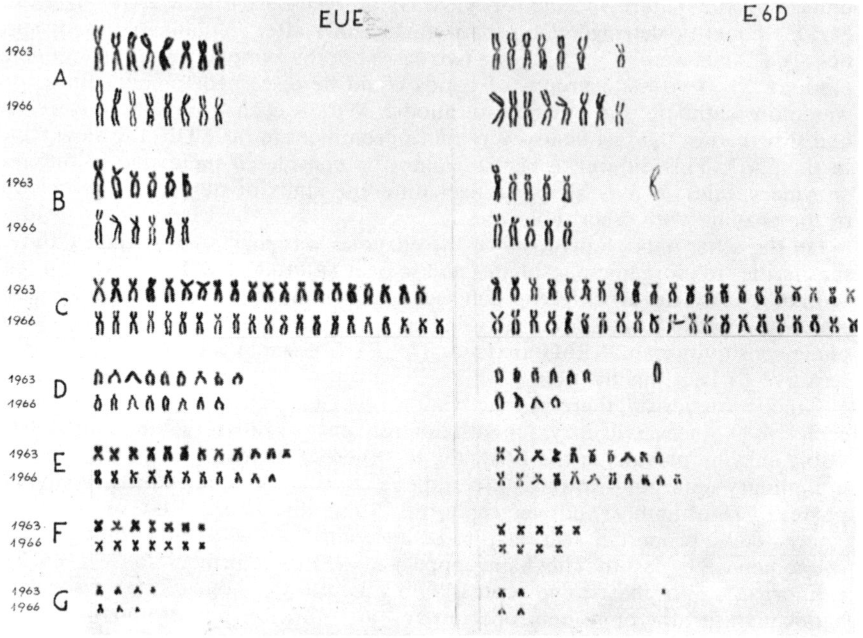

FIGURE 4. Karyotypes of EUE AP$^+$ line and E6D AP$^-$ subline from mitoses analyzed in different years.

isolations, showed a further reduction of the total number of chromosomes, although the number of G chromosomes remained consistently two. Therefore, the relationship between number of G chromosomes and AP activity, as originally described, is still valid for the present line and its clonal subline E6D. In addition, the response of these lines to the action of the organic phosphates and the steroid hormones has remained unchanged, although lower values of induction for E6D and of repression for EUE can be observed in respect to those found previously (see again TABLE 2). Cytologically, this study does not appear amenable to further analysis due to the limits of the karyotyping procedure, which does not enable us to specify which individual pair of chromosomes of the group 21–22 is actually involved in the control of AP synthesis.

One aspect of this study that can be thoroughly investigated concerns the physicochemical properties of the enzyme in the AP^+ and AP^- line. This would answer the question whether a single enzyme or different enzymes are produced in the two lines, under the control of one or more genes, respectively. To this end some properties of the enzyme of the EUE line and its clone E6D, with a low enzyme level have been analyzed (Santachiara-Benerecetti *et al.*, 1967).

Biochemical Characterization of Alkaline Phosphatase in EUE Lines and E6D Variant

One of the properties that first appeared to differ between the two lines is the binding of the enzyme to particulate cell structures. Such binding was found to be more firm in the case of E6D AP. In fact, when electrophoresis was carried out on extracts obtained by mechanical disruption of EUE and E6D cells, after the extracts had been diluted so that both contained the same number of enzyme units, a visible pattern specific for AP was observed only for the EUE. The E6D enzyme could be detected electrophoretically only after solubilization with butanol. The bands were multiple in the two cases but the zymograms did not coincide (FIGURE 5). Two main groups of bands could be discerned for both lines: one was more cathodic, the other more anodic. Within each group there were fast and slow bands, the fast bands were more prominent in the EUE, the slow bands in the E6D. This difference per se cannot be considered indicative of different enzyme species; it may simply reflect different kinds of degrees of association of the enzyme with other molecules.

On the other hand, a diversity of the enzymes was suggested by their different sensitivities to inorganic phosphates and to heat (FIGURES 6 & 7). Treatment with sodium phosphate at different concentrations inhibited the AP activity more effectively in the E6D extract than in the EUE, demonstrating the higher phosphate sensitivity of the E6D enzyme. The EUE enzyme was found to be more sensitive to heat inactivation.

Kinetic studies on thermal inactivation seem to indicate the presence within each line of at least two enzymes with different heat sensitivities; the more thermostable enzyme prevails in the E6D, the less thermostable one in the EUE. Some preliminary data point towards a certain relationship among sensitivity to phosphate, thermostability, and electrophoretical mobility of the EUE and E6D enzymes. These properties also seem to be correlated with the induction-repression phenomena. The fast moving bands appear to be more thermolabile, less sensitive to inorganic phosphates, and repressible by steroid hormones. The slow moving bands manifest the opposite properties and are inducible by hormones.

The bulk of the evidence suggests a qualitative difference, in addition to the quantitative ones, between the enzymes of the EUE and the E6D. Therefore,

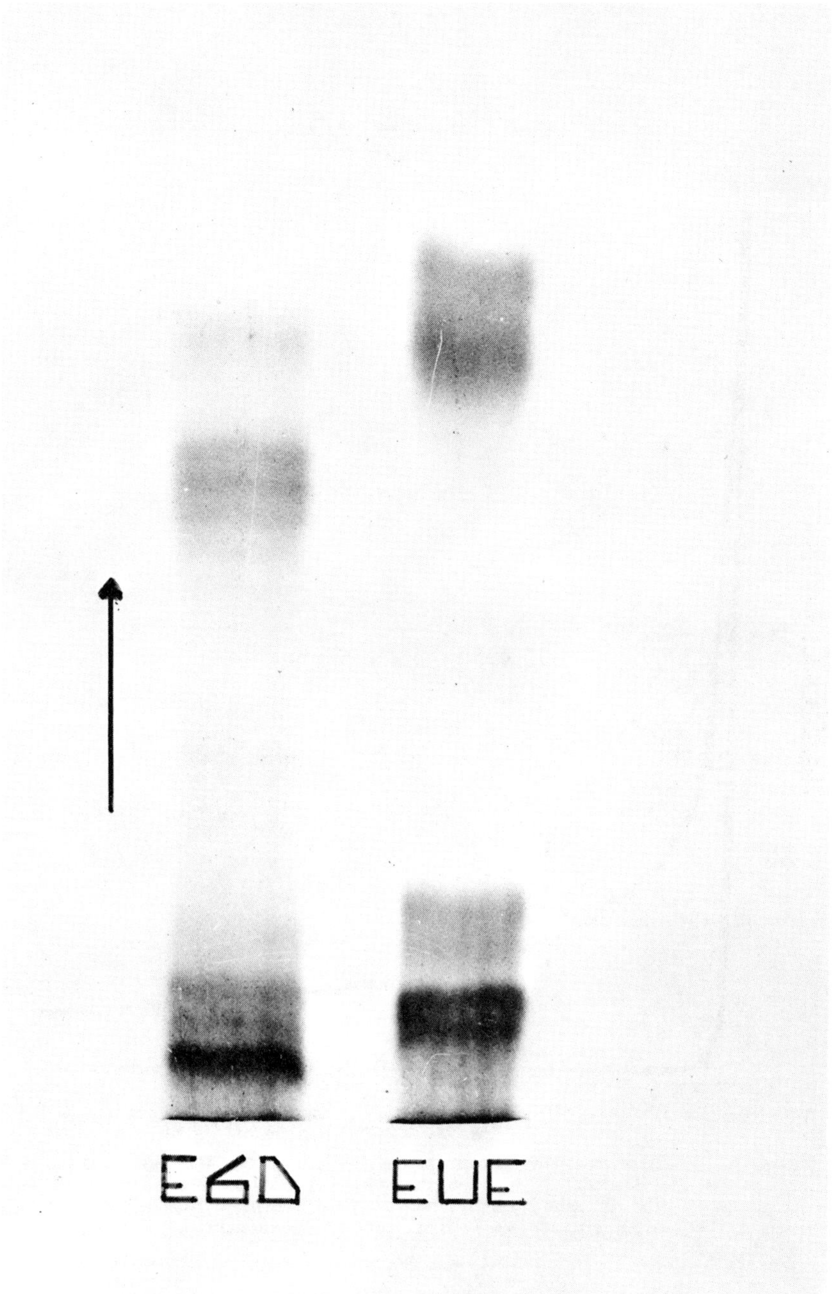

FIGURE 5. Starch-gel electrophoresis of AP of E6D and EUE extracts after butanol treatment. Samples of 0.05 ml adsorbed onto small pieces of Whatman 17 M filter paper were subjected to electrophoresis. Insertion is at the bottom of the figure. The arrow shows the direction of migration toward the anode.

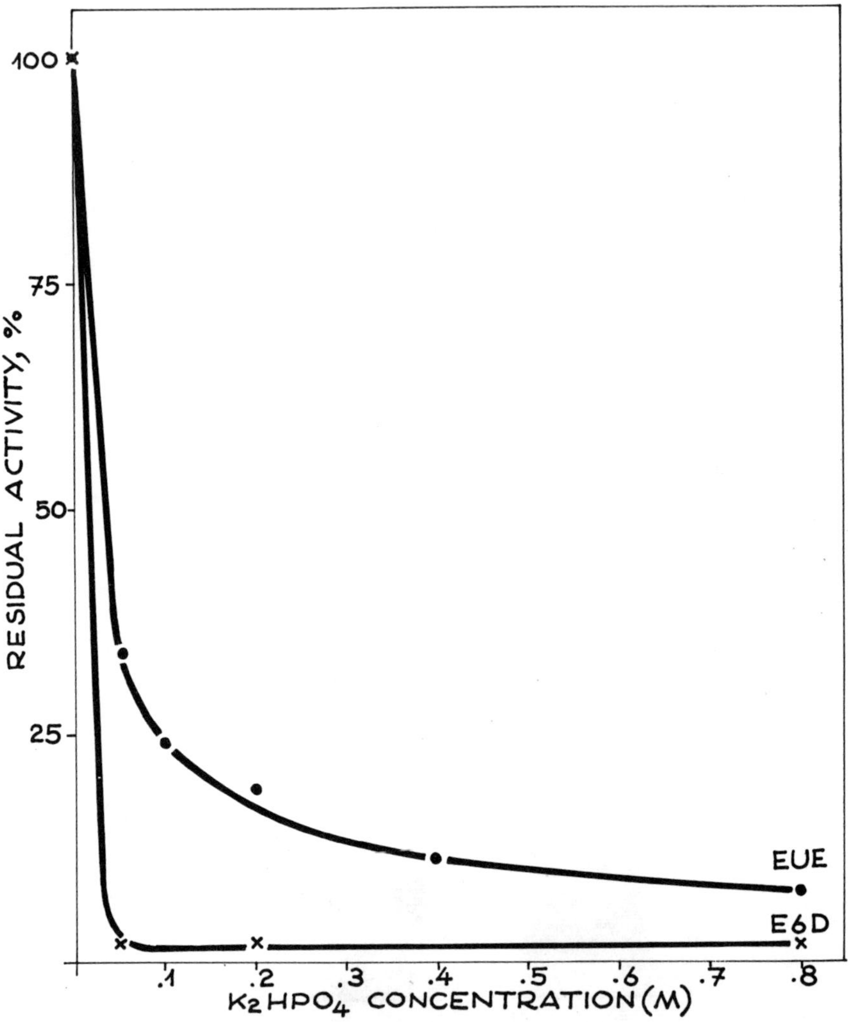

FIGURE 6. Effect of inorganic phosphate on AP activity of EUE (●——●) and E6D (x——x) extracts. The activity was determined on cell extracts, not treated with butanol, in the presence of the different K_2HPO_4 concentrations. The pH of incubation mixtures was unchanged. The values are expressed as percent of the activity of the sample without phosphate.

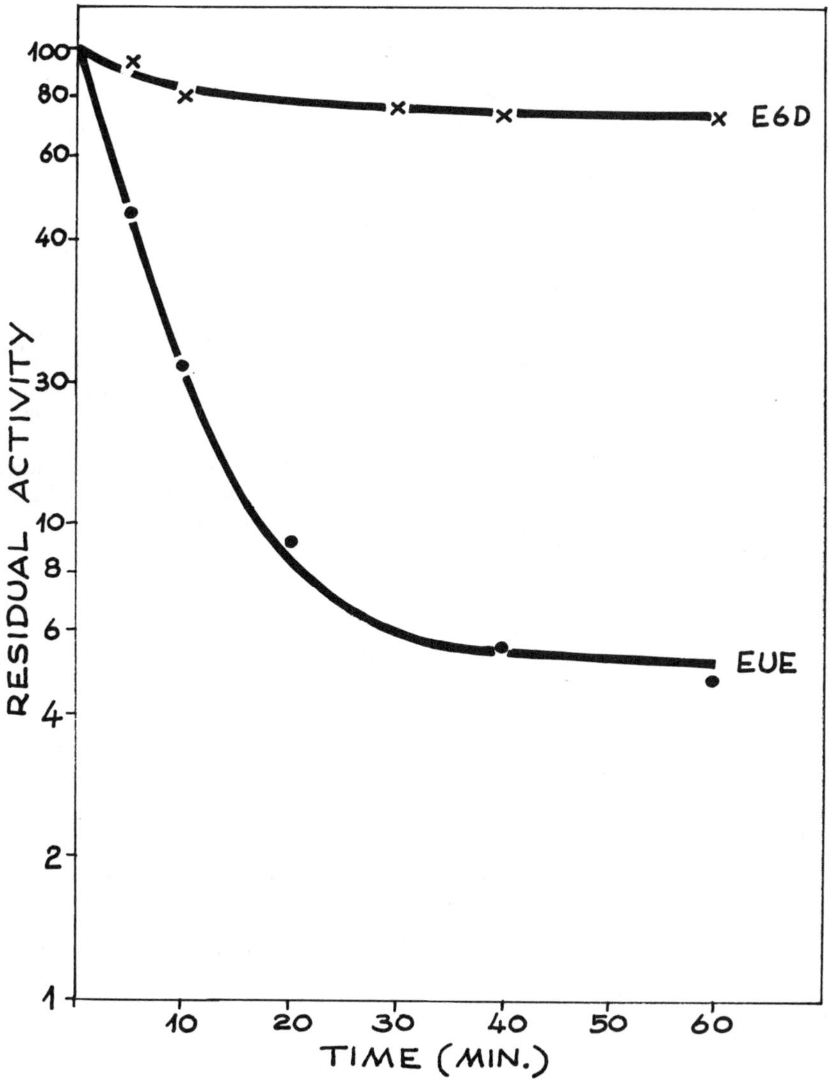

FIGURE 7. Time course of inactivation at 70° C of EUE (●——●) and E6D (x——x) AP. 0.2 ml aliquots of cells extracts were added to 0.8 ml of 0.05 M tris HCl buffer, pH 7.1, pretreated at 70° C and kept at this temperature for the indicated times. Controls were stored at 4° C. Residual activity measured after butanol treatment is expressed as the percent of control.

determination of the character by multiple alleles and/or loci has to be postulated. This does not change the hypothesis of the location of genes for AP on the G chromosomes. However, there is a question which of these genes are situated on the G chromosomes.

Possible Role of 8-Azaguanine in Increasing the Frequency of Alkaline Phosphatase Variants

Preliminary experiments indicated that the prolonged treatment of EUE cultures with 8-azaguanine to obtain resistant lines resulted in an increased frequency of clones with low levels of AP. Two lines, EUE AZA 10 and EUE AZA 100, resistant to 8-azaguanine at 10 μg/ml and 100 μg/ml, respectively, and showing a proportional reduction of IMP-pyrophosphorylase enzyme, were isolated from strain EUE. When these resistant lines appeared to be growing steadily, they were cloned and the colonies that developed scored for AP activity. An excess of negative colonies was found in both resistant variants.

The frequency of AP^- colonies varied greatly from one plating to another. Values in the range of 5–23 percent were observed when the cells were plated either in the absence or in the presence of 8-azaguanine. As the culture ages, the frequency of AP^- cells is progressively reduced. This can be explained by the lower growth rate of the negative variants.

Chromosomal analysis of the EUE AZA 10 and EUE AZA 100 lines showed a reduction in chromosomal number; this reduction was more pronounced in the lines resistant to a higher concentration of azaguanine (Nuzzo *et al.*, 1966). No information on the karyotypes is available at present; morphological analysis of the chromosomes is in progress in an attempt to identify the missing chromosomes. All these data, summarized in TABLE 3, would suggest either a selective advantage of AP^- cells toward the 8-azaguanine or a common mechanism for the production of the IMP-pyrophosphorylase deficient cells and AP^- cells.

Discussion

There is no doubt that variation of the basal levels of AP in the EUE line has a chromosomal determination. The fact that the reduction of AP activity is

TABLE 3

CORRELATION AMONG IMP-PYROPHOSPHORYLASE ACTIVITY, FREQUENCY OF AP^- VARIANTS AND MODAL CHROMOSOME NUMBERS IN EUE SUBLINES RESISTANT TO 8-AZAGUANINE

Cell Lines	EUE	EUE AZA 10	EUE AZA 100
IMP-pyrophosphorylase specific activities*	148 ± 13	27.1 ± 2.6	5.6 ± 5.0
Plating efficiency in HAT medium† Percent of control	100	95.85	0
Frequency of AP^- variants‡	0.008 (0.001–0.029)	0.076 (0.009–0.159)	0.23 (0.171–0.284)
Modal chromosome number	64	61	59

* mμmoles of hypoxanthine transformed per hour per mg of protein.

† Selective medium containing 0.1 μg/ml of aminopterin, 5 μg/ml each of hypoxanthine and thymidine.

‡ The values in parentheses are the confidence limits at 0.05 probability.

associated with a loss of chromosomes provides a simple explanation of the dynamics of the AP character in the EUE population. The relatively constant frequency of cells with low levels of AP in spite of their lower growth rate, requires that the variation from AP^+ to AP^- have a very high probability. The mitotic errors that bring about a reduction in chromosome number are probably much more frequent than those leading to an increase of chromosomes. In addition, a loss of all the members of a given pair is irreversible; this might have happened in the stable negative clones.

The identification of the G chromosomes as presumptive sites of genetic control of AP character is validated by the observation that these chromosomes, and only these, show a consistent correlation with the variations of the AP level in the EUE lines.

Since the variation in the basal activity of the enzyme is mostly due to changes in chromosome numbers, it is conceivable that any agent that affects the dynamics of the chromosome complement is likely to increase the probability of such variation. This might be the case for 8-azaguanine, which caused a remarkable effect on the distribution of chromosome numbers in cultures of EUE selected for resistance to the analogue. Induction of random variation in chromosome numbers coupled to selection of certain chromosomal variants may cause the accumulation of cells with a lower number of chromosomes, and thus with low levels of AP. The possibility that 8-azaguanine acts by inducing chromosomal changes is suggested by the observation that there is an increased frequency of polyploids, which divide by multipolar mitoses, in cultures treated with this agent. These mitoses either do not proceed to completion or give rise to cells that rapidly degenerate. But occasionally, when the distribution of chromosomes is proportionate at mitosis, viable cells may originate with chromosome numbers higher or lower than those of the parental cells. In this way a number of chromosomes can be randomly lost or gained in a single step. However, selection will stabilize those karyotypes that show the best adaptation to the culture conditions. In the case of 8-azaguanine, since the resistance has been shown to be dependent on the loss of an enzymic function (IMP-pyrophosphorylase) presumably the cells that have lost chromosomes have a better chance to survive the action of 8-azaguanine. The fact that AP deficiency is also dependent on a loss of chromosomes makes selecting for 8-azaguanine resistance parallel to selecting for low levels of AP. All the foregoing facts can adequately be interpreted by assuming a common mechanism of production of both 8-azaguanine resistant and AP^- variants, based on chromosomal changes. However, the final proof that the AP^- variants induced by 8-azaguanine treatment are hereditary is still to be found. In this respect the isolation and subculturing of these AP^- clones will be decisive. At the present stage of investigation, the regulatory or physiological nature of the enzymic variation cannot be excluded.

By analogy with azaguanine, other agents known for their capacity to induce chromosome losses, such as *p*-fluorophenylalanine (Morpurgo, 1961; Lhoas, 1961) and low doses of radiations (Nias & Ockey, 1965), might bring about an increase of AP^- variants through the mechanisms described above. Scoring for both AP^+ and chromosome numbers on azaguanine-resistant clones, also showed that the reduction of the total number of chromosomes per se does not cause a reduction in AP activity, since AP markedly positive clones with total chromosome numbers even lower than those observed in AP^- lines, could be found in the azaguanine resistant lines. This is further evidence in favor of the specificity of the cytological changes bringing about the enzyme variations.

The relationship between the small acrocentric chromosomes and levels of AP has been confirmed by control experiments performed more than two years later than the first analyses. To explain this relationship and its implications for the induction-repression phenomenon observed in the EUE line, we proposed a hypothetical model based on the Jacob and Monod operon system (1961), in which the structural AP gene(s) were under the control of two regulators, one producing an active repressor (R_2) and the other producing an aporepressor (R_1). The same effector was capable of interacting with both regulators, by inactivating the former and activating the latter. Accordingly, induction or repression should follow; the prevalence of one or the other effect is dependent upon the relative dosage of the three types of genes, namely, the structural, the R_1, and R_2 genes. It was further postulated that at least one type of these genes, the R_1 genes, was located on chromosome 21.

This model was based on the simplified assumption that a single enzyme species was produced by the AP^+ and AP^- lines. However, the recent physicochemical studies of the enzyme in the EUE and E6D line indicate that we are dealing with at least two different enzymes present in different proportions in the two lines. This requires that the previous model be modified by assuming that each regulator controls its own structural gene. In fact, one of the two presumptive enzymes, the one prevailing in the AP^- line, appears to be inducible; the other, prevailing in the AP^+ line, repressible. Therefore, the structural genes that determine the synthesis of these enzymes must involve two different control systems, one inducible and the other repressible. However, they have to be interlocked with one another by a common effector such as β-glycerophosphate or prednisolone. This would account for the observation that these substances induce the negative lines and repress the positive ones.

Four distinct genetic determinants would thus be recognized in this model: the structural gene that produces the fast moving enzymes (S_F), and which is controlled by a regulator gene that forms an aporepressor (R_F); and the structural gene for the synthesis of the slow moving enzyme (S_S) controlled by a regulator gene producing an active repressor (R_S). This model is illustrated in FIGURE 8.

The question now arises: which one of these genes can be located on the G chromosomes? From the model proposed, the only possibility is that the S_F gene is located on these chromosomes. This would account both for the observed dependence of the enzyme levels on the numbers of G chromosomes and for the induction-repression phenomenon as correlated with the constitutive levels of the enzyme.

In the absence of any affector, when the number of S_F genes increases, the activity also increases and the fraction of fast moving thermolabile enzyme increases. This is the case for the AP^+ lines. On the other hand, when the number of S_F genes decreases, the total activity also decreases and the slow moving thermostable fraction prevails.

In the presence of the affector (i.e., hormones, organic monophosphates) S_F genes will be repressed and S_S genes will be induced at the same time. According to the number of S_F genes, and thus the number of G chromosomes, induction or repression will be prevalent. Since the total enzyme activity is the result of two opposite processes, one determining an increase and the other a decrease in their respective enzyme activities, it is perfectly understandable why the induction of negative lines never brings the enzyme activity to the constitutive levels of the positive lines. The same reasoning applies to the repression of the positive lines, which never reduces the enzyme activity to the levels of the negative lines.

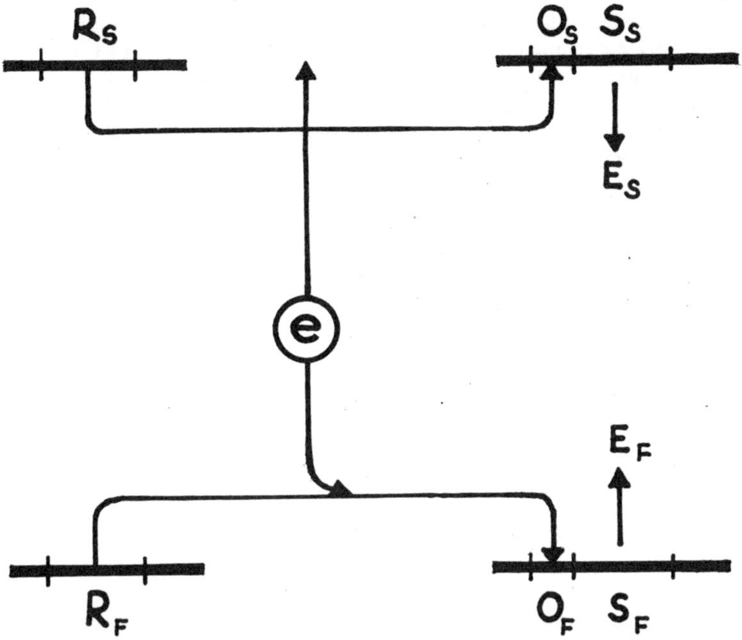

FIGURE 8. Hypothetical model for determination of AP variation in the EUE line.
S_S = structural gene for the slow moving enzymes
S_F = structural gene for the fast moving enzymes
R_S = regulatory gene producing an active repressor of S_S
R_F = regulatory gene producing an aporepressor for S_F
e = effector: organic monophosphate, or hormone.

All these variations in enzyme activity can be the result of a changed dosage of only one of the four genes considered, namely, the one located on the G chromosomes. But any one of the other three can undergo dosage changes, which may alter the proportion and amount of the two presumptive molecular species of the enzyme. This might explain the variation in specific activity which can be observed among lines with the same number of G chromosomes. The model here described is largely speculative and not unique, but it seems to be the simplest one that can be envisaged in order to account for most of the variables, which have been shown experimentally to be involved in the system. On the basis of this model, we suggest that the correlation between G chromosomes and AP is restricted to one component of the enzyme complex, which corresponds to the thermolabile and electrophoretically more mobile fraction. Further cytogenetical analyses might be carried out with this orientation.

SUMMARY

Clonal variation of alkaline phosphatase (AP) activity has been demonstrated previously in a human heteroploid line, the EUE, and a correlation between enzyme levels and karyotypes has been established. More recent studies indicate some changes in the composition of EUE cell populations which have resulted in two types of variants, namely, AP positive or weakly positive cells and AP negative cells. However, the observed positive correlation between the number of small acrocentric chromosomes and AP specific activities is still found valid for the actual line and its clonal derivatives. The cells have also retained their regulatory capacities since AP can still be either repressed or induced by organic phosphates and steroid hormones, depending on the basal activity levels.

The study of some properties of the AP extracted from the EUE parental line and from one clonal derivative with low activity revealed differences concerning their thermal stability, their sensitivity to inorganic phosphate, and electrophoretic mobility. The data so far suggest that there are several enzyme forms within each line and qualitative differences in addition to the quantitative ones between AP of EUE lines and its variant clones. However, the hypothesis of a gene-dosage effect to explain the differences in AP levels still holds, although the system becomes more complicated.

Further evidence for the association between changes in chromosome number and AP variation is the effect of 8-azaguanine on EUE cell population. A higher frequency of AP negative variants has been found among cells resistant to various doses of this compound; these variants show also a reduced chromosome number. Two hypotheses are considered: (1) 8-azaguanine acts as a selective agent for AP negative cells and (2) 8-azaguanine provokes random chromosome losses, thus increasing the frequency of AP negative cells.

Acknowledgments

We wish to express our thanks to Dr. J. J. Maio, Dr. A. Falaschi, and Dr. F. Scudo for their suggestions and criticisms. We also are indebted to Dr. I. Cesari for his assistance in the experimental work.

References

Alter, A. A., L. L. Stanley, M. Pourfar & G. Dobkin. 1963. Studies of leukocyte alkaline phosphatase in mongolism: a possible chromosome marker. Blood **22:** 165–177.

Beckman, L., G. Björling & A. Heiken. 1966. Human alkaline phosphatase and the factors controlling their appearance in serum. Acta Genet. **16:** 305–312.

Boyer, S. H. 1961. Alkaline phosphatase in human sera and placentae. Science **134:** 1002–1004.

Boyer, S. H. 1963. Human organ alkaline phosphatase: discrimination by several means including starch-gel electrophoresis of antienzyme-enzyme supernatant fluids. Ann. N. Y. Acad. Sci. **103:** 938–951.

Cox, R. P. 1965. Regulation of alkaline phosphatase in skin fibroblast cultures from patients with mongolism. Exp. Cell Res. **37:** 690–692.

Cox, R. P. & C. M. MacLeod. 1962. Alkaline phosphatase content and the effects of prednisolone on mammalian cells in cultures. J. Gen. Physiol. **45:** 439–485.

De Carli, L. & J. J. Maio. 1963. Isolation of clonal cell lines deficient in alkaline phosphatase from a human epithelioid strain. Mammalian Chrom. Newsletter **9:** 45.

De Carli, L., J. J. Maio & F. Nuzzo. 1963. Alkaline phosphatase activity and chromosome variation in human cells in culture. J. Nat. Cancer Inst. **31:** 1501–1509.

De Carli, L., J. J. Maio, F. Nuzzo & A. S. Benerecetti. 1964. Cytogenetics studies with alkaline phosphatase in human heteroploid cells. Cold Spring Harbor Symp. Quant. Biol. **29:** 223–231.

Gomori, G. 1958. Microscopic Histochemistry: Principles and Practice. The University of Chicago Press. Chicago, Ill.

Hsu, T. C. & D. S. Kellog. 1960. Primary cultivation and continuous propagation *in vitro* of tissues from small biopsy specimens. J. Nat. Cancer Inst. **25:** 221–234.

Jacob, B. & J. Monod. 1961. On the regulation of gene activity. Cold Spring Harbor Symp. Quant. Biol. **26:** 193–211.

King, M. J., E. M. Gillis & A. G. Baikie. 1962. Alkaline phosphatase activity of polymorphs in mongolism. Lancet **ii:** 1302–1305.

Lhoas, P. 1961. Mitotic haploidization by treatment of *Aspergillus niger* diploids with *para*-fluorophenylalanine. Nature **190:** 744.

MAIO, J. J. & L. DE CARLI. 1962. Distribution of alkaline phosphatase variants in a heteroploid strain of human cells in tissue culture. Nature **196:** 600–601.

MAIO, J. J. & L. DE CARLI. 1963. Induction and repression of alkaline phosphatase in human cultured cells by prednisolone, hydrocortisone and organic monophosphates. Biochem. Biophys. Res. Comm. **11:** 335–342.

MELLMAN, W. J., F. A. OSKI, T. A. TEDESCO, A. MACIERA-COELHO & H. HARRIS. 1964. Leukocyte enzymes in Down's syndrome. Lancet **ii:** 674–675.

MORPURGO, G. 1961. Somatic segregation induced by *p*-fluorophenylalanine. Aspergillus News Letter **2:** 10.

NIAS, A. H. W. & C. H. OCKEY. 1965. Change in chromosome number during continuous irradiation. Nature **206:** 840–841.

NUZZO, F., L. DE CARLI & B. CHIARELLI. 1961. Analisi morfologica degli assetti cromosomici in un ceppo di cellule umane stabilizzate *in vitro*. Atti Ass. Genet. It. **6:** 111–124.

NUZZO, F., J. MORROW & L. DE CARLI. 1966. Chromosomal changes associated with resistance to 8-azaguanine in a human heteroploid cell line (abst.). 1966 Conference on Mammalian Cytology and Somatic Cell Genetics. Saint Simon Island, U.S.A. Nov. 8–10, 1966.

SANTACHIARA-BENERECETTI, A. S., I. CESARI & L. DE CARLI. 1967. Some properties of alkaline phosphatase from a human cell strain and from a clonal derivative with low activity. J. Cell. Physiol. **69:** 169–176.

TEPLITZ, R. L. 1966. Regulation of leukocyte alkaline phosphatase and the Philadelphia chromosome. Nature **209:** 821–822.

TEPLITZ, R. L., R. B. ROSEN & M. R. TEPLITZ. 1964. Granulocytic leukaemia, Philadelphia chromosome, and leukocyte alkaline phosphatase. Lancet **ii:** 418–419.

TERNI, M. & G. B. LO MONACO. 1958. Coltura continua di cellule derivate da embrione umano. Lo Sperimentale **108:** 177–185.

TRUBOWITZ, S., D. KIRMAN & B. MASEK. 1962. The leukocyte alkaline phosphatase in mongolism. Lancet **ii:** 486–487.

ABNORMAL LEUKOKINETICS IN 21 TRISOMY*

W. J. Mellman, S. O. Raab, F. A. Oski, and T. A. Tedesco
Department of Pediatrics and Medical Genetics
University of Pennsylvania School of Medicine
Philadelphia, Pa.
and
Department of Medicine
Woman's Medical College of Pennsylvania
Philadelphia, Pa.

Granulocytes of some individuals with 21 trisomy have been noted to have increased enzyme activities. These increases have been used as evidence for locating specific gene determinants on chromosome 21. The first reports of increases in activities of certain leukocytic enzymes in mongoloid subjects have been generally confirmed, as well as extended to include other enzymes. However, certain clinical and experimental data have challenged this case for gene localization. An equally plausible explanation for the observed enzyme findings is that there is a physiological anomaly of the granulocyte of mongoloid subjects. This paper reviews some of the indirect evidence and presents some direct evidence that the granulocyte in mongoloid subjects is often kinetically atypical.

It should be recalled that anomalous granulocytes morphology, the association of mongolism and acute leukemia of childhood, and other abnormal leukocyte responses had been recognized before enzyme alterations were described. Teplitz and his associates[1] have reviewed defects in the evidence that a hypothetical gene for leukocyte alkaline phosphatase is located on chromosome 21. They pointed to the increase in this enzyme's activities in granulocytes of patients with chronic myeloid leukemia, when there is leukocytosis secondary to intercurrent infection or acute transformation of the leukemic state. Valentine and Beck[2] had previously described an increase in granulocyte alkaline phosphatase activity in nonleukemic patients with leukocytosis as a response to infection or inflammation.

Evidence that an enzyme's activity is significantly increased in the leukocytes of mongoloid individuals has been based on enzyme determinations in a group of mongoloid patients and a group of reasonably well-matched controls. Characteristically, there has been considerable overlapping of values for these two groups. This has been our experience with measurements of leukocyte galactose-1-phosphate uridyl transferase, an enzyme determination that shows virtually no overlap when the leukocytes of normal individuals are compared with those from heterozygotes for a mutant of galactosemia.[3] Certainly, for this enzyme, one would expect to observe unequivocal bimodality in the enzyme activity distributions of control and mongoloid leukocytes, if the gene dosage mechanism was operative. Furthermore, fibroblast cultures of tissues from individuals with 21 trisomy have failed to show increased activities of the enzymes that are so affected in the leukocytes of individuals with 21 trisomy. Nevertheless, genetic variants for both glucose-6-phosphate dehydrogenase (G-6-PD) and galactose-1-phosphate uridyl transferase have reduced activities in both leukocytes and fibroblast cell cultures from the same individuals.[4]

In 1964, we observed, in the leukocytes of mongoloid subjects, significant increases in the activities of three enzymes, one of which was G-6-PD. Since there is strong evidence that the gene determining G-6-PD is located on the X chromo-

* Supported in part by USPHS grants nos. HD–00588, HD–15545, AM–02231, HE–08955, and 3NO1 FR40.

some, this experiment compelled us to seek an alternative to the gene locus explanation to account for the elevated leukocyte enzyme levels in 21 trisomy. We further noted that the relative activities of all three enzymes when measured in the same leukocyte preparations were positively correlated, i.e., if one enzyme level was elevated over control levels, the other two enzyme levels tended to be correspondingly elevated.[5] This suggested that there might be a general alteration of leukocyte physiology.

We have studied the kinetics of the circulating granulocytes in a group of mongoloid adult males by the *in vitro* labelling technique of Mauer and his colleagues.[6] This method determines the total body and circulating granulocyte pools, as well as the rate of disappearance of the labelled granulocytes from the circulation ($t\frac{1}{2}$). The granulocyte pools of the six mongoloid subjects were similar to normal male adults, although five of the six had a significant shortening of their circulating granulocyte half-life (mongoloids 3.2 ± 0.96 hours; controls 6.5 ± 1.5 hours.) These data indicate that there is an increase in granulocyte turnover rate in mongoloid adults. With normal granulocyte pools and an increased turnover rate, the mean age of the granulocyte population must therefore be younger than normal. This increased granulocyte turnover was further confirmed by uric acid excretion measurements made at the time of the kinetic studies. For the six mongoloid individuals, there was an inverse correlation between the circulating half-life of the granulocytes and urine uric acid expressed as mg/kg/24 hours.[7] Parenthetically, we now suspect that this increased granulocyte turnover may explain the findings of elevated serum uric acids and urinary β-aminoisobutyric acid in mongolism, since both of these measurements can reflect nuclear degradation.

The elevated leukocyte enzyme levels observed in mongoloid individuals may simply indicate a younger circulating leukocyte population. In infectious leukocytosis, increased cell enzyme activity is also probably a function of cell age, but in contrast to mongolism, here the granulocyte pool size tends to be increasing, whereas the granulocyte half-life is normal or increased.[8]

Since most of the metabolic alterations have not been observed in all mongoloid subjects, we have attempted to determine if there is a consistent pattern of normal or abnormal cell function for a given individual over a period of time. The leukocyte galactose-1-phosphate uridyl transferase activity of four mongoloid and four nonmongoloid mental retardates from the same institution was measured weekly for four consecutive weeks. The assays were expressed in terms of the DNA content of the leukocyte preparations, as we have found this to be a more reliable estimate of cell numbers than direct cell counts of leukocyte suspensions.[9] FIGURE 1 shows that activities of certain individuals fluctuate weekly between normal and increased activity levels and suggests that anomalous cell metabolism may not always be in evidence. In the group of nonmongoloid retardates used as controls, there was one individual whose enzyme activity levels were consistently higher than those of the mongoloid subjects, indicating the nonspecificity of these enzyme elevations.

With direct evidence of an anomaly of granulocyte physiology that can account for many of the metabolic findings in mongolism, we are still faced with the need to relate this alteration in cell function to the extra chromosome 21. Before we can speak specifically of granulocyte turnover rates in 21 trisomy, we need information about the turnover rate of cells other than the granulocyte in this condition and kinetic studies in other trisomic states. If, in fact, we are dealing with a specific alteration of granulocyte kinetics, we might postulate that there is a specific gene that regulates granulocyte turnover on chromosome 21, or we

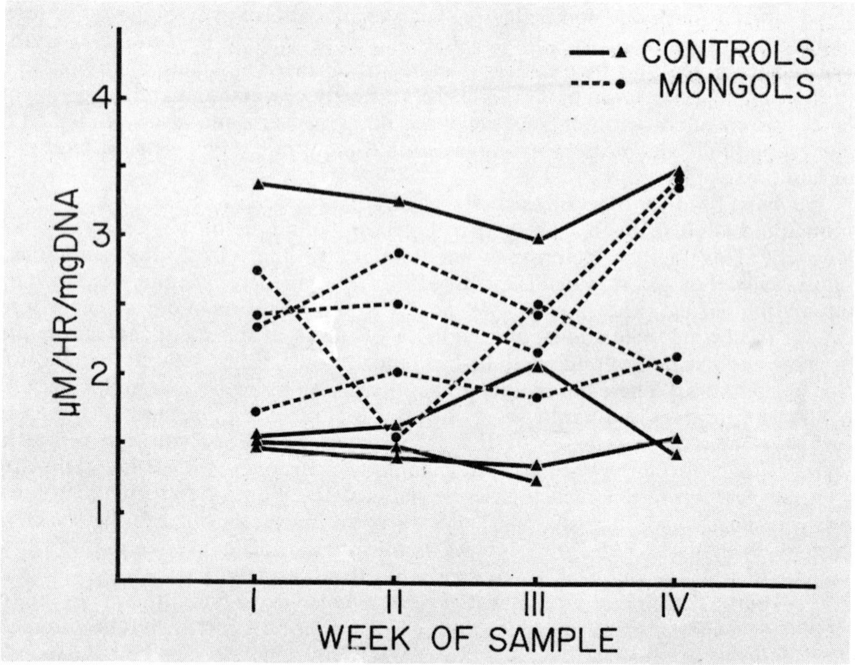

FIGURE 1. Results of galactose-1-phosphate uridyl transferase assays (μM UDPG consumed/hour/mg DNA) performed weekly on leukocytes from four mongoloid adult males and four nonmongoloid mental retardates. Lines connect the determinations performed on each individual subject over a four-week period.

might look for a more direct and perhaps nongenetic mechanism to account for the altered cell kinetics in 21 trisomy. Cell biologists have proposed a number of models of cell systems that can show altered kinetics in the presence of viruses or chemical stimulants of the cell cycle. Such alternative mechanisms need to be considered as possible explanations for the altered granulocyte kinetics in 21 trisomy before the concept of a gene regulator can be affirmed.

Acknowledgment

The authors appreciate the cooperation of the students and staff of the Elwyn Institute, Elwyn, Pa.

References

1. TEPLITZ, R. L., R. B. ROSEN & M. R. TEPLITZ. 1964. Lancet **ii:** 418–419.
2. VALENTINE, W. N. & W. S. BECK. 1951. J. Lab. Clin. Med. **38:** 39–55.
3. MELLMAN, W. J., T. A. TEDESCO & L. BAKER. 1965. Lancet **i:** 1395–1396.
4. HSIA, D. Y. Y., H. L. NADLER & L. SHIH. 1968. This monograph.
5. MELLMAN, W. J., F. A. OSKI, T. A. TEDESCO & H. HARRIS. 1964. Lancet **ii:** 674–675.
6. MAUER, A. M., J. W. ATHENS, H. ASHENBRUCKER, G. E. CARTWRIGHT & M. M. WINTROBE. 1960. J. Clin. Invest. **39:** 1481–1486.
7. MELLMAN, W. J., S. O. RAAB & F. A. OSKI. 1966. *In* Ciba Study Group no. 25: *Mongolism.* G. E. W. Wolstenholme & R. Porter, Eds. J. & A. Churchill. London.
8. ATHENS, J. W., O. P. HAAB, S. O. RAAB, D. R. BOGGS, H. ASHENBRUCKER, G. E. CARTWRIGHT & M. M. WINTROBE. 1965. J. Clin. Invest. **44:** 778–788.
9. TEDESCO, T. A. & W. J. MELLMAN. 1967. Exp. Cell Res. **45:** 230–232.

LEUKOCYTE ALKALINE PHOSPHATASE IN THE 21-TRISOMY (DOWN'S) SYNDROME

Aaron A. Alter and Stanley L. Lee

Maimonides Medical Center, Brooklyn, N. Y.

and

State University of New York, Downstate Medical Center Brooklyn, N. Y.

Low levels of alkaline phosphatase activity in neutrophilic leukocytes are a consistent finding in chronic granulocytic leukemia.[1-3] In 1960, Nowell and Hungerford[4] first reported deletion of part of the long arm of a small acrocentric chromosome in chronic granulocytic leukemia. This chromosomal abnormality, known as the Philadelphia (Ph^1) chromosome, has proven to be of important diagnostic value, since it is found in most cases of this type of leukemia and has not been demonstrated to occur in other diseases. If the gene determinant for leukocyte alkaline phosphatase activity is located on the deleted portion of the chromosome, which would then account for the decreased activity, a condition in which there is trisomy of the same chromosome should have an extra gene and, therefore, increased levels of leukocyte alkaline phosphatase activity.

In 1959, Lejeune *et al.*[5] reported trisomy of the number 21 chromosome in Down's syndrome, probably the same autosome which is partially deleted in chronic granulocytic leukemia. In order to test the hypothesis that the gene determining leukocyte alkaline phosphatase activity is located on the long arm of the number 21 chromosome, the enzyme activity was studied in a group of individuals with the 21-trisomy syndrome.

Leukocyte alkaline phosphatase activity was determined by a biochemical method[6] in a group of 58 individuals with the 21-trisomy syndrome, 41 of whom were under ten years of age. A group of 58 normal subjects of comparable ages were selected to serve as controls. Those persons who had evidence of fever, acute infection, or a hematological abnormality were excluded from consideration, because these conditions can alter the level of leukocyte alkaline phosphatase activity. Leukocyte alkaline phosphatase activity was expressed as LAPA (mg of phosphorus per 10^{10} neutrophils per hour).

Leukocyte alkaline phosphatase activity showed a statistically highly significant negative correlation with age in both the control and the study groups (FIGURES 1 & 2, TABLE 1). The mean leukocyte alkaline phosphatase activity per 10^{10} neutrophils for the 41 control children under ten years of age was 71 mg of phosphorus per hour, whereas for the subjects over ten years of age it was 29 mg per hour. This difference is significant at the 0.1 percent level of confidence (TABLE 1). The negative regression on age is also highly significant (TABLE 1 & FIGURE 1). For the trisomy-21 group, leukocyte alkaline phosphatase activity showed a statistically significant mean difference when comparing the subjects under ten years of age with those over ten years of age. The negative regression on age also proved to be highly significant (TABLE 1 & FIGURE 2).

By comparison, the mean phosphatase activity per 10^{10} neutrophilic leukocytes for the trisomy-21 group under ten years of age (89 mg of phosphorus per hour) was statistically greater than the age-corrected control subjects under ten years of age (66 mg of phosphorus per hour). This difference was significant at the 0.5 percent level of confidence (Fisher's t).

A significantly higher level of leukocyte alkaline phosphatase activity in a group

TABLE 1

ALKALINE PHOSPHATASE ACTIVITY PER 10^{10} NEUTROPHILS (LAPA)

Age of Subjects (years)	No. of Subjects	Mean Age	Mean LAPA	1 S. D. (Log Units)	Regression Coefficient (Log Phosphatase Units/Month)	Correlation Coefficient	Significance of Regression (Covariance)
Trisomy-21							
0–9	41	32 months	89*†	± .27	—.0025	—.315	.05>p>.02
10+	17	21 years	32‡	± .24	—.00074	—.38	.20>p>.10
Combined	58	7.9 years	71§	± .31			
Control group							
0–9	41	25 months	71†	± .21	—.0047	—.60	p<.001
10+	17	25 years	29‡	± .21	—.00050	—.47	p<.001
Combined	58	8.8 years	56§	± .25			
0–9	41	corrected to 32 months	66*				

* Difference between these means is significant at the 0.5 percent level of confidence.
† Difference between these means is significant at the 5 percent level of confidence.
‡ Difference between these means is not significant.
§ Difference between these means is significant at the 5 percent level of confidence.

of individuals with 21-trisomy syndrome has been reported by others[7–8] and supports the hypothesis that the gene controlling this enzyme is located on the long arm of the number 21 chromosome. Furthermore, it was anticipated that the 21-trisomy group would have a 50 percent greater level of enzyme activity than the control group because of increased gene dosage. This expected 3:2 ratio was found.

Despite the preceding findings, the genetic relationship of leukocyte alkaline phosphatase to the number 21 chromosome is not clear cut. Other white cell enzymes have been reported to be increased in Down's syndrome, such as galactose-1-phosphate-uridyl transferase, acid phosphatase, 5-nucleotidase,[9] and glucose-6-phosphate dehydrogenase.[10] It seems unlikely that the genes for all these white cell enzymes are located on the number 21 chromosome and suggests that individuals with 21-trisomy have a nonspecific increase of many, if not all, white cell enzymes.

The reporting of normal levels of leukocyte alkaline phosphatase activity[11] in patients with chronic granulocytic leukemia, although the Ph^1 chromosome still persists in the bone marrow, raises some doubts about locating the leukocyte alkaline phosphatase gene on the number 21 chromosome. During remission, however, the granulocytes in the peripheral blood are too mature to enter mitosis. Therefore, there is no way of showing that these white cells do not have the Ph^1 chromosome. There are reported cases of patients with classic chronic granulocytic leukemia without the Ph^1 chromosome in the bone marrow or peripheral blood, who have low levels of leukocyte alkaline phosphatase activity.[11] Paroxysmal nocturnal hemoglobinuria is a hematological disorder characterized by low levels of leukocyte alkaline phosphatase activity.[12] To date, cytogenetic studies have not revealed any abnormalities of the karyotype in this condition.[13,14]

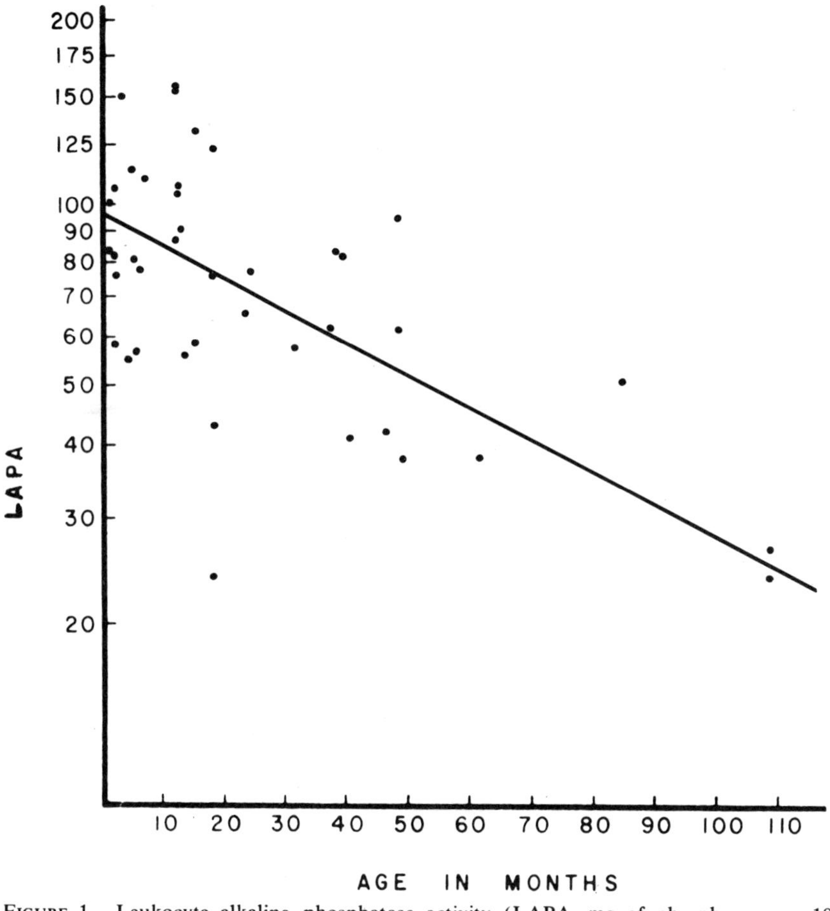

FIGURE 1. Leukocyte alkaline phosphatase activity (LAPA, mg of phosphorus per 10^{10} neutrophils) of control subjects plotted against age showing a significant regression.

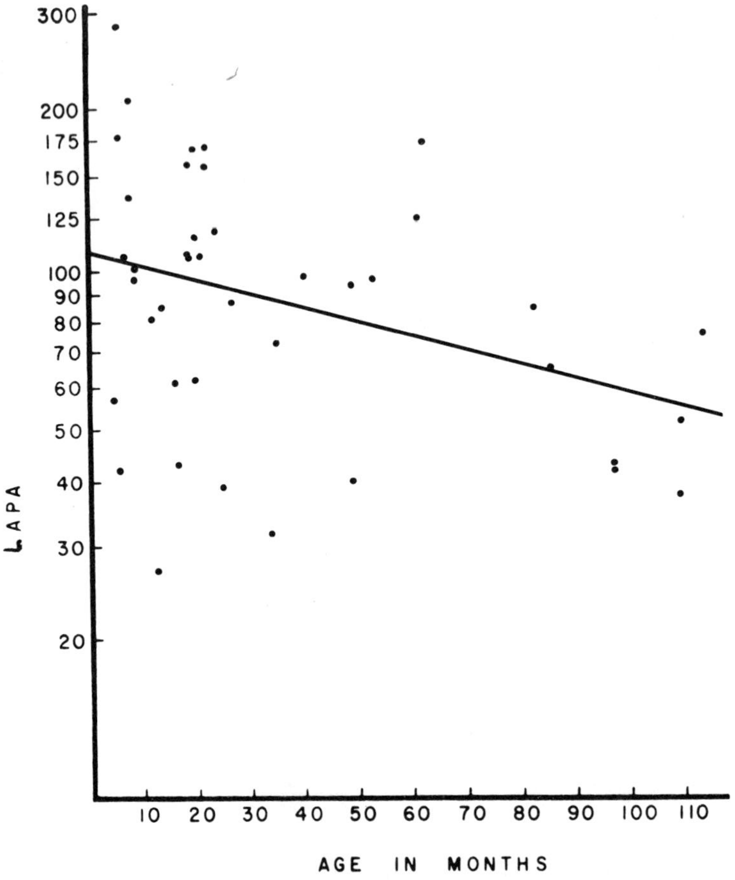

FIGURE 2. Leukocyte alkaline phosphatase activity (LAPA, mg of phosphorus per hour per 10^{10} neutrophils) of subjects with Down's syndrome plotted against age showing a significant regression.

In conclusion, although the level of leukocyte alkaline phosphatase activity has been shown to be significantly elevated in Down's syndrome, there are many observations that refute the hypothesis that the gene for leukocyte alkaline phosphatase is located on the number 21 chromosome.

References

1. Wachstein, M. 1946. Alkaline phosphatase activity in normal and abnormal blood and marrow cells. J. Lab. Clin. Med. **31:** 1–17.
2. Valentine, W. M. & W. S. Beck. 1951. Biochemical studies on leucocytes; I., phosphatase activity in health, leucocytosis and myeloctic leukemia. J. Lab. Clin. Med. **38:** 39–55.
3. Wiltshaw, E. & W. C. Moloney. 1955. Histochemical and biochemical studies on leucycyte alkaline phosphatase activity. Blood **10:** 1120–1131.
4. Nowell, P. C. & D. A. Hungerford. 1960. Chromosome studies on normal and leukemic human leukocytes. J. Nat. Cancer Inst. **25:** 85.
5. Lejeune, J., N. Gauthier & R. Turpin. 1959. Les chromosomes somatiques des enfants mongoliens. C. R. Acad. Sci. (Paris) **248:** 1721.
6. Alter, A. A., S. L. Lee, M. Pourfar & G. Dobkin. 1963. Studies of leukocyte alkaline phosphatase in mongolism: A possible chromosome marker. Blood **22:** 165.
7. Trubowitz, S., D. Kirman & B. Masek. 1962. The leucocyte alkaline phosphatase in mongolism. Lancet **ii:** 486.
8. King, M. J., E. M. Gillis & A. G. Baikie. 1962. Alkaline phosphatase activity of polymorphs in mongolism. Lancet **ii:** 661, 1302.
9. Rosner, F., B. H. Ong, R. S. Paine & D. Mahanand. 1965. Biochemical differentiation of trisomic Down's Syndrome from that due to translocation. New Eng. J. Med. **273:** 1356–1361.
10. Mellman, W. J., F. A. Aski, T. A. Tedesco, A. Macieracoehlo & H. Harris. 1964. Leucocyte enzymes in Down's Syndrome. Lancet **ii:** 674.
11. Block, J. J., P. P. Carbone, J. J. Oppenheim & E. Frei. 1963. The effect of treatment in patients with chronic granulocytic leukemia. Ann. Intern. Med. **59:** 629.
12. Tanaka, K. R., W. N. Valentine & R. E. Fredricks. 1960. Studies on leukocytic and erythrocytic enzyme in paroxysmal noctural hemoglobinuria. Clin. Res. **8:** 132.
13. Bottura, C. & I. Ferrari. 1962. Études chromosomiques dans quelques anemias hemolytiques. Acta Haemat. **28:** 20–24.
14. Beutler, E., E. W. Goldenberg, S. Ohno & M. Yettra. 1964. Chromosome-21 and paroxysmal noctural hemoglobinuria. Blood **24:** 160.

CONCLUDING REMARKS

Margaret A. Kelsall
Cleveland Psychiatric Institute, Cleveland, Ohio

Papers presented during the first session contained data on the incidence of chromosome anomalies. The need for additional studies on meiotic chromosomes, their chronology, chiasma formation and nondisjunction was emphasized and the absence of known autosomal linkage groups in man was recognized as a serious gap in information (Fraccaro *et al.*).

An extensive chromosome survey on 358 human abortuses indicated that the overall incidence of sex-linked and autosomal aberrations was 2.8 percent (Makino *et al.*). In this survey, the incidence of chromosome anomalies was lower in induced abortuses than in spontaneous abortuses; a long Y chromosome, which is frequently hereditary, was associated with mental retardation. No change in chromosomes was apparent in three rare ethnic groups from the area of Hokkaido, Japan (Makino *et al.*).

Phenotypic expressions in patients with a variety of sex chromosome anomalies and mosaicisms was described. This description included data on buccal smears and discussion of the activity of genes on the heterochromatin that develops by the late blastocyst stage (Morishima & Grumbach).

The familial inheritance of Down's syndrome, which is usually sporadic, was described as due to three main types of chromosomal aberrations: fertilization of a 21-disomic gamete, a translocation (21/22 or 15/21), or chromosomal mosaicism (Zellweger). Familial trisomy 21 in individuals with karyotypically normal parents indicates a familial tendency for ovogonial nondisjunction that increases with maternal age (Zellweger).

Disorders predisposing to cancer and the incidence of malignancies in many organs were considered in relation to age, the percentage incidence of histologically confirmed cancer in first degree relatives, and the occurrence of multiple primary neoplasms (Lynch *et al.*). An insignificant difference in incidences of cancer in families of children having acute leukemia compared with that in families of controls indicated a probable absence of genetic influences (McCullough *et al.*). Families of patients having the chromosomal aberrations that are present in constitutional (Franconi's type) aplastic anemia had a higher incidence of monocytic leukemia (Bloom & Diamond).

Autoantibodies, viruses, and radiation are etiological factors of interest in trisomies and other chromosome anomalies. Thyroid autoantibodies were found in significantly more mothers of patients with Down's syndrome than in women of comparable ages or in fathers of patients (Fialkow & Uchida). This high incidence is not specific for Down's syndrome because mothers of patients with gonadal dysgenesis also had an increased incidence of thyroid autoantibodies (Fialkow & Uchida). Among the pathogenic mechanisms considered was the possibility that the chromosome anomalies and the thyroid autoantibodies are two unrelated effects of a common cause, such as a viral agent (Fialkow & Uchida).

Effects of several viruses on variations in chromosomal aberrations are discussed in this monograph. Single breaks and gaps in chromosomes were frequent in patients after three to four days of infection with measles virus, whereas, chromosome fragmentation was the predominant effect *in vitro* (Aula *et al.*). No metaphase figures were observed in leukocytes obtained from patients during the acute stages of infectious hepatitis (Mella & Lang). Use of an indirect method indicated that a transferable factor in serum inhibited mitosis (Mella & Lang).

Viruses, cytotoxic drugs, and radiation did not cause chromosomal aberrations in 50 percent of the cultured cells from most patients with constitutional aplastic anemia (Bloom & Diamond). Endoreduplications and chromosome breaks were present in these cultures, but the chromosome number was normal (Bloom & Diamond). The frequency of these chromosome changes was considered specific for separating various congenital aplastic anemias (Bloom & Diamond). Polyploidy and endoreplications in cultures of leukocytes were the predominate changes that followed treatment of patients with cobalt-60, ^{131}I, and x-radiation (Nasjleti & Spencer).

Several trisomies of autosomal and sex chromosomes produce morphological changes in the nucleus of leukocytes. The nucleus of neutrophils in the blood of individuals with trisomy D(13–15) frequently had two projections extending between nuclear lobes and a number of nuclear projections (Huehns *et al.*). Similar types of projections were not found in E trisomy and Down's syndrome (Huehns *et al.*). The size of X chromosomes was directly correlated with the size of the drumsticks in nuclei of neutrophils; and the XXY karyotype lowered the incidence of drumsticks, but did not decrease the incidence of Barr bodies (Mittwoch).

Morphological changes are described in the limiting membranes in polymorphonuclear leukocytes of patients having the homozygous expression of the autosomal recessive genes that cause the Chediak-Higashi syndrome (Windhorst *et al.*) and those that cause Batten's syndrome (Donahue *et al.*). The morphological abnormality of the gigantic granules in leukocytes was related to the decreased resistance to infection in patients with the Chediak-Higashi syndrome. Immunological, phagocytotic and bactericidal properties of these leukocytes were normal (Windhorst *et al.*). In chronic granulomatous disease, a syndrome of recurrent and eventually fatal bacterial infection, the leukocytes had normal Krebs cycle activity, lactic acid production, glucose and glycogen metabolism during phagocytosis, but did not degranulate during this process (Holmes *et al.*). In patients with Batten's disease, the limiting membranes around azurophilic and specific granules were poorly defined in neutrophils, but well-defined trilaminar membranes were present in basophils, eosinophils, and mononuclear leukocytes (Donahue *et al.*). A high incidence of abnormal granules in leukocytes was found to be indicative of the carrier state in parents and siblings of children with Batten's syndrome (Merritt *et al.*).

The cytochemical assessment of leukocyte alkaline phosphatase activity (LAPA) is an inexpensive, simple, and accurate method for indicating hormonal changes, but cause and effect relations are not known. A consistent increase in LAPA occurs during pregnancy and the puerperium (Kaplow). A high LAPA index was considered a more reliable test for pregnancy than the *Rana pipens* and the Ortho human chorionic gonadotropin tests (Stubblefield). An increase of LAPA was evident two to three days after the administration of estrogen, whereas, this enzyme activity decreased after treatment with androgens (Rosner *et al.*). However, *in vitro* studies did not prove that either estrogens or androgens had a direct effect on LAPA (Rosner *et al.*).

Several papers in this monograph contain data on changes in LAPA during development and aging. The LAPA index increased during gestation until the 36th week when it stabilized (O'Kell). However, a normal decline in LAPA occurred from birth until the 15th day (O'Kell). This decrease was not altered by race, the RH_0 factor, the use of hormonal stimulation to induce labor, or the type of delivery (O'Kell). A sex difference in LAPA was not found until puberty; the level was higher in women than in men until the menopause (Rosner *et al.*). During ovulation, the normal diurnal fluctuation was altered (Kaplow).

Leukocyte alkaline phosphatase, extracted from isolated leukocytes with saline butanol, was studied by horizontal starch-gel electrophoresis. The three major enzyme bands are referred to as isozymes: "fast" (F), "intermediate" (I), and "slow" (S) (Lyons *et al.*). No difference was found in the isozymes of patients with Down's syndrome compared with normal controls, but the F band was never observed during the postpartum period in normal women (Lyons *et al.*).

A direct correlation usually exists between an absence, or a very low level, of LAPA in patients having chronic myeloid leukemia and the Philadelphia (Ph^1) chromosome. However, LAPA increases during intercurrent infection and active ulcerative colitis in children with chronic granulocytic leukemia (Rosen & Nishiyama). An elevated LAPA index also has diagnostic value as a possible indication of infection and inflammation in patients with chronic myeloid leukemia (Krauss).

Reports in the literature on increased LAPA levels during remissions following busulfan therapy were not confirmed. A low level of LAPA remained during busulfan-induced remissions in the childhood form of chronic granulocytic leukemia (Rosen & Nishiyama).

Several evaluations of LAPA in differentiating myeloproliferative syndromes are included in the monograph. The LAPA index was considered valueless in differentiating acute granulocytic leukemia and acute lymphocytic leukemia (Mitus & Kiossoglou). In addition, the absence of the Philadelphia chromosome and normal LAPA levels were found in occasional cases of chronic granulocytic leukemia (Mitus & Kiossoglou). The presence of the Ph^1 chromosome and low LAPA indicates an enzyme activity-gene-dosage correlation, but this correlation does not occur in atypical cases of chronic myeloid leukemia (Krauss). In addition, the levels of LAPA overlap in several myeloproliferative syndromes (Krauss).

LAPA levels are considered helpful, but not an absolute diagnostic criterion, in differentiating chronic granulocytic leukemia from leukemoid reactions, and polycythemia vera from secondary erythrocytosis (Mitus & Kiossoglou). In polycythemia vera, leukocyte zinc is increased, but no correlation between either zinc or magnesium values and enzyme activity was found in pregnancy, acute myelocytic leukemia, or other conditions having increased LAPA (Rosner *et al.*).

Significance of the leukocyte alkaline phosphatase index in many pathological conditions was reviewed (Kaplow). Other evaluations of the significance of LAPA included the following:

1. An elevated LAPA index does not parallel many indicators of stress, such as fever, leukocytosis and sedimentation rate (Kaplow).
2. Elevated LAPA levels are not correlated with all disorders characterized by the presence of toxic granules in the polymorphonuclear leukocytes (Rosner *et al.*).
3. The only direct correlation between levels of serum alkaline phosphatase and neutrophil LAPA occurs in hereditary hypophosphatemia (Kaplow).

A positive correlation between the number of small acrocentric chromosomes and alkaline phosphatase activity occurs in the original human heteroploid line and its clonal derivatives (De Carli *et al.*). This correlation indicated that the gene-dosage hypothesis is valid in explaining alkaline phosphatase activity in this experimental situation. The direct correlation between elevated LAPA and trisomy 21 in 41 children with trisomy 21 also substantiates the gene-dosage hypothesis (Alter & Lee).

Several suggestions were made to explain variation and regulation of LAPA during growth, pregnancy, bacterial infections; in trisomy 21 and other chromosome anomalies; and leukemias. These possibilities include the following: (1) a gene-dosage hypothesis for trisomy 21 in children (Alter & Lee) and strains of cultured leukocytes (De Carli *et al.*); (2) a complex interaction of genetic, hormonal, and physiological determinants (Rosen & Nishiyama); (3) aging of cells (Rosen & Nishiyama); (4) hormonal action on granules (Rosner *et al.*); (5) several granulocytic populations in blood (Mitus & Kiossoglou); and (6) a shorter half-life of granulocytes in Down's syndrome (Mellman *et al.*).

A second enzyme in polymorphonuclear leukocytes was the subject of several papers. Glucose-6-phosphate dehydrogenase (G-6-PD), which is sex-linked in man (Mellman *et al.*) and other animals (Yoshida *et al.*), is elevated in Down's syndrome (Mellman *et al.*). The elevated level of G-6-PD in mongolism was attributed to altered physiology, rather than to a gene determinant located on the trisomic chromosomes (Yoshida *et al.*). Three lines of evidence established that the genetic control of G-6-PD in white blood cells was the same as that in erythrocytes (Yoshida *et al.*). No difference in activities of G-6-PD, acid and alkaline phosphatases, or galactose-1-phosphate-uridyl transferase was found in cultured fibroblasts of patients with trisomy 21, 18, or D_1 (Hsia *et al.*).

Several papers contain information of value for experimental studies. The absence of LAPA in mice and a high level of LAPA in rats may be used to differentiate neutrophils in experiments using blood transfusions (Kaplow). The method of isolating the isozymes of leukocyte alkaline phosphatase (Lyons *et al.*) and the purification and crystallization of G-6-PD (B+) from red blood cells (Yosida *et al.*). will provide tools for enzymic and biochemical studies.

Doctor Kaplan and I want to express our appreciation to the speakers for their well-prepared papers and slides, the session chairmen for leading discussions, and Admiral Schanze and The New York Academy of Sciences for sponsoring this conference.

Printed in the United States of America